Primary Care for Paramedics

Edited by

**Georgette Eaton,
Alyesha Proctor**
and
Joseph St Leger-Francis

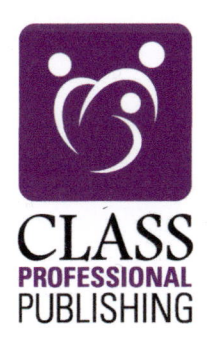

**CLASS
PROFESSIONAL
PUBLISHING**

Class Professional Publishing have made every effort to ensure that the information, tables, drawings and diagrams contained in this book are accurate at the time of publication. The book cannot always contain all the information necessary for determining appropriate care and cannot address all individual situations; therefore, individuals using the book must ensure they have the appropriate knowledge and skills to enable suitable interpretation. Class Professional Publishing does not guarantee, and accepts no legal liability of whatever nature arising from or connected to, the accuracy, reliability, currency or completeness of the content of *Primary Care for Paramedics*. Users must always be aware that such innovations or alterations after the date of publication may not be incorporated in the content. Please note, however, that Class Professional Publishing assumes no responsibility whatsoever for the content of external resources in the text or accompanying online materials.

Text © Georgette Eaton, Alyesha Proctor and Joseph St Leger-Francis 2023

All rights reserved. Without limiting the rights under copyright reserved above, no part of this publication may be reproduced, stored in or introduced into a retrieval system, or transmitted, in any form or by any means (electronic, mechanical, photocopying, recording or otherwise) without the prior written permission of the publisher of this book.

The information presented in this book is accurate and current to the best of the authors' knowledge. The authors and publisher, however, make no guarantee as to, and assume no responsibility for, the correctness, sufficiency or completeness of such information or recommendation.

Printing History
First published in 2023.

The authors and publisher welcome feedback from the users of this book. Please contact the publisher:

Class Professional Publishing,
The Exchange, Express Park, Bristol Road, Bridgwater TA6 4RR

01278 472 800
info@class.co.uk
www.class.co.uk

Class Professional Publishing is an imprint of Class Publishing Ltd
A CIP catalogue record for this book is available from the British Library

Paperback ISBN: 9781801610322
ePub ISBN: 9781801610339
ePDF ISBN: 9781801610476

Designed and typeset by PHi Business Solutions
Printed in the UK by Hobbs

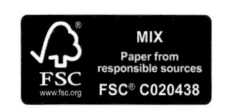

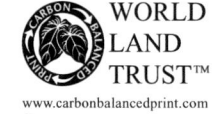

Contents

Foreword v
About the Authors vii

Introduction 1

Chapter 1 Professional Considerations 5
Georgette Eaton

Chapter 2 Consultation Skills and the Diagnostic Process 31
Tom Mallinson

Chapter 3 Decision-making Theory 55
Jaqualine Lindridge

Chapter 4 Laboratory Investigations 65
Colin Roberts

Chapter 5 Neurological Presentations 95
Chris McGregor and Georgette Eaton

Chapter 6 Mental Health Presentations 121
Anita Cawley

Chapter 7 Eyes, Ears, Nose and Throat Presentations 143
Ajay Bhatt and Georgette Eaton

Chapter 8 Respiratory Presentations 179
Marc Gildas Thomas

Chapter 9 Cardiovascular Presentations 209
Jessica Willetts

Chapter 10 Gastrointestinal and Hepatic Presentations 247
Ant Kitchener

Chapter 11 Genitourinary and Gynaecological Presentations 277
Sarah Brown and Elizabeth Steer

Contents

Chapter 12	Contraception and Sexual Health *Alyesha Proctor*	301
Chapter 13	Obstetric Presentations *Aimee Yarrington*	337
Chapter 14	Musculoskeletal Presentations *Sarah Jardine and Georgette Eaton*	365
Chapter 15	Dermatological Presentations *Vanessa Smeardon*	383
Chapter 16	Endocrine Presentations *Ant Kitchener*	421
Chapter 17	Palliative and End-of-Life Care Presentations *Karina Catley and Joseph St Leger-Francis*	439
Chapter 18	A Note on Assessing and Managing Chronic Pain *Jim Huddy and Keith Mitchell*	461
Chapter 19	Safeguarding Considerations *Karen Kitchener*	475
Chapter 20	Making Every Contact Count: Health Promotion in Primary Care *Andrew Hichisson*	493
Index		501

Foreword

There are many books and resources available that paramedics can use in their primary care roles, but what is special about this one is that the chapters have been written for paramedics by paramedics, or by doctors who understand what paramedics can do in primary care roles. My clinical role is in general practice, and over the years I have amassed a large collection of books which have helped me in my practice. I am thrilled to add this one to my library.

I am delighted to have been asked to write the foreword for this publication and have spent many a happy hour revising and learning new things throughout this process. This book will help paramedics new to primary care and those already in post, be it in community, specialist, first-contact or advanced paramedic roles. There is significant coverage of the domains and clinical presentations in Health Education England's *(Paramedic) A Roadmap to Practice* (HEE, 2021) within this book, which paramedic colleagues will find incredibly useful.

The book includes a range of topics you might come across whilst working within general practice, including those which, as paramedics, we may have limited knowledge of when transitioning into primary care roles; for instance, sexual health and contraception, and the wide array of skin complaints covered in the dermatology chapter. Chapters also discuss prescribing and paediatric presentations, providing a basis for further reading around both of these topics, if progressing through the *Roadmap*.

With the increasing opportunities for paramedics to work in non-traditional roles, this book will no doubt be useful not only to those currently in primary care, but also to those wishing to learn more about non-emergency presentations.

I hope you enjoy reading it as much as I did.

Helen Beaumont-Waters
*Head of Clinical Development
(Primary and Urgent Care),
College of Paramedics*

Reference

Health Education England (HEE) (2021) *First contact practitioners and advanced practitioners in primary care: (paramedic) a roadmap to practice*. Available at: https://www.hee.nhs.uk/sites/default/files/documents/Paramedics-FINAL%20(002).pdf (accessed 9 May 2023).

About the Authors

Editors

Georgette Eaton is now at the stage of her career that she has spent more time working in primary and urgent care roles, than she ever has in the back of an ambulance (though she still occasionally does). She currently holds two posts; one as the first paramedic National Institute for Health and Care Research (NIHR) Doctoral Research Fellow at the Nuffield Department of Primary Care Health Sciences, at the University of Oxford; the other as the clinical practice development manager for advanced paramedic practitioners in urgent care within London Ambulance Service NHS Trust (LAS).

Prior to this appointment, Georgette split her employment between clinical practice and education, balancing work as a specialist paramedic in urgent care across a range of primary care settings whilst being senior lecturer in Paramedic Science at Oxford Brookes University. Alongside this, she has been involved in the College of Paramedics since 2017 and is currently the trustee for research on their Board of Trustees.

She was a graduate paramedic from Coventry University in 2011 and after 'topping up' to Bachelor of Science (Hons) began practising as a specialist paramedic (then an emergency care practitioner). Georgette completed her first master's degree in Critical Care at Cardiff University in 2017 and her second in Education Research Design and Methodology at the University of Oxford in 2018. She is also the editor of *Law and Ethics for Paramedics*.

Alyesha Proctor is an advanced paramedic practitioner and independent prescriber working in general practice. Alyesha is also a fellow of the Higher Education Academy and previously worked as a senior lecturer in Paramedic Science at the University of the West of England. She is now an NIHR Clinical Doctoral Research Fellow, and her PhD aims to develop an intervention to support paramedics to safely assess and manage children with minor head injury. She has a passion for all aspects of prehospital care; however, her interests include the clinical decision-making processes that occur in the out-of-hospital setting, the interfaces between primary, secondary and ambulance care, the evaluation of prehospital interventions to reduce avoidable conveyance, paediatrics as a patient group and the impact of multidisciplinary teams in primary care.

Alyesha also has a keen interest in sexual health and contraception, as increasingly primary care practitioners are expected to have generalist knowledge on a range of sexual health and contraception issues. She is also co-editor of the forthcoming title, *Sexual Health and Contraception*.

About the Authors

Joseph St Leger-Francis is an advanced paramedic, educationalist and health leader splitting his time between caring for patients, leading system change and passionately educating medical and allied health students. Joe started his career working as a frontline paramedic for LAS before transitioning into advanced practice roles in the wider healthcare system to include intermediate care teams, minor injury units, emergency departments, general practice surgeries and now within integrated urgent care. Within these areas, Joe has focused his postgraduate studies on primary care therapeutics, developing specific interests in antibiotic resistance and mental health. Within his educational roles, Joe has worked across several universities teaching paramedic science, Bachelor of Medicine and Bachelor of Surgery programmes, and leading a Master of Science programme in advanced clinical practice. Joe has continuously championed learner engagement and satisfaction and has been awarded multiple fellowship grants to strategically implement radical learning pedagogies in creative and playful adult learning. In recent years, Joe has drawn from his experience across these various roles to gain strategic leadership positions and now acts as the lead for an integrated urgent care service in the south west of England.

Contributors

Ajay Bhatt is an advanced paramedic practitioner and clinical practice development manager for the advanced practice programme (urgent care) for LAS. He is also a supervision and assessment lead for the London Faculty for Advancing Practice, Health Education England. Ajay has worked in the NHS for 22 years in primary, secondary and prehospital care, as an emergency department paramedic and an emergency care practitioner, and now as an advanced practitioner. He has a special interest in clinical supervision and the development of advanced practitioners.

Sarah Brown has been a paramedic with LAS since 2012. Her specialist interests include women's health, maternity care and newborn care. This has led to her becoming the practice lead paramedic for maternity care for LAS. This role focused on providing safe and effective prehospital care to patients and families who contacted the ambulance service. Whilst in this role she contributed to the Joint Royal Colleges Ambulance Liaison Committee (JRCALC) guidelines around maternity health inequalities. She was recently appointed as a senior clinical lead for LAS and maintains her keen interests in women's health and health inequalities within her new role.

Karina Catley is the Macmillan paramedic lead for palliative and end of life care, for LAS. She started out her career in the Trust as a paramedic in 2013, and in 2016 continued in this role alongside a clinical educator position at Anglia Ruskin University teaching on undergraduate paramedic science courses. She completed a master degree in Palliative Care in 2020, where her research focused on paramedic use of electronic palliative care coordination systems for decision making with end-of-life care patients.

Anita Cawley is an advanced clinical practitioner (specialist paramedic) within the emergency department at Derriford Hospital, Plymouth, Devon. She joined the ambulance

About the Authors

service in 1994 as an ambulance care assistant. She qualified as a paramedic in 2006 and as a specialist paramedic in 2016. As well as working frontline, she has also worked in primary care and in an out-of-hours setting. Her undergraduate degree is in Health Studies and her master's degree is in Professional Development (2020). She is currently working to credential with the Royal College of Emergency Medicine.

Andrew Hichisson started his paramedic education in 2000 and was one of the first Institute of Healthcare Development (IHCD) and Bachelor of Science-trained paramedics to graduate from the University of Hertfordshire. His career has been predominantly spent with LAS in various different roles have been undertaken including advanced paramedic practice, practice education, and clinical leadership. He also has experience working in primary and urgent care settings as well as lecturing for undergraduate and postgraduate university courses. Andrew has a special interest in public health and is passionate about tackling health inequalities and inequities. As well as other postgraduate study, Andrew has completed his Master of Public Health qualification and published research relating to paramedic wellbeing and homeless populations.

Jim Huddy is a general practitioner (GP) in Cornwall and has developed an interest in chronic pain over the last five years. This started with writing local guidance and educational resources for use in primary care in collaboration with Dr Keith Mitchell (consultant in pain medicine, Royal Cornwall Hospital). Much of this was focused on safe prescribing and deprescribing of pain medications. More recently, Jim and Keith have teamed up with expert patients and social prescribers in Cornwall to broadcast the strategy of self-management of chronic pain as an alternative to medications. They are embarking on a five-year plan to make these alternatives better understood and more widely available in Cornwall.

Sarah Jardine is a principal lecturer and programme lead for the Master of Science in Advanced Paramedic Practice at the University of Hertfordshire. Sarah began her career as a physiotherapist, graduating from Coventry University in 1996. She worked in a variety of roles in and around Milton Keynes before travelling out to Australia to work there. When she returned to the UK, Sarah started working for Two Shires Ambulance Trust, now South Central Ambulance Service NHS Foundation Trust (SCAS), and qualified as a paramedic in 2004. She has worked for the university since 2007. Her teaching interests are varied but include patient assessment, musculoskeletal assessment and clinical reasoning. Sarah maintains dual registration with the Health and Care Professions Council.

Ant Kitchener is an advanced clinical practitioner with over 20 years' NHS experience across urgent, unscheduled and emergency care. Currently, he directs the senior leader portfolio for education at the East of England Ambulance Service NHS Trust (EEAST), coordinating educational delivery to over 3,500 learners and preceptors. He also works one session per week in general practice in Peterborough, as well as holding contracts at Cambridge University Hospitals as a senior advanced clinical practitioner.

Ant has worked in academia, and is a published author as well as a published researcher. He graduated from the University of Hertfordshire in Paramedic Science, and he holds one master's degree in Education and a second in Educational Leadership, as

About the Authors

well as a postgraduate diploma in Advanced Clinical Practice. He has a fellowship from the Higher Education Academy and was one of the first UK paramedic independent prescribers, following regulation of paramedic prescribing in England. As an academic he has taught across paramedicine, allied health, nursing, midwifery, advanced practice and non-medical prescribing at university level. He is currently a doctoral student at the University of Lincoln.

Karen Kitchener is an advance clinical practitioner, working in a general practice with the additional role as a children's safeguarding lead. She originally trained as a paramedic in 2007 after completing her Bachelor of Arts (Hons) degree in Criminology, before then training to become a paramedic with a diploma in Health in Paramedic Science. After seven years working frontline and supporting and mentoring student paramedics, as well as newly qualified paramedics, she moved into a community role as a community matron in 2014, working in many settings, managing and supporting healthcare practitioners, as well as patients, in the community. Her role then evolved to working in minor injuries units and accident and emergency departments before settling in the role within general practice, where she completed her Master of Science in Advanced Clinical Practice, taking on leadership roles to support staff and patients through their learning and health journeys.

Jaqualine Lindridge is Director of Quality at LAS. Jaqualine started her career in the ambulance sector in January 2000, qualifying as a paramedic in 2003 and later as an emergency care practitioner. After working in clinical and educational roles for a number of years, she progressed to a consultant paramedic role where her focus was on urgent care and clinical service development, including the establishment of an advanced paramedic practitioner in urgent care service. Jaqualine holds an undergraduate qualification in Healthcare Practice and a master's degree in Medical Ethics and Law. She continues to practise clinically.

Tom Mallinson started his career in London, with the IHCD Ambulance Aid and Paramedic qualifications alongside the University of Hertfordshire bachelor's degree in Paramedic Science. After working as a paramedic, practice placement educator and chemical, biological, radiological and nuclear (CBRN) responder for the LAS, he went on to read medicine at Warwick Medical School. He continued his studies with postgraduate qualifications in healthcare education, wilderness medicine and primary care. Tom is also a fellow of the Higher Education Academy and the Royal Geographical Society. He works as a prehospital care doctor and rural GP, as well as undertaking roles in healthcare education and with BASICS Scotland.

Chris McGregor is currently the head of education and learner experience at EEAST. Chris started his career in the ambulance service in 2008 having achieved his undergraduate degree in Human Biology and Physiology at the University of Glasgow. Chris worked in various clinical and operational roles before moving into higher education where he worked as a senior lecturer on paramedicine programmes in the EEAST region. Chris has studied to master-degree level in Education and achieved fellowship to the Higher Education Academy during his time in higher education institutes. In 2016, Chris returned to clinical practice to develop the paramedic function within the primary care setting and continues to work as an advanced practitioner and independent prescriber alongside his role at EEAST. Within his current role, Chris champions the importance of education in advancing and improving the services delivered by ambulance trusts, supporting new models of care and joined up working across the wider healthcare economy.

Keith Mitchell has worked as a pain consultant in Royal Cornwall Hospitals NHS Trust for 19 years. He is currently lead consultant for acute pain at the hospital. He is involved in provision of pain relief procedures in the emergency department, and the management of pain following trauma.

Colin Roberts is a GP in the South West, and associate professor in advanced clinical practice at Plymouth University. Colin has been a trainer of GPs and active in medical school education since the mid-1990s and is also a GP appraiser and mentor for advanced clinical practitioners (ACPs) and newly qualified GPs in practice. He has been an educator and enthusiast for advanced practice for 25 years, passionately believing in underpinning clinical skills and diagnostics with sound scientific knowledge. Colin maintains his clinical practice whilst assisting with the provision of high-quality ACP education at the university and is working towards greater integration of the paramedic ACP role in the community.

Vanessa Smeardon is a paramedic practitioner working in a general practice surgery in Bristol. She trained with LAS and obtained a Bachelor of Science (Hons) in Paramedic Science from the University of Hertfordshire in 2014. Following completion of her degree, she worked for South Western Ambulance Service NHS Foundation Trust (SWASFT), whilst maintaining a bank contract with LAS and working as an associate lecturer for Oxford Brookes University. In 2016 Vanessa moved into primary care, initially working as part of a complex care hub, undertaking home visits across a group of surgeries for patients with acute exacerbations of chronic conditions. The role also involved visiting nursing homes and undertaking anticipatory care planning. Since 2017, she has run primary care clinics in general practice surgeries, working as part of the urgent care team managing a range of undifferentiated conditions that present acutely in primary care. Throughout her time in primary care, Vanessa has developed an interest in dermatology and, through working alongside general practitioners with extended roles (GPwERs) in dermatology, has become experienced in managing skin complaints that commonly present in primary care. To complement her primary care role, Vanessa also became an independent prescriber in 2020 and is due to complete her master's degree in Advanced Clinical Practice in 2023.

Elizabeth Steer is the lead paramedic practitioner for a large general practice within Hertfordshire. She is also a senior lecturer for Paramedic Science at the University of Hertfordshire. Elizabeth was awarded a first-class Bachelor of Science in Paramedic Science in 2013 and went on to work as a paramedic for LAS. She then worked as part of a prevention-of-admission team for Hertfordshire Community Trust, where she developed a passion for palliative care and was awarded champion of champions for her work to highlight the importance of advanced care planning. Elizabeth is currently completing her master's in Advanced Clinical Practice and is the paramedic ambassador for the Hertfordshire and West Essex integrated community service training hub.

About the Authors

Marc Gildas Thomas is a senior lecturer within the paramedic science academic team at Swansea University. He is the programme director for paramedic sciences work-based learning and deputy programme director for the Bachelor of Science (Hons) Paramedic Science programme. Marc is an advanced paramedic practitioner holding an Master of Science in Advanced Clinical Practice with extensive experience working as part of multidisciplinary teams within emergency, prehospital, unscheduled and primary care environments as an emergency medical technician, paramedic, advanced paramedic practitioner and non-medical independent prescriber. In 2019, he became one of the first UK paramedics to qualify as a non-medical independent prescriber, being one of the first five advanced paramedic practitioners in Wales to achieve this. In addition to working for many years within the emergency medical service, Marc has worked within primary care for several years and has also been part of community-based multidisciplinary teams providing holistic care to people within their own homes normally associated with secondary care. In addition to writing academic articles, he is also a peer reviewer for some paramedic-specific publications. Marc is currently working towards a professional doctorate within Swansea University Medical School, researching the role and educational requirements of paramedics within primary care worldwide.

Jessica Willetts is an advanced paramedic in primary care. She has special clinical interests in frailty and cardiology. Jessica started working for the ambulance service in 2007 after a career in IT. Registering in 2010, she has worked for both EEAST and South East Coast Ambulance Service NHS Foundation Trust (SECAMB), where she qualified as a paramedic practitioner. In 2015, Jessica worked on an innovative pilot combining 999 response with a home-visiting service for GPs which received national attention. Jessica has worked in primary care since 2016, qualifying as an independent prescriber in 2019. In 2020, she was the main author of the competencies in the *First Contact Practitioners and Advanced Practitioners in Primary Care: (Paramedics) a Roadmap to Practice*, working with Health Education England and the College of Paramedics. Jessica has been involved in primary care network leadership and education, and is currently part of the practice senior management team. She greatly enjoys clinical work and learning alongside teaching, and is currently supporting a group of trainee advanced clinical practitioners through their course.

Aimee Yarrington has been a qualified midwife since 2003. She has worked in all areas of midwifery practice, from the high-risk consultant-led units to the low-risk, stand-alone midwife-led units. She left full-time midwifery practice to join the ambulance service, starting as an emergency care assistant and working her way up to paramedic, while always keeping her midwifery practice up to date. She has worked in several areas within the ambulance service, including the emergency operations centre and the education and training department. Her work towards improving the education of prehospital maternity care has led to her being awarded a fellowship award from the College of Paramedics. Aimee strives to improve the teaching and education for clinicians in dealing with prehospital maternity care.

Introduction

Georgette Eaton, Alyesha Proctor and Joseph St Leger-Francis

A lot has changed for the paramedic profession in the United Kingdom (UK) since its inception in the late 1990s. Registration with the Health and Care Professions Council (HCPC), requirements to undertake a pre-registration undergraduate degree (HCPC, 2021) and independent prescribing of medicines (NHS England, 2018) have all contributed to the professionalisation of paramedicine. Two decades on, paramedics are no longer only synonymous with the ambulance services but are embedded across a range of clinical, educational and leadership settings, and none more so than primary care.

The first paramedics took up roles in primary care in the early 2000s (College of Paramedics, 2021), with a further influx following the Additional Roles Reimbursement Scheme (ARRS) (NHS England, 2021). The NHS People Plan (NHS England, 2020) has outlined the significant role that allied health professionals play to support the demands that the NHS will face in the next ten years to deliver the ambitions of the NHS Long Term Plan (NHS England, 2019). Together with the General Practice Forward View (NHS England, 2016), these documents all outline a vision for the NHS where the professionals that deliver care will work in more multidisciplinary teams, take on more responsibility and autonomy and work more effectively within their professional roles. The shortage of general practitioners (GPs) (Majeed, 2017) is well documented and, together with the plans to create more multidisciplinary teams, under the ARRS (NHS England, 2021) paramedics are now being actively recruited as 1 of 12 additional roles to create multidisciplinary teams and boost accessible care within the community.

Whilst paramedics may not have been an immediately obvious choice for primary care due to their association with emergency response, it is this that gives the transferable skills required for primary care. Any person, of any age, with any presenting complaint may phone 999. It is this undifferentiated, undiagnosed case load that is found in primary care. Indeed, ambulance services in the UK have increasingly moved to an 'urgent and emergency' response service – with the oft-quoted 5% of 999 calls considered an emergency (NHS England, 2014) – and so the case mix for paramedics in the ambulance service has become increasingly similar to that in primary care. For paramedics, there is an increasing choice of employers, no longer limited to ambulance services. It is no wonder that paramedics may seek employment in a clinical setting that offers further clinical development, an absence of night shifts and more regular access to facilities (Eaton et al., 2018).

With the movement of paramedics into primary care roles only set to increase, the education and support for this professional group to work effectively in primary care needs

Introduction

careful attention (Eaton et al., 2021). For paramedics working in primary care in England, Health Education England (HEE) have set out a development roadmap and associated competencies and capabilities expected of paramedics working in English primary care (HEE, 2021). There is nothing similar that exists yet for paramedics employed in Northern Ireland, Scotland or Wales – however, given the shared registration with the HCPC and the similarities that would exist within primary care settings across the devolved nations of the UK, it is reasonable to assume that capabilities and competences outlined within this 'roadmap' are suitable for all UK paramedics in primary care.

How This Book Works

Edited by paramedics for paramedics, this book closely follows the expected case presentations for paramedics working in primary care, as set out by HEE (2021). Each clinical chapter sets out the core clinical skills expected for paramedics in primary care, outlining regular case presentations or clinical conditions within each system with a structured approach of:

- Structured history taking
- An appropriate examination or assessment
- Well-evidenced differential diagnosis and suggested management or support plan
- Appropriate therapies for supply, administration or prescription
- Consideration of suitable and appropriate referrals.

Each clinical chapter ends with a case study concerning the chapter contents, written to aid reflection.

Throughout the book, in addition to images used to demonstrate specific areas of learning, the below icons are used to draw attention to specifically important areas within the text:

Red Flag: Identifies red flags pertinent to particular conditions.

Clinical Pearl: Important points to remember which may be experience- or evidence-based or things you wish you had known ages ago!

Clinical Rules and Tools: When these are presented in the text, we invite you to consider the supporting research evidence and what the sensitivity or specificity of the tool is.

Further Reading: Resources pertinent to the particular area being discussed.

Introduction

> **Caution:** Considerations, common mistakes or cryptic signs that may be missed or cause a negative outcome.

> **Social Prescribing:** Considerations for involvement of social prescribing link workers in the management of the patient.

Georgette Eaton begins in Chapter 1, exploring the professional issues many paramedics will encounter working in primary care, covering the paramedic scope of role in this setting, the provision of clinical supervision and dealing with occupational stress when working in primary care. Tom Mallinson (a dual-registered GP and paramedic) lends his voice to outlining the consultation techniques and medical models in Chapter 2, which is developed further in Chapter 3 by Jaqualine Lindridge in her discussions of risk mitigation and management in decision-making theory. In Chapter 4, Colin Roberts, an academic general practitioner, uses his expertise to present a concise understanding of relevant laboratory investigations within primary care – much of which will be used throughout the clinical chapters in the remainder of the text.

Chapter 5 kicks off the first clinical chapter regarding neurological assessment, jointly authored by Chris McGregor and Georgette Eaton, followed by Anita Cawley discussing mental health presentations in Chapter 6. Georgette returns again in Chapter 7 with Ajay Bhatt to outline presentations to the eyes, ears, nose and throat. Respiratory presentations are covered in Chapter 8 by Marc Gildas Thomas, followed by Jessica Willets discussing cardiovascular presentations in Chapter 9 and Ant Kitchener covering presentations affecting the gastrointestinal and hepatic organs in Chapter 10. Sarah Brown and Elizabeth Steer outline common case presentations for the genitourinary and gynaecological systems in Chapter 11, and Alyesha Proctor covers contraception and sexual health in Chapter 12, before obstetric presentations are covered by Aimee Yarrington, a dual-registered paramedic and midwife, in Chapter 13. Sarah Jardine, a physiotherapist, works with Georgette Eaton in Chapter 14 to outline musculoskeletal presentations, followed by some reading to make you itch in Vanessa Smeardon's overview of dermatological presentations in Chapter 15. Ant Kitchener lends his voice again to endocrine presentations you may expect to see in primary care in Chapter 16. Chapter 17 is our last clinical chapter, which gives an overview of dying and the symptom management for patients at the end of their life, authored by Karina Catley and Joseph St Leger-Francis.

As we approach the end of the text, Jim Huddy, a GP and lead for chronic pain, and Keith Mitchell, consultant in pain medicine, combine their voices in an engaging manner in Chapter 18 to provide a narrative note concerning the principles of assessment and management of chronic pain. Written by Karen Kitchener, Chapter 19 outlines important considerations concerning safeguarding, and the text ends with a final note from Andrew Hichisson on the importance of using our consultations in primary care for health promotion, and making every contact count.

Learning from the experience of the authorship team, each with their own clinical interest, we cover the cases that paramedics may expect to see in primary care. No single book can

Introduction

replace the clinical practice guidance for individual clinical scenarios; however, we hope this book provides an introduction and a point of reference for further resources to consider when faced with new case presentations in primary care.

References

College of Paramedics (2021) The journey of the College. Available at: https://collegeofparamedics.co.uk/COP/About_Us/The_Journey_of_the_College.aspx (accessed 17 January 2023).

Eaton, G., Mahtani, K. and Catterall, M. (2018) The evolving role of paramedics – A NICE problem to have? *Journal of Health Services Research and Policy* 23(3).

Eaton, G., Wong, G., Tierney, S. et al. (2021) Understanding the role of the paramedic in primary care: A realist review. *BMC Medicine* 19(1).

Health and Care Professions Council (HCPC) (2021) HCPC increases the education threshold for paramedics. Available at: https://www.hcpc-uk.org/news-and-events/news/2021/hcpc-increases-the-education-threshold-for-paramedics/ (accessed 30 January 2023).

Health Education England (HEE) (2021) First contact practitioners and advanced practitioners in primary care: (Musculoskeletal) A roadmap to practice. Available at: https://www.hee.nhs.uk/our-work/allied-health-professions/enable-workforce/ahp-roadmaps/first-contact-practitioners-advanced-practitioners-roadmaps-practice (accessed 30 March 2023).

Majeed, A. (2017) Shortage of general practitioners in the NHS. *BMJ* 358: j3191.

NHS England (2014) The Keogh urgent and emergency care review. Available at: https://www.nhs.uk/NHSEngland/keogh-review/Documents/UECR.Ph1Report.FV.pdf (accessed 27 February 2023).

NHS England (2016) General practice forward view. Available at: https://www.england.nhs.uk/publication/general-practice-forward-view-gpfv/ (accessed 1 March 2023).

NHS England (2018) Paramedic prescribing. Available at: https://www.england.nhs.uk/ahp/med-project/paramedics/ (accessed 30 January 2023).

NHS England (2019) The NHS long term plan. Available at: www.longtermplan.nhs.uk (accessed 30 January 2023).

NHS England (2020) We are the NHS: People Plan for 2020/2021 – Action for us all. Available at: www.england.nhs.uk/ournhspeople (accessed 30 January 2023).

NHS England (2021) Expanding our workforce. Available at: https://www.england.nhs.uk/gp/expanding-our-workforce/ (accessed 30 January 2023).

Professional Considerations

Georgette Eaton

Introduction

Whilst primary care may offer a new frontier for paramedics to practise, the professional responsibilities and expectations remain little different regardless of the clinical environment. However, there do exist professional issues that are more relevant to primary care than in other clinical settings that paramedics may be employed within.

In an exploration of professional practice, the Health and Care Professions Council (HCPC) determined that, whilst professionalism is context, profession and patient dependent, the overarching standards within registration offered suitable benchmarks across the range of professions, and settings within these professions, that the HCPC covers (HCPC, 2012). Whilst the concept of professionalism starts with registration, and ongoing regulation, the role it has in day-to-day practice relates more to the level of competence held by the clinician, the quality of care given and the pride and passion in the delivery of that care (Scottish Government, 2012). It is this pride and passion that is considered to be one of the foremost behaviours across today's National Health Service (NHS). Unlike ambulance services and hospital trusts, few primary care providers list a string of core behaviours, expressed as values, that employees are expected to demonstrate. Because of this, and the different models of commissioning that exist within primary care, professionalism within such settings is likely determined by the inherent individual values within the clinician's character (Sudron, 2022), by the internalised values, attitudes and ethical behaviour that are personal to them. Therefore, professionalism begins with the individual paramedic and then extends to practice that reflects the occupational or organisation's behaviours (Stern et al., 2005). So, as we approach professionalism in a clinical setting that is now 'open' and encouraging of paramedics, the need for individuals to be aware of their internalised values – their needs, preferences, wishes, personal expressions and judgements (Fulford, 2011) – is fundamental to ensure the success, and development, of paramedics in this area of practice.

> 💡 Take a moment to reflect on your values. What are your preferences, your beliefs, your needs? What underlying principles make you the person you are?

CHAPTER 1 Professional Considerations

Scope of Practice

The HCPC defines scope of practice as:

> The area or areas of your profession in which you have the knowledge, skills and experience to practise lawfully, safely and effectively, in a way that meets our standards and does not pose any danger to the public or to yourself.
>
> (HCPC, 2014: 4)

The College of Paramedics has since issued their own *Scope of Practice* document to provide members with clear and definitive information outlining the fundamental principles, standards and guidelines underpinning scope of practice (College of Paramedics, 2021). This document outlines that a scope of practice describes the breadth of activities currently carried out by the profession, as well as the activities undertaken by individual paramedics. Individual scope of practice must exist within the scope of practice of the profession as a whole. Unlike in the ambulance service, there is currently no UK-wide document that outlines guidance and scope of practice for paramedics working in primary care. Of the devolved nations, only Health Education England (HEE) has outlined a set of capabilities – the skills, knowledge and behaviours which people bring to the workplace – for how paramedics may work in primary care (HEE, 2019b) and the underpinning training and education to work in this setting (HEE, 2021). However, recognising that the paramedic working in primary and urgent care must be adaptable and not constrained by protocols for practice, it is likely that these documents produced by HEE will not fit all paramedics in all primary care settings – and perhaps not outside of England. What both documents do, however, is outline the expectations for paramedics to safely and effectively manage service users across the lifespan, whilst retaining responsibility and accountability for their own practice. Thus, these capabilities, and the education requirements alongside the scope of practice they present, have been recommended by both the Royal College of General Practitioners (RCGP) and the College of Paramedics as the model to which paramedics work in primary care. Given this endorsement, it is hard to ignore the influence of these capabilities in practice.

The Core Capabilities Framework

HEE's (2019b) model outlines 14 capabilities across four separate domains:

Domain A: Person-centred collaborative working

- Capability 1: Communication
- Capability 2: Person-centred care
- Capability 3: Working with families and carers
- Capability 4: Referrals and integrated working
- Capability 5: Law, ethics and safeguarding

Domain B: Investigation, assessment, advice and clinical impression or diagnosis

- Capability 6: History taking and consultation skills
- Capability 7: Physical and mental health assessment
- Capability 8: Investigations and diagnosis

Scope of Practice

Domain C: Condition management, treatment and prevention
- Capability 9: Treatment and care planning
- Capability 10: Pharmacotherapy
- Capability 11: Health promotion and lifestyle interventions

Domain D: Leadership and management, education and research
- Capability 12: Leadership and management
- Capability 13: Education
- Capability 14: Research.

Each capability sets out what a paramedic in the primary care setting should be able to do and is underpinned by the clinical knowledge to promote health and to diagnose and manage the care of people. Rather than being used in isolation, they are designed to be interpreted together across the domains. For some capabilities, paramedics will be required to expand their scope of practice from the ambulance service, for example in the requesting and interpretation of blood tests. The HCPC is clear on this also:

> If you want to move outside of your scope of practice, you should be certain that you are capable of working lawfully, safely and effectively. This means that you need to exercise personal judgement by undertaking any necessary training or gaining experience, before moving into a new area of practice.
>
> (HCPC, 2014: 4)

As well as setting out these capabilities, HEE also outlines how individual paramedics' fulfilment of the capabilities should be demonstrated and assessed via their *First Contact Practitioners and Advanced Practitioners in Primary Care: (Paramedic) A Roadmap to Practice* (HEE, 2021). For paramedics in England, this offers an academic or portfolio route (the latter aimed at paramedics who have been employed in primary care for some time) to ensure that paramedics have the relevant training, education and support to be safe in general practice, and subsequently be named as first contact practitioners or advanced practitioners. The aim is similar to the credentialling undertaken by advanced clinical practitioners in emergency medicine (RCEM, 2021), with options to join a subsequent directory or register after.

For the devolved nations, it is currently only the HCPC that requests evidence of competence obtained through continuing professional development, rather than any formal assessment or portfolio (HCPC, 2018b). This leaves a lot of scope for paramedics working in primary care in Northern Ireland, Scotland and Wales to develop their own portfolio of evidence in relation to these competencies. The nature of this will depend upon the context or setting where the framework is used and how paramedics have been supervised and have developed their capability. However, such a portfolio is a requirement for completion of national examinations, such as the College of Paramedics' Diploma in Primary and Urgent Care.

Titles

What is in a name? For paramedics working in primary care, largely a lot of confusion. Whilst the College of Paramedics sets out specific nomenclature against its career

CHAPTER 1 Professional Considerations

framework (Figure 1.1), this is little adopted in primary care. A recent scoping review found that paramedics working in primary care operate under a variety of titles, from emergency care practitioner to paramedic practitioner, to community paramedic, to advanced paramedic practitioner and everything in between (Eaton et al., 2020). This is problematic for paramedics, employers and, most importantly, patients. When a patient sees their general practitioner (GP), they know exactly what to expect, based on years of similar encounters. Should they need to see a GP whilst on holiday somewhere else in the UK, they will expect and see a similar type of consultation, and a doctor within the same title and the same broad role. This is not so for paramedics. How would the patient know that the specialist paramedic they saw in Oxfordshire is the same as the community paramedic their relative attends in the Outer Hebrides, is the same as the advanced paramedic their relative saw in Wales and is the same as a first contact practitioner paramedic they once saw when visiting London – save for an explanation at the start of the consultation? The role of the paramedic in primary care is increasingly important and prevalent, and it is therefore important that there is a standardisation in title across the UK. This will help give confidence to patients being treated by paramedics, as well as to GPs and other professionals working alongside such a highly skilled allied healthcare professional.

> What is your job title? Does is accurately represent your academic attainment and level of practice? Does it mean the same to you as it does to others who hold the same title?

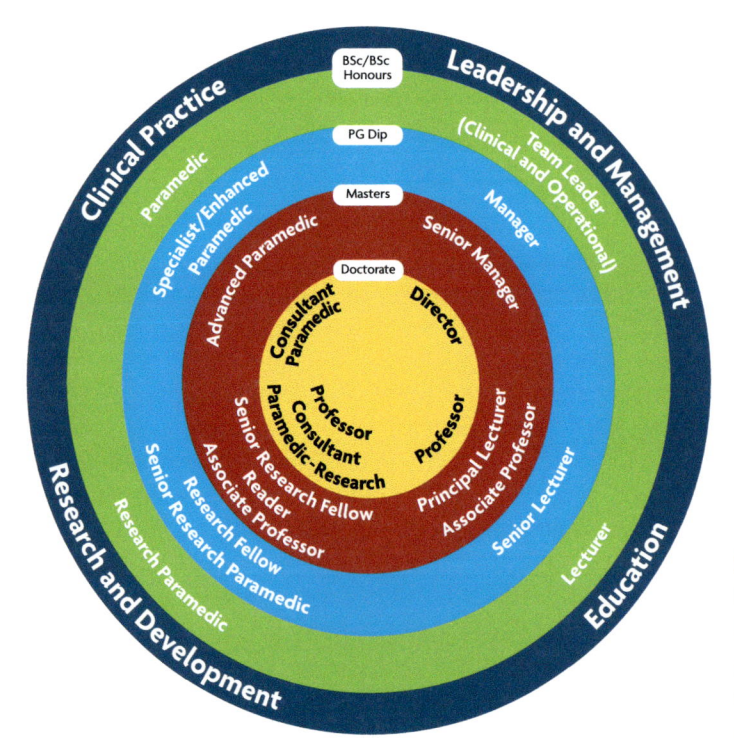

Figure 1.1 The College of Paramedics Paramedic Career Framework.

Source: College of Paramedics (2023). Reproduced with kind permission.

Career Progression

For paramedics, career progression is synonymous with education. The College of Paramedics has long associated clinical progression with academic attainment (College of Paramedics, 2023) and HEE have more recently set the expectation that those working in advanced clinical roles will have completed a relevant master's degree (HEE, 2019a), which is the focus of their multi-professional advanced practice register. Scope of practice is inextricably linked with these education standards, and independent prescribing is recommended to only be undertaken at master-degree level by advanced paramedics (College of Paramedics, 2018).

> Blaber, A. et al. (2018) *Independent Prescribing for Paramedics*.
> This text offers a comprehensive overview of the legislation related to paramedic prescribing and is a fundamental text for paramedics in prescribing roles, including in primary care.

Therefore, additional education is fundamental for paramedics working in primary care if they are to fulfil and excel in all functions of their role (Eaton et al., 2021; HEE, 2021). Notwithstanding this, the roles undertaken by advanced paramedics are determined by the needs of the employer and how they require the level of practice to be deployed within their setting.

Paramedics have been steadily moving into primary care settings over the last decade, with an anticipated increase associated with the Additional Roles Reimbursement Scheme in England, which offers a financial benefit for the employment of paramedics in this setting (NHS England, 2019). However, with this movement into primary care, it is likely that many paramedics will be faced with employers who do not fully understand the paramedic role and all that it can offer. The onus will therefore be on the individual paramedic to outline the capabilities that are fundamental to their role and, if practising in England, relating it to HEE's frameworks (HEE, 2019b) and roadmaps (HEE, 2021).

> Do you have a scope of practice document within your workplace? Does it adequately reflect the work you undertake?

Indemnity Insurance

On 1 April 2019, state-backed GP indemnity schemes were launched in England (Clinical Negligence Scheme for General Practice – CNSGP) and Wales (General Medical Practice Indemnity – GMPI). Previously, GPs and practice staff, such as paramedics, were required to arrange and fund their own clinical negligence cover. GP contractors and their staff, including salaried GPs, locums, nurses, paramedics, clinical pharmacists and other practice staff, are all included in this scheme (BMA, 2020) as long as they are providing NHS services.

Healthcare professionals are required to hold appropriate clinical negligence indemnity cover to meet the costs of claims and damages awarded to patients arising out of negligence (DHSC, 2019). Should a patient seek compensation for injury or illness as a result of the care provided, clinical negligence indemnity cover will pay for the compensation costs and legal fees arising as a result of incidents of clinical negligence.

CHAPTER 1   Professional Considerations

> ❗ It is your professional responsibility as a paramedic to ensure you have appropriate medical negligence indemnity cover for your practice.

As this scheme covers paramedics employed in general practice, the provider has a duty to arrange suitable cover; this should be provided to you in writing. For paramedics engaged as self-employed contractors, it is likely that individual indemnity protection will be required.

Supervision

It is in the public's and patients' interests that there is clear evidence of an effective, robust, transparent and fair system for clinical supervision for paramedics in primary care. As well as ensuring paramedics continue to demonstrate what is expected in the *Standards of Proficiency – Paramedics* (HCPC, 2014), it is important to ensure that effective clinical supervision and pastoral support are given to achieve the supervision outcomes required to work at an advanced level, and for completion of independent prescribing programmes. Within the paramedic undergraduate curriculum (College of Paramedics, 2018), and across other professions in healthcare, clinical supervision is viewed as a cornerstone within the development of practice and is associated with effectiveness of care (Snowdon et al., 2017). Patient safety correlates directly with opportunities for learning and a culture that promotes clinical excellence; therefore the provision of supervision is an important element of employment within primary care.

Responsibilities for Supervision

The provision of effective supervision within primary care is shared between employers, clinical supervisors and individual paramedics.

Employer Responsibilities

Employers have a duty to provide clinical supervision within the workplace. The Care Quality Commission (CQC) (2013) outlines that there must be suitable arrangements in place to ensure registered clinicians are supported to enable them to deliver care and treatment to people who use services safely and to an appropriate standard. Part of ensuring such suitable arrangements is that the environment and culture for clinical supervision is safe, open and provides a good standard of care and experience for patients.

> ❗ Does your employer set out supervision for you in your role in primary care? Whilst there currently exists no standard for the provision of supervision for paramedics in primary care, the most appropriate supervision arrangements will be determined by a number of factors, including experience, the type of work carried out and individual needs (Skills for Care, 2007). The governance system for supervision must continuously encourage improved quality and outcomes for those patients cared for by the paramedic.

Supervisor Responsibilities

The General Medical Council (GMC) defines a clinical supervisor as:

> A trainer who is selected and appropriately trained to be responsible for overseeing a specified trainee's clinical work and providing constructive feedback during a training placement.
>
> (GMC, 2023)

Thanks to the RCGP, primary care has benefited from robust training resources and systems to support physicians as they transition from GP training to qualified GP. More recently, the RCGP launched its First5 initiative to support GPs in the first five years after Membership of the Royal College of General Practitioners (MRCGP) examinations through to revalidation. As well as systems in place to support GP training, there is also a quality management system in place to ensure standardisation across their membership (RCGP, 2020).

Paramedics working in primary care would undoubtedly benefit from supervision by these GP trainers. Clinical supervision can take several forms. The primary type of supervision is direct supervision, where the clinical supervisor oversees all activities that are being performed by the paramedic and continuously provides them with feedback and guidance. This form of supervision is a required element of independent prescribing modules, as well as other clinical practice modules. Indirect supervision may take the form of retrospective review of documentation, case-based discussion or evaluation of a recorded consultation. In this, whilst the clinical supervisor is not present, they are contactable if required for support and to provide direct supervision as necessary.

Clinical supervisors should have the necessary knowledge and skills for their role and receive the support and resources they need to deliver effective education and training (HEE, 2018).

Supervision, and mentorship, is a requirement of registration (HCPC, 2018c). It is, therefore, also expected that paramedics may be a clinical supervisor within their practice. As a clinical supervisor, paramedics should expect to receive the support, resources and time required to meet their own requirements to provide excellent clinical care; this in turn will enable the supervisor to provide feedback to learners on their professional practice.

Paramedic Responsibilities

Building on the *Standards of Proficiency – Paramedics* (HCPC, 2014), individual paramedics working in primary care have the main responsibility to ensure that they make the most of their clinical supervision and develop into well-rounded and safe clinicians.

Duty of Candour

As well as supporting a culture of safety that supports organisational and personal learning, all healthcare employers must promote a culture that encourages candour, openness and honesty at all levels.

The duty of candour is a statutory duty to be open and honest with patients and their families when something goes wrong that appears to have caused, or could lead to, significant harm in the future (UK Government, 2014). The statutory duty was introduced in

CHAPTER 1   Professional Considerations

November 2014 for NHS bodies such as trusts and foundation trusts in England and was extended in April 2015 to cover all other care providers registered with the CQC (2015). Similar legislation is supported by the Care Inspectorate in Scotland (Scottish Government, 2018) and the Healthcare Inspectorate in Wales (National Assembly for Wales, 2019). However, this is currently not supported by Northern Ireland, where the Department of Health Northern Ireland (2020) is reviewing the implementation of such a duty in light of a published report where deaths occurred due to hyponatraemia (O'Hara Inquiry, 2020).

Duty of Candour in Primary Care in England

The principle of the duty of candour is that care organisations have a general duty to act in an open and transparent way in relation to care provided to patients. The statutory duty applies to both organisations and 'registered persons', such as paramedics and doctors in primary care.

The key principles as outlined in the duty of candour are:

1. Care organisations have a general duty to ensure that an open and honest culture exists throughout their organisation, and that they act in an open and transparent way in relation to care provided to patients.
2. For registered persons (such as paramedics or general practitioners), a notifiable patient safety incident has a specific statutory meaning: it applies to incidents where something unintended or unexpected has occurred in the care of a patient and appears to have resulted in:
   - Changes to the structure of the body (for example, amputation following arterial occlusion)
   - Impairment (of sensory, motor or intellectual function) that has lasted or is likely to last for 28 days continuously
   - Prolonged pain or prolonged psychological harm. The pain or psychological harm must be, or be likely to be, experienced continuously for 28 days or more
   - Shortening of their life expectancy
   - Their death, where this relates to the incident and is not simply due to the natural progression of the illness or condition
   - Or where the patient requires treatment by a healthcare professional in order to prevent death or the adverse outcomes listed above.
3. If a notifiable patient safety incident occurs, the organisation must tell the patient (or their representative) about it in person as soon as reasonably practical. Following the initial notification, the patient must be given written notification, including details of any further enquiries into the incident and the outcome of these enquiries. The organisation must keep copies of correspondence with the patient. Failure to inform the patient may amount to a criminal offence.
4. As well as notification to the patient, general practices and other primary care services must submit all notifications to the CQC.
5. The organisation is required to provide a written apology to the patient (or their representative).
6. There is a statutory duty to provide reasonable support to the patient. Reasonable support could be giving emotional support to the patient following a notifiable patient safety incident or providing an interpreter to ensure discussions are understood.

This legislation also mandates that organisations have clear governance procedures for reporting and investigating incidents. If these are followed, it is unlikely that a notifiable patient safety incident will be overlooked. In any event, paramedics must always follow their ethical duty, irrespective of whether the statutory duty applies.

Ethical Duty

A 'duty of candour' is familiar to most paramedics, at least in principle. Under *The Standards of Conduct, Performance and Ethics* (HCPC, 2018c), paramedics have an ethical duty to tell patients when things have gone wrong, apologise and try to put things right. Whilst more recently revised, such standards have been in place for paramedics since regulation began in the early 2000s.

An area of difficulty may be deciding whether an incident reaches the threshold for notification under the statutory duty. The HCPC (2018c) *Standards* outline a low threshold for notification – when 'something has gone wrong'. However, as outlined above, the statutory duty is much higher and more complex.

For those incidents that do not meet the definition of a notifiable patient safety incident, individual paramedics need to be ethically and morally comfortable with the decision they have made and follow local governance procedures to navigate the incident to a positive outcome.

> Ensure every patient and relative receives the assessment and treatment you would like those you love to receive. If you would expect your loved ones to receive a higher standard of care, are you practising in an ethical way that meets the standards of your registration?

Occupational Stress in Primary Care

The term 'workload' is a hypothetical construct which has been developed from human factors psychology and reflects the perceived margin between task demands and an individual's coping capacity (Macdonald, 2006). In the domain of occupational stress, however, workload is further equated with job demand and the performance of repetitive tasks. Various occupational factors contribute to general practitioner burnout, including lack of support, increased patient demands and increased administration needs, both in terms of documentation and audit (Hall et al., 2019). Work environments which are high demand (such as long hours, high work volume and pressure), or which have low levels of job control (such as autonomy or use of skills) or of job resources (such as support, or physical resources), have long been known to contribute to occupational stress, burnout and ill-health (Karasek, 1979). Occupational stress, and the ensuing burnout and ill-health, in healthcare professionals is associated with poorer patient safety outcomes, such as increased risk of adverse events, near misses and prescription errors (Avery et al., 2012; Hall et al., 2016; Salyers et al., 2017). It is important for paramedics in primary care to have a very real understanding of the possibility of occupational stress in this environment and to consider how it can be effectively managed.

Burnout

Primary care has long been associated with practitioner stress and burnout (McManus et al., 2011; O'Connor et al., 2000; Orton et al., 2012). With workforce shortages (Gibson et al., 2015), an alarming number of GPs considering leaving the profession (BMA, 2017) and the impact of the recent COVID-19 pandemic, the pressures on primary care are very clear. It is in part due to these reasons that paramedics are able to move into primary care, where they cover the gaps created by the workforce so well due to their generalist approach (Eaton et al., 2018). However, with the current workforce challenges still remaining, it is likely that paramedics will suffer the same feelings of burnout and stress within this setting unless it can be managed appropriately.

Recognising Burnout

Despite the fact that paramedics are expected to recognise the signs of stress in their patients, it can be difficult to do so when directly experiencing them. Indicative signs such as muscle tension, feeling overwhelmed, eating too much or little or being irritable (NHS, 2022) can easily be overlooked or put down to time of day, personal factors or just a 'one-off'. However, stress – and burnout – can manifest in a myriad of different, subtle ways, as outlined in Box 1.1.

BOX 1.1   Symptoms of Burnout

Physical symptoms	Mental symptoms
• Headaches or dizziness • Muscle tension or pain • Stomach problems • Chest pain or a faster heartbeat • Sexual problems	• Difficulty concentrating • Struggling to make decisions • Feeling overwhelmed • Constantly worrying • Being forgetful
Changes in behaviour	**Changes in attitude towards role**
• Being irritable and snappy • Sleeping too much or too little • Eating too much or too little • Avoiding certain places or people • Drinking or smoking more	• Emotional exhaustion (exhausted after a clinical day and unable to recover despite time off work) • Depersonalisation (manifests as a negative, detached response to duties and complaining about patients and their problems) • Cynicism (lost ability to care, empathise and connect with patients and colleagues) • Doubt (questioning personal competence and the quality of work undertaken, including whether the role makes any difference)

Source: Drummond (2014).

Primary care research has previously highlighted that when faced with burnout, GPs try to preserve care quality at a greater personal cost to themselves (Hall et al., 2019), and it is likely that paramedics working in the same environment adopt such a culture. However, this is not an effective mechanism to cope with burnout. Recognising the underlying cause and applying both organisational and personal treatment mechanisms is an effective way to manage burnout.

Managing Stress and Burnout

Research that specifically focuses on how paramedics manage stress in the ambulance service has previously outlined that paramedics prefer informal coping strategies, such as cognitive mechanisms and peer support (Mildenhall, 2012). In the absence of any other research focusing specifically on paramedics in primary care, it can be considered likely that such mechanisms are also suitable for this setting too.

The GMC has outlined an 'ABC of doctors' core needs'. It suggests that when these core needs are met, doctors experience better well-being and improved health and are more motivated. The following needs can apply just as well to paramedics as to doctors:

> **A** – Autonomy: Having some control within work and acting consistently with both life and work values in mind
> **B** – Belonging: Feeling valued and respected, and being connected to and caring of others in the workplace
> **C** – Competence: Feeling clinically effective and well supported to deliver high-quality care.
>
> (GMC, 2019: 15)

Even if just one core need is not met, this can have a negative impact and contribute towards feelings of burnout. In order to effectively monitor stress and burnout, the way these elements are managed needs to be considered.

Identifying Triggers

Identifying what triggers stress can help in anticipating problems and thinking of ways to solve them. Even if these situations cannot be avoided, being prepared and understanding their impact can help in regaining some control and a sense of autonomy.

> 💡 Take time to reflect on events and feelings that contribute to you feeling stressed. Consider discussing these with someone you trust.

Organising Time

With booked appointments in narrow time slots, it can be difficult to keep to time in primary care, and this has long been found to contribute to feelings of stress in this healthcare setting (Gibson et al., 2015). Efforts focused on workplace redesign has previously been outlined as one way to effectively manage clinician burnout in primary care (Hall et al., 2016). Therefore, engaging with employers to make adjustments to how

CHAPTER 1 Professional Considerations

days are structured may be one way to prioritise tasks and to effectively manage time without feeling overloaded.

Occupational Changes

Other occupational characteristics that may help in the workplace include reducing administrative work, hiring more administrative staff and providing a more supportive environment (Hall et al., 2019). This may not be achievable in some practices, due to workspace and financial constraints. However, all settings can foster a more positive and supportive team culture both informally (such as communal tea breaks) and formally (such as mentoring systems) (Patel et al., 2019). If not already in place, these should be given serious consideration among practice staff and managers to assist paramedics experiencing burnout.

Accept What Cannot Be Changed

Within the NHS, paramedics working in primary care are a small but important cog in an intricate mechanism of gears, cogwheels and other working components. There are aspects of care that we can very much have an impact on, and there are other aspects that we cannot change – such as treatments that are approved within the NHS by the National Institute of Clinical Excellence (NICE) or waiting times for review by specialist consultants. Whilst not easy to do, accepting what cannot be changed and focusing on what can is an effective tool in managing burnout.

Developing Resilience

As well as workplace redesign, efforts focused on clinician self-care are incredibly important in managing the feelings of burnout (Patel et al., 2019). Developing emotional resilience is not just about the ability to bounce back but is also the capacity to adapt in the face of challenging circumstances whilst maintaining stable mental well-being. Resilience does not come naturally to everyone and is something that small steps can be taken to achieve. Mind (2017) has outlined several tips to build and maintain emotional resilience, as outlined in Box 1.2.

BOX 1.2 Tips to Develop Resilience

Lifestyle changes	Look after physical health
There are some general changes that you can make to your lifestyle that could help you feel more able to cope with pressure and stressful situations: • Be straightforward and assertive • Develop interests and hobbies • Find balance in your life • Regularly use relaxation techniques	Looking after your physical health can help you to look after your mental health and reduce feelings of burnout and stress. These include having enough sleep, being physically active and eating healthily

Give yourself a break	Build a support network
• Be kind to yourself • Forgive yourself when you have made a mistake or have not achieved something you planned for • Reward your achievements • Take a break with a change of scenery	Remember that if you are stressed, you do not have to cope alone. Your support network may include: • Friends and family • Peer support • Specialist websites and organisations • Support at work (practice manager) • Your own GP
Improve mental well-being	**Improve self-esteem**
• Build positive relationships • Embrace new experiences or try something new • Give (volunteering or being part of a wider group helps build more connections to those around you) • Learn how to relax and unwind • Take time for yourself	• Be kind to yourself • Focus on the good things • Learn to be assertive • Look after yourself • Set yourself a challenge

Source: Mind (2017).

> Mind (2017) Developing resilience [online].
> Mind, the mental health charity, has excellent information to assist in the management of stress, anxiety and other symptoms of ill-health related to burnout.

Infection Prevention and Control

Infection prevention and control is a key priority for the Department of Health and Social Care, reinforced by the Health and Social Care Act, 2008 (UK Government, 2008). The policy (NHS England and NHS Improvement, 2019) on the standard infection control precautions and related guidance states that infection prevention and control is a mandatory requirement across all healthcare providers and outlines ten standard infection control precautions (SICPs) that need to be considered in all clinical practice settings.

Standard Infection Control Precautions

There are ten elements of SICPs:

- Patient placement or assessment for infection risk
- Hand hygiene
- Respiratory and cough hygiene
- Personal protective equipment (PPE)

CHAPTER 1 Professional Considerations

- Safe management of care equipment
- Safe management of the care environment
- Safe management of linen
- Safe management of blood and body fluids
- Safe disposal of waste (including sharps)
- Occupational safety or managing prevention of exposure (including sharps).

SICPs are the basic infection prevention and control measures necessary to reduce the risk of transmitting infectious agents from both recognised and unrecognised sources of infection. Sources of (potential) infection include blood and other body fluids, secretions or excretions (excluding sweat), non-intact skin or mucous membranes and any equipment or item in the care environment that could have become contaminated. To protect effectively against infection risks, SICPs must be implemented and monitored by all staff.

Infection Control

Standard precautions should be applied during all working practices to protect patients and staff from infection. All blood and body fluids are capable of transmitting infection. Controlling the spread of infection within clinical practice requires standard precautions at the basic minimum level of hygiene to be applied throughout all contact with blood and body fluids from any source. Body fluids include:

- Blood
- Breast milk
- Faeces
- Peritoneal fluid
- Semen
- Urine
- Vaginal fluids
- Vomit.

Hand Hygiene

During patient contact, staff should be 'bare below the elbows' and cuts or abrasions should be covered with a waterproof dressing. Hands should also be visibly clean from dirt.

Hand hygiene refers to the process of hand decontamination where there is physical removal of dirt. This includes the removal of bodily fluids and the destruction of micro-organisms from the hands. During clinical practice, hands can become contaminated by handling equipment, by direct contact with a patient or by contact with the general environment. Whilst hands may look visibly clean, micro-organisms are always present and hand hygiene is the single most important way to prevent the spread of infection. To achieve this, hands should be washed regularly with the correct technique (Mathur, 2011). Figure 1.2 outlines the correct technique for handwashing. You should wash your hands when visibly soiled, otherwise use a handrub. The duration of the entire procedure is 40–60 seconds.

Infection Prevention and Control

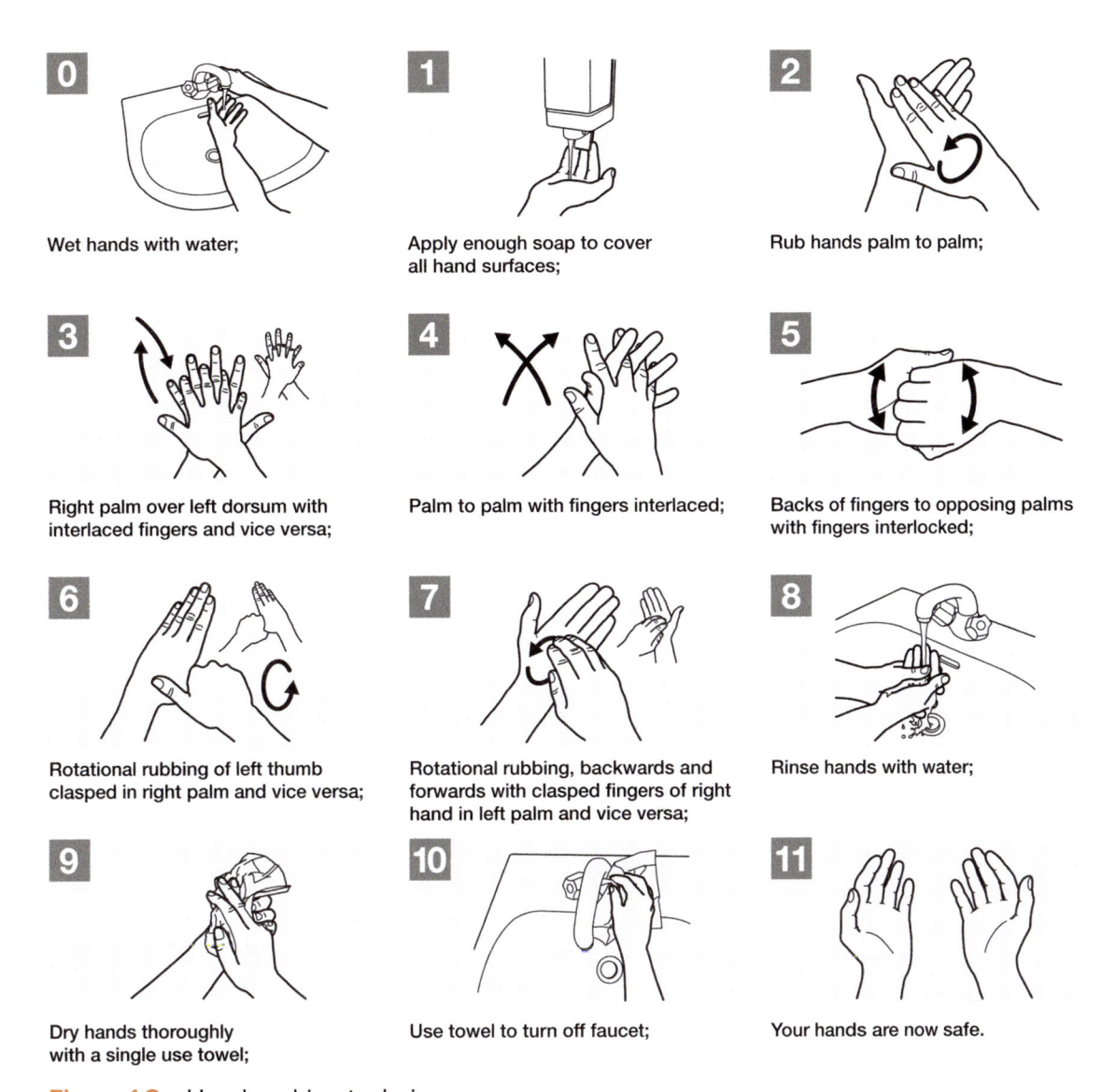

0 Wet hands with water;	1 Apply enough soap to cover all hand surfaces;	2 Rub hands palm to palm;
3 Right palm over left dorsum with interlaced fingers and vice versa;	4 Palm to palm with fingers interlaced;	5 Backs of fingers to opposing palms with fingers interlocked;
6 Rotational rubbing of left thumb clasped in right palm and vice versa;	7 Rotational rubbing, backwards and forwards with clasped fingers of right hand in left palm and vice versa;	8 Rinse hands with water;
9 Dry hands thoroughly with a single use towel;	10 Use towel to turn off faucet;	11 Your hands are now safe.

Figure 1.2 Handwashing technique.
Source: WHO (2009).

Hands should be washed before and after contact with a patient and before and after all clinical procedures, using liquid soap from refillable, wall-mounted dispensers. Hands should be wet under warm running water. Apply liquid soap and rub all parts of the hands and wrists thoroughly, then rinse and dry using disposable paper towels. Antimicrobial solutions are not recommended for routine handwashing, as they dry the skin which can cause damage. They are, however, recommended for use prior to an invasive procedure, such as minor surgery.

CHAPTER 1   Professional Considerations

Alcohol handrubs are of particular value where handwashing facilities are limited or not available, such as during home visits. However, these products are only effective if hands are physically clean and as such should be applied to dry, visibly clean hands. It is important to wash hands which are visibly contaminated prior to its application. Alcohol handrub is not effective when dealing with a patient with suspected norovirus (viral gastroenteritis) or *Clostridium difficile* (Jabbar et al., 2010). Therefore, handwashing with liquid soap and warm running water is essential when treating any patient known to have had diarrhoea within the last 48 hours. Patients should be encouraged to use alcohol handrub when entering and leaving the primary care setting.

Decontamination of Equipment

Decontamination of reusable medical equipment after use on a patient is an essential part of routine infection control to prevent the transmission of infection.

For items used on intact skin and non-infectious patients, cleaning is essential before disinfection or sterilisation is carried out. Detergent wipes or neutral detergent, warm water and single-use cloths should be used for the cleaning of any reusable medical equipment, such as the examination couch, stethoscope, blood pressure cuff or anything that has been in contact with intact skin. Disinfection follows cleaning for items used on non-intact skin, such as mucous membranes, or where contact has occurred with body fluids or known or suspected infectious patients. For this reason, a majority of instruments which would have had this contact are now disposable, such as otoscope covers. For instruments that need to be disinfected, disinfectants can be in the form of wipes or of chlorine-releasing tablets, liquids or granules.

Each general practice will have a local policy and procedure regarding the management of:

- Blood and body fluid spillages
- Cleaning
- Decontamination of equipment
- Disposal of waste
- Isolation of patients
- Laundry
- Sharps injury.

It is prudent for paramedics to understand their local policy and procedure regarding such management.

Invasive Devices

Invasive devices are devices which, in whole or in part, penetrate inside the body, either through a body orifice or through the surface of the body. Examples of invasive devices common in primary care include vascular access devices, urinary catheters, subdermal contraceptive implants and intrauterine devices. Paramedics must have demonstratable competency in the insertion and management of invasive devices, as well

Infection Prevention and Control

as in the application of the aseptic technique required to undertake each specific procedure (Harrogate and District NHS Foundation Trust, 2017a).

Personal Protective Equipment

Workwear requirements differ across primary care settings. Regardless of whether paramedics wear work-issued uniforms or their own clothes, the Code of Practice on the prevention and control of infections and related guidance outlines the importance of using PPE, such as a disposable apron, to prevent contamination of the clinician's clothing.

It is a professional standard for paramedics to 'maintain a safe working environment' (HCPC, 2014). Workwear worn by staff when carrying out their duties should be clean, be fit for purpose and support good hygiene. Workwear should be laundered separately from other clothing on a hot-wash cycle at the highest temperature that the fabric will tolerate. It should then be dried thoroughly, as tumble drying or ironing will further reduce the small number of micro-organisms present after washing. It is not good practice to wear neck ties or lanyards during direct patient care. Ties have previously been shown to be contaminated by pathogens (Nurkin, 2004), and it is likely that lanyards that are rarely laundered can have the same level of contamination.

Aprons

Disposable aprons are impermeable to bacteria and body fluids and protect the areas of maximum potential contamination on the front of the body. A disposable apron should be worn whenever body fluids or other sources of contamination are likely to soil the front of workwear, and especially when:

- Undertaking an aseptic technique
- Undertaking a procedure on a patient with a known or suspected infection
- Decontaminating equipment or the environment.

Disposable aprons should be removed and disposed of after each task, particularly after completion of a dirty task and before a clean task begins. Hand hygiene should be performed after removing the apron (NHS England and NHS Improvement, 2019).

Eye Protection

A face visor or safety glasses should be worn when there is a risk of splashing body fluids to the face and eyes, and a splash-resistant surgical mask should be worn when there is a risk of splashing body fluids to the nose or mouth (NHS England and NHS Improvement, 2019). This applies both to diagnostic and procedural skills during primary care assessment, as well as to patients who attend with coughs and sneezes. Both these items are required to be worn together for specific occasions, such as in a pandemic (WHO, 2014). Normal prescription glasses do not provide adequate protection. Reusable items, such as non-disposable goggles, face shields and visors, must be decontaminated after each use.

CHAPTER 1 Professional Considerations

Face Masks

There are several different face masks suitable for different situations, as outlined in Table 1.1.

For FFP1, FFP2, FFP3 and respirator masks, the fit of the masks is critically important and every user should be fit-tested for a seal check and trained in application and removal.

Disposable masks should be removed or changed:

- Before each patient contract
- If the mask's integrity is breached, for example, from moisture build-up after extended use or from gross contamination with blood or body fluids.

Table 1.1 Mask Types

Type of mask	Description and level of protection
Fluid-resistant face masks	Worn to protect patients from the operator as a source of infection, e.g. when performing surgical procedures or epidurals or inserting a central vascular catheter (CVC). Masks should be well-fitting and fit for purpose, fully covering the mouth and nose.
Protective masks: FFP1	Filtering efficiency of 80%, useful to protect against non-toxic substances (such as those used in DIY).
Protective masks: FFP2	Filtering efficiency of 94%. During the COVID-19 pandemic, the WHO recommended the minimum of an FFP2 mask for offering protection.
Protective masks: FFP3	Filtering efficiency of 99%. Offers the highest protection from breathing in hazardous substances in the environment. The mask can protect from a variety of toxins, such as asbestos, bacteria and viruses.
Respirator masks	A respirator mask with disposable filters providing more than a 99% filtering efficiency is rarely required in general practice. Advice on the wearing of these masks during an influenza pandemic is issued by Public Health England (2020).

Source: HSE (2022).

Gloves

If contact with blood, body fluids, non-intact skin or mucous membranes is anticipated or the patient has a known infection, disposable gloves should be worn that are appropriate to the task (NHS England and NHS Improvement, 2019). Clinical gloves must be powder-free and should be nitrile or vinyl material in case of latex allergy or sensitivity.

Gloves must be worn as single-use items and changed between each different task on a service user. Hands must be washed or alcohol handrub applied immediately before putting on and after removing each pair of gloves. Many gloves will develop micro-punctures very quickly and will no longer perform their barrier function.

Glove integrity can be impaired with substances such as isopropanol, ethanol, oil and disinfectant, thus washing or using an alcohol-based handrub on gloves is considered unsafe practice (Harrogate and District NHS Foundation Trust, 2017a).

Infection Prevention and Control

Applying Personal Protective Equipment

The correct order for putting on PPE is as follows:

1. Perform hand hygiene.
2. Pull apron over the head and fasten at back of waist.
3. Secure mask ties at back of head and neck. Fit flexible band to nose bridge.
4. Place eye protection over eyes.
5. Put on gloves and extend to cover wrists.

This is outlined in Figure 1.3.

- **Perform hand hygiene before putting on PPE**

1 Apron
Pull over head and fasten at back of waist.

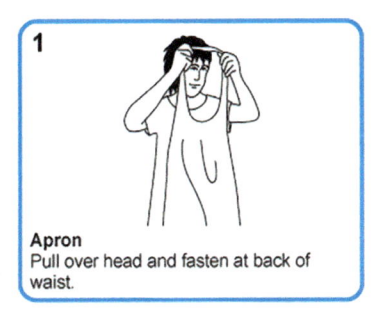

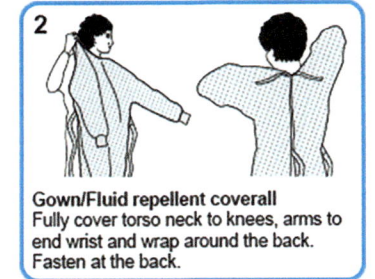

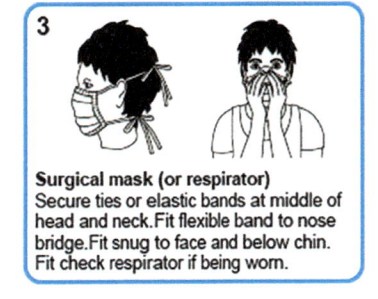

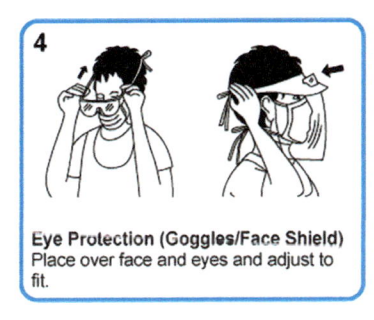

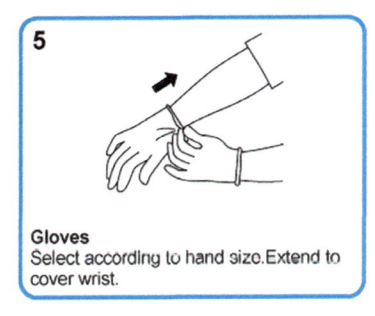

2 Gown/Fluid repellent coverall
Fully cover torso neck to knees, arms to end wrist and wrap around the back. Fasten at the back.

3 Surgical mask (or respirator)
Secure ties or elastic bands at middle of head and neck. Fit flexible band to nose bridge. Fit snug to face and below chin. Fit check respirator if being worn.

4 Eye Protection (Goggles/Face Shield)
Place over face and eyes and adjust to fit.

5 Gloves
Select according to hand size. Extend to cover wrist.

Figure 1.3 Applying PPE.
Source: Image supplied by kind permission of Antimicrobial Resistance and Healthcare Associated Infection Scotland, a service provided by NHS National Services Scotland. Image correct as of November 2022.

To minimise the risk of cross- or self-contamination, there is a correct order for removing PPE too, which is as follows:

1. Gloves, which are potentially the most contaminated item of PPE, must always be removed first. Grasp the outside of the glove with the opposite gloved hand and peel off.
2. Hold the removed glove in the gloved hand. Slide the fingers of the ungloved hand under the remaining glove at the wrist and peel off.
3. Unfasten or break apron ties. Pull apron away from neck and shoulders, lifting over the head and touching the inside of the apron only. Fold or roll into a bundle.
4. Handle eye protection only by the headband or the sides.

CHAPTER 1 Professional Considerations

5. Unfasten the mask ties – first the bottom, then the top. Remove by handling ties only.
6. Perform hand hygiene immediately after removal.
7. All PPE should be removed before leaving the area and disposed of as healthcare waste.

This is outlined in Figure 1.4.

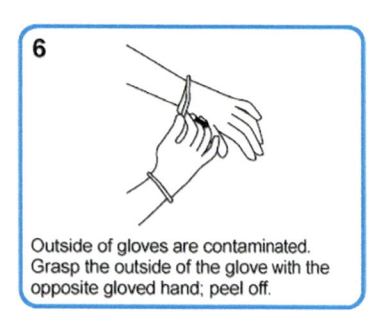

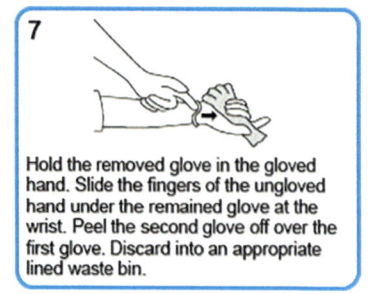

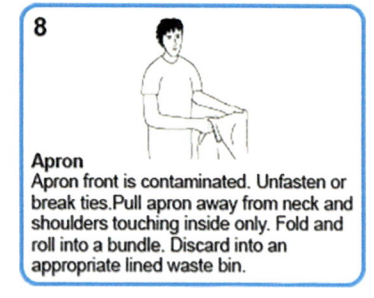

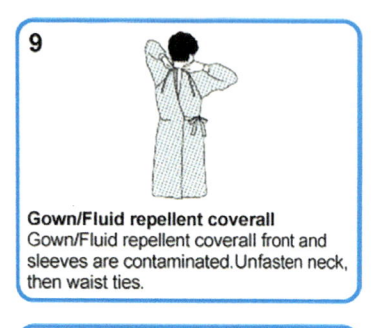

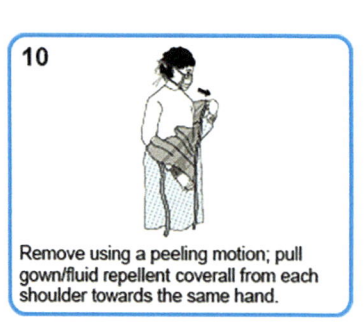

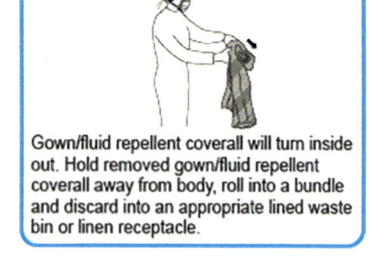

6
Outside of gloves are contaminated. Grasp the outside of the glove with the opposite gloved hand; peel off.

7
Hold the removed glove in the gloved hand. Slide the fingers of the ungloved hand under the remained glove at the wrist. Peel the second glove off over the first glove. Discard into an appropriate lined waste bin.

8
Apron
Apron front is contaminated. Unfasten or break ties. Pull apron away from neck and shoulders touching inside only. Fold and roll into a bundle. Discard into an appropriate lined waste bin.

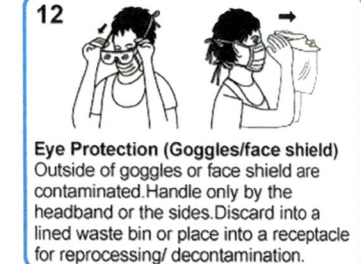

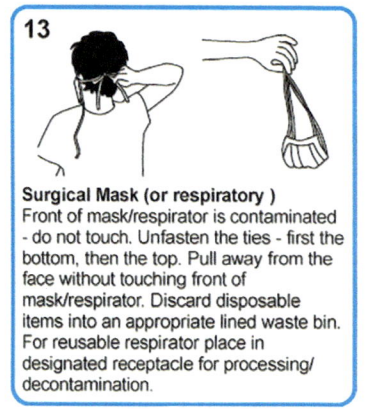

9
Gown/Fluid repellent coverall
Gown/Fluid repellent coverall front and sleeves are contaminated. Unfasten neck, then waist ties.

10
Remove using a peeling motion; pull gown/fluid repellent coverall from each shoulder towards the same hand.

11
Gown/fluid repellent coverall will turn inside out. Hold removed gown/fluid repellent coverall away from body, roll into a bundle and discard into an appropriate lined waste bin or linen receptacle.

12
Eye Protection (Goggles/face shield)
Outside of goggles or face shield are contaminated. Handle only by the headband or the sides. Discard into a lined waste bin or place into a receptacle for reprocessing/ decontamination.

13
Surgical Mask (or respiratory)
Front of mask/respirator is contaminated - do not touch. Unfasten the ties - first the bottom, then the top. Pull away from the face without touching front of mask/respirator. Discard disposable items into an appropriate lined waste bin. For reusable respirator place in designated receptacle for processing/ decontamination.

- **Perform hand hygiene immediately on removal.**
- **All PPE should be removed before leaving the area and disposed of as healthcare waste.**

Figure 1.4   Removing PPE.

Source: Image supplied by kind permission of Antimicrobial Resistance and Healthcare Associated Infection Scotland, a service provided by NHS National Services Scotland. Image correct as of November 2022.

Infection Prevention and Control

Exposure Management

Sharps Management

General practices and their employees have legal obligations under the Health and Safety (Sharp Instruments in Healthcare) Regulations (HSE, 2013). All employers are required to ensure that risks from sharps injuries are adequately assessed and that appropriate control measures are in place, and employees should demonstrate safe use and disposal of sharps. Syringes and needles should be discarded as one unit. Needles must not be re-sheathed, and sharps are to be disposed of at the point of use.

Procedure Following a Splash or Inoculation Injury

All primary care services will have a local guidance document regarding the management of splash or inoculation injuries experienced by staff, including paramedics. All such injuries must be reported to the practice manager, with attendance at the nearest emergency department and an occupational health review. The following principles are generic across England:

- In the event of a splash injury to eyes, nose or mouth, rinse the affected area thoroughly with copious amounts of running water.
- In the event of a bite or skin contamination:
  - Wash the affected area with liquid soap and warm running water
  - Dry and cover with a waterproof dressing.
- In the event of a needlestick or sharps injury:
  - Encourage bleeding of the wound by squeezing under running water (do not suck the wound)
  - Wash the wound with liquid soap and warm running water and dry (do not scrub)
  - Cover the wound with a waterproof dressing
  - If a needlestick or sharps injury has occurred from an item which has been used on a patient (source), the patient may consent to a blood sample being taken to test for hepatitis B, hepatitis C and HIV (HSE, 2013).

At the emergency department:

- A blood sample will be taken to check your hepatitis B antibody levels and immunoglobulin will be offered if they are low. The blood sample will be stored until results are available from the patient's blood sample. If the source of the sharps injury is unknown, you will also have blood samples taken at 6, 12 and 24 weeks for hepatitis C and HIV.
- If the patient (source) is known or suspected to be HIV positive, post-exposure prophylaxis (PEP) treatment will be offered. This should ideally commence within 1 hour of the injury and is not recommended beyond 72 hours after the first exposure (Cresswell et al., 2022).

CHAPTER 1 Professional Considerations

Chapter Summary

The professional responsibilities and expectations of paramedics remain little different regardless of the clinical environment. However, there do exist professional issues that are more relevant to primary care than to other clinical settings that paramedics may be employed in, and these are particularly concerned with scope of practice, supervision and the duty of candour. Maintaining fitness to practise is important regardless of the clinical setting, and since primary care has long been associated with occupational stress for clinicians, paramedics should be aware of how they may manage stress and build personal resilience. There are particular infection control practices that are perhaps more relevant to primary care than to other employment types, and paramedics must be familiar with their local guidance and policies and procedures regarding this.

References

Avery, A., Barber, N., Ghaleb, M. et al. (2012) *Investigating the Prevalence and Causes of Prescribing Errors in General Practice: The PRACtICe Study*. London: General Medical Council.

Blaber, A., Morris, H. and Collen, A. (2018) *Independent Prescribing for Paramedics*. Bridgwater: Class Professional Publishing.

British Medical Association (BMA) (2017) Quarterly tracker survey: Current views from across the medical profession Quarter 2, June 2017. London: British Medical Association. Available at: https://www.bma.org.uk/what-we-do/viewpoint-surveys (accessed 28 January 2023).

British Medical Association (BMA) (2020) Medical Indemnity: State backed GP indemnity. Available at: https://www.bma.org.uk/advice-and-support/medical-indemnity/medical-indemnity/state-backed-gp-indemnity-scheme (accessed 30 January 2023).

Care Quality Commission (2013) Supporting effective clinical supervision. Available at: https://work-learn-live-blmk.co.uk/wp-content/uploads/2018/04/CQC-Supporting-information-and-guidance.pdf (accessed 27 January 2023).

Care Quality Commission (2015) Duty of candour guidance. Available at: https://www.cqc.org.uk/sites/default/files/20210421%20The%20duty%20of%20candour%20-%20guidance%20for%20providers.pdf (accessed 27 January 2023).

College of Paramedics (2018) *Practice Guidance for Paramedic Supplementary and Independent Prescribers*. Bridgwater: College of Paramedics.

College of Paramedics (2021) Scope of practice. Available at: https://collegeofparamedics.co.uk/COP/ProfessionalDevelopment/Scope_of_Practice.aspx (accessed 30 January 2023).

College of Paramedics (2023) Post Registration – Paramedic Career Framework. 5th edn. Available at: https://collegeofparamedics.co.uk/COP/ProfessionalDevelopment/post_reg_career_framework.aspx (accessed 26 April 2023).

Cresswell, F., Asanati, K., Bhagani, S. et al. (2022) UK guideline for the use of HIV post-exposure prophylaxis 2021. *HIV Medicine* 23(5): 494–545.

Department of Health & Social Care (DHSC) (2019) Clinical negligence indemnity consultation. Available at: https://assets.publishing.service.gov.uk/government/uploads/system/uploads/attachment_data/file/777469/Clinical_negligence_indemnity_consultation.pdf (accessed 30 January 2023).

References

Department of Health Northern Ireland (2020) Get involved in duty of candour. Available at: https://www.health-ni.gov.uk/articles/ihrd-get-involved-duty-candour (accessed 30 January 2023).

Drummond, D. (2014) *Stop Physician Burnout: What to Do When Working Harder Isn't Working*. New York: Heritage Press Publications.

Eaton, G., Mahtani, K. and Catterall, M. (2018) The evolving role of paramedics – a NICE problem to have? *Journal of Health Services Research and Policy* 23(3): 193–195.

Eaton, G., Wong, G., Williams, V. et al. (2020) Contribution of paramedics in primary and urgent care: A systematic review. *British Journal of General Practice* 70(695): e421–e426.

Eaton, G., Wong, G., Tierney, S. et al. (2021) Understanding the role of the paramedic in primary care: A realist review. *BMC Medicine* 19(1): 145.

Fulford, K.W.M. (2011) The value of evidence and evidence of values: Bringing together values-based and evidence-based practice in policy and service development in mental health. *Journal of Evaluation in Clinical Practice* 17(5): 976–987.

General Medical Council (GMC) (2019) Caring for doctors. Caring for patients. Available at: https://www.gmc-uk.org/-/media/documents/caring-for-doctors-caring-for-patients_pdf-80706341.pdf (accessed 30 January 2023).

General Medical Council (GMC) (2023) Approval of trainers. Available at: https://www.gmc-uk.org/education/how-we-quality-assure-medical-education-and-training/approving-medical-education-and-training/approval-of-trainers (accessed 27 January 2023).

Gibson, J., Checkland, K., Coleman, A. et al. (2015) Eighth national GP worklife survey. Available at: https://www.research.manchester.ac.uk/portal/en/publications/eighth-national-gp-worklife-survey(a76ed99e-c54e-4ba4-a20e-ce432322689e)/export.html (accessed 6 April 2020).

Hall, L., Johnson, J., Watt, I. et al. (2016) Healthcare staff wellbeing, burnout, and patient safety: A systematic review. *PLoS One* 11(7): e015901.

Hall, L., Johnson, J., Watt, I. et al. (2019) Association of GP wellbeing and burnout with patient safety in UK primary care: A cross-sectional survey. *British Journal of General Practice* 69(684): e507–e514.

Harrogate and District NHS Foundation Trust (2017a) Hand hygiene policy for general practice. Available at https://www.hdft.nhs.uk/services/infection-prevention-control/ (accessed 27 January 2023).

Harrogate and District NHS Foundation Trust (2017b) Community Infection Prevention and Control Guidance for General Practice: Invasive Devices [GP09]. Available at: https://www.infectionpreventioncontrol.co.uk/content/uploads/2018/12/GP-09-Invasive-devices-December-2017-Version-1.00.pdf (accessed 27 January 2023).

Health and Care Professions Council (HCPC) (2012) *Education Annual Report*. Available at: https://www.hcpc-uk.org/globalassets/resources/reports/education/education-annual-report-2012.pdf?v=636785009160000000 (accessed 27 January 2023).

Health and Care Professions Council (HCPC) (2014) *Standards of Proficiency – Paramedics*. London: HCPC.

Health and Care Professions Council (HCPC) (2018a) Fitness to practice annual report 2018. Available at: https://www.hcpc-uk.org/resources/reports/2018/fitness-to-practise-annual-report-2018/ (accessed 30 January 2023).

Health and Care Professions Council (HCPC) (2018b) *Our Standards for CPD*. London: HCPC.

CHAPTER 1 Professional Considerations

Health and Care Professions Council (HCPC) (2018c) Standards of conduct, performance and ethics. Available at: https://www.hcpc-uk.org/standards/standards-of-conduct-performance-and-ethics/ (accessed 27 January 2023).

Health and Safety Executive (HSE) (2013) Health and safety (sharp instruments in healthcare) regulations. Available at: https://www.hse.gov.uk/pubns/hsis7.htm (accessed 30 January 2023).

Health and Safety Executive (HSE) (2022) Face masks: When and how to wear one. Available at: https://www2.hse.ie/conditions/covid19/preventing-the-spread/when-to-wear-face-covering/ (accessed 30 January 2023).

Health Education England (HEE) (2018) Enhancing supervision for postgraduate doctors in training. Available at: https://www.hee.nhs.uk/sites/default/files/documents/Handbook_Update_Film.pdf (accessed 30 January 2023).

Health Education England (HEE) (2019a) Advanced clinical practice. Available at: https://www.hee.nhs.uk/our-work/advanced-clinical-practice/what-advanced-clinical-practice (accessed 30 January 2023).

Health Education England (HEE) (2019b) Core capabilities framework. Available at: https://www.hee.nhs.uk/sites/default/files/documents/Paramedic%20Specialist%20in%20Primary%20and%20Urgent%20Care%20Core%20Capabilities%20Framework.pdf (accessed 30 January 2023).

Health Education England (HEE) (2021) First contact practitioners and advanced practitioners in primary care: (Paramedic) A roadmap to practice (issue July). Available at: https://www.hee.nhs.uk/sites/default/files/documents/Paramedics-FINAL%20(002).pdf (accessed 30 January 2023).

Jabbar, U., Leischner, J., Kasper, D. et al. (2010) Effectiveness of alcohol-based hand rubs for removal of Clostridium difficile spores from hands. *Infection Control & Hospital Epidemiology* 31(6): 565–570.

Karasek, R. (1979) Job demands, job decision latitude, and mental strain: Implications for job redesign. *Administrative Science Quarterly* 24: 285–308.

Macdonald, W. (2006) The impact of job demands and workload on stress and fatigue. *Australian Psychologist* 38(2): 102–117.

Mathur, P. (2011). Hand hygiene: Back to the basics of infection control. *The Indian Journal of Medical Research* 134(5): 611–620.

McManus, I., Jonvik, H., Richards, P. et al. (2011) Vocation and avocation: Leisure activities correlate with professional engagement, but not burnout, in a cross-sectional survey of UK doctors. *BMC Medicine* 9(1): 100.

Mildenhall, J. (2012) Occupational stress, paramedic informal coping strategies: A review of the literature. *Journal of Paramedic Practice* 4(6): 318–328.

Mind (2017) Stress: Managing stress and building resilience. Available at: https://www.mind.org.uk/information-support/types-of-mental-health-problems/stress/developing-resilience/#collapse5c1d9 (accessed 30 January 2023).

NHS (2022) Stress. Available at: https://www.nhs.uk/conditions/stress-anxiety-depression/understanding-stress/ (accessed 30 January 2023).

NHS England (2019) A five-year framework for GP contract reform to implement The NHS Long Term Plan. Available at: https://www.england.nhs.uk/wp-content/uploads/2019/01/gp-contract-2019.pdf (accessed 8 September 2020).

NHS England and NHS Improvement (2019) National policy on hand hygiene and PPE. Available at: https://www.england.nhs.uk/wp-content/uploads/2019/03/Standard-infection-control-precautions-national-hand-hygiene-and-personal-protective-equipment-policy.pdf (accessed 18 November 2022).

References

Nurkin, S. (2004) Is the clinician's necktie a potential fomite for hospital acquired infections? *104th General Meeting of the American Society for Microbiology*. American Society for Microbiology, New Orleans, USA, 23–27 May 2004.

O'Connor, D.B., O'Connor, R.C., White, B.L. et al. (2000) The effect of job strain on British general practitioners' mental health. *Journal of Mental Health* 9(6): 637–654.

O'Hara Inquiry (2020) Report of the inquiry into hyponatraemia related deaths. Available at: http://www.ihrdni.org/inquiry-report.htm (accessed 30 January 2023).

Orton, P., Orton, C., Gray, D.P. et al. (2012) Depersonalised doctors: A cross-sectional study of 564 doctors, 760 consultations and 1876 patient reports in UK general practice. *BMJ Open* 2(1): e000274.

Patel, R.S., Sekhri, S., Bhimanadham, N. et al. (2019) A review on strategies to manage physician burnout. *Cureus* 11(6): e4805.

Public Health England (2020) Explanation of the updates to infection prevention and control guidance. Available at: https://www.gov.uk/government/publications/wuhan-novel-coronavirus-infection-prevention-and-control/updates-to-the-infection-prevention-and-control-guidance-for-covid-19 (accessed 30 January 2023).

Royal College of General Practitioners (2020) Training and examinations. Available at: https://www.rcgp.org.uk/training-exams/training.aspx (accessed 30 January 2023).

Royal College of Emergency Medicine (RCEM) (2021) The guide to RCEM emergency care ACP credentialing. Available at: https://rcem.ac.uk/wp-content/uploads/2021/11/The_guide_to_Emergency_Care_ACP_credentialing_v3_July2021_final.pdf (accessed 30 January 2023).

Salyers, M.P., Bonfils, K.A., Luther, L. et al. (2017) The relationship between professional burnout and quality and safety in healthcare: A meta-analysis. *Journal of General Internal Medicine* 32(4): 475–482.

Scottish Government (2012) Professionalism in nursing, midwifery and the allied health professions in Scotland: A report to the coordinating council for the NNMAHP contribution to the healthcare quality strategy for NHS Scotland. Available at: https://webarchive.nrscotland.gov.uk/3000/https://www.gov.scot/resource/0039/00396525.pdf (accessed 30 January 2023).

Skills for Care (2007) Supervision. Available at: https://www.skillsforcare.org.uk/Leadership-management/managing-people/supervision/Supervision.aspx (accessed 30 January 2023).

Snowdon, D.A., Leggat, S.G. and Taylor, N.F. (2017) Does clinical supervision of healthcare professionals improve effectiveness of care and patient experience? A systematic review. *BMC Health Services Research* 17(1): 786.

Stern, D.T., Frohna, A.Z. and Gruppen, L.D. (2005) The prediction of professional behaviour. *Medical Education* 39(1): 75–82.

Sudron, C. (2022) Professional regulation and accountability. In Eaton (ed) *Law and Ethics for Paramedics*. 2nd edn. Bridgwater: Class Professional Publishing, pp. 13–28.

UK Government (2008) Health and Social Care Act 2008: Code of practice on the prevention and control of infections. Available at: https://www.gov.uk/government/publications/the-health-and-social-care-act-2008-code-of-practice-on-the-prevention-and-control-of-infections-and-related-guidance (accessed 30 January 2023).

World Health Organization (2009) Hand hygiene. Available at: https://www.who.int/teams/integrated-health-services/infection-prevention-control/hand-hygiene/training-tools (accessed 30 January 2023).

CHAPTER 1   Professional Considerations

World Health Organization (2014) Infection prevention and control of epidemic- and pandemic-prone acute respiratory infections in health care. Available at: https://apps.who.int/iris/bitstream/handle/10665/112656/9789241507134_eng.pdf;jsessionid=15EBA8A01894DA1E4B985114DFD7E647?sequence=1 (accessed 30 January 2023).

Legislation

Health and Social Care (Quality and Engagement) (Wales) Act.
The Duty of Candour Procedure (Scotland) Regulations 2018.
The Health and Social Care Act 2008 (Regulated Activities) Regulations 2014.

Consultation Skills and the Diagnostic Process

Tom Mallinson

Introduction

There are many consultation models, and it has been said that while all are flawed, they can influence and improve our practice. They provide a scaffolding on which to build an empathetic working relationship with our patients, their carers and their family members. Whichever consultation model or strategy we adopt, we must be able to adapt both our verbal and non-verbal communication styles to the individual in front of us. In many circumstances, this means adjusting to a patient's needs and preferences and being attuned to individual issues such as varying levels of health literacy, and someone's abilities in relation to both spoken and written English. There is a legion of models to guide consultations in medicine, and only a selection is presented in this text. It may be that you find a structure which works well for you, or that a combination of the models presented here suits your personality and communication style.

The Medical Model (The Hospital Clerking Model)

This is the backbone of all medical history taking and is the consultation model which is most often utilised when admitting patients to hospital or seeing them in the emergency department (Figure 2.1). It represents a disease-centred model, which focuses on identifying a medical problem and treating it. This consultation model provides a core structure for obtaining information and aims to provide a comprehensive overview of the patient's pathophysiological and pharmacological situation.

However, it has a number of key limitations: it is not patient centred by nature, which risks lack of buy-in from the patient; it does not seek to elicit the patient's thoughts or feelings in relation to their medical situation; and nor does it aim to place the presenting complaint in its psycho-social context. It also contains little in the way of prompts to ensure safe practice and appropriate diagnostic decision making.

Some of these limitations can be mitigated with the use of communication techniques, but it is likely that in primary care, the medical model alone is insufficient. Active listening and reflective listening strategies for example can encourage patients to 'tell their story' to a greater degree even when using the Medical Model, and this may allow an insight into the psycho-social context of a biological complaint (Table 2.1). It is also useful to consider the Reflective Listening Cycle as a core communication skill, which can be applied to any other model or framework (Figure 2.2).

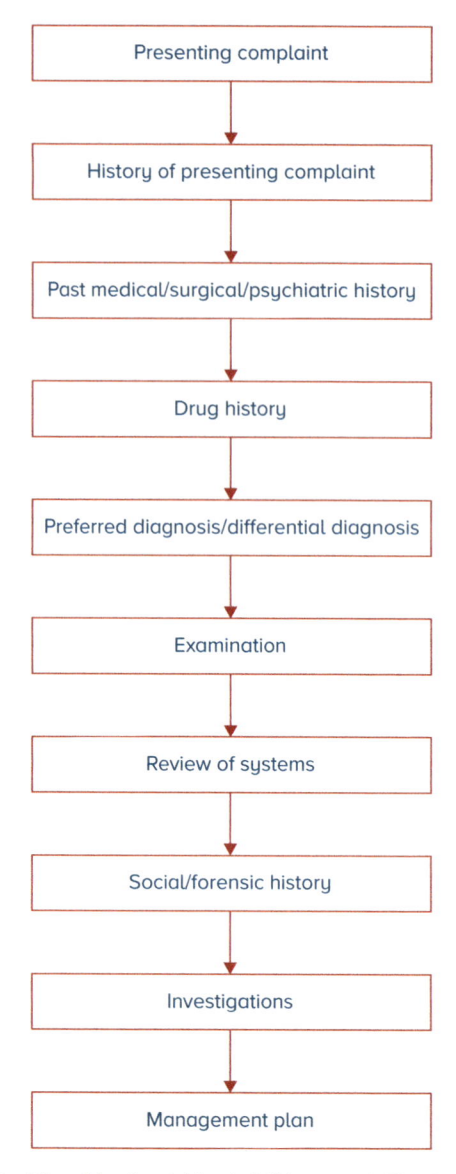

CHAPTER 2 Consultation Skills and the Diagnostic Process

```
Presenting complaint
        ↓
History of presenting complaint
        ↓
Past medical/surgical/psychiatric history
        ↓
Drug history
        ↓
Preferred diagnosis/differential diagnosis
        ↓
Examination
        ↓
Review of systems
        ↓
Social/forensic history
        ↓
Investigations
        ↓
Management plan
```

Figure 2.1 The Medical Model (Hospital Clerking Model).

Whichever model is used, it is essential to avoid common consultation pitfalls, such as early interruptions, becoming distracted by your notes or computer or premature closure (also known as anchoring), where an early diagnosis may overshadow subsequent data received and lead you to an incorrect diagnosis.

> 💡 Interrupted patients are less likely to disclose further details, and you may miss important information.

The Bio-Psycho-Social Model (The RCGP Model)

Table 2.1 Active and Reflective Listening Techniques

Active listening techniques	Reflective listening techniques
• Frequent clarification • Nodding • Using pacing cues (e.g. phrases like 'uh huh', 'yeah' etc.) • Maintaining eye contact • Mirroring the patient's body language • Allowing the patient to finish a sentence or thought (resisting interrupting) • Summarising key points • Asking probing questions	• Repeating and paraphrasing • Expressing your understanding (e.g. phrases like 'I see' or 'I understand') • Seeking confirmation • Non-judgemental approach • Drawing out implicit feelings

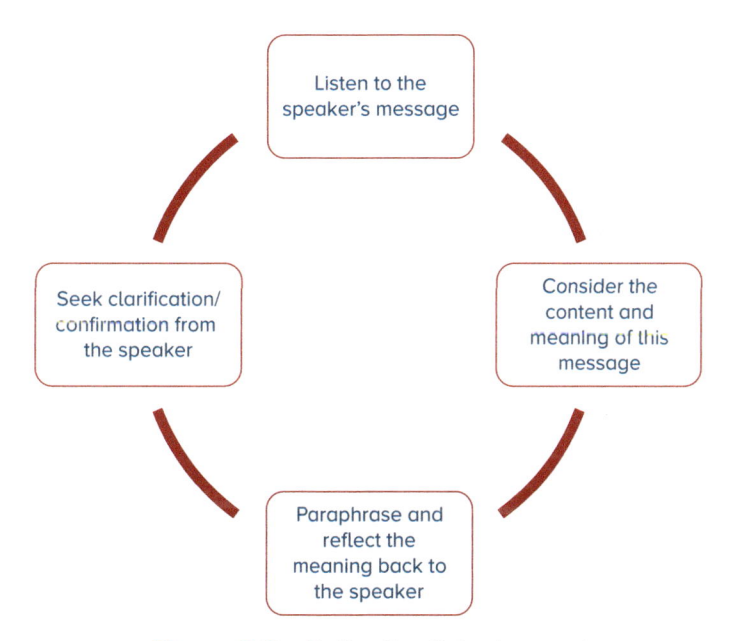

Figure 2.2 Reflective listening cycle.

The Bio-Psycho-Social Model (The RCGP Model)

When applying the Medical Clerking Model into primary care, there are a number of important considerations, most notably the need to include an integration of the biological, psychological and social aspects of a patient's experience. This is also referred to as the

CHAPTER 2 Consultation Skills and the Diagnostic Process

triple-diagnosis or triaxial model, as these three aspects will overlap and influence the patient's presentation. It is sometimes considered the standard Royal College of General Practitioners (RCGP) model (RCGP, 1972). The other notable difference is that primary care in the United Kingdom is based around a system of very short appointment times, which do not allow time for the full history taking advised in the Medical Clerking Model. In most primary care consultations, the clinician will also have access to the patient's notes and medical records, therefore only a brief clarification of issues around past medical history or concordance with documented medication regimes will be needed.

> This model can be a gateway to consider potential social prescribing interventions through building a clearer picture of what matters to the patient.

There are a number of ways in which we can elicit the psychological and social aspects of a patient's illness experience, with active and reflective listening being two core techniques. Another strategy is to enquire specifically about the patient's Ideas, Concerns and Expectations (ICE), which reminds the clinician to gain the patient's views during the consultation (Table 2.2). ICE has however been criticised as overly formulaic and antithetical to building rapport with your patients (Snow, 2016), and it should certainly not be used in a checklist fashion. Another way of considering the patient's agenda is through Helman's list of patient questions, known as Helman's Folk Model (Helman, 1981). Helman proposed that patients attend a healthcare provider with seven key questions: three *whys* and four *whats*. Initially, a patient comes to ask *what* is happening, *why* is it happening, *why* is it happening to me and *why* now. Then, once those have been addressed to some extent, and perhaps after a diagnosis is given, *what* would happen if I did nothing, *what* are the wider effects if nothing is done about this (perhaps in terms of employment or strain on relationships) and, finally, *what* should I do about it.

Table 2.2 Example Questions for ICE

Components of ICE	Example phrases
Ideas	• 'Did you have any thoughts about what was going on?' • 'Have you had any thoughts about what's causing this?'
Concerns	• 'Was there anything specific you were worried this might be?' • 'What's your biggest worry about this problem?'
Expectations	• 'Was there anything specific you hoped to gain from the consultation today?' • 'What would be your preferred plan of action today?' • 'Did you have any thoughts on how we might handle this issue?'

Consultation Structure

> 💡 The Medical Model is the cornerstone of medical history taking but is not always a suitable model for consultations in primary care, where the psycho-social needs of the patient may need to be explored in more detail.

Consultation Structure

Many consultation models focus on a specific structure or framework for the conduct of a consultation beyond simply guiding what topics should be covered. Three of the most widely used are Pendleton's, Neighbour's and the Calgary-Cambridge Model.

Pendleton's Model

In 1984, Pendleton, Schofield, Tate and Havelock published their model (Pendleton et al., 1984), which focuses on a number of tasks for the clinician to complete during the course of a consultation, with two of these being overarching goals for the encounter (Figure 2.3). The first of these tasks is directed at identifying why the patient is attending, and in terms of the Medical Model would include the presenting complaint, the history of the presenting complaint and the aetiology of the presenting complaint. It also incorporates gaining an insight into the patient's ideas, concerns and expectations and the effect of this presenting complaint on aspects of their life such as work, relationships and psychological well-being. This is quite a lot to cover, and it is perhaps a bit ambitious to include all of this under one 'task'; further discussion of a specific model to aid the diagnostic process is discussed later in this chapter.

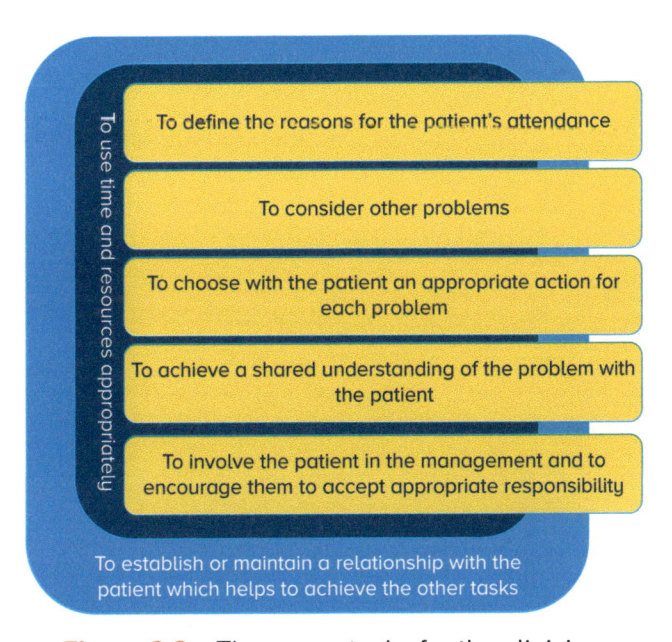

Figure 2.3 The seven tasks for the clinician.

- To define the reasons for the patient's attendance
- To consider other problems
- To choose with the patient an appropriate action for each problem
- To achieve a shared understanding of the problem with the patient
- To involve the patient in the management and to encourage them to accept appropriate responsibility
- To use time and resources appropriately
- To establish or maintain a relationship with the patient which helps to achieve the other tasks

CHAPTER 2 Consultation Skills and the Diagnostic Process

The second task, considering other problems, covers both ongoing problems – perhaps something you discussed at a previous consultation – and addressing modifiable risk factors for ill-health (for example, obesity, smoking, alcohol intake). The third task relates to the formulation of a plan for the future, and emphasises that this is a shared decision-making process, with the aim of formulating a plan acceptable to both clinician and patient. Roger Neighbour provides some tips for this in relation to his 'hand-over' checkpoint in the next section.

The final two tasks are over-arching and will need to be considered during both consultations and your longer-term care for this patient. The first of these highlights the need to use both time and resources appropriately. One example of this may be the safe and appropriate use of telephone triage consultations and another may be the concept of 'realistic medicine', which incorporates shared decision making with open acknowledgement that all of us working in healthcare are working with limited resources (Calderwood, 2019). The final task relates to the development of a relationship with your patient, which is beneficial both during a single consultation, and in the longer term with respect to primary care looking after people from cradle to grave.

While Pendleton's Model is widely taught, it has also been criticised for being too in-depth for a 10–20-minute consultation as is standard in UK primary care, and for risking dwelling on irrelevant tasks for a consultation which otherwise would be quick and fairly focused (for exmaple, a patient with a cut hand may not appreciate significant time spent delving into their modifiable risk factors).

> Realistic Medicine (2023) Working together to provide the care that's right for you [online].
> RCGP (2022) WPBA assessments: Consultation Observation Tool (COT) [online].

Neighbour's Model

In 1987, Roger Neighbour formulated his consultation model, which consisted of five main checkpoints. His model is often represented as fingers on a hand to aid recall (Figure 2.4). It is a simpler model of the mechanics of a consultation than Pendleton's seven tasks and is easy to remember during a consultation.

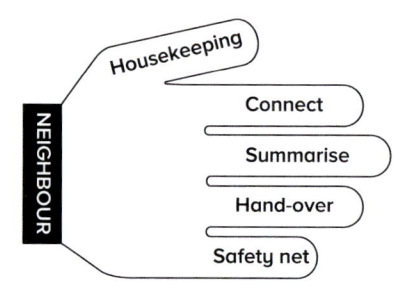

Figure 2.4 Neighbour's consultation model.

Neighbour commences (and concludes) with the idea of 'housekeeping', which is similar to the 'setting' heading in the SPIKES mnemonic discussed later (Table 2.4) but has a greater focus on personal readiness. Neighbour highlights that as a clinician (and human) we have needs and limitations: we may be hungry, frustrated or desperate for a toilet visit, and such issues should be addressed before commencing the next consultation. We could perhaps compare Neighbour's 'housekeeping' with Reid's heading of 'self' as presented in his STEP-UP mnemonic of the Zero Point Survey, and the mnemonic of IMSAFE. Table 2.3 presents an easy means to remember various factors which may adversely affect clinician performance (Reid, 2013; Reid et al., 2018).

After ensuring the clinician is prepared for a new consultation, Neighbour invites us to 'connect' with our patient. This serves as a cue to build rapport with the patient, not just at a superficial level but in a way which will facilitate the growth of genuine empathy and understanding. This relates strongly with the concept of narrative medicine discussed later. Building rapport is also one aspect of the consultation that is seriously restricted when undertaking remote consultations, and this is discussed later.

While the next checkpoint is entitled 'summarise', it also encapsulates the core diagnostic process of a consultation, that being assessing the patient's problem and seeking to reach a diagnosis. The keyword of summarise is here to remind us to ensure that we have accurately understood the patient's reasons and motivation for attendance, and that their ideas, concerns and expectations have been identified and addressed. Neighbour advises that an effective way of demonstrating (and checking) one's

Table 2.3 IMSAFE Mnemonic

I	Illness	Awareness and mitigation of any illness you may be experiencing which may affect your performance
M	Medication	Avoidance of medications which may limit your practice
S	Stress	Reflect on your stress levels, be that in general or from the last consultation
A	Alcohol	Hopefully this is not a concern, and it should go without saying that alcohol should not be part of your day of clinical work
F	Fatigue	Tiredness affects our cognitive abilities and can lead to emotional lability; if in doubt, it is best to take a break
E	Emotion & Eating	If the last consultation prompted strong or upsetting emotions for you, it is best to take a few minutes to gather your thoughts before seeing the next patient
		A hungry clinician is liable to make errors; this serves as a reminder (and excuse) to have a snack

CHAPTER 2   Consultation Skills and the Diagnostic Process

understanding is through summarising or repeating back to the patient the information they are giving you. This reiteration should include emotional and 'medical' issues, and it provides an opportunity for the patient to correct anything you have missed or misunderstood, before you move on to the next stage.

The 'hand-over' checkpoint highlights the stage of the consultation when the clinician and the patient cooperate to formulate a management plan. This stage may involve a degree of negotiation and the clinician may utilise a number of techniques to facilitate an agreeable outcome. These may include presenting explanations using the Shingles Technique, named after the roofing material rather than the dermatological disorder, where an overlapping series of explanations leads, almost inexorably, to a set conclusion (Figure 2.5). Other influencing techniques may also be used, such as reframing or shepherding, one example of which is 'My friend John …'. In this technique, John is an ephemeral imaginary third party but the concept facilitates the use of phrases such as 'I had another patient like you who …' or 'Some patients get really worried when they have headaches …'. This sidesteps a direct approach of 'Were you worried this headache was something really serious?', which can inadvertently imply that you as a clinician are concerned that a serious pathology is at work, and leaves the patient open to explain their own thoughts. Once agreement has been reached about the way forward, the consultations can be drawn to a close. Neighbour's last checkpoint is to remind us at the end of consultations to safety net our patients appropriately, and document any advice given. Safety netting is discussed more fully later.

Neighbour (1987) also advanced the idea of being fully attentive to the patient, in an attempt to pick up on their 'minimal cues', these being tell-tale signs (verbal or non-verbal) that provide an insight into the patient's inner thoughts, and which may lead to uncovering a hidden agenda or a topic the patient is keen to avoid. He also discussed the concept of 'doctor as catalyst', meaning the role of the clinician in a consultation is to facilitate change and assist with problem solving. He highlights the importance of the patient having a strong buy-in to any plan or diagnosis, and in his

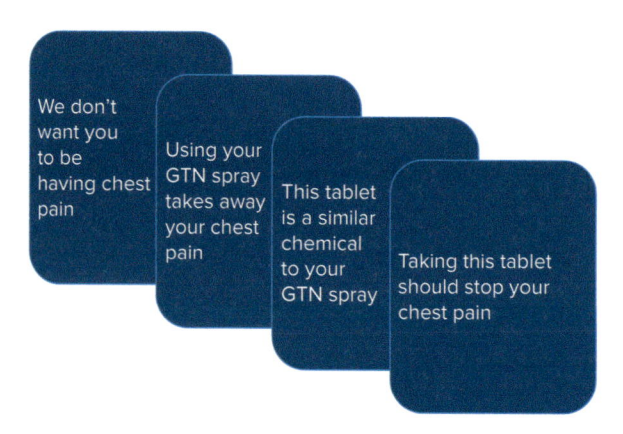

Figure 2.5   Shingles technique.

work discusses various approaches to negotiating, influencing and gift-wrapping ideas, concepts and plans during a consultation, which are beyond the scope of this text to fully explore.

> Neighbour, R. (2012). Models of the Consultation [Online].
> My e-Learning → General Practice 2012 Curriculum → 2.01a_10 → Models of the Consultation

Calgary-Cambridge Model

The Calgary-Cambridge model is perhaps the best approach to use as a framework for teaching consultation skills and it aims to be highly practical in nature (Silverman et al., 1998). This model is useful in terms of giving structure and flow to a consultation and is widely advocated for general practice registrars sitting their Membership of the Royal College of General Practitioners (MRCGP) examinations. In its fullest form, this model is very thorough, with over 70 individual points to cover, which is a challenge in a traditional 10–20-minute consultation.

The core framework as presented in Figure 2.6 is more manageable, with two overarching goals of maintaining the structure and flow of the consultation and developing rapport and a therapeutic relationship with the patient during your time with them. Alongside these two goals are the more chronological stages of a standard consultation: initiating a session, gathering information, physical examinations, explanation and planning and finally closing the session. In this way, the Calgary-Cambridge model is perhaps reminiscent of the Medical Model discussed earlier, in that it suggests a fairly strict journey from one stage to the next. This is perhaps why it is considered a useful model to teach clinicians who are new to primary care consultations (Kurtz and Silverman, 1996).

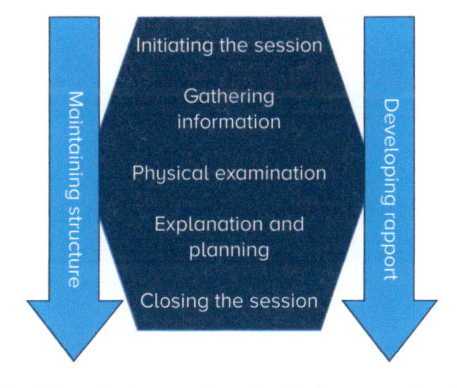

Figure 2.6 The Calgary-Cambridge consultation model.

CHAPTER 2   Consultation Skills and the Diagnostic Process

> 💡 While these models provide options for a clinician during a consultation, they should never be used as checklists, as each consultation is unique.

Recently Developed Consultation Models

There are a number of newer or less well-known consultation models, which may each have something to offer for becoming an expert practitioner in primary care, and it is certainly worth spending some time reading around consultation skills as part of your onward continuing professional development.

A recently developed model, narrative medicine (Charon, 2001), is perhaps best described as a combination of the bio-psycho-social approach and the patient-centred approach, but with a focus on the journey the patient and the clinician are taking separately and together. It takes full advantage of the reflective listening techniques touched upon earlier (Table 2.1) and encourages the clinician to listen to the patient as a 'story teller', with the hope of encouraging the clinician to empathetically embrace the patient's narrative, to fully understand the origin of their ideas, worries and questions related to their health in the broadest sense. In this sense, it is reminiscent of Helman's Folk Model and his list of questions that all patients want to ask and receive answers to (Helman, 1981). Narrative medicine directs us to consider the interpersonal interactions occurring all around us, which influence us as clinicians and also the patients we serve. Such interactions can come in many forms, such as:

- Clinician and patient
- Clinician and colleagues
- Clinician and society
- Clinician and their family
- Patients and other patients
- Patients and their family.

Considering such interpersonal connections is perhaps more important now than ever, with the increasing popularity and necessity of remote consultations, which by their nature limit our ability to connect to others on a personal level.

The BARD model proposed by Warren (2002) is another way of framing the relationship between the clinician and the patient. BARD stands for:

- **B**ehaviour
- **A**ims
- **R**oom
- **D**ialogue.

It aims to highlight that there is individual variation between clinicians and that their personality traits will influence a consultation. Furthermore, it discusses that in the same way that every consultation is unique, the clinicians' techniques and attitudes will vary each time. While some consultations may benefit from the injection of a little humour, others certainly would not and it is essential to modify your behaviour to suit the patient and the conversation. Warren also advocates clarity around the presence of aims and priorities for a consultation, although acknowledges that these may not all be covered in a single session. Like many other models, Warren also highlights that the physical environment, and the clinician's place within that setting, is important to the dynamics of a consultation. Lastly, the BARD model reminds us about dialogue, and the importance of a conscious choice of words, tone and language in relation to building rapport with a patient.

Even more recently, the FRAYED Model has been developed, which seeks to provide guidance for clinicians dealing with challenging consultations (Mirza, 2016). FRAYED stands for:

- **F**act finding
- **R**efuse request
- **A**cceptable alternative
- **Y**ield (or don't yield)
- **E**nd encounter
- **D**ocument diligently.

Within this model, you can see many aspects covered in older models, for example fact finding is a common thread to nearly all models both in terms of medical questions and seeking hidden agendas and the psycho-social background of a patient's experience. Refuse request and acceptable alternative are perhaps already encompassed by Neighbour when he discusses negotiation, shepherding and influencing. The reminder to document diligently is of course a useful one and is likely to be familiar to those of us with a prehospital background, where the mantra 'if you didn't write it, it didn't happen' is still alive and well, despite it not aligning with the reality of legal investigations: a number of cases have highlighted that a lack of documentation is insufficient to form a *prima facie* case of poor conduct against a clinician (Przybylska, 2018).

Remote Consultations

Telephone and Video Consultations

Remote consultation strategies bring with them increased uncertainty and risk, and it is an evolving field (Abbs et al., 2020). As such, we must be mindful to avoid the use of unvalidated clinical tests performed in this new medium of consultations. The widespread use of the unvalidated Roth Score during the COVID-19 pandemic – initially advocated by multiple organisations, including the RCGP, despite a lack of clear evidence base for its use in this way – is an example of how easily we can all fall into such a trap.

A number of frameworks and models have been suggested to assist clinicians working predominantly in this new media. The DR SAMOSA model has been suggested to facilitate effective telephone consultations (Box 2.1) due to perceived limitations of other models in this modality (Tahir and Mirza, 2018); however, it could be argued the model is a little simplistic and adds little to standard communication skills and models. It is perhaps more appropriate to use tried and tested consultation techniques, with adjustments as needed when consulting on the telephone. The main challenge (aside from undertaking an examination) of consulting remotely is how to achieve a connection at a personal level, and how to promote the idea of 'digital warmth' to gain a good rapport when speaking on the telephone or on a video call. Neighbour reminds us that during remote consultations we

CHAPTER 2 Consultation Skills and the Diagnostic Process

must ensure we are focused on the task at hand and make the encounter personal to the patient, avoiding falling into rehearsed phrases or expressions (Neighbour, 2020a). He also reminds us that some of the cornerstones of face-to-face consultation do not translate well to the remote consultation, such as the use of silence, and that the use of pacing cues ('uh huh', 'yeah', 'okay') and affirmative interjections may be even more important.

> **BOX 2.1 DR SAMOSA: A Mnemonic for Telephone Consultations**
>
> **D:** Documentation
> **R:** Rapport
> **S:** Speak Clearly
> **A:** Active Listening
>
> **M:** Mini-management Plan
> **O:** Opportunistic Health Promotion
> **S:** Summarise and Safety Net
> **A:** Alternative Access

- Be very sure to clarify who you are talking to by checking demographic details, and always endeavour to speak directly to the patient.
- Check that the patient is in an environment where they are free to talk and will be comfortable discussing their health issues.
- Aim to establish the reason for the consultation early.
- Aim to rapidly detect those patients for whom a face-to-face appointment will be required.

There are of course many other hints and tips related to specific types of remote consultation; for example, in video consultations, to achieve eye contact one must remember to look into the webcam rather than at the patient's face. There are of course technical challenges; for example, when using systems with a time delay the normally helpful pacing cues may end up being miss-timed and may act as interruptions to the flow of the consultation (Neighbour, 2020b).

> Abbs et al. (2020) *Remote Consultations Handbook*.
> The RCGP has endorsed this handbook covering remote consultations in detail, which is available online and is also an accredited educational resource. This includes further discussion around topics such as undertaking physical examinations remotely, which are extremely helpful.

The Psychology of Consultations

There are also a number of key concepts from the fields of psychology and counselling which have direct relevance to primary care consultations, and a grounding in health psychology is clearly beneficial when one considers developing any therapeutic relationship.

A leading voice in both health psychology and general practice is the psychoanalyst Michael Balint (Balint, 1957). Balint has developed ideas such as 'doctor as drug', where there is therapeutic benefit in the consultation itself; the concept of 'collusion of anonymity' which is experienced by a patient when they feel they are being passed from one specialist to another, with none of them truly assuming responsibility for the patient as a whole person; and the theory of 'transference and counter-transference' during consultations (Balint and Balint, 1939; Denness, 2013). Balint Groups also exist as a forum for clinicians (traditionally doctors) to gather and discuss cases which have played on their mind as a result of their emotional impact on the clinician, a concern related to the consultation or the outcome experienced by the patient (Salinsky, 2009).

Balint also delved into the idea of patient regression during a consultation, which relates to the work of Berne, who described the three states of mind one can occupy: parent, adult or child. This concept from Berne, called 'transactional analysis', can be a useful tool for assessing dysfunctional consultations (Denness, 2013) and is an interesting concept when considering patients who present with a strong external locus of control.

Consultation Models in Practice

Whichever framework you choose to utilise to structure your consultations, it must be remembered that in general, the goal of a consultation is to safely manage the patient's concerns, expectations and medical conditions. Therefore, to be an effective clinician, you need to be able to seamlessly incorporate the diagnostic process into your consultations. Any consultation model used must also not feel artificial or forced to the patient, as this is an easy way to derail a burgeoning therapeutic relationship.

> It can be a useful educational experience to purposefully utilise a single consultation model for an entire session, or day, and reflect on how it altered your interactions with patients.

Breaking Bad News

Breaking bad news is one of the most challenging aspects of a successful consultation and performing this skill badly may cause significant damage to a developing therapeutic relationship and has the potential to cause psychological harm to both clinician and patient.

Much of the literature related to breaking bad news comes from our colleagues in oncology (Baile et al., 2000), and while this provides some helpful insights into this challenging aspect of consultation, breaking bad news in an oncology clinic is a very different setting to primary care. Furthermore, the 'bad news' in question in primary care may not be as extreme as a terminal diagnosis. In general practice, it may be something seemingly more benign, such as discussing a patient's weight, that their lifetime risk of a heart attack is significant or that you want to refer them for a specific investigation. The SPIKES protocol (Table 2.4) can be a useful prompt for considering the many factors which contribute to breaking bad news effectively.

CHAPTER 2   Consultation Skills and the Diagnostic Process

Table 2.4   The SPIKES Protocol for Breaking Bad News

S	Setting up and starting	Preparing yourself and the environment for the consultation, ensuring privacy and that you are free from interruptions Introducing yourself and outlining your role in the consultation
P	Perception	Gain an insight into the patient's perspective; what do they already know?
I	Invitation	Ask the patient what information they would, and would not, like to know
K	Knowledge	Using appropriate language, explain the diagnosis, prognosis and management options available
E	Emotions	Acknowledge and respect the patient's emotional responses and be aware of your own emotions during the consultation
S	Strategy/ summary	Reiterate the key points, and check understanding Plan a strategy for moving forwards

Source: Adapted from Baile et al. (2000).

> 💡 It is challenging to anticipate which pieces of information a patient may consider as bad news; it is wise to tread carefully when proposing any diagnosis or prognosis.

Breaking bad news can also take the form of discussing a move away from a very interventionalist pathway of invasive tests, repeated investigations and treatments with a heavy side-effect burden, towards a direction of travel focusing on symptom control. This is perhaps most notable in cases of palliative care but may also form part of the discussion for any incurable disorder which needs to be managed in terms of symptom control, such as irritable bowel syndrome or asthma. In such cases, the concept of Divergence of Care (Figure 2.7) is a useful communication strategy for discussing this dichotomy, and is one

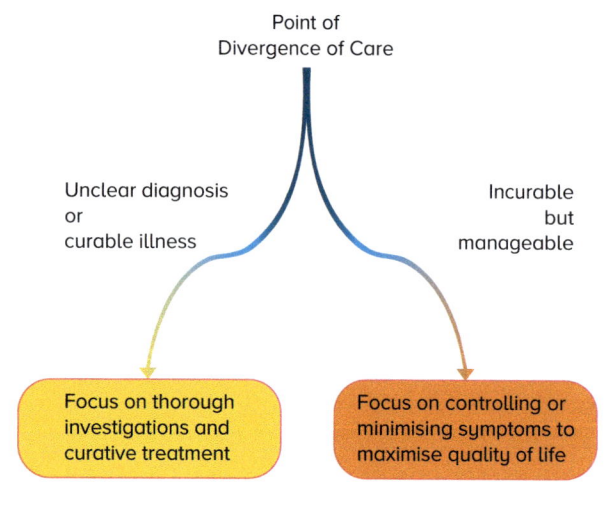

Figure 2.7   The Divergence of Care theory.

which may be revisited at a later date if required. You might for example revisit the point of divergence for a patient with a chronic disease diagnosis when a new investigation becomes available or for a patient with an advanced (presumed incurable) disease if a new or experimental treatment is now accessible to them.

At difficult times, such as when breaking bad news, we know that patients often do not remember the details of what is said. However, they will remember how you made them feel, and fostering an effective clinician–patient relationship when breaking bad news keeps the metaphorical door open for the patient to return to you at a later date if they wish to discuss anything further. As with any consultation, we must remember that whatever model, aid memoire or formula we use, we are having a conversation with another human being, and it is this interpersonal connection and humanity which facilitates communication and the development of a therapeutic relationship.

> 💡 Discussing a transition from a curative to a symptom-control approach can be facilitated using the Divergence of Care model.

Making a Diagnosis

Murtagh's Diagnostic Model

Murtagh provides us with a clear model to guide the formation of a diagnosis in primary care (Murtagh, 2011; Murtagh et al., 2018). The model lacks a number of the prompts to facilitate a smooth and efficient consultation discussed previously, focusing instead on the diagnostic process. Murtagh asks five questions of the clinician, in relation to the problem presented to them by the patient:

1) What is the most likely diagnosis?
2) What serious pathology must not be missed in this case? (Red flags)
3) What conditions could be easily missed in this case? (Red flags)
4) Could the patient have one of the 'masquerades' commonly encountered in clinical practice?
5) Is the patient trying to tell me something? (Yellow flags or hidden agenda)

> 📖 Silverston (2020) SAFER diagnosis.

Most Likely Diagnosis

The most likely diagnosis (probability diagnosis) is based on the known epidemiology of the patient and population in relation to the presenting complaint being demonstrated (Murtagh et al., 2018). An example of this would be three patients with a red,

CHAPTER 2 Consultation Skills and the Diagnostic Process

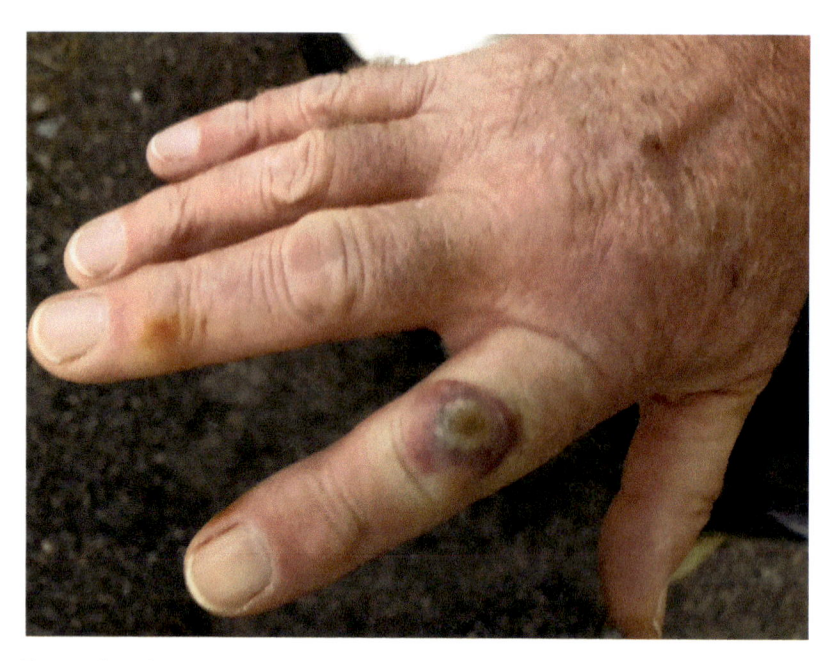

Figure 2.8 Example of red, ulcerated lesion on the dorsum of hand.

angry-looking ulcerated lesion on the dorsum of their hand with associated lymphangitis (Figure 2.8):

- One is a young sheep farmer in the Scottish Highlands
- The second is a 40-year-old refugee recently arrived in the UK from Algeria
- The third is an 80-year-old woman who avoids seeking medical attention.

For the first patient, the probability diagnosis here is orf, caused by a parapox virus. Perhaps you will already know that the local lambs are not feeding well this year, and that local farmers are having a hard time bottle feeding lambs.

For the second patient, cutaneous leishmaniasis is a highly likely cause based on their travel and social history, and would need to be ruled out.

And for the last, a carcinoma would have to be strongly suspected (either squamous cell or basal cell) with or without secondary infection.

> The use of Diagnostic Triads can also be beneficial in narrowing down a diagnosis. For example, if a patient attends with nasal congestion, with a past medical history of asthma and a documented allergy to aspirin, this may pique your suspicion of nasal polyps being the diagnosis here based on Samter's Triad.
> There are also tetrads, pentads and pathognomic signs and symptoms which can all help in formulating a diagnosis.

What Serious Pathology Should Not Be Missed?

This is to remind the clinician that for the presenting complaint there is likely to be a serious possible diagnosis or sequelae that should never be missed. Furthermore, due to the nature of primary care, the diagnostic focus is often on ruling out serious conditions, rather than reaching a firm diagnosis for the presenting complaint.

A headache for example could be caused by raised intracranial pressure, or a hoarse voice may be a laryngeal tumour. In both cases, a less sinister pathology is far more likely but the serious condition must be ruled out (with a degree of certainty). In these examples, specific red-flag questions (see below) should be asked to probe whether these concerning causes of the presenting complaint could be present. In addition to these serious and potentially fatal conditions not to miss, there are a number of conditions which may be less serious but are very easy to miss.

What Conditions Could Be Easily Missed?

This is a prompt to consider serious and life-threatening conditions associated with the presenting complaint that can be easily missed (Table 2.5). These can be neatly summarised using the acronym VICE: Vascular, Infection, Cancer, Endocrine. This acts to remind us that seemingly simple presentations can be caused by life-threatening conditions; it is likely that a mixture of general and complaint-specific red-flag questions in addition to a thorough examination will be required to rule out some of these easily missed conditions.

General Red Flags

While there are specific red flags for certain presenting complaints, Murtagh (2011; Murtagh et al., 2018) also advocates six quick questions to be asked during routine consultations to elicit common red flags:

1) How is your general health (any tiredness, fatigue or weakness)?
2) Do you have a fever or night sweats?
3) Have you unintentionally lost any weight?

Table 2.5 Examples of Easily Missed Diagnoses

Presenting complaint	Easily missed diagnoses
Headache	<ul><li>Intracranial haemorrhage</li><li>Meningitis</li><li>Raised intracranial pressure</li><li>Temporal arteritis</li></ul>
Abdominal pain	<ul><li>Abdominal aortic aneurysm</li><li>Ectopic pregnancy</li><li>Mesenteric infarction</li><li>Myocardial infarction</li></ul>
Sore throat	<ul><li>Ludwig's angina</li><li>Mediastinitis</li><li>Quinsy</li></ul>

CHAPTER 2   Consultation Skills and the Diagnostic Process

4) Have you noticed any unusual lumps or bumps?
5) Do you have persistent pain anywhere?
6) Have you noticed any unusual bleeding?

Red flags are essential questions (or examination findings) for many presenting complaints, and it is important to be aware of these in your day-to-day practice; these will be discussed throughout this book. Red flags can also be used as red-flag safety nets, as discussed later.

> Mallinson, T. (2016). The importance of red flags [Online].
> My e-Learning → Paramedics (PRM) → Clinical decision making for paramedics → The importance of red flags

Masquerades

Murtagh (2011) tells us that there are 14 key masquerades (Table 2.6), these being important diagnoses which may be initially missed or overlooked. He starts with seven first-line masquerades, which are common conditions which are commonly missed. These are conditions worth considering frequently in your consultations. He adds to these seven second-line masquerades which are the rarer diagnoses which often go undiagnosed for some time. Some of these, such as HIV, can be ruled out with a simple and cheap test, while others may require more detailed investigation or detailed history taking to unearth. It is worth bearing all 14 in mind when consulting in primary care.

Table 2.6   Murtagh's Masquerades

First-line	Second-line
1) Depression	1) Baffling bacterial infections (e.g. tuberculosis, cerebral abscesses or endocarditis)
2) Diabetes	2) Baffling viral or protozoal infections (e.g. Epstein-Barr virus, dengue or malaria)
3) Drugs (iatrogenic, over-the-counter or recreational)	3) HIV/AIDS
4) Anaemia	4) Malignancy (e.g. lymphoma, leukaemia or myeloma)
5) Endocrine disorders (e.g. hypothyroidism or adrenal insufficiency)	5) Chronic kidney disease
6) Spinal dysfunction – pain syndromes	6) Connective tissue disorders (e.g. rheumatoid arthritis, systemic lupus erythematosus or giant cell arteritis)
7) Urinary tract infection	7) Neurological disorders (e.g. multiple sclerosis)

Yellow Flags

The term 'yellow flags' is used both to indicate important psycho-social factors to the current illness which may be predictive of slow recovery or long-lasting disability (Box 2.2), and also to highlight anything else the patient may wish to discuss but is perhaps unsure how to go about starting the conversation. This is often termed the patient's 'hidden agenda' in UK practice, a term which is perhaps unhelpful in that it implies a degree of deception on the patient's part. While this is usually an unfair assumption, as clinicians we must be aware that some patients may lie to us for a number of reasons, perhaps due to embarrassment, to avoid feeling judged, for secondary gain or because they don't want to openly disagree with their clinician's diagnosis or treatment plan. Patients most often lie about their dietary and exercise habits, sexual activities and concordance with treatments (Vogel, 2019).

These yellow flags may be volunteered spontaneously by the patient (for example, an allusion to a sibling's cancer diagnosis highlighting your patient's own fears) or through targeted questioning – such as in the ICE model discussed previously. Yellow flags may be even more subtle than this, and require a number of consultations to fully elucidate, to allow time for the patient to gain trust in you as a clinician and for you to gain a better holistic understanding of the patient's situation.

BOX 2.2 Yellow Flags

- Poor concordance with treatment
- Catastrophising
- Failure to return to work
- Fixation on a specific cause or diagnosis
- External locus of control
- Allusions to risk-taking behaviours

> The Bradford VTS (Vocational Training Scheme) website is an excellent resource for all things primary care, especially consultation skills: https://www.bradfordvts.co.uk.

Formulating a Management Plan

Discussing a management plan for a patient in primary care is often far more complex than within secondary care. There will likely be a higher degree of uncertainty, increased use of non-medical interventions such as counselling or exercise programmes, as well as the use of time as a diagnostic tool. All of these need to be effectively communicated to the patient to ensure patient buy-in.

We know that the use of clinical rules and tools or decision aids is effective in allowing patients to reach informed decisions about their care. However, in primary care, it is

CHAPTER 2   Consultation Skills and the Diagnostic Process

likely that patients will be multi-morbid with a degree of polypharmacy, which makes it challenging to find a decision aid which encompasses more than a single issue. Therefore, there may be more than one tool applicable to a patient's case. If we consider an elderly patient with atrial fibrillation requiring anticoagulation, we could easily apply two or three separate decision aids which may simply muddy the water and cause confusion. The HAS-BLED tool may indicate someone is at high risk of a significant haemorrhage if prescribed anticoagulants, while the CHA_2DS_2-VASc may demonstrate a high risk of stroke if not prescribed them.

> **HAS-BLED** – Calculates bleeding risk for patients taking oral anticoagulants (with better accuracy than the ATRIA, OBRI or $HEMORR_2HAGES$ tools).
> **CHA_2DS_2-VASc** – Calculates yearly risk of stroke, with an associated recommendation in relation to anticoagulation (see p. 216).

Any discussion of onward management can benefit from the clinician being open and honest about their rationale for any test or treatment, or indeed for using time as a diagnostic tool (watchful waiting). It can be helpful to have a framework as a reminder of the range of management options open to you, while in hospital a useful aide memoir is:

- Bedside tests
- Blood tests
- Imaging
- Special tests.

This is perhaps less useful in primary care, where something a little broader may be more appropriate. The RAPRIOP mnemonic is a useful cue in relation to the breadth of management options available (McAvoy, 1992), and can certainly be a helpful prompt that sharing information and explanations with a patient is part of your management plan (Table 2.7).

Table 2.7   RAPRIOP Mnemonic for Formulating a Management Plan

R	Reassurance and explanation
A	Advice and counselling
P	Prescribing
R	Referral
I	Investigation
O	Observation and follow-up
P	Prevention

Source: Adapted from McAvoy (1992).

> Whenever possible, a patient should be facilitated to arrange their own onward referral and management. This facilitates patient autonomy and allows them control over factors such as appointment times. This may be particularly useful for referrals to services such as physiotherapy and dietetics, where the patient will need a fair amount of motivation to get the most from these services.

Safety Netting

Safety netting is a term used in multiple consultation models and refers to the consultation technique of highlighting that a worsening of symptoms may occur and signposting how and when to seek help in the future (Neighbour, 1987). It can also provide an excellent opportunity to acknowledge any uncertainties you may have and to highlight Neighbour's 'what ifs' and what to do if deterioration were to occur. Neighbour (1987; Neighbour, 2018) might encourage us all to ponder three questions to inform our safety netting before we conclude any consultation:

- If my diagnosis is correct, what do I expect to happen?
- How will I know if this does not happen?
- What should then be done?

There are considered to be four distinct types of safety netting (Table 2.8) and it is usual for aspects from more than one of these categories to be used in every consultation, with most patients receiving a combination of two or more of the four categories.

> You should be safety netting every patient you see; if you get into the habit of doing this (and documenting it) it will serve you well.

Table 2.8 Types of Safety Netting

Type	Rationale	Example statement
General	This is a general worsening statement, which we should be giving to nearly every patient we encounter. In general, we always want to empower the patient to contact healthcare services if things get worse, or they are concerned	'If you feel any worse, or things don't get better, get back in touch with us.'

(Continued)

Type	Rationale	Example statement
Logistical	This is a useful approach for visitors to the area, those with little experience of the health service or anyone where onward deterioration or concern is likely Inclusion of specific contact details can be hugely beneficial	'If you are concerned, or things get worse, there are a number of ways of getting help. If you think something life threatening is happening, you should phone 999 and ask for an ambulance; if you are very concerned, you can attend the emergency department; if you think it is urgent but not life threatening, you can contact the out-of-hours GP service; if you think it can wait for an appointment with us, you can phone the surgery and come back and see us.'
Red flag	These highlight key ways in which a patient's condition may worsen and what to do if this occurs More usually, these red flags will have been covered during the consultation and highlighted as important, so a statement reminding the patient of these may be sufficient	'I would be concerned if you developed numbness around your groin and back passage, weakness in your legs, pain going below your knee, had any trouble going to the toilet etc. and I would want you to seek help immediately.' or 'If you developed any of those specific issues we discussed, I would want you to seek help immediately.'
Risk	A useful form of safety netting for patients who have decided to deviate significantly from your suggested management plan, e.g. someone with chest pain and dyspnoea refusing hospital admission Risk-based safety-netting statements may be fairly clear and direct	'I'm concerned we aren't doing everything we should be for you, and the risk is that you might become seriously unwell or die. If you change your mind, please attend the hospital straight away.' While giving such a direct message may seem out of character for a primary care encounter, if there is a risk of death or of a missed serious diagnosis such as cancer, this should be clearly communicated to the patient, to ensure they are able to make an informed decision

> Two useful resources in relation to providing an appropriate level of detail to allow patients to make an informed decision are presented in the case of Montgomery v Lanarkshire Health Board [2015] SC 11 [2015] 1 AC 1430, and the discussion of this ruling by Chan, S. et al. (2017) Montgomery and informed consent: Where are we now?

Chapter Summary

In summary, this chapter has introduced a range of consultation models and discussed key points within each framework to aid the consultation. Having an awareness of multiple consultation models provides more options for a clinician during any consultation. However, such models and frameworks should never be used as checklists, as each consultation is unique. Health psychology underpins our interactions with patients, and an understanding of this area can help in challenging consultations. During the consultation, consideration of red and yellow flags and of masquerades can ensure that key (often detrimental) presentations are not missed, and it is imperative that all patients receive a documented safety net of some kind.

References

Abbs, A.D., Hyams, A. and Ahmed, Z. (2020) *Remote Consultations Handbook*. 2nd edn. Arc. Available at: https://www.nasgp.org.uk/resource/remote-consulting-handbook/ (accessed 27 January 2023).

Baile, W., Buckman, R., Lenzi, E. et al. (2000) SPIKES – A six-step protocol for delivering bad news: Application to the patient with cancer. *Oncologist* 5(4): 302–311.

Balint, A. and Balint, M. (1939) On transference and counter-transference. *The International Journal of Psychoanalysis* 20: 223–230.

Balint, M. (1957) *The Doctor, His Patient and the Illness*. London: Churchill Livingstone.

Calderwood, C. (2019) *Personalising Realistic Medicine: Chief Medical Officer for Scotland's Annual Report 2017–2018*. Chief Medical Officer Directorate, Scottish Government.

Chan, S., Tulloch, E., Cooper, E.S. et al. (2017) Montgomery and informed consent: Where are we now? *British Medical Journal* 357: j2224.

Charon, R. (2001) Narrative medicine: A model for empathy, reflection, profession, and trust. *Journal of the American Medical Association* 286(15): 1897–1902.

Denness, C. (2013) What are consultation models for? *InnovAiT* 6(9): 592–599.

Helman, C.G. (1981) Disease versus illness in general practice. *The Journal of the Royal College of General Practitioners* 31(230): 548–552.

Kurtz, S.M. and Silverman, J.D. (1996) The Calgary–Cambridge Referenced Observation Guides: An aid to defining the curriculum and organizing the teaching in communication training programmes. *Medical Education* 30(2): 83–89.

Mallinson, T. (2016) The importance of red flags. eLearning for Health. College of Paramedics. Available at: https://portal.e-lfh.org.uk/LearningContent/Launch/752747 (accessed 12 February 2023).

McAvoy, B. (1992) Patient management. In Fraser, R.C. (ed) *Clinical Method: A General Practice Approach*. 2nd edn. Oxford: Butterworth Heinemann, pp. 6–72.

Mirza, D. (2016) *The FRAYED Consultation Model for Doctors Dealing with Unreasonable Demands from Difficult Patients: A Communication Skills Guide for Stressed GPs on How to Survive Doctor-Patient Conflict*. Bromley: Better Doctor Training Ltd.

Murtagh, J. (2011) Diagnostic modelling in general practice. *Australian Medical Student Journal* 2(1): 46–47.

CHAPTER 2 Consultation Skills and the Diagnostic Process

Murtagh, J., Rosenblatt, J., Coleman, J. et al. (2018) *John Murtagh's General Practice*. 7th edn. Sydney: McGraw-Hill Education.

Neighbour, R. (1987) *The Inner Consultation*. Oxford: Radcliffe Medical Press.

Neighbour, R. (2012) Models of the Consultation. eLearning for Health. Royal College of General Practitioners. Health Education England. Available at: https://portal.e-lfh.org.uk/LearningContent/Launch/63548 (accessed 12 February 2023).

Neighbour, R. (2018) Safety netting: Now doctors need it too. *British Journal of General Practice* 59(568): 872–874.

Neighbour, R. (2020a) Creating 'digital warmth' in remote consultations, with Roger Neighbour. Available at: https://www.youtube.com/watch?v=VAQE9RTgLGc (accessed 20 March 2021).

Neighbour, R. (2020b) Top tips for GP video consultation during COVID-19 pandemic. Available at: https://www.youtube.com/watch?v=W5zsEpka2HE (accessed 20 March 2021).

Pendleton, D., Schofield, T., Tate, P. et al. (1984) *The Consultation: An Approach to Learning and Teaching*. Oxford: Oxford University Press.

Przybylska, S. (2018) If it's not written down, it didn't happen. Available at: https://www.2harecourt.com/training-and-knowledge/if-its-not-written-down-it-didnt-happen/ (accessed 6 October 2019).

Realistic Medicine (2023) Working together to provide the care that's right for you. Available at: https://www.realisticmedicine.scot/ (accessed 27 January 2023).

Reid, C. (2013) Making things happen. *SMACC Conference*. Sydney, Australia. Available at: https://vimeo.com/66596623 (accessed 6 October 2019).

Reid, C., Brindley, P., Hicks, C. et al. (2018) Zero point survey: A multidisciplinary idea to STEP UP resuscitation effectiveness. *Clinical and Experimental Emergency Medicine* 5(3): 139–143.

Royal College of General Practitioners (RCGP) (1972) *The Triaxial Model of the Consultation*. London: Royal College of General Practitioners.

Royal College of General Practitioners (RCGP) (2022) WPBA assessments: Consultation Observation Tool (COT). Available at: https://www.rcgp.org.uk/gp-training-and-exams/training/workplace-based-assessment-wpba/assessments (accessed 30 January 2023).

Salinsky, J. (2009) Very short introduction to Balint Groups. Available at: https://balint.co.uk/about/introduction/ (accessed 20 March 2021).

Silverman, J.D., Kurtz, S.M. and Draper, J. (1998) *Skills for Communicating with Patients*. Oxford: Radcliffe Medical Press.

Silverston, P. (2020) SAFER diagnosis: A teaching system to help reduce diagnostic errors in primary care. *British Journal of General Practice* 70(696): 354–355.

Snow, R. (2016) I never asked to be ICE'd. *British Medical Journal* 354: i3729.

Tahir, A. and Mirza, D. (2018) *The 'DR SAMOSA' Consultation Model for Telephone Triage: A Guide for Primary Care Clinicians*. London: SAGE Publications.

Vogel, L. (2019) Why do patients lie to their doctors? *Canadian Medical Association Journal* 191(4): E115.

Warren, E. (2002) *An introduction to BARD: A new consultation model*. Update 5.9: 152–154.

Decision-making Theory

3

Jaqualine Lindridge

Introduction

Clinical decision making is a core skill for paramedics in any clinical setting. Good clinical decision making is essential to safe and effective healthcare, and requires a combination of cognitive skills, knowledge and experience. Developing good clinical decision-making skills requires clinicians to learn from their experiences; part of this is learning to recognise patterns, but moreover in primary care paramedics must develop their critical-thinking skills and learn to evaluate and apply evidence alongside best-practice guidelines. Primary care requires the paramedic to make decisions in a context of ever-increasing complexity, and to work as a core member of the multi-disciplinary team. In order to make these decisions effectively, it is helpful for primary care paramedics to consider how decisions are made, and what influences them.

Clinical Decisions

Clinical decisions are broadly made in an iterative cycle which consists of four stages: the data collection stage, the generation of hypotheses stage, the testing of hypotheses stage and the review, reflect and revise stage (Figure 3.1).

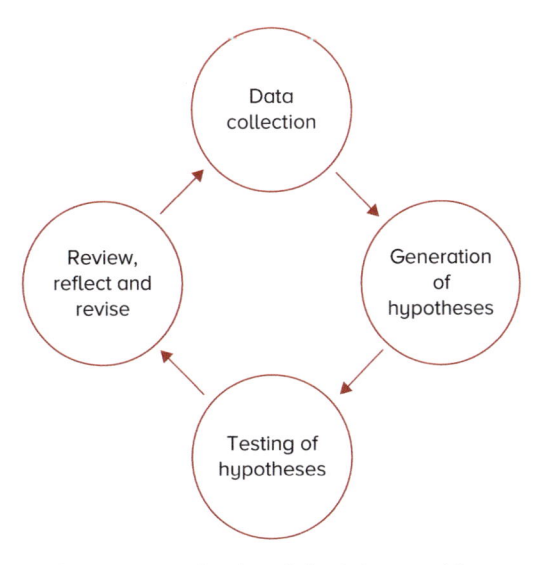

Figure 3.1 Cycle of decision making.

CHAPTER 3   Decision-making Theory

The data-collection stage consists of gathering information about the patient's presentation, focused largely on taking a history, establishing the patient's preferences and priorities, referring to clinical records and beginning a physical examination. This leads to the formation of hypotheses and the generation of differential diagnoses and the beginnings of care planning. These hypotheses are then tested, with further techniques of examination or with the use of investigations, the results of which are used to reflect on the 'fit' of the working diagnosis and management plan. This process typically takes place on a continuum in an iterative fashion until the diagnosis and management plan that is the best fit for the patient is established.

> Collen, A. (2022) *Decision Making in Paramedic Practice*.
> The book goes into a range of decision-making models in more detail.

Theoretical Approaches to Decision Making

There are a number of theoretical approaches to clinical decision making. One of the most popular was advanced by a leading psychologist in the field of decision making, Professor Daniel Kahneman. Dual process theory consists of two models of decision making: one based on intuition and the other based on reasoning (Kahneman, 2003). These are labelled system 1 and system 2 respectively (Stanovich and West, 2000), in an effort to style them more neutrally and remove the influence of the words themselves. System 1, or intuitive, decisions are 'fast, automatic, effortless, [and] associative', whereas system 2, or reasoned, decisions are more rational in that they are 'slower, serial, effortful, and deliberately controlled' (Kahneman, 2003: 1451). It is this dual process theory which has been thought to be responsible for clinical decision making (Norman et al., 2014).

> Kahneman, D. (2012) *Thinking, Fast and Slow*.
> See for further reading on the dichotomy of system 1 and system 2 thinking.

Although often attributed to 'experienced' clinicians and characterised as 'gestalt', intuitive approaches to decision making, such as heuristics, have also been labelled as prone to serious cognitive error, due to their construct requiring information to be ignored in the decision-making process in an effort to speed up decision making (Norman et al., 2014; Tversky and Kahneman, 1974). However, another view is that heuristics produce more accurate results than more complex strategies, depending on the environment in which they are used (Gigerenzer and Gaissmaier, 2011). This view is reinforced by Gary Klein (2008), who proposes the theory of naturalistic decision making (NDM) as a real-world alternative, particularly outside of laboratory environments and in conditions characterised by uncertainty and time pressure. Nonetheless, biases associated with intuitive, or system 1, thinking continue to be associated with errors of clinical decision making, particularly around diagnostic error. For example, biases such as framing, the development of diagnostic momentum, premature diagnostic closure and search satisficing have been associated with missed diagnoses of cauda equina syndrome and pulmonary embolism (Croskerry et al., 2013).

Cognitive Biases in Practice

There are potential biases which arise from many aspects of clinical practice, and life in general. Healthcare frequently involves hand-offs of care between different clinicians and different services, be that out-of-hours to in-hours, general practitioner or practice nurse to paramedic, ambulance crew to paramedic and so on. This means that patients frequently come with working diagnoses and assumptions which may 'frame' the case in the clinician's mind and contribute to the development of 'diagnostic momentum' which may blinker the clinician in exploring further differential diagnoses, ultimately risking 'premature diagnostic closure' (Croskerry et al., 2013). Linked to this is the potential for any early ideas on diagnosis or culprit organ system to act as an 'anchor' which limits further decision making, for example an early assumption of peptic ulcer disease which anchors decision making and inhibits consideration of important cardiovascular disorders. These forms of 'search satisficing' can limit the opportunity to fully explore clinical presentations and identify the most appropriate course of action to recommend (Croskerry et al., 2013).

Born of NDM, recognition-primed decision theory is a fusion of intuition and analysis and is based on the premise that people use their previous experiences to 'rapidly categorize situations' (Klein, 2008: 457). This leads to the development of an internal library of patterns which can be used to inform the selection of options on how to react to a given scenario and allow for rapid decision making to occur.

The variables in clinical decision making are usually thought of as predominantly rational in nature. Diagnoses are usually formed based on patient presentations, predictive values and likelihoods. However, issues such as affect and attitude to risk are also important. There is an inverse relationship between the severity of perceived risk and how beneficial a given activity is perceived to be (Slovic et al., 2005). This is commonly referred to as the 'affect heuristic', with unfavourable feelings towards a particular activity resulting in a 'high risk and low benefit' judgement. Fear plays an important role in the prediction of harm, and the affective responses which contribute to decision making tend to take place rapidly, and to a degree unconsciously, particularly where the focus is on negative rather than positive stimuli.

Whilst the emphasis on clinical decision making is often assumed to centre on the clinical facts and patient choice, there are other influencing factors which clinicians should be alert to. These can be extrinsic or intrinsic to the decision maker and include issues such as the context of the decision and any resource limitations, for example whether the patient is being seen in the context of out-of-hours or in-hours primary care and the ease of access to supportive care services. Individual-level, intrinsic issues such as physical or cognitive fatigue will also play an important role and are not to be underestimated.

> Understanding the psychology of decision-making may improve diagnostic accuracy and reduce the negative effects of uncertainty.

CHAPTER 3 Decision-making Theory

Risk and Decision Making

Most paramedics qualifying in the UK will have spent the majority of their pre-registration clinical training in an ambulance trust practice environment. This practice environment will have set the scene for issues such as risk appetite and framed how many different patient presentations are conceptualised. Clinical practice in the ambulance trust setting tends to occur in a reactionary manner, with arguably more binary clinical decisions which focus on the immediate needs of the patient, particularly in respect of the need to provide immediate urgent or emergency interventions or to otherwise escalate care. There are some similarities to out-of-hours here; however, on the whole primary care is far more concerned with caring for patients in a more holistic and long-term manner. One key difference in how this can influence decision making manifests in how time can be used as a risk-management strategy. In the urgent and emergency care setting, interventions tend to be immediate, whereas in primary care 'watching and waiting' over days and weeks represents a far more useful strategy.

Qualitative research exploring paramedic decision making has identified a number of issues influencing the decisions of paramedics in clinical practice, including a number of factors which drive risk-averse behaviours. This research has identified a strong theme of the fear of sanctions as a key influencing factor (Burrell et al., 2013; O'Hara et al., 2015; Porter et al., 2007; Simpson et al., 2017), as well as perceptions of vulnerability and lack of confidence in employer support (Rees et al., 2017). Whilst this research is largely born of the emergency ambulance setting in the UK and Australia, it is relevant here in that it suggests that paramedics transitioning to practice in primary care may need to reflect on their own concerns as part of that transition and that clinical supervisors in primary care should recognise there may be a professional need to support this process.

Risk and Perceived Risk

How we perceive risk is important. As discussed earlier, our conceptions of risk are influenced by a number of factors beyond the mathematical probabilities of any given event arising or not, including how immediately our mind conceptualises something of concern. Consider a common case:

> An 82-year-old man lives alone. He presents out-of-hours with minor skin infection which has developed around a small laceration on his ankle and for which he needs oral antibiotics. He is frail, but systemically well. His flat is very cluttered, and you are worried about the risk of him falling. You refer him to hospital for treatment and ask social services to assist with making his home safer.

In this case, there is a concern that the man will fall if he remains in his own home, which drives the decision to admit him to hospital. The anticipated outcome is likely to be a brief stay in hospital and a return to a safer home environment. However, now consider an alternative outcome:

> Whilst an inpatient, a man goes on to develop a series of hospital-acquired infections and deteriorates significantly. He is discharged to a nursing home on a Fast-Track pathway for palliative care and dies there 10 weeks after being admitted to hospital. He never went home.

Risk and Decision Making

It is essential to ensure that the preferences and choices of individuals are fully taken into consideration when supporting service users to make their decisions, and that the value of proposed activities and management plans is fully explored. Consider what the patient is likely to gain physically, psychologically and socially (RCOT, 2018).

Complexity and Uncertainty

Patients in primary care frequently present with a background of psychosocial problems as well as mental and physical co-morbidities. Clinicians working in primary care frequently have a relatively short space of time within which to make a care decision and may need to coordinate the patient's care in association with a variety of other professionals, something which has been highlighted as a potential contributory factor in patient safety incidents (Vincent and Amalberti, 2016). The presence of multi-morbidity increases the uncertainty and complexity of the clinical consultation, more so in primary care than urgent and emergency care settings as the requirements for ongoing and more holistic care are greater in this practice setting. It is essential that paramedics have a keen understanding of working with patients who have complex needs, whether those needs are mental, psychosocial or physical in nature. Paramedics transitioning from practice in the urgent and emergency care settings, where the emphasis may have been more on acute-on-chronic exacerbation of long-term conditions, or their influence on injury, will find that care of patients in primary care involves a far greater degree of ongoing and holistic care.

Managing uncertainty is another essential skill for paramedics working in primary care. Patients frequently present with undifferentiated problems, and the diagnosis is often initially unclear, particularly when patients first present. There are multiple zones of uncertainty to consider, yours and those of the patient, and potentially those of their families and carers. Dealing with uncertainty generally requires a good understanding of relevant clinical evidence, how to access it and how to use it to consider the probabilities of any given differential diagnosis. Strategies to assist paramedics in primary care to deal with uncertainty can be extrapolated from those aimed at primary care physicians. These include approaches to practice which will already be familiar to paramedics and include 'meticulous' assessment of the presentation and exclusion of red flags and alarming diagnoses. Shared decision making is also emphasised, which will be discussed in more detail in the next section. Here, establishing a trusting relationship with patients is vital, as is accessing the support of the multi-disciplinary team. Returning to some of the theory discussed earlier, there are a number of pitfalls associated with uncertainty and complexity which are particularly relevant to paramedics as they step into primary care (O'Riordan et al., 2011). O'Riordan further suggests that clinical trainers refer to a helpful list of common diagnostic pitfalls associated with complexity. These urge attention to ensuring clinicians have enough knowledge and skill to make the decisions they are required to make, and to ensuring that possibilities are fully explored, avoiding premature diagnostic closure. These are pitfalls worth thinking about during consultations, but also in reflective practice and case debriefs.

CHAPTER 3 Decision-making Theory

Shared Decision Making

Shared decision making is increasingly recognised as a cornerstone of good clinical practice and is enshrined in UK law within the Health and Social Care Act (2012), which introduced the now famous phrase 'no decision about me, without me' into everyday language in the NHS. Shared decision making is a building block of person-centred care, which focuses on the needs of the individual rather than of the service and aims to ensure that patients are fully informed on the options available to them and are able to participate fully and as an equal partner in their health and care decisions.

Whilst the emphasis on shared decision making in UK legislation is relatively new, it originally arises from a number of more longstanding sources, not least the ethical principles which underpin clinical practice. The moral requirement to respect patients' autonomy is at the forefront of deontological clinical ethical frameworks; for examples, see: Beauchamp and Childress (2013); Gillon (1994); Sokol and Bergson (2005). Whilst it is relatively uncontentious that a clinician should respect the autonomy of their service users, the key here is working with service users to ensure that they develop sufficient understanding of the information they need to make the relevant healthcare decision. This will be a familiar principle for those accustomed to working with patients who lack mental capacity; however, it is pertinent for any and all patients, particularly those with vulnerabilities or who experience low health literacy.

Shared decision making is a collaborative approach which recognises the expert and complementary contributions of both the healthcare professional and the patient. Healthcare professionals are expected to provide information on the effectiveness of treatment and management options, and what the anticipated harms and benefits might be. Patients bring expert knowledge about themselves, their life and circumstances, as well as their attitudes towards risk, their conceptions of illness and their values and preferences. Whilst it is recognised that the extent to which people wish to take an active role in healthcare decision making varies considerably, service users should always be afforded the opportunity to choose how much they wish to engage. It is not appropriate to assume that a patient would not want to be involved in making their own healthcare decisions, including where they have chosen a low-involvement approach previously.

Shared decision making is appropriate for many healthcare scenarios but is particularly suited to decisions where there is equipoise in respect of the treatment options or trade-offs between factors such as length and quality of life and where the decision rests on the values and preferences of the service user concerned. Decisions such as this are frequently made in primary care, particularly in cases where patients have multiple co-morbidities and in the context of polypharmacy. Patients must be advised of all the suitable options and supported to make their decision based on an open and collaborative discussion. As in all aspects of care, it is important to document shared decision making carefully, including making a record of the risks and benefits discussed and the stated views of the service user in respect of their values and preferences.

Person-centred Care and Informed Consent

Decision making in the context of healthcare does not occur transactionally and represents contributions from the clinician and the patient. It is a long-held principle of good clinical

Person-centred Care and Informed Consent

practice that patients should receive adequate information to enable them to make decisions, and this is enshrined in the standards of conduct, performance and ethics which all paramedics must adhere to as Health and Care Professions Council registrants. The case of *Montgomery v Lanarkshire Health Board* (2015) was a landmark case in medical consent law in the UK and provided definitive legal strength for patients to demand information according to their own terms and wants.

Nadine Montgomery was a pregnant woman with diabetes and of small stature. In advance of the birth of her son, it was known he was going to be a large baby, as is common in the context of maternal diabetes. Mrs Montgomery was not advised by her obstetrician, Dr McClelland, that this increased the risk of shoulder dystocia. Unfortunately, this complication arose during delivery and her son received a hypoxic brain injury which led to cerebral palsy. In court, Mrs Montgomery argued that had she been advised of this risk, she would have asked for a caesarean section. Dr McClelland argued that she did not feel a caesarean section was in her patient's best interests and did not advise her of the risk of it occurring as she anticipated that this would influence her to request a caesarean section. In court, Dr McClelland attempted to rely on the legal precedents set by *Bolam v Friern Hospital Management Committee* (1957) and *Sidaway v Board of Governors of the Bethlem Royal Hospital* (1985), in that a reasonable obstetrician in her position would have made the same decision. However, Mrs Montgomery won her case on appeal and was awarded in excess of £5 million in damages after the court found that information which the patient was likely to find important could not reasonably be withheld. In essence, what *Montgomery* established was that clinicians could no longer approach providing information to patients for the purpose of consent based on what *clinicians* thought the patient should know. It became necessary in law to disclose any risks which a reasonable person in the patient's position would consider significant enough to be disclosed.

> 💡 Shared decision making and person-centred care are the cornerstones of practice in the primary care environment, with informed decision making at the heart of each consultation.

Other relevant sources of law, such as the Mental Capacity Act (2005), which is relevant to England and Wales, the Mental Capacity Act (Northern Ireland) 2016 and the Adults with Incapacity (Scotland) Act (2000), also enshrine requirements to share information with patients in order to gain consent for clinical assessment and interventions. This legislation requires functional tests to be made of the ability of people who may lack capacity to understand, retain and use relevant information in the process of making a decision in regard to their healthcare (or other relevant decision). Where patients are not able to make decisions for themselves, it is essential to liaise with those close to them to try and gain an understanding of what is relevant and important to them. Some patients have nominated proxy representatives, such a person holding a lasting power of attorney for health and welfare (England and Wales) or welfare guardianship (Scotland). Where such representatives exist, they must be included in decision making, and should receive the same level of information sharing as the patient themselves would have received.

CHAPTER 3 Decision-making Theory

Chapter Summary

In summary, this chapter has introduced theories of decision making and conceptions of risk and perceived risk, and has discussed decision making in the context of complexity and uncertainty. The models of shared decision making and person-centred care have been discussed, along with the legal framework for informed consent in contemporary clinical practice. Decision making is a core skill for paramedics and is developed in primary care in the context of increased complexity and uncertainty. Decisions are increasingly shared with patients, with both parties contributing to and sharing in the decision-making process. The increased complexity of primary care holds opportunities and risks for paramedics in this area of clinical practice, with important areas to consider for those developing their practice in this field.

References

Beauchamp, T.L. and Childress, J.F. (2013) *Principles of Biomedical Ethics.* 7th edn. Oxford: Oxford University Press.

Burrell, L., Noble, A. and Ridsdale, L. (2013) Decision-making by ambulance clinicians in London when managing patients with epilepsy: A qualitative study. *Emergency Medicine Journal* 30(3): 236–240.

Collen, A. (2022) *Decision Making in Paramedic Practice*. 2nd edn. Bridgwater: Class Professional Publishing.

Croskerry, P., Singhal, G. and Mamede, S. (2013) Cognitive debiasing 1: Origins of bias and theory of debiasing. *BMJ Quality & Safety* 22(Suppl 2): ii58–ii64.

Gigerenzer, G. and Gaissmaier, W. (2011) Heuristic decision making. *Annual Review of Psychology* 62(1): 451–482.

Gillon, R. (1994) Medical ethics: Four principles plus attention to scope. *British Medical Journal* 309: 184.

Kahneman, D. (2003) Maps of bounded rationality: Psychology for behavioral economics. *American Economic Review* 93(5): 1449–1475.

Kahneman, D. (2012) *Thinking, Fast and Slow*. London: Penguin.

Klein, G. (2008) Naturalistic decision making. *Human Factors* 50(3): 456–460.

Norman, G., Sherbino, J., Dore, K. et al. (2014) The etiology of diagnostic errors: A controlled trial of system 1 versus system 2 reasoning. *Academic Medicine: Journal of the Association of American Medical Colleges* 89(2): 277–284.

O'Hara, R., Johnson, M., Siriwardena, A.N. et al. (2015) A qualitative study of systemic influences on paramedic decision making: Care transitions and patient safety. *Journal of Health Services Research & Policy* 20(1 Suppl): 45–53.

O'Riordan, M., Aktürk, Z., Ortiz, J.M.B. et al. (2011) Dealing with uncertainty in general practice: An essential skill for the general practitioner. *Quality in Primary Care* 19(3): 175–181.

Porter, A., Snooks, H., Youren, A. et al. (2007) 'Should I stay or should I go?': Deciding whether to go to hospital after a 999 call. *Journal of Health Services Research & Policy* 12(Suppl 1): S1–32-8.

Rees, N., Rapport, F., Snooks, H. et al. (2017) How do emergency ambulance paramedics view the care they provide to people who self harm? Ways and means. *International Journal of Law and Psychiatry* 50: 61–67.

Royal College of Occupational Therapists (RCOT) (2018) *Embracing risk; Enabling Choice. Guidance for Occupational Therapists.* London: RCOT.

Simpson, P., Thomas, R., Bendall, J. et al. (2017) 'Popping nana back into bed' – A qualitative exploration of paramedic decision making when caring for older people who have fallen. *BMC Health Services Research* 17(1): 299.

Slovic, P., Peters, E., Finucane, M.L. et al. (2005) Affect, risk, and decision making. *Health Psychology* 24(4s): S35–40.

Sokol, D.K. and Bergson, G. (2005) *Medical Ethics and Law: Surviving on the Wards and Passing Exams.* London: Trauma Publishing.

Stanovich, K.E. and West, R.F. (2000) Individual differences in reasoning: Implications for the rationality debate? *Behavioral and Brain Sciences* 23(5): 645–665.

Tversky, A. and Kahneman, D. (1974) Judgment under uncertainty: Heuristics and biases. *Science* 185(4157): 1124–1131.

Vincent, C.D. and Amalberti, R. (2016) *Safer Healthcare: Strategies for the Real World.* Cham: Springer Open.

Legislation

Adults with Incapacity Act (Scotland) 2000.
Health and Care Social Act 2012.
Mental Capacity Act (England and Wales) 2005.
Mental Capacity Act (Northern Ireland) 2016.

UK Case Law

Bolam v Friern Hospital Management Committee [1957] 1 WLR 582.
Montgomery v Lanarkshire Health Board [2015] SC 11 [2015] 1 AC 1430.
Sidaway v Board of Governors of the Bethlem Royal Hospital [1985] AC 871.

Laboratory Investigations

4

Colin Roberts

Within This Chapter
- Principles of ordering and interpretation
- The full blood count and inflammatory markers
- Urea and electrolytes

Introduction

This chapter will focus on the common blood tests that paramedics will request and interpret in primary care, aiming for understanding and looking to develop a routine approach to this difficult, often neglected area. Blood tests can be a challenging area to master. Ultimately, testing patients falls into different categories and it is critical to understand the differences. These are:

- The routine monitoring of chronic disease
- When testing a hypothesis, either acutely or chronically
- As a reassurance for clinicians and patients alike.

This chapter is not exhaustive and will focus on introducing basic knowledge, as it is important to understand basic pathology on a solid base of a functional or normal anatomy and physiology.

Principles of Ordering and Interpretation

Before pitching into the interpretation of blood tests, it is important to understand the rationale behind why they were requested. By considering this question, clinicians can ensure they *think* before ordering the tests and ensure that the interpretation has a clear purpose. It is important to remember where testing fits into the diagnostic pathway. If chronic disease or the effects of treatment are not being routinely monitored, then a hypothesis is being tested. This is arrived at from pre-encounter information, first impressions and history taking.

CHAPTER 4   Laboratory Investigations

Arriving at a differential or working diagnosis at this point directs both examination and laboratory tests. The hypothesis is being tested, so that it can be confirmed or refuted. In reality, a picture is being built, but you must bear the following potential outcomes in mind:

- The test confirms the diagnosis: move on to management.
- The test does not confirm the diagnosis: think again.
- There are *unexpected* abnormal results, which force the clinician to revisit the patient and the problem.

> Before ordering tests, you need a rationale for what you order, and you must accept responsibility for those results. Ask yourself 'Can I justify this test in this patient?'.

Hence, a position is moved to where scattergun testing is avoided. If it is clear why tests are being ordered both in practice and in note keeping, then the skill of interpretation will follow. Negative test results are both common and helpful. If a hypothesis is being logically tested, then they rule out certain diagnoses, aiding in the progress to an answer for the patient.

> Think before you order, and the interpretation of the result flows from this clear, logical thought process.

Clinicians often worry about missing rare diagnoses in patients. This, of course, drives scattergun testing. In primary care, the accepted adage is that 'common things occur commonly'. Whilst the presence of rare disease presentations should be considered, if rarity were tested in each patient, every time, labs would be overloaded.

> Lam, J.H., Pickles, K., Stanaway, F.F. et al. (2020) Why clinicians overtest: Development of a thematic framework.
> The concept of overusing diagnostic testing is a subject of much research. Lam et al. outline a few considerations regarding why clinicians may do this.

Reference Ranges

Before learning to interpret a test result, the reference range should be understood. Without this understanding, accuracy is lost in the assessment.

For example, to develop a reference range for haemoglobin in adult males:

- Take 100 humans (all men), all of whom are healthy and well.
- Measure their haemoglobin levels.
- Create a range (lowest to highest).
- Apply 95% confidence level: we are confident that this is an accurate range from bottom to top for 95% of results.

Principles of Ordering and Interpretation

- This range will exclude the bottom 2.5% and the top 2.5%.
- They are now 'out of range' but are clearly not unwell or abnormal.

You need to be aware of this as it could lead to a misjudgement, most likely to be an overreaction to a result.

Patient Factors When Interpreting Results

There are a number of further factors you need to consider and build in as part of your routine:

- What is the context of the test?
  - If you can see or determine the origin of the test, you can assess the result according to this.
- Is this a repeat test and do you have access to previous results?
  - You can track changes, balance your response to patterns and put the result into context.
- Can you identify a pattern?
  - A new, abnormal test will assist in diagnosis and direct next steps. A recurrent abnormal test leads us elsewhere.
- Has the patient just had surgery or an intervention?
- Is this a complex patient with many co-morbidities?
- Is the patient symptomatic?

The Tests and You

There are many factors which practitioners need to consider. Learning the skill of ordering and interpretation needs time, and exposure to results in a structured, protected and supervised way.

When learning a new skill, clinicians need cognitive space. This requires cognitive resources, time and often to be left alone. Without this environment you may struggle to learn, and the chance of making mistakes is higher. Blood results are often hidden work, left to the end of the day, popping up out of hours when the lab phones through a result or a variety of other scenarios.

Think hard about your own experience and ability and pay heed to the following tips:

- If you order a test and do not see the result, try and look it up – this is great learning.
- If you are not sure about a result, do not just file it. Speak to someone!
- You will learn more from asking than just filing, and the more experienced practitioners around you are your best resource.
- How far out of range is it? We all have instincts about abnormal results ranging from Novice to Expert. Trust your instinct and listen to it. Ask for advice, whether acutely or the next day.
- Is this an important blood test? If I leave it, could there be a serious consequence?
- Results are talked about in groups (urea and electrolytes, liver function tests). What is the pattern within the group?

When learning to interpret results, you need time, information, an environment where you can concentrate, and access to advice. It is a process you are learning and there are many pitfalls. You will see common things frequently, but never act on uncertainty by filing when you are unsure.

CHAPTER 4 Laboratory Investigations

The Full Blood Count and Inflammatory Markers

This section will address the following common and critical tests which are performed in assessing infection and inflammatory problems. These are:

- Full blood count (FBC)
- C-reactive protein (CRP)
- Plasma viscosity (PV)
- Erythrocyte sedimentation rate (ESR).

What Is Blood?

An average adult male weighing 70 kg will have an average of 5 to 6 litres of blood made up of 45% cells and 55% plasma (water, salts, hormones, nutrients, elements of the immune system) (Thibault et al., 2006). Blood carries oxygen and nutrients to tissues and metabolic waste products away from tissues. It is involved in homeostasis, helping to control body temperature and other physiological processes and is fundamental to the immune response. It is also a transport mechanism for hormones and medication.

Bone Marrow

Bone marrow is the site of haematopoiesis (the formation of blood cells). Other organs are involved in haematopoiesis, namely the spleen, liver, lymph nodes and thymus gland.

In adults, blood cells are formed in the bone marrow of long bones, the ribs and the spine.

Red Blood Cells (Erythrocytes)

The transport of oxygen from the lungs to the body tissues uses haemoglobin. This complex protein binds to oxygen in areas of high concentration (the lungs) and releases it in the tissues where it is needed. Red blood cells live for 120 days and are then filtered out by the spleen (Guyton and Hall, 2011). Iron, Vitamin B12 and folic acid are needed for the creation of red blood cells.

Platelets

Platelets are the building blocks of clots. They are formed in the bone marrow and live for close to 10 days (Lebois and Josefsson, 2016). They are activated in the clotting cascade, causing them to adhere to each other and staunch the blood flow.

White Cells

Most white blood cells mature in the bone marrow. They are fundamental to our immune system, patrolling looking for infection, abnormal proteins and abnormal cells and activating the immune response when it is needed. We measure mature cells in the bloodstream; we will discuss the varieties below.

Full Blood Count (FBC)

In the vast majority of acute cases, and in the monitoring of all chronic disease, the FBC is ever-present. It is used as a diagnostic aid, as reassurance and in monitoring disease.

The Full Blood Count and Inflammatory Markers

The FBC has a range of components, but for immediate assessment four elements should be focused on:

- Haemoglobin (Hb): the concentration of haemoglobin in the blood
- Mean cell volume (MCV): the average volume or size of the red cells
- Platelets (Plt): the number of platelets
- White cell count (WCC): the number of white blood cells.

Haemoglobin

Range: < 130 g/dl in males, < 115 g/dl in females (Murphy, 2014).

Low haemoglobin levels are common, especially in menstruating women, but can be a sign of other disease processes (Guyton and Hall, 2011). High haemoglobin levels are less common. They are often driven by low oxygen levels, for example in those living at high altitudes or with COPD. Occasionally, bone marrow disorders can overproduce red blood cells (Guyton and Hall, 2011).

Anaemia, a low haemoglobin, is a common finding in disease. It is seen acutely, in haemorrhage or as a function of chronic disease or chronic bleeding. Patients with significant anaemia may be pale or have cardiovascular dysfunction, low blood pressure or tachycardia. Remember that in chronic cases the patient will accommodate to the haemoglobin as it falls (Mayo Clinic, 2023). The bone marrow and the 'building' of red blood cells depend on many factors. The bone marrow is sensitive and a true reflection of health.

Low Haemoglobin

Step 1: How low is it and how rapidly has this developed?
Step 2: Look at the MCV which can be one of three things.

If the MCV is low (< 88), then this is microcytic (the cells are small) anaemia. This means that the bone marrow does not have enough iron to create full-size cells to maintain the cycle of replacement, so it churns out smaller cells as it tries to keep pace. Iron deficiency is the most common cause (WHO, 2023).

Again, logically, if a patient is iron deficient it can be from one of three reasons:

- Losing more iron than they consume: this bleeding is either obvious (menorrhagia, melaena) or as an occult process (bleeding from bowel pathology).
- Consuming enough iron but not absorbing it: some patients have malabsorption problems – think Coeliac disease or Crohns disease (the absorptive organ, the bowel, is diseased) – or they simply do not absorb iron with ease.
- Not eating enough: common in children, anorexia, unbalanced vegan diets and other dietary deficiencies (Gupta et al., 2016).

If the MCV is raised (> 98), then this is macrocytic (the cells are large) anaemia. The causes of macrocytic anaemia can be divided into megaloblastic macrocytic anaemia and non-megaloblastic macrocytic anaemia.

Megaloblastic red blood cells are large and ovoid in shape, due to abnormalities in their production. Inhibition of DNA synthesis due to a deficiency of vitamin B12 or folate interferes with the process and creates these abnormalities. Left untreated, this can lead also to problems with platelet and red blood cell production. This is common (Guyton and Hall, 2011).

CHAPTER 4 Laboratory Investigations

Non-megaloblastic red blood cells are typically round and occur for a variety of reasons. Direct bone marrow toxicity with alcohol leads to large cell formation, while liver disease causes deposition of lipids in red blood cell walls, enlarging their surface area. In this setting, B12 and folate are likely to be normal (Imashuku et al., 2012).

If the MCV is normal (88–98), then this is normocytic (the cells are normal sized) anaemia.

The bone marrow is sensitive to age and chronic disease processes where the production of red blood cells is reduced. This is commonly seen in chronic kidney disease, chronic heart failure, chronic pulmonary disease and the auto-immune diseases, for example rheumatoid arthritis (Begum and Latunde-Dada, 2019). The complication here is that with these patients, often elderly with co-morbidities, there are frequently many issues contributing to the result.

Checking haematinics is important as a baseline and to test your hypothesis:

- Ferritin: Most iron is in the liver, the bone marrow or the red blood cells. Only 2% of iron is measured as ferritin in the blood (Guyton and Hall, 2011). If this is low, you can rest assured that the iron stores in the body are significantly depleted.
- B12: Absorbed in the stomach and critical for blood production and health of the nervous system. Low B12 due to autoimmune destruction of the B12 receptors in the stomach is pernicious anaemia.
- Folate: Absorbed in the small bowel. Often a feature of Crohn's disease or coeliac disease where small bowel pathology reduces folic acid absorption and, hence, levels drop in the circulation.

Platelets (Thrombocytes)

Platelets are the building blocks of blood clots. The clotting cascade is a complex series of events driven by clotting factors (produced by the liver) which ultimately leads to platelets clumping together and staunching the flow of blood. Platelet counts can be too high (thrombocytosis), normal or low (thrombocytopenia). A patient with too many platelets risks clotting and may present as deep vein thrombosis or pulmonary embolism.

Of real importance is watching raised platelets. If platelets are high (> 400), then there are a number of potential causes (NICE, 2021a):

- Platelets are also a marker of inflammation so can commonly be raised in infections or in inflammatory disorders (for example, rheumatoid arthritis, coeliac disease).
- They can be raised in the early stages of cancer (paraneoplastic).
- If a patient has had a splenectomy, then there is no spleen to store platelets, which results in all platelets in the bloodstream.
- Cancers like leukaemia and other bone marrow disorders (for example, primary thrombocythemia) can also present this way.

If platelets are low (< 150), then there are two possible causes (NICE, 2021a):

- Impaired platelet production in bone marrow failure: drugs (for example, chemotherapy), infection (for example, Eptein Barr Virus), leukaemia, lymphoma, vitamin B12 and folate deficiency, liver diseases
- Increased use of platelets: autoimmune disorders, pregnancy, coagulation disorders, chronic bleeding, post surgical.

The Full Blood Count and Inflammatory Markers

The interpretation of the result is context driven. Why was the test done and, in reality, how low is the number as a major judgement around bleeding risk? Remember to take advice and look at past results.

White Cells (Leucocytes)

High numbers of white blood cells (leucocytosis > 10 x 10^9/L) are commonly seen in practice (Guyton and Hall, 2011). The test is often done in infection or as a screening tool. If you are familiar with the FBC, you will know it features a list of white cell types detailing relative numbers of each type. We shall list these first to orientate us to interpretation:

- Neutrophils are the most common and most numerous. They react to bacteria and are the first line of defence here. They will be raised in bacterial infection. In chemotherapy, where the bone marrow is suppressed as a side effect of the treatment, you should be alert to neutropaenia. Here, too few neutrophils leave the patient open to rapid and overwhelming bacterial infection.
- Lymphocytes tend to react to viruses and come in different forms. B lymphocytes and T lymphocytes (COVID-19) are the most common.
- Monocytes assist in bacterial infection.
- Basophils or eosinophils are a marker of allergy and parasite infection (worms in the bowel).
- Blast cells are immature cells and may represent a blood cancer, leukaemia. Be assured that if they are present the specialist services will see them on a test and alert you.

Common scenarios for raised WCC are:

- Immune system disorders (for example, Crohn's, Grave's)
- Infection (specific to the type of infection)
- Leukaemia (as blast cells)
- Medications (for example, corticosteroids)
- Pregnancy
- Smokers
- Stress.

Common scenarios for low numbers of white blood cells are:

- Bone marrow irradiation
- Drug toxicity
- Infections (for example, HIV and sepsis)
- Lymphoma.

> Fever, body aches and pains and rigors (shivering) are signs of infection, but remember that both high and low white blood cell counts can present with infection. If a significant immune system response is occurring, you will see raised white cells; if the body is unable to respond you may not see a raised white cell count, which is equally significant according to the context.

CHAPTER 4 Laboratory Investigations

Inflammatory Markers

The inflammatory processes are designed to fight off infection and foreign proteins. The inflammatory response creates the environment for the elements of the immune system to go to work. Once the system is activated, the ideal is that the tissues have an increased blood supply and the blood vessels open up to allow fluid, inflammatory proteins and cells into the tissues and then deal with the problem.

This presents as:

- Heat as the blood vessels open up
- Swelling as the fluid from the plasma in the blood enters the tissues, carrying with it inflammatory mediators and white cells
- Redness as a consequence of increased blood flow
- Pain as nerve endings in the tissues are compressed by the fluid, increasing tissue pressure.

This is the underlying process in the majority of conditions; you can apply it to infection, injury and autoimmune processes. We have discussed the importance of white blood cells; now we will look at particular inflammatory markers.

C-reactive Protein (CRP)

This is a familiar test, which is seen in a number of acute situations. CRP is an inflammatory protein released by the liver in the acute phase of inflammation. Its job is to activate white blood cells and, conveniently, it is released in amounts proportional to the severity of the disease process. Hence, it can be used to measure the degree of the inflammatory response, climbing rapidly in the early stages of the illness and equally rapidly reducing once treatment is initiated or natural resolution occurs.

Plasma Viscosity (PV)

Another measure of inflammatory response is the viscosity. Essentially, what is being looked at is the amount of inflammatory protein in the blood plasma. Clearly, the greater the inflammatory process the more inflammatory proteins will be found in the bloodstream and hence the thicker (more viscous) the blood plasma will be. It is this thickness which is measured. The difference between this marker and CRP is that it tends to gradually increase and gradually reduce (Figure 4.1). This makes it less effective in the acute phase at monitoring the severity but very useful in more chronic conditions such as Crohn's disease or rheumatoid arthritis.

One particular condition where it can be highly elevated is multiple myeloma, where a viscosity of greater than two is found at diagnosis (NICE, 2022a). This reflects the amount of protein that is released by the tumour cells in the bone marrow (paraproteins).

- If > 1.72 and < 2 then you cannot know what the issue is, only that there is one.
- If > 2 then assume Myeloma until disproved.

Erythrocyte Sedimentation Rate (ESR)

Although less common now, you may see this result. Essentially, as the inflammatory process progresses the red blood cells become more adhesive to each other and that stickiness is measured. Again, this is non-specific, akin to PV.

Urea and Electrolytes

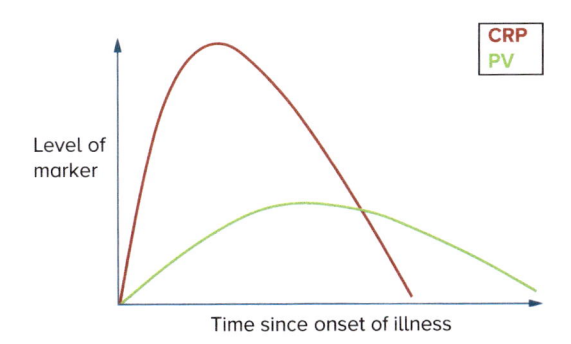

Figure 4.1 Difference between PV and CRP.

D-Dimer

The d-dimer is frequently tested in current medical practice. It is important to recognise that this test measures one of the products of blood clotting. The degree of this in the bloodstream will give you an indication that significant clotting has been taking place. However, it again is non-specific, often being elevated in cellulitis (Maze et al., 2013).

The two conditions that are tested with this are deep vein thrombosis and pulmonary embolism. Logically, using d-dimer to support the diagnosis in both conditions is rational. However, it is not a discriminatory test and should you be considering a diagnosis of pulmonary embolism in practice, question whether taking a d-dimer to rule it out is good practice. In reality, this condition needs more detailed imaging. Hence, if you consider it a diagnostic possibility, then using a d-dimer to exclude the diagnosis is not accurate.

> In DVT, however, the combination of a Wells score and a d-dimer would allow for accurate diagnosis in primary care. For more information on the Wells score, see pp. 221–222 in Chapter 9 – Cardiovascular Presentations.

Urea and Electrolytes

This test is commonly encountered, and the result is commonly abnormal for a multitude of reasons. The focus here will be on renal function, and it may be more accurate to think of this as a renal function test.

There are usually two kidneys, which sit at the back of the abdominal cavity lateral to the spine at the level of the lower ribs. The kidney has a range of functions:

- Filtering the blood: to remove waste products (urea and creatinine, drugs, proteins, *et cetera*)
- The maintenance of fluid and electrolyte balance in the body
- A major role in the control of blood pressure
- Via erythropoietin, the kidney stimulates the production of red blood cells
- Activation of vitamin D.

CHAPTER 4   Laboratory Investigations

Acute Kidney Injury

This is the loss of kidney function, leading to the retention of urea and other nitrogenous waste products and dysregulation of extracellular volume electrolytes. It is not uncommon now to see test results which raise the possibility of this diagnosis. It is characterised by a rise in serum creatinine of at least 50% within the previous 7 days in tandem with a fall in urine output (NICE, 2021b). So, it is important to look out for rising creatinine readings with a reduction in urine flow and eGFR. There are multiple causes of this, but, increasingly, it is a consequence of significant illness in patients with coincidental impaired renal function (NICE, 2021b). The causes can be categorised into:

- Pre-renal: anything which significantly affects renal blood flow
    - Volume depletion, oedematous states, hypotension, cardiovascular causes, renal hypoperfusion
- Renal: intrinsic renal disease
    - Glomerular disease, tubular disease, acute interstitial nephritis, vascular disease, eclampsia
- Post-renal: obstruction of urine flow
    - Stones, blood clots, bladder tumour, pelvic malignancy.

The likelihood increases with these risk factors (NICE, 2021b):

- Age, particularly over 65
- Chronic kidney disease
- Co-morbidities such as diabetes or cardiac failure
- Hypovolaemia
- The use of iodinated contrast in imaging
- Nephrotoxic medications.

Clinical symptoms or signs:

- Drop in urine output, nausea and vomiting, dehydration, confusion
- Hypertension, abdominal mass indicative of urinary retention, fluid overload
- Indications of vascular disease, emboli DIC, pallor, rash, bruising.

Assessment:

1. Ask about their drug history, urinary symptoms and PMH
2. Look for signs of infection or sepsis, heart failure, fluid status, palpable bladder, systemic disease (pre-renal, renal or post-renal)
3. Carry out:
    - Urinalysis, blood tests
    - Consider radiology where appropriate.

Management:

1. Stop nephrotoxic drugs where appropriate
2. Monitor creatinine and electrolytes
3. Identify and treat and other causes
4. Treat the acute complications.

Chronic Kidney Injury

This is 'a reduction in kidney function or structural damage (or both) present for more than 3 months, with associated health implications' (NICE, 2021b). Monitoring and categorising of renal function is conducted in a number of conditions, looking particularly at the eGFR. It is important to remember that this is an 'estimate' of the renal function, not an absolute. Detecting deterioration of real function early means that we can intervene with risk factor modification and management. Similar to with acute kidney injury, the causes can be categorised as below:

- Pre-renal: arteriopathic renal disease, hypertension, diabetes, hypercalcaemia
- Renal: glomerulonephritis
- Post-renal: retention due to tumours, prostate issues, congenital problems.

Table 4.1 illustrates the five stages of kidney disease. This highlights that early detection is important, particularly in cardiovascular disease. Close and careful management of blood pressure, cholesterol and other lifestyle factors which influence vascular disease will inhibit disease progression (NICE, 2022b).

Table 4.1 Stages of Chronic Kidney Disease

Stage	Description	eGFR	Kidney function
1	Possible kidney damage (e.g. protein in the urine with **normal** kidney function	90 or above	90–100%
2	Kidney damage with **mild** loss of kidney function	60–89	60–89%
3a	**Mild to moderate** loss of kidney function	45–59	45–59%
3b	**Moderate to severe** loss of kidney function	30–44	30–44%
4	**Severe** loss of kidney function	15–29	15–29%
5	Kidney **failure**	Less than 15	Less than 15%

Source: National Kidney Foundation (2022).

CHAPTER 4   Laboratory Investigations

Electrolytes

The testing and monitoring of electrolyte levels is critical. All of these are electrically active substances and they are important in the usual functioning of neurological and muscular tissue. Some are more critical than others, especially in terms of sudden disruption of nervous or muscular tissue, particularly cardiac muscle. We are going to look at the common tests we do, focusing particularly on low sodium levels as a way to logically approach the reasoning behind the different scenarios we identify.

Sodium

Range: 133–146 mmol/L (Guyton and Hall, 2011).

Sodium is critical to the functioning of electrically active tissue. It is particularly critical for the nervous system, and an approach which is based upon scientific knowledge is needed to understand the processes at play. In essence, the critical factor to understand is that sodium lives an extracellular existence. It is found in fluid compartments in the body.

It lives outside of cells and hence we have three compartments in the body where it could be:

- The blood
- The urine
- The fluid around the cells.

So, when assessing patients with sodium abnormalities, a question should be: 'Where is the sodium?'. Remember, you are testing blood levels, and blood plasma is only one of the compartments in which it could be found. Various disease processes will force sodium in and out of these different compartments, and it is important to understand these mechanisms so you can work out the disease process at play and how to intervene.

You also need to ask yourself:

- Is there enough sodium in the body?
- Is it being lost or not taken in?
- Is it being diluted with water?

Logically, sodium is either:

- Within the normal range
- Too high: Hypernatraemia
- Too low: Hyponatraemia.

Hyponatraemia

This is a sodium level of < 133 (Ball, 2013). This is likely to be the commonest scenario you encounter. It is also the most complex one to follow in terms of the diagnostic possibilities, but try and use this as a way of building your knowledge about how to approach these problems. Remember, this is all about fluid.

Clinical symptoms:

- Typically asymptomatic until quite severe.

Neurological symptoms, if very severe and acute:

- Cerebral oedema
- Coma.

Non-specific symptoms:

- Nausea
- Headache
- Fatigue
- Confusion (NICE, 2020b).

Clinical assessment should include:

- Capillary refill
- Skin turgor
- Pulse
- Blood pressure
- JVP
- Mucous membranes
- Urine output (NICE, 2020b).

Scenario 1: The patient has a reasonably low blood volume, as much of the fluid and sodium is in the tissues as oedema.

- Heart failure – venous pressure forces fluid into tissues
- Cirrhosis – less ALB in the blood, so fluid is lost into the tissues
- Nephrotic syndrome – kidneys are losing protein and hence there is less of it in the blood.

Here, the sodium and water are in the tissue compartment because of the disease processes detailed above. The kidneys are attempting to absorb more water and sodium, but these are continually lost into the tissue space.
The water and sodium end up in the tissues and the urine is concentrated.

Scenario 2: The kidneys are losing salt because they are failing or because they are being driven to do so.

- Renal failure – with failure, the ability to re-absorb sodium from the urine deteriorates
- Diuretic use – forcing sodium into the urine to encourage water to follow.

This is not similar to scenario 1, where the patients may well be oedematous and the sodium is either forced into or trapped in the urine or in the tissues.

Scenario 3: The patient is consuming a large amount of fluid that is diluting their blood.
Normally, we compensate for increased fluid intake by preventing water reabsorption and increasing urine flow. In this scenario, the drinking habits of the patient overwhelmed this mechanism.
Continually drinking high levels of fluid results in dilution of the blood. This is known as primary polydipsia, commonly seen in the elderly population with their 'tea and toast diet'.
The body has enough sodium; this is simply over-dilution with water. The answer is to encourage fluid restriction to correct the low sodium.

CHAPTER 4 Laboratory Investigations

Scenario 4: The pituitary gland is producing too much anti-diuretic hormone (ADH) and this acts to increase water absorption from the urine when it is not needed, hence the sodium is diluted.

This introduces the concept of hormonal control in fluid balance in the body. SIADH (syndrome of inappropriate anti-diuretic hormone) is one of these mechanisms.

There are a number of causes, including primary brain injury and malignancy. One of the commonest causes is head injury in the elderly, often unwitnessed falls.

ADH is one of the compensatory mechanisms needed to increase water reabsorption in the kidneys. If the body is creating too much ADH, too much water will be absorbed from the urine, which will dilute the blood, reducing the sodium level.

Before treatment, it is important to exclude hypoaldosteronism as the cause. This is another of the compensatory mechanisms, and fluid restriction, which is the way to manage this, can lead to serious consequences (see scenario 6).

The body has enough sodium; this is simply over-dilution with water. Fluid restriction is effective here, but beware of AKI.

Scenario 5: There is accumulation of sodium in the urine that cannot be reabsorbed.

The transporter mechanism in the kidney is designed to move water and sodium back and forth in the tubules. This is under hormonal control. Aldosterone production, from the adrenal glands, is driven by the pituitary gland (centrally controlling hormonal systems). Aldosterone recovers sodium from the urine and hence brings water back with it. Remember, these hormonal systems are perpetually in a balanced state, working all of the time to maintain electrolytes in the correct concentration.

So, logically there are two potential problems here:

- Adrenal insufficiency: Addison's disease, where too little aldosterone is created
- Hypopituitarism: reduced production of messenger hormones leading to poor aldosterone production.

There is reabsorption of water in the kidney but not of sodium, diluting the blood and concentrating the urine. This scenario can present in crisis. When rapid sodium and water reabsorption from the urine to maintain blood pressure is needed, particularly in times of infection, we are unable to achieve that and hence can become rapidly hypotensive. This is an Addisonian crisis.

The body has enough sodium; this is simply over-dilution with water.

Scenario 6: As a normal response to vomiting or excessive sweating. It is electrolytes as well as water that is lost, leading to a hyponatraemia.

The sodium has been lost in vomit or sweat and the kidneys are trying to absorb water and sodium from the urine to compensate. It is important to carry out a fluid assessment, as this can help determine the severity of the dehydration. The urine is concentrated in this scenario. Rehydration with saline should resolve the hyponatraemia.

The body is sodium deficient and needs replacement.

Scenario 7: Patients can also develop pseudohyponatraemia. The role of sodium in holding water in the blood (osmotic effect) has been replaced by fats, sugar or protein. Hence, sodium is lost in the urine to compensate for these other substances having taken over its role.

This would include:

- Lipids – hyperlipidaemia
- Glucose – hyperglycaemia
- Proteins – myeloma.

Often, the presentation in this scenario is related to the underlying condition, which once resolved will lead to resolution of the sodium levels in the blood.

Hypernatraemia

This is a sodium level of > 146. This is less common but, knowing the mechanisms, you can work out what might be behind this scenario. There are two possibilities:

There is decreased total body water relative to sodium:

- Water loss: GI loss (severe diarrhoea), dermal (burns) or urinary loss
- Inadequate water intake: diabetes insipidus, this is rare and has a number of causes.

There is too much sodium:

- Iatrogenic: excess IV saline administered
- Hyperaldosteronism: driving salt reabsorption from the urine
- Excess salt ingestion.

Symptoms (these depend on degree of hypernatremia):

- Thirst
- Weakness
- Lethargy
- Irritability
- Tremor
- Ataxia
- Confusion
- Seizures
- Coma.

> If sodium is > 155 mmol/L, seizure and coma can result – and these patients should be considered a medical emergency (Ranjan et al., 2020).

On examination:

- Cool peripheries
- Decreased skin turgor
- Dry mouth
- Hypotension
- Low JVP
- Prolonged capillary refill time
- Tachycardia.

CHAPTER 4 Laboratory Investigations

Management (Ranjan et al., 2020):

- Prevent further water losses
- Replace water lost – a third of the deficit per 24 hours
- Check serum sodium every 12–24 hours – to prevent it falling by more than 8 mmol/L in 24 hours.

Potassium

Range: 3.5–5.3 mmol/L (Guyton and Hall, 2011).

As with sodium, it is important to understand where potassium is in the body and how its movements are managed. Potassium is found both inside and outside of cells, and hence there are three compartments where it could be:

- The blood
- The cells
- The fluid around the cells.

Again, it is an essential electrolyte for normal muscle and neurological function. Potassium has the potential to create catastrophic and unpredictable cardiac arrhythmias, particularly in an elevated state. Our possibilities are:

- Within the normal range
- Too high: hyperkalaemia
- Too low: hypokalaemia.

So, you should be asking: Is there enough potassium in the patient's body? Is it being lost or not taken in? Has it been moved into the cells and hence is not being seen in the bloodstream?

This might seem inconsequential, but the body has an ability to move potassium rapidly from the blood into the cells, and then back again, hence we can see a rapid shift in potassium levels in the bloodstream.

Hypokalaemia

Low potassium is common and of less concern than raised potassium. There are various scenarios which might create this result:

- Increased loss: via the kidneys, the GI tract or the skin (many causes of each)
- Transcellular shift: the movement of potassium away from where it should be (into cells)
- Decreased intake: malnutrition, failures of TPN or inadequate replacement when on IV fluids and NBM.

Management

1. Potassium replacement – amount and urgency depend on severity
   Rate of change, existence of risk factors, ongoing losses?
2. < 2.5 mmol/L then will likely need admission.

Urea and Electrolytes

Complications of Treatment
- Cardiac arrythmias
- Iatrogenic hyperkalaemia
- Muscle weakness
- Changes in renal function.

> The management of potassium is full of risk. Catastrophic cardiac arrythmias are unpredictable and so management should be considered carefully, with appropriate advice sought and safety netting in place.

Further Investigations
Further tests will help when looking for patterns:

1. Sodium: if sodium is also low, this suggests significant fluid loss OR thiazide diuretic use
2. Magnesium: accompanies hypokalaemia and will need concurrent correction
3. Blood sugar: remember diabetes
4. ECG: important to determine if this is affecting cardiac function. Typical findings when < 3 mmol/L are flat T waves, ST depression and prominent U waves (Nickson, 2020).

Symptoms and Signs
It is generally asymptomatic. Symptoms may include weakness, fatigue, muscle cramps and constipation. It is also very important to be aware of the risk of abnormal heart rhythms, especially in those with pre-existing heart disease.

When < 2.5 mmol/L, there may be serious neuromuscular complications, including (Cleveland Clinic, 2022):

- Weakness and paralysis
- Respiratory failure (involvement of the muscles)
- Ileus
- Paraesthesia
- Tetani.

Hyperkalaemia

Special care needs to be taken with raised potassium levels. The potential to create fatal cardiac arrhythmia is always present.

Causes
- Renal: acute or chronic kidney injury is the predominant cause which was addressed earlier in the text
- Increased circulation of potassium:
  - Administration of supplements (exogenous; from without)
  - Tumour lysis syndrome and rhabdomyolysis (endogenous; from within). Here, rapid cell breakdown in chemotherapy or when patients are lying on the floor for long periods of time will release potassium into the bloodstream from damaged cells.

CHAPTER 4 Laboratory Investigations

- Shift from intracellular to extracellular space:
  - This is the scenario in diabetic ketoacidosis (DKA), acidosis of other causes and occasionally medication.
  - In DKA, the concern is often the level of blood sugar when in fact what needs analysis and very close monitoring is the potassium level.

DKA

> ANY acidosis will force potassium out of cells and into the blood. Insulin forces potassium back in. The management here is based around blood sugar, BUT potassium must be monitored very closely.

Pseudohyperkalaemia

In patients who have been difficult to bleed, there will be blood cell damage when the sample was taken, again releasing potassium into the sample but not being representative of the blood level. It is very important to determine whether or not the result is true.

It can be false in the case of (Kerr et al., 1985):

- Prolonged tourniquet time
- Test tube haemolysis
- Use of the wrong anticoagulant
- Excessive cooling of the specimen
- Length of storage
- Marked leukocytosis and thrombocytosis
- Sample while the patient was receiving IV K+.

> Levels above 6 mmol/L are dangerous and require immediate review and treatment (Rodan, 2017).

Symptoms

These are typically non-specific and include weakness and fatigue. Patients can also present with:

- Muscular paralysis
- Shortness of breath
- Cardiac symptoms.

Investigations

- Repeat any unexpected result to confirm, as there can be intervening factors giving false results.
- Check urine output and other electrolytes.
- ABG – metabolic acidosis causes a transcellular shift.
- Capillary blood glucose and plasma glucose.
- Check their medications – specifically for digoxin, methotrexate, ciclosporin and theophylline.
- ECG changes are more likely when there is a rapid rise in potassium, for example with an AKI.

Urea and Electrolytes

> Patients with elevated potassium of 6 and above need hospital admission and monitoring, and there is no alternative.

Calcium

Range (adjusted): 2.2–2.6 mmol/L (Guyton and Hall, 2011).
Calcium is essential for:

- Muscle contraction
- Nerve conduction
- Bone strength
- Cell replication.

> Calcium is carried in the blood by ALB and, hence, with altered levels of ALB the result will change (as in liver failure, as the liver makes ALB). The result you are given by the lab has been adjusted to allow for this.

The level of blood calcium is monitored by the parathyroid glands (situated within the thyroid) and they produce parathormone or calcitonin to increase or decrease calcium levels in the blood. This is via a 'negative feedback loop', as outlined in Figure 4.2. If blood calcium falls, it stimulates the parathyroid gland to release PTH (parathyroid hormone). This acts on bone, the kidney and the small intestine. Bone releases calcium directly into the bloodstream. The kidney reabsorbs more calcium and converts more vitamin D into its active form, which causes the GI tract to absorb more calcium. If blood calcium increases, the parathyroid gland instead releases calcitonin which causes the opposite effect.

Hypercalcaemia

This is a serum calcium level of > 2.6 mmol/L (Guyton and Hall, 2011).
We do see this relatively commonly and it is usually as a consequence of increased cell activity removing calcium from bones. Responsible cells in bone are osteoclasts.

Causes

- Hyperparathyroidism: the most common cause; too much parathyroid hormone
- Malignancy: a number of mechanisms
- Medications: thiazide diuretics – increased resorption in the kidney
- Increased intake: supplements cause increased GI uptake.

Symptoms

- Bone pain. The bone is being stripped away and released into the blood
- Muscle weakness
- Formation of kidney stones
- Constipation
- Impaired brain function

CHAPTER 4 Laboratory Investigations

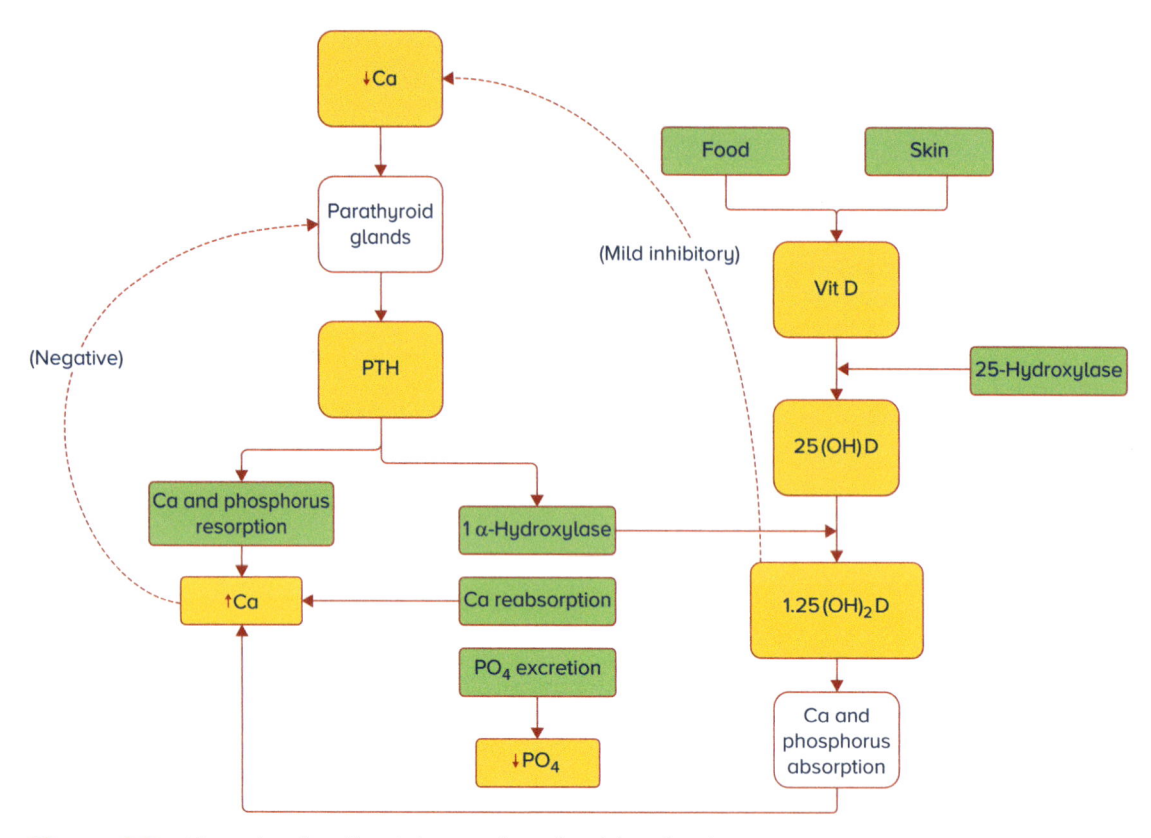

Figure 4.2 Negative feedback loop related to blood calcium.

> 💡 This can be remembered as bones, groans, stones, thrones and psychiatric moans.

Management
If less than 3.5 and the patient is asymptomatic, then this can be monitored and the underlying causes addressed.

> 🚩 If severe over 3.5 mmol/L, they need specialist monitoring (NICE, 2019).

Hypocalcaemia
This is a serum calcium level of < 2.2 mmol/L (Guyton and Hall, 2011).
  The two main causes are:
- Too little calcium intake from the diet
- Loss of calcium from the blood.

84

Causes

- Loss of the parathyroid gland due to surgery (thyroidectomy), after disease of the gland or via autoimmune destruction
- Magnesium deficiency can create a coincidental hypocalcaemia
- Low levels of vitamin D can also cause this: poor diet, lack of sunlight, renal failure
- Kidneys or bowels are not resorbing it
- Tumour lysis and acute pancreatitis – both of these release negatively charged ions that bind with the positively charged calcium ions in the blood.

Symptoms

> Use the mnemonic CATS:
> - **C**onvulsions
> - **A**rrhythmias
> - **T**etany
> - **S**eizures.

Signs

These signs occur because the neurones are more excitable:

- Chovsteks signs – tap the facial nerve and there will be twitching of the muscles at the corner of the mouth
- Trousseau's sign – BP cuff pressure on the nerve causes spasm of the hand.

Investigations

1. Confirm the hypocalcaemia is TRUE
2. Check their PTH
3. Magnesium levels
4. Urea and creatinine: to check renal function
5. Vitamin D deficiency.

Treatment

- Oral calcium if mild
- Active vitamin D if there is renal failure
- If severe, give IV calcium gluconate.

> Think and apply logic and work with what is common.

CHAPTER 4   Laboratory Investigations

Magnesium

Range: 0.7–1.0 mmol/L (Guyton and Hall, 2011).

Magnesium is involved in many aspects of physiology within the body – a very extensive list.

The concentration is a reflection of dietary intake and the ability of the body to retain it through the kidneys and the GI tract. Most of it resides in the cells, so the relationship between deficiency and plasma level is not strong.

Hypomagnesaemia

This means low levels of magnesium. It is commonly found in scenarios where electrolytes are abnormal. Potassium and calcium are two examples, so it is difficult to pin down what is actually down to raised magnesium levels.

Causes

This is typically caused by malabsorption syndromes. However other causes are:

- Malnutrition
- Chronic alcoholism
- Side effect of PPIs or other medications
- Renal disease
- Diabetes.

Hypermagnesaemia

This means high levels of magnesium. This is commonly seen in patients with late-stage renal disease who are taking medications containing Mg – ordinarily, excess would be excreted but with kidney damage this does not occur.

Causes

- Lithium therapy
- Dialysis
- Hypercalcaemia
- Hypothyroidism
- Addison's disease.

Symptoms

- Nausea and vomiting
- Hypotension
- Facial flushing
- Weakness
- Respiratory depression
- Bradycardia.

Liver Function Tests

Liver function tests are frequent and often perceived as difficult to interpret. There are a range of conditions which affect the liver, and it is important to understand the tests you are performing and what they indicate and then to look at the patterns within the testing which will help towards diagnosis. If you apply the principle of commonality and think about what is actually seen in practice, you can find your own logical approach.

It is important to remember the functions of the liver. These are wide-ranging and critical. It is a waste disposal unit, a storage device, a crucial part of the immune system, a metaboliser (all of the absorbed material from the bowel passes through the liver) and crucial to clotting.

The common tests are:

- Bilirubin (Br)
- Alanine transaminase (ALT)
- Aspartate aminotransferase (AST)
- Alkaline phosphatase (ALP)
- Gamma GT (GGT)
- Albumen (ALB).

ALB is included because it is a direct measure of the liver's synthetic function. One of the features of liver failure is oedema. ALB sits in the bloodstream, working to prevent loss of fluid to the tissues (osmotic pressure) and, hence, if less is made, the ability to hold fluid in the bloodstream is lost, which transfers to the tissue spaces and manifests as oedema.

Before you interpret any liver function tests, remember that problems with the liver can occur prior to it, within the liver structure itself or after the liver in the biliary tree.

ALT and AST

The transaminases, particularly ALT, are important markers of liver disease. AST is also released from muscle and is less specific. Their role is to assist the liver in creating glucose. They sit within hepatocytes, essentially within the very structure of the liver. There is always a degree of cell turnover within every organ and hence levels of these enzymes can always be measured in the bloodstream. It then follows that high levels of ALT signify damage to liver cells.

Causes of damage to liver cells and a rise in AST and ALT:

- Non-alcoholic fatty liver disease
- Alcoholic liver disease
- Paracetamol overdose
- Hepatitis.

ALP

This enzyme is found in the membrane of liver cells in the biliary tree. It indicates a post-hepatic problem should it be elevated. Hence, if there are elevated levels of ALP in liver testing, it is likely (as biliary problems are common) to be an obstructive problem which is preventing the flow of bile. This then backs up into the biliary tree and back into the bloodstream.

One of the major pitfalls here is that ALP is also released by bone, placenta, kidney and the intestines. The commonest trap to fall into is to see an isolated raised ALP and assume it is coming from the liver. In the late middle-aged male or female, we must consider metastatic disease. Both prostate and breast cancer metastasise to the bone and the ALP we see in the bloodstream may be coming from there.

CHAPTER 4 Laboratory Investigations

Hence, if the ALP is raised, firstly look at the Br and if this is raised, this is a hepatic cause. If the Br is not raised, then look elsewhere. A GGT, which is also specific to the biliary tree, can be requested and if elevated promotes a hepatic source for the ALP.

Br

The liver breaks down the products of red cell destruction arriving from the spleen. Its job is to create bile to assist fat digestion from some of these breakdown products. Br is tested because it indicates where the problem might be.

When raised levels are seen, patterns can be worked out which explain the origins. Logically, there are three scenarios to consider, and these map to the causes of jaundice:

- There is accelerated breakdown of red blood cells, as seen in haemolysis. This overwhelms the liver and hence these salts find themselves in the circulation. This is not a liver problem, and patients present with severe anaemia and jaundice.
- There is very significant liver damage, as in acute hepatitis or paracetamol overdose where the liver is unable to metabolise bile salts and they are released into the bloodstream in higher amounts. Jaundice will be present.
- There is a problem with the drainage of bile, either secondary to gallstones or more sinister causes such as pancreatic carcinoma. When the outflow of bile is prevented, it backs up into the liver and then back into the bloodstream.

Table 4.2 and Table 4.3 map changes in the various blood test results to particular diagnoses. One thing to bear in mind is that the pattern you are looking for is which element rises first. The more advanced the problem, the more likely it is that other tests will be elevated at a later date. For example, a cancer in the head of the pancreas will create raised ALP and Br to begin with but, as backpressure affects the liver itself, the AST and ALT will rise as liver cells are damaged.

What the eagle-eyed will spot is that in chronic liver damage the tests may well all be normal. This is testament to the incredible ability of the liver to cope. This is false reassurance, as it is not atypical for the liver to 'decompensate' and suddenly lose the ability to function.

Looking at some potential diagnoses, you will see that there is a range of scenarios to consider to consolidate your understanding. Be logical, and to begin with look at commonality. There are many conditions that affect the liver.

Table 4.2 Changes in Blood Test Results to Certain Diagnoses

	Pre-hepatic (haemolysis)	Acute hepatocellular damage (hepatic)	Chronic hepatocellular damage (hepatic)	Post-hepatic (biliary)
ALT	Normal	Very raised	Normal or slight increase	Normal or slight increase
ALP	Normal	Normal or slight increase	Normal or slight increase	Very raised
Br	Raised	Normal or slight increase	Normal or slight increase	Very raised

Urea and Electrolytes

Table 4.3 Changes in Blood Test Results to Certain Diagnoses

Pre-hepatic (haemolysis)	Acute hepatocellular damage (hepatic)	Chronic hepatocellular damage (hepatic)	Post-hepatic (biliary)
Haemolytic anaemia	Paracetamol overdose	Alcoholic liver disease	Pancreatic carcinoma
Malaria	Infectious hepatitis, particularly hepatitis A	Non-alcoholic fatty liver disease	Gallstone disease
Certain medications, anti-TB drugs	Certain medications	Chronic hepatitis, typically hepatitis B or C	Cholangiocarcinoma

Thyroid Function Tests

Range:

- TSH: 0.4–4 mU/L
- Free T4: 9–25 pmol/L (Guyton and Hall, 2011).

The thyroid regulates the rate of metabolism in the body, determining how hard cells of the body are working to carry out their specific function. It is the commonest hormone deficiency, and it is important to understand the physiology. The thyroid is like the drummer in the band; all the cells of the body respond to the rate it sets and without it they grind to a halt. This is not a rapid process unless the thyroid has been surgically removed.

The regulation of thyroid hormone production is under the control of the hypothalamic-pituitary-thyroid (HPT) axis, the mechanism by which thyroid hormone production is increased or decreased according to central nervous system monitoring. Levels of thyroxine in the body are measured by receptors within the brain. TRH (thyrotrophin releasing hormone) is released by the hypothalamus and acts on the anterior pituitary gland. The anterior pituitary then releases TSH (thyroid stimulating hormone), which acts on the thyroid gland itself, regulating production of T4 and T3. There is constant balancing at play as the brain measures the levels of T4 in the blood and acts to increase or decrease the TSH as a response. This is outlined in Figure 4.3.

Specifically, the thyroid plays a crucial role in:

- Metabolism
- Body temperature
- Keeping energy and mood stable
- Maintaining heart rate
- Regulating gut motility
- Maintaining periods and fertility.

In understanding abnormal thyroid function tests, these principles can be applied.

CHAPTER 4 Laboratory Investigations

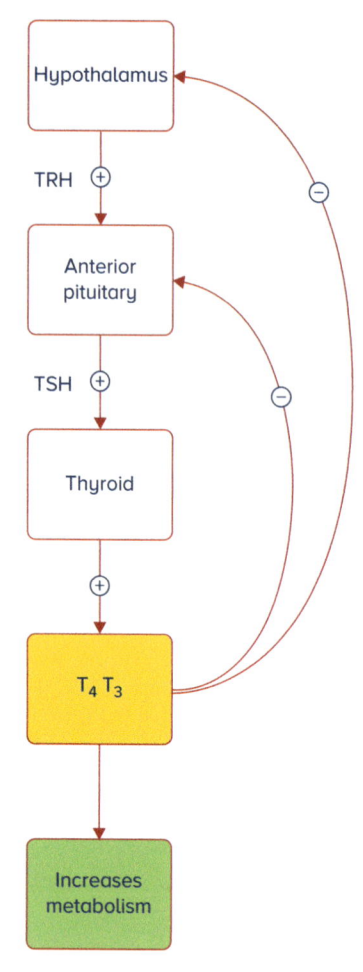

Figure 4.3 Hypothalamic-pituitary-thyroid (HPT) axis.

Hypothyroidism (Under-functioning)

Range:

- TSH: > 4
- Free T4: < 9 (Guyton and Hall, 2011).

In this scenario, the thyroid gland is under-producing thyroxine. The commonest, acquired, cause is Hashimoto's thyroiditis where the body produces antibodies which destroy the thyroid gland. This is insidious and presents with typical symptoms of thyroid underactivity.

Patients will often complain of tiredness, feeling cold, weight gain, muscle pain, dry skin, constipation and low mood. It is incredibly common within families as an inheritable problem (NICE, 2021c).

> Remember that the development of hypothyroidism is a long-term problem. You are looking for trends in the blood test; often you will only be given a TSH result. You need to look at the problem holistically; this is not just a blood test but needs to be taken and interpreted in the context of the patient's symptoms. This is incredibly important when addressing changes according to annual testing.

Hyperthyroidism (Over-functioning)

Range:

- TSH: < 0.5
- Free T4: > 24 (Guyton and Hall, 2011).

In this scenario, the thyroid gland is over-producing thyroxine. The commonest, acquired, cause is Grave's disease, where the body produces antibodies which mimic thyroid-stimulating hormone, leading to over-release of T4 and hence avoiding the feedback loop. Patients will often complain of feeling hot, agitated and having diarrhoea, and occasionally of having palpitations and feeling anxious. Their sleep is also affected (NICE, 2021c). This group needs specialist management and referral to thyroid services.

Subclinical Hypothyroidism and Hyperthyroidism

Range:

- TSH: 4–10
- Free T4: 9–25 (NICE, 2021c).

This group will often have a slightly elevated TSH and will often be asymptomatic. Here it is important to ask about family history and potentially to request a thyroid auto-antibody test which may well predict their future trajectory. Any treatment here will need specialist involvement.

Chapter Summary

Developing skill and confidence in ordering and interpreting blood tests requires time and patience, the use of supportive resources and, crucially, understanding of the underlying physiology and the impact pathology on these systems. Building knowledge and adhering to a rational and logical approach is critical. The FBC, haematinics and inflammatory markers, renal function, calcium metabolism, liver function and thyroid testing are a starting point, and the use of local guidelines and further reading in enhancing depth of understanding is encouraged.

CHAPTER 4 Laboratory Investigations

Case Study

You see a 40-year-old man complaining of a two-month history of abdominal pain.

History
PC: Abdominal pain.
HxPC: He tells you the pain is in the epigastric region and is intermittent. He had a similar episode last year, which was relieved by omeprazole. The pain usually lasts for 1 hour at night, and can wake him in the night. Spicy foods worsen the symptoms and he feels tired all the time.
PMHx: None, normally fit and well.
SHx: Smoker, 10–15 per day for 25 years. Drinks alcohol 30 units per week.
DHx: No regular medicines.

Examination
- Mild tenderness in the epigastrium.
- All other observations within healthy ranges.

Blood Results
- Haemoglobin: 10.2
- MCV: 71
- WCC: 8.9
- Platelets: 350
- Ferritin: 6 mg/L
- The blood film is reported as showing microcytic, hypochromic red cells.

Preferred Diagnoses
- Peptic ulcer

The blood count shows anaemia with a low MCV, indicating a microcytic anaemia. The low ferritin shows an iron-deficiency anaemia. The most common cause of iron-deficiency anaemia in a man is gastrointestinal blood loss. The abdominal pain is consistent with a peptic ulcer.

Management
- The potential diagnosis should be confirmed with endoscopy.
- The patient should be tested for Helicobacter pylori (HP).
- Depending on results, the patient should commence on a Proton-pump inhibitor (PPI) medication such as omeprazole (stool sample first, as PPI will affect the results), and antibiotics if HP test is positive.

References

Arias, C.F. (2017) How do red blood cells *know* when to die? *Royal Society of Open Science* 4: 160850.

Ball, S.G. (2013) How I approach hyponatraemia. *Clinical Medicine Journal (London)* 13(3): 291–295.

Begum, S. and Latunde-Dada, G.O. (2019) Anemia of Inflammation with an emphasis on chronic kidney disease. *Nutrients* 11(10): 2424.

Cleveland Clinic (2022) Low potassium levels in your blood (hypokalemia). Available at: https://my.clevelandclinic.org/health/diseases/17740-low-potassium-levels-in-your-blood-hypokalemia (accessed 28 January 2023).

Gupta, P.M., Perrine, C.G., Mei, Z. et al. (2016) Iron, anemia, and iron deficiency anemia among young children in the United States. *Nutrients* 8(6): 330.

Guyton, A. and Hall, J. (2011) *Guyton and Hall Textbook of Medical Physiology*. 12th edn. Philadelphia, PA: Saunders, Elsevier.

Imashuku, S., Kudo, N., and Kaneda, S. (2012) Spontaneous resolution of macrocytic anemia: Old disease revisited. *Journal of Blood Medicine* 3: 45–47.

Kerr, D.J., McAlpine, L.G., and Dagg, J.H. (1985) Pseudohyperkalaemia. *British Medical Journal* 291(6499): 890–891.

Lam, J.H., Pickles, K., Stanaway, F.F. et al. (2020) Why clinicians overtest: Development of a thematic framework. *BMC Health Services Research* 20: 1011.

Lebois, M. and Josefsson, E.C. (2016) Regulation of platelet lifespan by apoptosis. *Platelets* 27(6): 497–504.

Mayo Clinic (2023) Anemia. Available at: https://www.mayoclinic.org/diseases-conditions/anemia/symptoms-causes/syc-20351360 (accessed 30 January 2023).

Maze, M.J., Skea, S., Pithie, A. et al. (2013) Prevalence of concurrent deep vein thrombosis in patients with lower limb cellulitis: A prospective cohort study. *BMC Infectious Diseases* 13: 141.

Murphy, W.G. (2014) The sex difference in haemoglobin levels in adults — Mechanisms, causes, and consequences. *Blood Reviews* 28(2): 41–47.

National Institute for Health and Care Excellence (NICE) (2019) Clinical Knowledge Summaries: Hypercalcaemia. Available at: https://cks.nice.org.uk/topics/hypercalcaemia/ (accessed 28 January 2023).

National Institute for Health and Care Excellence (NICE) (2020a) Venous thromboembolic diseases: Diagnosis, management and thrombophilia testing [NG158]. Available at: https://www.nice.org.uk/guidance/ng158/chapter/recommendations#diagnosis-and-initial-management (accessed 28 January 2023).

National Institute for Health and Care Excellence (NICE) (2020b) Clinical Knowledge Summaries: Hyponatraemia. Available at: https://cks.nice.org.uk/topics/hyponatraemia/ (accessed 28 January 2023).

National Institute for Health and Care Excellence (NICE) (2021a) Clinical Knowledge Summaries: Platelets: What are the causes of thrombocytosis? Available at: https://cks.nice.org.uk/topics/platelets-abnormal-counts-cancer/background-information/causes-of-thrombocytosis/ (accessed 28 January 2023).

National Institute for Health and Care Excellence (NICE) (2021b) Clinical knowledge Sumaries: Acute kidney injury: How should I respond to AKI warning stage test results? Available at: https://cks.nice.org.uk/topics/acute-kidney-injury/diagnosis/responding-to-aki-warning-stage-test-results/ (accessed 30 January 2023).

CHAPTER 4 Laboratory Investigations

National Institute for Health and Care Excellence (NICE) (2021c) Clinical Knowledge Summaries: Hypothyroidism: When should I suspect a diagnosis of hypothyroidism? Available at: https://cks.nice.org.uk/topics/hypothyroidism/diagnosis/diagnosis/ (accessed 28 January 2023).

National Institute for Health and Care Excellence (NICE) (2022a) Clinical Knowledge Summaries: Multiple myeloma: When should I suspect multiple myeloma? Available at: https://cks.nice.org.uk/topics/multiple-myeloma/diagnosis/when-should-i-suspect-multiple-myeloma/ (accessed 28 January 2023).

National Institute for Health and Care Excellence (NICE) (2022b) Clinical Knowledge Summaries: Chronic kidney disease: When should I suspect chronic kidney disease? Available at: https://cks.nice.org.uk/topics/chronic-kidney-disease/diagnosis/diagnosis/ (accessed 28 January 2023).

National Kidney Foundation (2022) Stages of chronic kidney disease. Available at: https://www.kidney.org/professionals/explore-your-knowledge/how-to-classify-ckd (accessed 27 January 2023).

Nickson, C. (2020) Life in the Fast Lane: Hypokalaemia. Available at: https://litfl.com/hypokalaemia/ (accessed 28 January 2023).

Palmieri, F., Gomis, P., Ruiz, J.E. et al. (2021) ECG-based monitoring of blood potassium concentration: Periodic versus principal component as lead transformation for biomarker robustness. *Biomedical Signal Processing and Control* 68(3): 102719.

Ranjan, R., Lo, S.C., Ly, S. et al. (2020) Progression to severe hypernatremia in hospitalized general medicine inpatients: An observational study of hospital-acquired hypernatremia. *Medicina (Kaunas)* 56(7): 358.

Rodan, A.R. (2017) Potassium: Friend or foe? *Pediatric Nephrology* 32(7): 1109–1121.

Thibault, L., Beauséjour, A., de Grandmont, M.J. et al. (2006) Characterization of blood components prepared from whole-blood donations after a 24-hour hold with the platelet-rich plasma method. *Transfusion* 46(8): 1292–1299.

World Health Organization (WHO) (2023) Anaemia. Available at: https://www.who.int/health-topics/anaemia#tab=tab_1 (accessed 28 January 2023).

Neurological Presentations

Chris McGregor and Georgette Eaton

Within This Chapter

- Altered neurology
- Confusion
- Facial palsy
- Headache
- Memory problems

Long-term conditions
- Epilepsy
- Multiple sclerosis
- Myalgic encephalomyelitis

Introduction

Neurological presentations can take many forms in primary care environments, ranging from acute presentations to complex patients with long-term neurological conditions. It is estimated that each clinical commissioning group (CCG) has on average 59,000 patients living with a neurological condition (NHS England, 2016) and so the neurological presentation is likely within primary care, both as acute presentations and the ongoing care for those with chronic neurological conditions.

With the time constraints of a face-to-face primary care consultation usually set at around 10–20 minutes, and telephone consultations being increasingly used, the vast majority of clinical suspicion is going to be gleaned from excellent consultation skills. It is essential to use every minute of the consultation to gather information on neurological function, as a lengthy, in-depth neurological assessment may not be possible.

> If you work from a list and a patient is booked in with a neurological complaint (dizziness, severe headache, visual trouble), your assessment could start in the waiting room. Where you may normally use call boards in your workplace, this may be a good opportunity to personally call the patient and then use this time to assess gait, mobility, balance and coordination and even speech on the way back to the clinic room.

CHAPTER 5 Neurological Presentations

It is also important to consider that patients may present with overlapping conditions. Cardiovascular conditions, diabetes or chronic respiratory conditions may cause some symptoms that may appear neurological in nature, such as neuropathy or altered sensation. Equally, long-term neurological conditions can affect other systems and may need to be considered as differential diagnoses, such as neuropathic bladder in patients with Parkinson's disease. Again, this just goes to highlight the importance of sound consultation skills when operating in such a challenging and fast-paced environment.

Assessment

For autonomous clinicians working in primary care, the main function of a neurological assessment is to identify any red flags and to increase or decrease clinical suspicions identified during the initial history taking. There are eight main elements to neurological examination, though realistically as part of a primary care initial-screening test it is unlikely that each examination will be undertaken unless clearly indicated to confirm (or refute) a diagnosis.

Mental Status

- Mini Mental State Examination
- Speech (language) tests include checking for fluency in speech during conversation; for comprehension by giving a simple command that crosses the brain's midline (for example, asking the patient to move their right index finger to their left ear and stick their tongue out); and for repetition by asking the patient to repeat a simple phrase – such as 'baby hippopotamus'.

Cranial Nerves

Examination of the cranial nerves (Table 5.1) is an integral and important part of a complete neurological examination. Each test should be completed in full.

Table 5.1 Overview of Cranial Nerve Examination

Cranial nerve		Type	Function	Possible tests (in primary care)
I	Olfactory	Sensory	Sense of smell	History taking; use of alcohol swab
II	Optic	Sensory	Sense of sight	Patient covers one eye. Clinician holds up fingers. Ask patient to count fingers (repeat for other eye) Check peripheral – clinician wiggles finger in peripheral field. Work in X shape. Bring towards centre. Assess at which point patient can see movement

Assessment

Cranial nerve		Type	Function	Possible tests (in primary care)
III	Oculomotor	Motor	Eye movement and pupil constriction	Patient holds head still. Follow letter 'H' shape with eyes only (check III, IV & VI together with 'H' test) Check pupil response (direct and consensual)
IV	Trochlear	Motor	Downward gaze	Downward part of 'H' test
V	Trigeminal	Sensory and motor	S – facial sensation M – Chewing	Ask patient to open mouth wide then clench jaw while clinician palpates muscles of jaw Touch cheeks and lower jaw line to assess for sensation
VI	Abducens	Motor	Lateral eye movement	Lateral eye movement on 'H' test
VII	Facial	Sensory and motor	S – portion of taste M – facial muscle movement	History taking regarding taste. Ask patient to smile. Raise eyebrows. Blow out cheeks. Squeeze eyes closed. Look for weakness/symmetry
VIII	Vestibulocochlear	Sensory	Hearing and balance	History taking regarding hearing. Rub fingers close to each ear
IX	Glossopharyngeal	Sensory and motor	Taste sensation	History taking regarding taste. Ask patient to say 'Ah', and inspect uvula. Check for symmetry of soft palate during movement
X	Vagus	Sensory and motor	S – gag reflex and stretch receptors M – influences heart rate, involved in voice production	Ask patient to swallow and cough
XI	Spinal (accessory)	Motor	Shoulder movement, head turning and movement of viscera	Evaluate muscle strength against resistance. Shrug shoulders (trapezius). Turn head to left and right against resistance
XII	Hypoglossal	Motor	Tongue movement	Ask patient to stick tongue out. Move tongue to left and right, and up and down

CHAPTER 5   Neurological Presentations

Power

Methodically assess the power of each joint. Each joint must be stabilised and isolated to ensure it can be accurately measured. One side at a time should be examined, then compared to the other, assessing for weakness. The Medical Research Council (MRC) muscle power assessment scale (Table 5.2) can be used to score muscle strength.

Table 5.2   MRC Scale of Muscle Strength

Score	Description
0	No contraction
1	Flicker or trace of contraction
2	Active movement, with gravity eliminated
3	Active movement against gravity
4	Active movement against gravity and resistance
5	Normal power

Tone

Assess tone in the muscle groups of the shoulder, elbow, wrist, upper and lower leg, and the ankles. One side at a time should be examined, then compared to the other, assessing for abnormalities such as spasticity, rigidity, cogwheeling or hypotonia.

Reflexes

Assess the reflexes (knee, biceps and triceps, ankle and jaw) using a tendon hammer and ensure the patient is completely relaxed. If the reflex is absent, using a reinforcement manoeuvre such as asking the patient to clench their teeth whilst tapping the tendon can help confirm this.

Sensory Assessment

Sensation should be checked by contrasting a sharp object (such as a neurotip) with a soft object (such as cotton wool). Sensation should be checked across both the spinothalamic track (pain and temperature) and the dorsal column (vibration sense and proprioception); one from each section should be performed.

Coordination

A range of assessments can be used to inform an assessment on coordination, including the finger-to-nose test, dysdiadochokinesia and the heel-to-shin test.

Gait

Ask the patient to walk and then turn and walk back whilst you observe their gait, paying attention to stance, stability and turning. A tandem heel-to-toe gait will also help exacerbate any underlying steadiness, making it easier to identify more subtle ataxia.

Presentations in Primary Care

Altered Neurology

Aetiology

Altered neurology refers to abnormal function of the body, such as an altered gait, altered power, altered tone, altered sensitivity or speech changes. This may be manifested by weakness, tremor, paraesthesia or aphasia, as some common examples. Altered neurology is typically caused by a focal neurological deficit, such as a problem with nerve, spinal cord or brain function. The type, location and severity of the problem can indicate which area of the brain or nervous system is affected.

> Lowth, M. (2020) Abnormal gait [online].
> This has an excellent outline of the different types of abnormal gait, and the relevant considerations for assessment and management.

History and Examination

Focal neurological deficits affect a specific location, such as the left side of the face, right arm or tongue. Vision and hearing problems are also considered focal neurological deficits, and common problems associated affecting eyes and ears are outlined in Chapter 7 – Eyes, Ears, Nose and Throat Presentations (pp. 143–178). History and examination, therefore, should be focused on ruling out common, immediately life-threatening conditions. This should include checking the pupils, reflexes, motor response, meningeal signs and vital signs, looking for evidence of meningitis, stroke, epilepsy or a mass effect (such as tumour, infarct, bleed or abscess) (Gray and Gavin, 2005).

The patient should be asked specifically about the speed of onset and about any associated symptoms – including the presence of other neurological deficits, such as difficulty with speech or swallowing (bulbar symptoms), breathing difficulties, visual disturbance, pain or twitching of the muscles.

Management

Depending on the presenting complaint, and the degree of neurological deficit, conditions to consider as a differential diagnosis are listed below:

- Botulism
- Guillian-Barré
- Metabolic disorders
- Motor neurone disease
- Multiple sclerosis
- Myasthethia gravis
- Spinal cord disease
- Vasculitic neuropathy.

CHAPTER 5   Neurological Presentations

Each of these has a relevant management and treatment pathway outlined in the NICE Clinical Knowledge Summary on the subject.

> Any patient with bulbar symptoms or shortness of breath should be referred to hospital immediately.

Confusion

Aetiology

Confusion is a non-specific, non-diagnostic term to describe a patient with disorientation, impaired memory or abnormal thought process. It does not have a single aetiology, but often has multiple different and potentially interacting aetiologies (Vasilevskis and Ely, 2016).

History and Examination

Taking a history directly from the patient with confusion may not be possible; however, this can yield really helpful insight as to whether delirium could be a factor if the patient is seeing/hearing/experiencing anything else. General conversation during history taking can be helpful as well to assess the patient's current mental state and provide gentle re-orientation if required.

> A collateral history (such as from family, friends and care staff) can be very helpful to confirm or refute the version of events from the patient, but this should be carefully navigated to not exclude the patient's version.

As well as vital signs, a relevant neurological examination and considering sources of infection, there is a standard set of further investigations which are often referred to as a 'confusion screen'. This panel of investigations is useful for identifying or ruling out common causes of confusion, as outlined in Table 5.3.

Management

Importantly, the new onset of confusion should prompt the paramedic to investigate the underlying cause, and this will determine the management approach.

> NICE (2023) Delirium: prevention, diagnosis and management [online].

Presentations in Primary Care

Table 5.3 Diagnostic Testing for Confusion

	Test	Conditions under consideration
Blood tests	B12 + folate/haematinics	B12 or folate deficiency
	Calcium	Hypercalcaemia
	Coagulation/INR	Intracranial bleeding
	HbA1c	Diabetes
	Liver function tests	Liver failure with secondary encephalopathy
	Thyroid function tests	Hypothyroidism
	Urea and electrolytes	Hyponatraemia; hypernatraemia
Urinalysis	Urinalysis	Bacteria urinary tract infection (alongside evidence of supra-pubic tenderness/dysuria/offensive urine/positive urine culture)
Imaging	CT scan	Concern about intracranial pathology (bleeding, ischaemic stroke, abscess)
	Chest X-ray	Lung pathology (pneumonia, pulmonary oedema, cancer)

Facial Palsy

Aetiology

The exact cause of facial palsy is unknown but it is likely to be caused by inflammation or oedema to the facial nerve. Although relatively uncommon, Bell's palsy accounts for the biggest proportion of diagnosis associated with facial weakness or paralysis (Baugh et al., 2013).

History

In the acute setting, a sudden onset of facial weakness and neurological deficit must be managed as an emergency. Once confirmed as facial palsy, the primary care management will centre around symptom care and medicine management.

Examination Findings

The following symptoms can suggest facial palsy as a diagnosis in the absence of any other possible differential:

- Rapid onset (less than 72 hours)
- Facial muscle weakness (almost always unilateral) involving the upper and lower parts of the face
- Ear and postauricular region pain on the affected side
- Difficulty chewing, dry mouth and changes in taste

CHAPTER 5 Neurological Presentations

- Incomplete eye closure, dry eye, eye pain or excessive tearing
- Numbness or tingling of the cheek or mouth
- Speech articulation problems, drooling
- Hyperacusis.

Investigations

If symptoms have not begun to improve after three weeks of treatment, further investigations may be required. Consider referring patients to specialist ear, nose and throat (ENT) consultants or neurologists for onward management. It may also be beneficial to refer patients to an ophthalmologist for any specialist eye investigations or care.

Management

Facial palsy can be managed using oral corticosteroids, typically using either a set dose for a period of ten days or an initial higher dose for the first five days followed by a reduction dose over the remaining five days.

> ! Eye care is vitally important in this patient group. Consideration should be given for prescribing tear replacement or lubricants. Patients who are unable to close their eyes at night should be advised to tape them closed using microporous tape and protect them from sunlight by wearing sunglasses when needed.

> 📖 NICE (2019) Clinical Knowledge Summaries: Bell's palsy [online].

Headaches

Headaches are by far the most common neurological complaint seen in primary care. The World Health Organization (WHO) reports that in any given year almost half the world's population will experience headaches of some description (WHO, 2022). The aetiology of headaches can roughly be subdivided into two groups:

Primary Headache

When the problem lies with the pain-sensitive structures within the head, such as vascular structures, muscles, nerves or chemical interactions. Headaches in this group include cluster headaches, tension headaches and migraines.

Secondary Headache

When there is an additional underlying issue contributing to the headache. There are extensive lists of reasons for secondary headaches, ranging from brain tumours through to alcohol-induced headaches (hangovers).

> Initial assessment of headaches should prioritise ruling out the presence of red flags (NICE, 2022a). Patients presenting with any of the following may warrant urgent referral or admission for further tests:
>
> - Worsening headache with fever
> - Sudden-onset headache reaching maximum intensity within five minutes
> - New-onset neurological deficit
> - New-onset cognitive dysfunction
> - Change in personality
> - Impaired level of consciousness
> - Recent (typically within the past three months) head trauma
> - Headache triggered by cough, valsalva (trying to breathe out with nose and mouth blocked) or sneeze
> - Headache triggered by exercise
> - Orthostatic headache (headache that changes with posture)
> - Symptoms suggestive of giant cell arteritis
> - Symptoms and signs of acute narrow-angle glaucoma
> - A substantial change in the characteristics of their headache
> - Compromised immunity (for example, IV immunosuppressant drugs)
> - Age under 20 years and history of malignancy
> - A history of malignancy known to metastasise to the brain
> - Vomiting without any other obvious cause.

Tension-type Headaches

Aetiology
This is the most common type of headache encountered by primary care clinicians. It can result from muscle contractions in the head or neck, increased stress or tension, overuse of computers or driving long distances.

History
Patients will often report that the headache is central or frontal and describe it like a pressure or a band around the head, sometimes associated with neck or shoulder tightness. It is generally not severe enough to affect day-to-day activities and is usually bilateral in nature, often with no other associated symptoms. They are usually episodic, but if they occur more than 15 times a month for at least three months in a row they are considered chronic tension-type headaches.

Examination Findings
Tension-type headaches will not cause any neurological deficit. Any other underlying findings (such as hypertension, anxiety, depression) should be considered and managed on a case-by-case basis, as these may be contributing to the presenting complaint (Collins, 2022).

CHAPTER 5 Neurological Presentations

Investigations
For reoccurring complaints, patients should be asked to keep a headache diary for up to eight weeks.

Management
Acute: Consider aspirin, paracetamol or non-steroidal anti-inflammatory drug (NSAID) where appropriate for treatment. Do not use opioids for acute tension-type headaches.
Chronic: Alongside pain management, can consider referral for acupuncture as prophylactic treatment.
Lifestyle advice: Should be related to the social history and may include smoking cessation; reduced alcohol intake; balanced diet and eating regular meals; remaining hydrated; reduced caffeine intake; and good sleep hygiene.

> NICE (2021c) Headaches in over 12s: Diagnosis and management [online].

Medication-overuse Headaches (Rebound Headaches)

Aetiology
Caused by overuse of pain relief being taken to treat the initial headache; commonly this is overuse of paracetamol (BASH, 2010).

History
Similar to tension-type headaches, patients will often report the headache is central or frontal and describe it like a pressure or a band around the head. Often starts early in the day and persists throughout, but episodes tend to spike as pain relief wears off and headache reoccurs.

Examination Findings
Medication-overuse headaches will not cause any neurological deficit. Patients may present with associated nasal congestion, neck pain or restlessness, and report poor sleep habits. Medication reviews will highlight overuse of medication, so encourage patients to be honest with answers.

Investigations
With a reoccurring headache, patients should be asked to keep a headache diary for up to eight weeks. The diary may help to highlight medication overuse; however, if medication overuse is strongly suspected, then manage immediately and use the headache diary to monitor results.

Management
Advise patients to immediately stop taking overused medication for at least one month. Explain that headaches may get worse initially. Arrange follow-up appointments within one to two weeks for review. Continue with headache diary.

Presentations in Primary Care

> If overused medication is a strong opioid, then specialist input for withdrawal may be required.

Cluster Headaches

Aetiology

Aetiology is not fully understood, but cluster headaches have been found to be more common in 30- to 40-year-olds and are more prevalent in males (Dowson, 2015). Higher occurrences in family groups are suggestive of a genetic link. Over-activity of certain areas of the brain – mainly the hypothalamus – results in severe sudden onset. Specific triggers are often involved, such as strong smells or excessive alcohol intake. Diagnosis is achieved by reviewing symptoms and elimination of other neurological conditions.

History

Cluster headaches are characterised by a sudden onset and usually last between 15 minutes and 3 hours. They can have a frequency of once per day up to eight times per day and last for a period of weeks to months. Once resolved, patients can often go months or even years without another attack.

Pain is typically:

- Extremely severe
- One sided
- Sharp or piercing in nature
- Located around one eye.

Patients may also notice erythema to the affected eye and nasal congestion on the affected side (BASH, 2010).

Examination Findings

Patients are often agitated and distressed due to the severity of the pain. However, symptoms can vary and can include the presence of neurological deficit, photophobia and unequal pupils. The patient's baseline observations will also likely be deranged due to the severity of the pain.

Investigations

In patients without a formal diagnosis of cluster headaches, several of their symptoms will be red flags and warrant admission to hospital for further tests to assess the need for neuroimaging and specialist management.

> In patients with known diagnosis of cluster headaches, it is important to assess their normal attack symptoms and use this as the basis for your clinical decision making. If severe, or if abnormal for the patient, then admission or urgent referral is likely needed.

CHAPTER 5 Neurological Presentations

Management
Ongoing management of the symptoms of cluster headaches is usually initiated by secondary care specialists. For acute bouts of cluster headaches, this includes:

- Short burst of oxygen therapy delivered at high flow rate of 12–15 litres per minute via a non-rebreather face mask for 15–20 minutes
- Subcutaneous or nasal triptan to people aged over 18 years – various options are available
- Verapamil is used as a preventative medication and again is initiated by specialists.

Giant Cell Arteritis (Temporal Arteritis)

Aetiology
Giant cell arteritis is caused by inflammation of the temporal arteries, resulting in reduced blood flow through the vessels. As this condition is a form of vasculitis, the inflammation can affect other arteries such as the posterior ciliary arteries, leading to visual disturbance. Prevalence is higher in the over 50s, and although uncommon it can lead to serious long-term symptoms (Mukhtyar, 2018).

History
Patients will often report that the headache is unilateral and located around the temporal area. Headaches tend to be sudden in onset and may have associated tenderness if the temporal area is palpated. It is possible for the patient to experience jaw claudication and discomfort around the temporal mandibular joint, and they may also report visual disturbance in the days prior.

Examination Findings
On assessment, the most common presentation will be sudden onset of temporal headache with tenderness. On inspection, thickening or nodularity of the arteries may be seen with some erythema. Over half the patients with giant cell arteritis will complain of associated jaw pain and also scalp tenderness. General muscle aches may be found in up to 40% of these cases, and around 20% of patients will present with visual disturbance in one or both eyes.

Investigations
Depending on the red flags present, it may be necessary to admit the patient for further investigations to rule out other neurological complaints such as cerebral vascular accidents or transient ischemic attacks.

Within primary care, the main investigation is urgent bloods to look for raised erythrocyte sedimentation rate (ESR), raised C-reactive protein (CRP) and raised platelets.

Management
When there is a high clinical suspicion of giant cell arteritis, urgently refer patients for a temporal artery biopsy. Positive results confirm diagnosis, although a negative does not exclude it completely.

Presentations in Primary Care

> ⚠️ Patients with any visual impairment must be seen by an ophthalmologist the same day. However, in primary care, acute onset of visual disturbance may warrant admission for neuroimaging depending on the duration of symptoms.

If there is no visual impairment, refer for urgent specialist assessment usually to rheumatology or general medicine.

Initial treatment is a high dose of oral corticosteroids. Unless contraindicated, this should be started the same day when there is a strong suspicion of giant cell arteritis. Once diagnosed, the specialist will often arrange a shared care agreement with primary care to monitor a reducing dose of corticosteroids, often over a number of years.

> 📖 NICE (2020) Clinical Knowledge Summaries: Giant cell arteritis.

Migraines

Aetiology

Although not fully understood, migraines are thought to be caused by a combination of environmental and genetic factors (Collins, 2022). In up to 60% of cases, there are family links. Migraines can be classed as 'migraines with aura' or 'migraines without aura'.

Typical migraines tend to include the phases shown in Table 5.4.

Migraines can be episodic or chronic in nature; they can also be commonly triggered by changes in hormone levels, so should be suspected in females who are complaining of headaches two to three days before the start of their menstrual cycle.

History

If it is the first time a patient has presented with a migrainous headache, then clinical suspicion of a diagnosis of migraine will be based on history taking and also examination

Table 5.4 Migraine Phases

Phase	Characteristics
Prodrome	Can occur one to two days prior to the onset of the pain. Can include poor concentration, fatigue and neck stiffness
Aura	If patient has a typical aura, this usually occurs approximately no more than an hour before the onset of pain
Headache	The pain phase. Can last 2–72 hours
Postdrome	Can last for up to 48 hours after pain has subsided. Can include changes in mood and fatigue

findings. The history observed will also assist with differentiating between migraines with and without auras.

Migraine with aura can be diagnosed in a person presenting with at least two attacks fulfilling the following criteria:

- One or more typical fully reversible aura symptoms, including:
  - Visual symptoms such as zigzag lines and/or scotoma – visual aura is the most common type of aura
  - Sensory symptoms such as unilateral pins and needles or numbness
  - Speech and/or language symptoms such as dysphasia.
- At least three of the following:
  - At least one aura symptom spreads gradually over at least five minutes
  - Two or more aura symptoms occur in succession
  - Each individual aura symptom lasts 5–60 minutes
  - At least one aura symptom is unilateral
  - At least one aura symptom is positive
  - The aura is accompanied, or followed within 60 minutes, by headache
  - Headache must not be better accounted for by another diagnosis.

Migraine without aura can be diagnosed in a person presenting with at least five attacks fulfilling the following criteria:

- Headache lasting 4–72 hours in adults or 2–72 hours in adolescents.
- Headache with at least two of the following characteristics:
  - Unilateral location (more commonly bilateral in children)
  - Pulsating quality – may be described as 'throbbing' or 'banging' in young people
  - Moderate or severe pain intensity
  - Aggravation by, or causing avoidance of, routine activities of daily life (for example, walking or climbing stairs)
- Headache with associated symptoms, including at least one of:
  - Nausea and/or vomiting
  - Photophobia (sensitivity to light) and phonophobia (sensitivity to sound)
  - Headache must not be better accounted for by another diagnosis.

Examination Findings

As with all neurological presentations, if a patient presents with acute onset of neurological deficit with no clear history of migraines, then this must be treated as an emergency. Some patients will have clear neurological symptoms linked to their typical migraine pattern and therefore can be managed in the primary care setting.

Investigations

Investigations will be guided by the results of the neurological examination and any findings that need further assessment. Also investigating and managing any abnormalities in baseline observation is important. If no concerning red flags are present, then further investigations of the symptoms may be required. An eight-week headache diary can be

Presentations in Primary Care

useful in further understanding the headache symptoms; it can also help identify potential triggers.

Referral to an optometrist can be useful to help rule out any potential triggers or underlying causes.

Baseline bloods can be useful to help identify any potential triggers such as anaemia or raised HbA1c.

Management
Acute Symptoms
Consider aspirin (if over 16), paracetamol or NSAID where appropriate for treatment. Do not use opioid for acute headaches. Children with migraines tend to respond well to these treatments alongside trigger avoidance. In adults, if these alone do not achieve relief then consider an oral triptan only, or in combination with paracetamol or NSAID. Treatment should be started as early in the headache phase as possible. Triptans should not be started when symptoms are still in aura phase.

Prophylactic Management
There are several considerations for managing the frequency and intensity of a migraine. There should also be consideration for managing associated conditions that can trigger migraines, such as depression, anxiety and sleep apnoea. Once diagnosed and fully investigated, migraines can be managed using several prophylactic medications. If patients are getting little relief from medication regimes, then onward referral to specialists may be required.

> NICE (2022a) Clinical Knowledge Summaries: Migraine [online].

Memory Problems
Aetiology
Memory loss can be caused by either damage or disease to the brain (Gazzaniga et al., 2009), and a thorough investigation is required to determine the cause and arrange appropriate treatment.

History and Examination
Include in the history the onset, and whether this is acute (for example, infection or trauma) or insidious (for example, due to degenerative disease); this will help set the cause of the examination. Ascertain the impact that symptoms have on activities of daily life (ADLs), and also on relationships with family or friends. A medication history (including prescribed medicines, over-the-counter (OTC) medicines and alternative medicines) will be important, as some commonly prescribed medicines are associated with an increased

CHAPTER 5   Neurological Presentations

anticholinergic burden (anticholinergic drugs, benzodiazepines and opioids) and therefore cognitive impairment.

Examination should include a full neurological examination, as well as a cardiovascular examination (considering hypertension or arrythmias). Blood tests should include:

- Full blood count (FBC)
- ESR
- CRP
- Urea and electrolytes (U&E)
- Calcium
- HbA1c
- Liver function tests (LFTs)
- Thyroid function tests (TFTs)
- Serum B12 and folate levels.

Other investigations that may be appropriate include urinalysis, chest X-ray, electrocardiogram (ECG), syphilis serology and HIV testing.

> Cognitive testing may be used. It is important to use a validated brief structured cognitive instrument, such as:
>
> - The ten-point cognitive screener (10-CS)
> - The six-item cognitive impairment test (6CIT)
> - The six-item screener
> - The Memory Impairment Screen (MIS)
> - The Mini-Cog
> - Test Your Memory (TYM).
>
> Whichever test is used, it should be the one also used within local referral pathways and units to aid comparison.

Management

Mild cognitive impairment should be discussed (without provoking undue anxiety) and monitored with regular follow-ups to determine any progression. There is evidence that healthy brain activities such as regular exercise, word games and socialisation all benefit patients with mild memory loss (Wang et al., 2020).

If there is concern regarding dementia, then referral to the memory clinic or community old-age psychiatry service is recommended.

> NICE (2018) Dementia: Assessment, management and support for people living with dementia and their carers [online].
> NICE (2021b) Clinical Knowledge Summaries: Suspected dementia [online].

Long-term Conditions

Within the primary care setting, a large percentage of patients will have numerous long-term conditions, including patients with chronic neurological symptoms. As well as managing any acute illness, awareness regarding deteriorating neurological function linked to their condition should be maintained. In addition, consider the patient in the context of the wider multidisciplinary team and local services, including healthcare professionals such as:

- Speech and Language Therapy (SALT): For management of swallow function, difficulties in eating, risk of choking or aspiration
- Dieticians: Can help manage any patients with increased frailty, ensuring access to build-up drinks or nutritional advice
- Physiotherapists: Can help with physical rehab and management of any mobility or gait issues
- Occupational therapists: Can assist with ensuring the home is safe and assessing for any specific aids such as raised seats, support in bathroom, *et cetera*.
- Charity or support groups: Ensure patients and relatives have information on local groups who can support them and avoid any feelings of isolation
- Social prescribers or link workers: Can support families with ongoing care, assess for any financial support or help to engage with respite care.

> Anticholinergic medication is commonly prescribed in primary care, but it has been found to increase the prevalence of cognitive impairment, dizziness, confusion and falls in the older adult population. When assessing older adults presenting with vague neurological symptoms, it is essential to carry out a medication review and use a scoring tool to gauge their anticholinergic burden. Simple medication changes could have a considerable beneficial impact on a patient's symptoms and quality of life.

Epilepsy

Aetiology

Epilepsy is defined as a neurological condition resulting in recurrent seizures. Seizures are caused by disturbed or chaotic neuronal activity in the brain and can affect patients in many ways.

History

Seizures can be subdivided into two broad categories:

- Focal seizures – localised to one hemisphere of the brain. Focal seizures can be localised or widely distributed. Patients who suffer with focal seizures can retain either awareness or loose awareness.
- Generalised seizures – affect bilateral networks within the brain. Can result in many presentations. Can be further divided into motor seizures or non-motor seizures (absent).

CHAPTER 5   Neurological Presentations

Management

Many patients with epilepsy will have already been fully assessed by neurologists and have an epilepsy specialist nurse in place to help with ongoing care. These patients tend to have shared care agreements to allow management in the community alongside access to specialists in secondary and tertiary care.

Any patient who presents in primary care following their first seizure should be urgently referred to the relevant specialist team. The patient and their family or carers should be provided with information on how to manage any suspected seizure in the interim and when to seek emergency care.

Most contact with this patient group will centre on regular reviews and management of changing symptoms.

When reviewing these patients, the following areas should be considered:

- Ensure a relevant specialist contact is in place and known to patient.
- Discuss seizure control and any recent changes.
- Discuss daily impact of epilepsy on day-to-day life.
- Ensure family or carers understand how to manage symptoms and administer any emergency drugs prescribed for the patient.
- Review any adverse effects and compliance issues with anti-epileptic drugs.
- Ensure any female patients of childbearing age understand they must seek specialist advice if considering getting pregnant whilst taking anti-epileptic medication.

Although initiating anti-epileptic medication will be undertaken by specialist care, it is important to have an overview of the drug groups and specific information regarding these treatments. The Medicines and Healthcare products Regulatory Agency (MHRA, 2017) outlines three categories for anti-epileptic drugs:

- Category 1: Phenytoin, carbamazepine, phenobarbital, primidone
- Category 2: Valproate, lamotrigine, perampanel, rufinamide, clobazam, clonazepam, oxcarbazepine, eslicarbazepine, zonisamide, topiramate.
- Category 3: Levetiracetam, lacosamide, tiagabine, gabapentin, pregabalin, ethosuximide, vigabatrin, brivaracetam.

> NICE (2021a) Clinical Knowledge Summaries: Epilepsy.

Multiple Sclerosis

Aetiology

Multiple sclerosis (MS) is an autoimmune-mediated disorder that affects the central nervous system. Causes of MS are multifactorial and include genetic predisposition together with environmental factors such as exposure to infectious agents, vitamin deficiencies and smoking. These agents can trigger a cascade of events in the immune system which lead to neuronal cell death accompanied by nerve demyelination and neuronal dysfunction (Ghasemi et al., 2017).

Long-term Conditions

> Four disease courses have been identified in MS: clinically isolated syndrome (CIS), relapsing-remitting MS (RRMS), primary progressive MS (PPMS) and secondary progressive MS (SPMS). Further reading is available from the National MS Society (2017) Types of MS.

History and Examination

MS is characterised by neurological symptoms such as visual changes, ascending sensory disturbance or weakness, problems with balance and dizziness. A diagnosis of MS is made by a neurologist, and a detailed history regarding experiences of altered neurology should be explored in patients whom you suspect would benefit from referral.

> Assess for the presence of Lhermitte's sign. This is the sense of electricity that shoots down the spine, often out through the arms and legs as well, when the neck is flexed forward (Khare and Seth, 2015).

Before referring a person suspected of having MS to a neurologist, alternative diagnoses should be excluded by performing blood tests, including:

- Calcium
- FBC
- Glucose
- HIV serology
- Inflammatory markers (ESR and CRP)
- LFTs
- Renal function tests (RFTs)
- TFTs
- Vitamin B12.

> Patients who have a diagnosis of MS will usually seek support from their neurologist if they experience symptoms of deterioration or new neurological changes. If such patients present to primary care, ensure other causes of altered neurology have been considered and excluded.

Management

Management for MS will depend on each individual's experiences of the condition, but will typically involve steroids. Initiation of any medication will be undertaken by specialist care, led by the neurologist.

CHAPTER 5 Neurological Presentations

> MS patients may also benefit from input from social prescribing link workers, who can support them to access exercise, smoking-cessation and support-group activities (NICE, 2022b).

Myalgic Encephalomyelitis

Aetiology

Myalgic encephalomyelitis, also called chronic fatigue syndrome or ME/CFS, is a long-term condition with a wide range of symptoms, the aetiology of which is unknown. Current hypotheses consider that an inflammatory response affecting the central nervous system, immune system and endocrine system may be the cause, alongside a wide range of environmental triggers (Cortes Rivera et al., 2019).

The National Institute of Health and Care Excellence (NICE) (2021d) outlines that ME/CFS should be suspected if:

- The following persistent symptoms are present for a minimum of six weeks in adults and four weeks in children and young people:
  - Debilitating fatigue that is worsened by activity, is not caused by excessive cognitive, physical, emotional or social exertion and is not significantly relieved by rest
  - Post-exertional malaise after activity in which the worsening of symptoms:
    o is often delayed in onset by hours or days
    o is disproportionate to the activity
    o has a prolonged recovery time that may last hours, days, weeks or longer
  - Unrefreshing sleep or sleep disturbance (or both), which may include:
    o feeling exhausted, feeling flu-like and stiff on waking
    o broken or shallow sleep, altered sleep pattern or hypersomnia
  - Cognitive difficulties (sometimes described as 'brain fog'), which may include problems finding words or numbers, difficulty in speaking, slowed responsiveness, short-term memory problems and difficulty concentrating or multitasking
- Reduced ability to engage in occupational, educational, social or personal activities from pre-illness levels
- Symptoms are not explained by another condition.

History and Examination

Both the history taking and assessment must be holistic (including symptoms and history, comorbidities, overall physical and mental health), with a relevant neurological and physical examination to determine or exclude the presence of other neurological symptoms. Symptoms should be assessed for their impact on psychological and social well-being.

In considering other differentials, investigations may include:

- CRP
- Calcium and phosphate

- Coeliac screening
- Creatine kinase
- ESR or plasma viscosity
- FBC
- Folate
- HbA1c
- LFT
- Serum ferritin
- TFT
- U&E
- Urinalysis for protein, blood and glucose
- Vitamin B12
- Vitamin D
- 9am cortisol.

Management

> If ME/CFS is suspected, referral to an appropriate specialist team is required, depending on local pathways. For children and young people, consider seeking advice from a paediatrician. The specialist team will work with the person to develop a personal care plan, which may require input from primary care services, such as social prescribing link workers.

> The ME Association has a range of resources and patient stories that can help support understanding of this complex condition.

Chapter Summary

Although this chapter only highlights a few neurological presentations common to primary care, it should serve to highlight the importance of excellent history taking alongside structured focused assessment models in all neurological complaints. As well as maintaining a high index of clinical suspicion, local referral pathways available to you should be utilised when necessary. It may be important to regularly follow up with this patient group and monitor patterns and trends in symptoms. Confident management and a well-rounded approach to patient care can make a considerable difference to these patients.

CHAPTER 5 Neurological Presentations

Case Study 1

You are working a routine session in primary care, when a 25-year-old female presents with altered sensation to her leg and foot.

History

PC: Altered sensation, described as tingling, to left leg and foot.
HxPC: Sudden onset whilst walking last week, with the sensation notable from the knee, radiating medially to the medial aspect of the foot and toe. The patient reports no reduction in power or function.
PMHx/SHx: Anxiety; previous labyrinthitis.
DHx: None.
SHx: Works as a spinning and yoga instructor in a local gym.
FHx: Father has coeliac disease, sister has diabetes mellitus (type 1) and mother has lupus.
ROS: Denies recent illness; has experienced feelings of tiredness but thought had been overdoing it at work.

Examination

- You notice that her gait is normal on walking into the room, with normal coordination and balance. The altered sensation is isolated to the left lower leg and foot.
- She is unable to detect a cotton bud or soft sensation, and reports the neurotip as less sharp when compared to the previous side.
- The sensory loss is isolated to the L4 dermatome only, and only on the left side.
- There has been no back pain, bladder or bowel disturbance or recent trauma. Lhermitte's sign is positive.

Preferred Diagnosis

- Further investigation required.

Differential Diagnoses

- MS
- ME/CFS.

Management

- Referral for blood tests.
- Ask the patient to keep a diary of development of symptoms (worsening or easing).
- Review appointment within two weeks.
- Discussion with clinical supervisor regarding possible differentials.

Case Study 2

A 34-year-old presents in a primary care clinic with recurrent headaches over a four-week period. They are concerned as both a parent and grandparent have suffered strokes, and it is unusual for the patient to experience headaches of this nature.

History

PC: Frontal headache. 5/10.
HxPC: Recurrent over period of three to four weeks. Relieved slightly by analgesics. Denies any visual disturbance or neurological deficit. No noted fever or illness.
PMHx/SHx: Anxiety.
DHx: Escitalopram.
SHx: Works in finance. Busy role. Commutes daily. Non-smoker. Moderate alcohol consumption. Denies recreational drug use. Generally fit – enjoys running.
FHx: Father and paternal grandmother both have had CVA in their 60s.
ROS: Recently seen private consultant regarding knee injury preventing him from running or exercising.

Examination

- Primary survey unremarkable, appears comfortable and engaged.
- No notable neurological deficit. Cranial nerves intact. No photophobia. Pupils appear normal and reactive.
- No additional symptoms indicated – headache is frontal and unfamiliar.
- States he was prescribed co-codamol 30/500 by private consultant for knee pain. Not helping as he needs to be able to mobilise well to get to and from work. Has been taking OTC medication alongside this as well as using topical treatments. Unable to confirm frequency of medication use.

Preferred Diagnosis

- Medication-overuse headache.

Differential Diagnoses

- Acute migraine
- Stress-induced headache
- Tension headache
- Hypertension.

Management

- Consider referral for ECG in practice, and set up routine observation of blood-pressure monitoring.
- Educate patient regarding medication-overuse headaches – discuss drug types and overlap with prescribed and OTC medications.
- Request that all pain relief medication is stopped for at least 1 month – caution around knee pain and consider continuation of topical NSAIDS.

CHAPTER 5 Neurological Presentations

- Encourage patient to keep headache diary and note of any medication use.
- Give realistic timeframes (up to 1 month) for improvements to be evident.
- Review appointment within two weeks as check point – consider review of knee here also.

References

Baugh, R.F., Basura, G.J., Ishii, L.E. et al. (2013) Clinical practice guideline: Bell's palsy. *Otolaryngology – Head and Neck Surgery* 149(3 Suppl): S1–S27.

British Association for the Study of Headache (BASH) (2010) Guidelines for all healthcare professionals in the diagnosis and management of migraine, tension-type headache, cluster headache, medication-overuse headache. Available at: https://bash.org.uk/wp-content/uploads/2012/07/10102-BASH-Guidelines-update-2_v5-1-indd.pdf (accessed 28 January 2023).

Collins, T. (2022) Migraine headache in adults. *BMJ Best Practice*. Available at: https://bestpractice.bmj.com/topics/en-gb/10 (accessed 28 January 2023).

Cortes Rivera, M., Mastronardi, C., Silva-Aldana, C.T. et al. (2019) Myalgic encephalomyelitis/chronic fatigue syndrome: A comprehensive review. *Diagnostics (Basel, Switzerland)* 9(3): 91.

Dowson, A. (2015) The burden of headache: Global and regional prevalence of headache and its impact. *The International Journal of Clinical Practice* 69(182): 3–7.

Gazzaniga, M., Ivry, R. and Mangun, G. (2009) *Cognitive Neuroscience: The Biology of the Mind*. New York: W.W. Norton & Company.

Ghasemi, N., Razavi, S. and Nikzad, E. (2017) Multiple sclerosis: Pathogenesis, symptoms, diagnoses and cell-based therapy. *Cell Journal* 19(1): 1–10.

Gray, J. and Gavin, C. (2005) The ABC of community emergency care. Assessment and management of neurological problems. *Emergency Medicine Journal* 22: 440–445.

Khare, S. and Seth, D. (2015) Lhermitte's sign: The current status. *Annals of Indian Academy of Neurology* 18(2): 154–156.

Lowth, M. (2020) Abnormal gait. Available at: https://patient.info/doctor/abnormal-gait#:~:text=Gait%20in%20cerebellar%20disease&text=There%20may%20be%20associated%20cerebellar,also%20arise%20from%20multiple%20sclerosis (accessed 28 January 2023).

Medicines and Healthcare products Regulatory Agency (MHRA) (2017) *Antiepileptic drugs: Updated Advice on Switching between Different Manufacturers' Products*. London: Medicines and Healthcare products Regulatory Agency.

Mukhtyar, C. (2018) Giant cell arteritis. *BMJ Best Practice*. Available at: https://bestpractice.bmj.com/topics/en-gb/177 (accessed 28 January 2023).

National Institute of Health and Care Excellence (NICE) (2018) Clinical Knowledge Summaries: Dementia: Assessment, management and support for people living with dementia and their carers. Available at: https://cks.nice.org.uk/topics/dementia/management/suspected-dementia/ (accessed 28 January 2023).

National Institute of Health and Care Excellence (NICE) (2019) Clinical Knowledge Summaries: Bell's palsy. Available at: https://cks.nice.org.uk/topics/bells-palsy/ (accessed 28 January 2023).

National Institute of Health and Care Excellence (NICE) (2020) Clinical Knowledge Summaries: Giant cell arteritis. Available at: https://cks.nice.org.uk/topics/giant-cell-arteritis/ (accessed 28 January 2023).

National Institute of Health and Care Excellence (NICE) (2021a) Clinical Knowledge Summaries: Epilepsy. Available at: https://cks.nice.org.uk/topics/epilepsy/ (accessed 28 January 2023).

References

National Institute of Health and Care Excellence (NICE) (2021b) Clinical Knowledge Summaries: Suspected dementia. Available at: https://cks.nice.org.uk/topics/dementia/management/suspected-dementia/ (accessed 28 January 2023).

National Institute of Health and Care Excellence (NICE) (2021c) Headaches in over 12s: Diagnosis and management [CG150]. Available at: https://www.nice.org.uk/guidance/cg150 (accessed 28 January 2023).

National Institute of Health and Care Excellence (NICE) (2021d) Myalgic encephalomyelitis (or encephalopathy)/chronic fatigue syndrome: Diagnosis and management [NG206]. Available at: https://www.nice.org.uk/guidance/ng206/chapter/Recommendations#suspecting-mecfs (accessed 28 January 2023).

National Institute of Health and Care Excellence (NICE) (2022a) Clinical Knowledge Summaries: Migraine. Available at: https://cks.nice.org.uk/topics/migraine/ (accessed 28 January 2023).

National Institute of Health and Care Excellence (NICE) (2022b) Multiple sclerosis in adults: management [NG220]. Available at: https://www.nice.org.uk/guidance/ng220 (accessed 28 January 2023).

National Institute of Health and Care Excellence (NICE) (2023) Delirium: Prevention, diagnosis and management [CG103]. Available at: https://www.nice.org.uk/guidance/cg103 (accessed 27 January 2023).

National MS Society (2017) Types of MS. Available at: https://www.mssociety.org.uk/about-ms/types-of-ms (accessed 28 January 2023).

NHS England (2016) Patient experience survey for people living with a neurological condition in England. Available at: https://www.england.nhs.uk/blog/alex-massey/ (accessed 28 January 2023).

Vasilevskis, E. and Ely, E. (2016) Chapter 226: Causes and epidemiology of agitation, confusion, and delirium in the ICU. In Webb, A., Angus, D., Finfer, S. et al. (eds) *Oxford Textbook of Critical Care*. 2nd edn. Oxford: Oxford University Press: 1073–1075.

Wang, Y., Pan, Y. and Li, H, (2020) What is brain health and why is it important? *BMJ* 371: m3683.

World Health Organization (WHO) (2022) Headache disorders. Available at: https://www.who.int/news-room/fact-sheets/detail/headache-disorders (accessed 28 January 2023).

Mental Health Presentations   6

Anita Cawley

Within This Chapter
- Acute anxiety
- Bereavement
- Depression
- Panic
- Paranoid personality disorder
- Post-natal mental health issues
- Stress
- Substance misuse
- Suicidal ideation
- Visual or auditory hallucinations
- The importance of social prescribing

Introduction

In recent years, a consensus of evidence has highlighted mental ill health to be one of the main causes of overall disease burden worldwide (Vos et al., 2013). Alarmingly, in the last decade, depression alone has been noted as the second leading cause of years lived with disability worldwide, beaten only by those living with lower back pain (Mental Health Foundation, 2016). As a presentation, mental ill health is complex, multifactorial and often poorly understood, making effective assessment and management challenging and leading to frustrations for both patients and healthcare providers. On top of this, mental health services in the UK continue to suffer from workforce sustainability issues, placing considerable strain on services to provide adequate care to this population. Sadly, this is demonstrated globally by statistics from the World Health Organization (WHO), who estimate that a staggering 35–50% of individuals in developed countries and 76–85% of those in developing areas who suffer severe mental ill health receive little to no treatment (Demyttenaere et al., 2004).

CHAPTER 6 Mental Health Presentations

Importantly, the management of mental ill health is not just concerned with prescribing medications but also with how patients can be better supported in the community by their surgery, and by third- and voluntary-sector organisations providing social prescribing initiatives. More and more frequently, this kind of joined-up approach and signposting role falls to the paramedic in primary care.

With the national shortage of GPs, NHS England (2016) has set an ambitious target to recruit an additional 5,000 'other staff', which includes mental health workers and other allied health professionals. Importantly, this NHS England (2016) report recognised the diversity of the current workforce that already includes paramedics who have the unique ability to provide patient care in any environment, without the constraints of standardised protocols. This gap requires that practitioners identify and work within their own limitations (HCPC, 2014).

Paramedics employed in primary care settings are often presented with patients experiencing a mental health crisis. Commonly, appointments will last 10–20 minutes, depending upon the requirements of the individual surgery, and within this time the clinician will need to decide whether or not the patient is at high risk of harm. If a decision is made that the patient is at high risk of harm, then they will need to be assessed by a mental health professional in a timely manner. It also might be possible to signpost these patients to another specialist mental health organisation for initial help and guidance. This task is extremely difficult and requires careful consideration.

Paramedics working in primary care settings should be confident in conducting a mental health assessment and considering any differential diagnosis, and should be competent in forming a management plan. Depending upon the policies of individual surgeries, this may need to be discussed with a senior clinician in the practice.

Assessment

Some general principles of assessment include:

- Despite time constraints, allow the patient to talk without the feeling of being hurried.
- Try and put yourself in their shoes; remain non-judgemental and empathetic.
- Try and keep an 'open', welcoming position; try and avoid typing notes as the patient speaks.

Mental Capacity Testing in Primary Care

It is not within the remit of this chapter to provide an in-depth guide for how to assess capacity, but to simply offer practical suggestions for how clinicians can carry out a safe and effective assessment within a restricted timescale, as mentioned above. It is important to note that in an ideal setting time would not be a factor, but the reality is that paramedics are increasingly placed under pressure to see, treat and manage

Assessment

patients within the 10–20-minute allocated slot. For consultations concerning mental ill health, this will need to include evaluation of the patient's ability to consent to treatment, application of the relevant legislation and engagement of the patient in shared decisions with regards to their care. Relevant legislation exists across the United Kingdom (UK) to protect and empower people who lack the capacity to make their own decisions about their care and treatment (Mughal, 2014). Mental capacity should always be presumed until proven otherwise and every adult has a right to make his or her own decisions, even if these are considered to be unwise.

> Mental Capacity Act (England and Wales) 2005
> Mental Capacity Act (Northern Ireland) 2016
> Adults with Incapacity (Scotland) Act 2000
> The underpinning legislation utilised to assess mental capacity is determined by which nation the paramedic is working in.

Patients experiencing mental health problems often appreciate continuity in their care; however, in the realities of practice this is not always possible. Due to the nature of the presentation, patients often present in crisis to 'on-the-day' clinics and are therefore more likely to see different practitioners. Once a treatment plan is in place, it is advisable to book a follow-up appointment with their own doctor or mental health practitioner. This supports the development of a good therapeutic relationship that may offer some continuity. Follow-up appointments are vital to ensure patient improvement and to monitor any noticeable declines and medication adherence, whilst also providing positive support and encouragement (NICE, 2011b).

Mental State Examination

The Mental State Examination (MSE) requires highly developed observation skills and provides the clinician with a really good idea of the patient's psychological state at that moment in time. The key components of this examination are appearance, attitude, behaviour, mood, affect, speech, thought process, thought content, perception, cognition, insight, and judgement.

The MSE allows you to obtain a cross-sectional description of the patient's mental state, which when combined with the general medical history, enables a holistic picture of the patient's concerns. This is a rapid assessment which collects both objective and subjective information and facilitates overall decision making (Murray et al., 1997).

CHAPTER 6   Mental Health Presentations

Clinical Assessment Tools

GAD Score

The GAD score is a self-administered patient questionnaire, used as a screening tool and severity measure for generalised anxiety disorder (GAD) – from which it gets its name.

Over the past two weeks, how often have you been bothered by any of the following problems? Please circle your answers.

GAD-7	Not at all	Several days	More half the days	Nearly every day
1. Feeling nervous, anxious or on edge	0	1	2	3
2. Not being able to stop or control worrying	0	1	2	3
3. Worrying too much about different things	0	1	2	3
4. Trouble relaxing	0	1	2	3
5. Being so restless that it's hard to sit still	0	1	2	3
6. Becoming easily annoyed or irritable	0	1	2	3
7. Feeling afraid as if something awful might happen	0	1	2	3
Add the score for each column				

Total score (add your column scores):

If you checked off any problems, how difficult have these made it for you to do your work, take care of things at home or get along with other people? (Circle one)

Not difficult at all   Somewhat difficult   Very difficult   Extremely difficult

PHQ-9

This is a self-administered patient questionnaire which is used to monitor the severity of depression and response to treatment.

Over the past two weeks, how often have you been bothered by any of the following problems? Please circle your answers.

PHQ-9	Not at all	Several days	More than half the days	Nearly every day
1. Little interest or pleasure in doing things	0	1	2	3
2. Feeling down, depressed or hopeless	0	1	2	3
3. Trouble falling or staying asleep or sleeping too much	0	1	2	3
4. Feeling tired or having little energy	0	1	2	3
5. Poor appetite or overeating	0	1	2	3
6. Feeling bad about yourself or that you are a failure or have let yourself or your family down	0	1	2	3

7. Trouble concentrating on things, such as reading the newspaper or watching television	0	1	2	3
8. Moving or speaking so slowly that other people could have noticed. Or the opposite, being so fidgety or restless that you have been moving around a lot more than usual	0	1	2	3
9. Thoughts that you would be better off dead or of hurting yourself in some way	0	1	2	3
Add the score for each column				

Total score (add your column scores):

If you checked off any problems, how difficult have these made it for you to do your work, take care of things at home or get along with other people? (Circle one)

Not difficult at all   Somewhat difficult   Very difficult   Extremely difficult

SAD PERSONS

The SAD PERSONS scale is based on ten of the major risk factors for suicide (Patterson et al., 1983). It was developed initially as a clinical assessment tool for medical professionals and, although it has sensitivity, it is considered to be of low clinical value. Therefore, it should be used as an aid as opposed to a decision-making tool. The score is calculated out of ten, with yes/no questions all achieving one point for a positive response.

- S: Sex = male
- A: Age < 19 or > 45 years
- D: Depression
- P: Previous attempt
- E: Excess alcohol or substance use
- R: Rational thinking loss
- S: Social support lacking
- O: Organised plan
- N: No spouse
- S: Sickness

The score is then calculated as follows:

- 0–4: Low
- 5–6: Medium
- 7–10: High.

Although these assessment tools might be useful to help structure or encourage a wider discussion of a person's needs, they should not be used in isolation to decide who should receive further treatment or support — or who is most at risk. This is because risk assessment tools do not accurately predict future risk of self-harm or suicide. Research studies have

CHAPTER 6   Mental Health Presentations

shown that tools are only accurate in their assessment of future risk in about 5% of cases, which mean that risk assessment tools fail to predict future risk 95% of the time.

In summary, the NICE guidelines (2022b) on the management of self-harm state that:

- Risk assessment tools and scales should not be used to predict future suicide or risk of future self-harm.
- Risk assessment tools and scales should not be used to determine who should and should not be offered treatment and who should be discharged.
- Risk assessment tools may, however, be considered to help structure, prompt, or add detail to a broader assessment.

Presentations in Primary Care

Acute Anxiety

Aetiology

In 2013, 8.2 million people in the UK suffered with anxiety-related health illnesses, with women being twice as likely to be affected (Fineberg et al., 2013).

History and Examination

In considering a diagnosis of anxiety for any patient, attention should be given to their history and symptoms. Anxiety can present in many ways, often with the patient presenting on multiple occasions with differing symptoms.

Symptoms can include:

- Abdominal pain
- Constant worrying
- Nausea
- Palpitations
- Restlessness
- Sleep deprivation
- Tachycardia
- Tachypnoea.

Symptoms can also be subtle or be masked by a 'physical' co-existing illness, and patients with long-term conditions may also have underlying psychosocial issues.

> Whereas anxiety manifests as feelings of helplessness, depression is associated with hopelessness, involving low mood, social isolation and lack of motivation. Both can lead to suicidal ideation. It is therefore imperative that the clinician is able to recognise this and reduce the risks of the patient coming to harm.

There are numerous 'toolkits' available to assist decision making for common mental health presentations. The GAD-2 scale concentrates on the patients' feelings and their ability to control them and is considered the most appropriate scoring tool (NICE, 2020b).

Management

With symptoms of anxiety, it is very common for patients to attend the surgery frequently and patients will sometimes feel that medication is the answer. In some cases this is true, but some medications come with adverse side effects which can often exacerbate the problem.

> Self-help measures can be more effective and should always be discussed as an option. In the digital world we live in, there is a multitude of downloadable apps available to help with anxiety and many are free to use. There are also a growing number of social prescribing initiatives that can support patients who are prepared to accept self-care and support as a treatment option.

Bereavement

Aetiology

Whereas grief is the emotional and psychological reaction to any loss, which is not limited to death, bereavement is the reaction experienced to the death of a loved person (Melhem, 2011). Bereavement is one of life's major stressors, and paramedics within primary care are quite often called upon to help the bereaved.

The five stages of grief, consisting of denial, anger, bargaining, depression and acceptance, are well known. It is through this cycle that a person will grieve for their loss but is able to carry on living their life (Tonkin, 1996). For some people, the processing of feelings of grief is acute and prolonged, and they can remain in this painful state for long periods of time, which in turn can affect their daily activities and considerably affect their mental health.

History and Examination

Patients experiencing bereavement and grief may present in many different ways, and the history should be sympathetic to the presenting reasons surrounding the grief. Ascertaining the presence of the following symptoms can be a helpful way to open up conversation during the consultation:

- Anger
- Crying
- Depression or low mood
- Fear
- Frustration
- Guilt
- Pain
- Regret
- Relief
- Sadness
- Shock
- Tiredness.

CHAPTER 6 Mental Health Presentations

Management

Management of the condition will depend on the reasons underpinning the person's experience of grief.

> NICE (2016) End of life care for infants, children and young people with life-limiting conditions: Planning and management [online].
> NICE (2018a) Preventing suicide in community and custodial settings [online].
> Specific National Institute for Health and Care Excellence (NICE) guidance may provide useful information if the person is experiencing the loss of a child (NICE, 2016) or the loss of someone who has taken their own life (NICE, 2018a).

> A social prescriber link worker can be an excellent resource to assist with local community support groups for those who have been bereaved. Other sources of help and support include Cruse Bereavement Support and Mind.

Depression

Aetiology

WHO states that globally 264 million people, of all ages, suffer with depression, with major depression more commonly seen in females (Monroe et al., 2014).

History and Examination

Depression can be debilitating, with symptoms ranging from everyday sadness to suicidal ideation. Depression can present as mild, moderate or severe.

Whilst there is no defined assessment for depression, either the validated tool PHQ-9 or HAD scale (for mixed anxiety and depression screening) are often advocated (NICE, 2020b).

> Both the PHQ-9 and GAD questionnaires are completed by the patient. It is not always possible, due to time constraints, to complete these during the consultation. However, it is important to provide a copy to the patient to complete and return, and it is worth recommending to them that they sit and complete it in the waiting room so they can hand it into reception after their consultation. This will aid future consultations and it provides a good base for monitoring purposes. These tools can also be set up as templates within some ICT systems and it is worth requesting them to be added, as it can save valuable time.

Presentations in Primary Care

A descriptor of the impact of symptoms on the individual's daily life is used to differentiate between mild, moderate and severe depression. It is important to keep in mind that the causes of depression can be multi-factorial, with the involvement of social, psychological and biological causes. This is the main reason that it is vital for the clinician to take a good, structured history, especially when asking about the patient's family history of mental health. Patients who have a first-degree family member with, or prior experience of, depression are up to ten times more likely to develop depression (Goodwin and Jamison, 2007). Other recognised predictors include a recent major life event and a personal history of depressive episodes (Monroe et al., 2014).

Presentations of severe self-neglect, social withdrawal and isolation should raise your concerns, and should be explored in the examination.

Management

NICE (2022a) advocates a stepped-care model for the detection and management of depression. If prescribing anti-depressants, it is good practice to initially prescribe one month's supply and book a follow-up appointment for one week later (even if a telephone call). This is to check compliance with the medication, explore the presence of side effects and evaluate if their mood or feelings have worsened.

Panic

Aetiology

Panic disorder is part of the anxiety disorder group, and is classified as recurrent, abrupt surges of intense fear or intense discomfort which reach their peak in 10–15 minutes and can last for approximately 30–45 minutes (Carvalho and McIntyre, 2017).

> 💡 Panic disorders are differentiated from panic attacks by the frequency of episodes. A panic attack is an individual event, classically with tachypnoea, chest tightness and paraesthesia.

Panic disorder also causes the patient to continuously worry even when not having an attack, which can affect their daily life, sometimes resulting in increased contact with healthcare services.

History and Examination

Patients may present with various signs and symptoms, which may include:

- Chest pain or palpitations
- Dizziness
- Lack of focus or concentration
- Shortness of breath or rapid breathing
- Sweatiness
- Tingling sensation or light headedness
- Trembling
- Unsettled behaviour.

CHAPTER 6   Mental Health Presentations

> 💡 Since some physical conditions can mimic panic disorders, it may be prudent to undertake routine blood tests to exclude an organic or pharmacological cause.

Management

Different treatments will suit different people, and so discussion with the patient regarding the available options is paramount. Whatever is decided, the chosen treatment should be available promptly. Psychological treatment, medication and self-help have all been shown to be effective in treating panic disorder; however, studies of different treatments have found that the benefits of psychological treatment lasted the longest (NICE, 2020b).

> 📖 NICE) (2020b) Generalised anxiety disorder and panic disorder in adults: Management [online].
> This NICE clinical guideline outlines stepped care for people with panic disorder and should be followed during management of panic disorder in adults.

Paranoid Personality Disorder

Aetiology

Paranoid personality disorder (PPD) belongs with other types of personality disorders. The aetiology of personality disorders is unknown, but evidence suggests that there is a link to childhood physical, emotional or sexual abuse or emotional neglect (Cleary and Raeburn, 2019).

It is widely accepted that PPD can be split into one of three clusters:

Cluster A
Behaviour: Odd or eccentric
Disorders: Paranoid, schizoid and schizotypal personality disorders

Cluster B
Behaviour: Dramatic, erratic and emotional
Disorders: Antisocial, borderline, histrionic, narcissistic personality disorders

Cluster C
Behaviour: Avoidant, dependent
Disorders: Obsessive-compulsive personality disorders

History and Examination

Whilst each personality disorder will present with particular characteristics, a person with PPD will generally lack trust in others and be suspicious of their intentions. There would be concerns, without good reason, that they were at risk of harm. They would be hypervigilant, experience anger and jealousy, demonstrate poor hygiene and appear detached and isolated (Williams, 2013). The consultation should seek to explore the presence of these characteristics.

> It is accepted that PPD is more closely related to experiences of trauma than other mental health disorders. Therefore, a sensitive approach to questioning around social and family history, including childhood experiences, may be appropriate during the consultation (Lee, 2017).

Management
PPD is unlikely to be managed solely in primary care due to the specialist nature of the treatment required. A collaborative approach with the local mental health services is needed, to determine the appropriate treatment plan between psychological treatment and medication. If the patient presents in crisis, then an assessment needs to be undertaken to establish the level of risk to the person or to others.

Post-natal Mental Health Issues

Aetiology
The Royal College of Obstetricians and Gynaecologists (2017) reports that as many as one in five women will develop a mental illness during pregnancy or within the first year post delivery. The three main disorders are:

- Baby blues: This usually consists of mild mood changes, lasting for a few days.
- Puerperal psychosis: This usually develops within the first two weeks of giving birth. Symptoms can include hallucinations, delusions, low or manic mood, fear or suspicion, confusion or acting out of character.
- Postnatal depression: Often thought to be 'baby blues', but post-natal depression usually lasts longer than two weeks. Symptoms can include low mood, lack of energy, sleep deprivation and lack of enjoyment or interest.

History and Examination
Mental well-being should be enquired about at each appointment with the person carrying the child during pregnancy and after birth, and all paramedics should seek to ensure that such conversations are had in an open way, focusing on the dialogue of the person and their concerns.

> During the consultation, if it has not already been established, the family history (for example, whether a grandmother, mother or sister had experienced mental health problems during or after pregnancy) of the person carrying the child should be ascertained. It is also important to acknowledge and understand the impact that pregnancy and birth can have on their partner, especially if they are experiencing mental health problems, and exploring this during the consultation can ensure the appropriate supportive packages are facilitated.

CHAPTER 6 Mental Health Presentations

During this conversation, a number of key points should be considered (Royal College of Psychiatrists, 2018):

- Problems with feeding the child
- Anxiety about the health of the child
- Lack of enjoyment being with the child, or other external influences
- Changes in appetite and eating habits
- Sleeplessness (even when the child is sleeping)
- Psychotic symptoms (auditory hallucinations, unusual beliefs).

Management

In all cases, a collaborative approach is necessary between the patient, the health visitor or midwife and the primary care clinician. Information provided to the patient should be culturally relevant and only discussed with their partner or carer with their consent.

If needed, paramedics should seek more detailed advice about the possible risks of mental health problems or the benefits and harms of treatment in pregnancy and the postnatal period from a secondary mental health service (preferably a specialist perinatal mental health service). This might include advice on the risks and possible harms of taking psychotropic medication while breastfeeding or how medication might affect the patient's ability to care for their baby.

> NICE (2020a) Antenatal and postnatal mental health: Clinical management and service guidance [online].
> This outlines the clinical management of patients with antenatal and postnatal mental health issues.

Stress

Aetiology

Stress is the adverse reaction people have to excessive pressures or other types of demand placed on them (NICE, 2017). Stress occurs when the hypothalamus in the brain is triggered; it transmits signals to the pituitary gland and the adrenal medulla, both of which are part of the autonomic nervous system (ANS), which is the part of the peripheral nervous system (PNS) that maintains homeostasis. From here, the body activates its fight or flight response (Porth and Matfin, 2008). There are many causes of stress such as financial, emotional, work, personal and health, and it is the body's reaction to feeling threatened or under pressure or the feeling of being unable to cope. Stress affects people in different ways, and their individual abilities to deal with the situation also differ.

History and Examination

The history will vary from patient to patient; however, signs and symptoms may have a common theme:

- Anxiety
- Behavioural changes

Presentations in Primary Care

- Chest pains or palpitations
- Depression or low mood
- Frustration
- GI upset
- Headaches
- Increased use of alcohol or drugs
- Irritableness
- Sadness
- Sleep deprivation.

This list is not exhaustive as there may be many other symptoms that patients present with. At times, patients may experience stress over long periods of time (chronic stress), which may develop into generalised anxiety or post-traumatic stress disorder (PTSD) (Mind, 2022).

> NICE (2018b) Post-traumatic stress disorder [online].
> This guideline provides further information on PTSD.

Management

There is no definitive treatment for stress. However, paramedics may wish to actively monitor patients who present with stress, to ensure early capture of deterioration and referral to appropriate services.

> A psychologically focused debriefing is not recommended as a management or preventative option for stress.

An individual trauma-focused cognitive behaviour therapy (CBT) intervention should be offered to adults who have acute stress disorder or clinically important symptoms of PTSD. These interventions include:

- Cognitive processing therapy
- Cognitive therapy for PTSD
- Narrative exposure therapy
- Prolonged exposure therapy.

Eye movement desensitisation and reprocessing (EMDR) therapy should be offered to adults with a diagnosis of PTSD (or clinically important symptoms of PTSD) who have presented more than three months after a non-combat-related trauma.

Venlafaxine or a selective serotonin reuptake inhibitor (SSRI) such as sertraline may be considered for patients with PTSD who have a preference for drug treatment. Benzodiazepines should not be offered, to prevent deterioration of stress to chronic stress or PTSD, and antipsychotics should only be started with specialist input.

CHAPTER 6   Mental Health Presentations

Substance Misuse

Aetiology

It is estimated that one in 12 adults (aged 15–59) has a substance use disorder, equating to approximately 2.7 million individuals, with heroin and cocaine being the most problematic (NHS Digital, 2017). Alcohol-use disorders are thought to affect 4% of the people in England aged between 16 and 65, and they typically coexist with other mental health disorders (NICE, 2011a). Another consideration is that of prescription drug dependence, where patients may have initially taken the drug as treatment but have subsequently become reliant on it. This is particularly prevalent in medications such as anti-depressants, opiates, benzodiazepines and gabapentoids but in reality can be experienced with any medication.

History and Examination

This is likely to differ between dependencies but a thorough history taking is imperative. Clinicians need to ask direct questions surrounding the patient's lifestyle, including alcohol and drug usage.

ASSIST-Lite (Alcohol, Smoking and Substance Involvement Screening Tool – Lite) is a shortened version of the ASSIST screening tool which was developed for WHO by an international group of researchers. Its function is to help detect and manage substance use and related problems in healthcare settings.

> Two versions of ASSIST-Lite have been developed. One version is specifically adapted for use in mental health settings; the other is for use in all other health and social care settings. Paramedics in general practice will require this latter, general tool.

Both tools help to determine the risks with substance and alcohol use and can provide a printable report.

Management

Managing patients with substance use disorder can often be complex, with occasions where patients will need to have their medications managed by primary care physicians with a specialist interest in drugs and alcohol. Paramedics need to be mindful that patients may have a long history of substance use and may find it difficult to reduce or completely detox from the medications.

> Patients also need to be made aware of potential consequences on employment, family, driving competency and housing that may arise from substance misuse. Liaison with local social prescribing link workers may identity local groups that can help in the navigation of these issues.

Suicidal Ideation

Aetiology

It is imperative that practitioners recognise that patients suffering with depression do and will succeed in completing suicide. In 2018 alone, there were 6,507 registered suicides in the UK compared to 5,821 in 2017 (ONS, 2022). Three-quarters of this number were men and this has been a common theme since the 1990s (Fineberg et al., 2013).

History and Examination

It is challenging to assess a person's risk of suicide in primary care, especially as not all aspects of their suicidal thought can be explored fully within the timescales permitted. Nevertheless, it is essential that the practitioner adopt a system where they can uncover those patients at high risk of suicide and use this short assessment to try to prevent any adverse outcomes. Risk behaviour can change over time but common causes for changes include delirium, drugs and alcohol and disorders of the mind. When assessing risk, consideration should also be given to any previous risk behaviour, as it is highly likely that it will happen again (Flewett, 2010).

> When evaluating patients for potential suicidality, refer to the three 'Is'. Does the patient have a problem they see as intolerable (I can't stand it), interminable (It will never end) or inescapable (I cannot get away from it)? This will help guide the consultation and determine the management risks.

Scores such as SAD PERSONS (Patterson et al., 1983) can assist with building a clinical picture, although they are not deemed to have good predictive ability and should not be relied upon (Runeson et al., 2017).

Patients with active plans for suicide must be referred immediately to the local crisis team, with local police support as necessary.

Management

The appropriate use of medication is an important tool both in treating a specific psychiatric illness and in reducing excess negative feelings (sadness, anxiety or shame) that contribute to suicidal thoughts. The four primary agents used to help suicidal patients are benzodiazepines, antidepressants, antipsychotics and mood-stabilising drugs.

During the consultation, the paramedic needs to establish whether or not the patient can be safely discharged. If deemed safe to be discharged, the patient should be provided with the tools and strategies for how to deal with their current feelings. If they are not deemed to be safe and they need an emergency referral to their local mental health team, it is vital that this referral is initiated immediately.

The patient may well still be discharged from the surgery, but this needs careful consideration. The main things to consider in this scenario are:

- Is there someone who can stay with the patient?
- Is the correct telephone number on their records?
- Have they been provided with strategies that may be useful?

CHAPTER 6 Mental Health Presentations

If there is no way of safeguarding the patient, then an assessment within the emergency department may be necessary.

> These consultations are never easy, and are often uncomfortable for both the clinician and the patient. Nevertheless, the situation needs to be explored as much as is possible to ensure that the safest, most appropriate resources are accessed in a timely manner.

Visual or Auditory Hallucinations

Aetiology

Although hallucinations have been a hallmark of mental illness for centuries, they are not always pathological. Clinical aspects of visual or auditory hallucinations include schizophrenia, affective disorders, postpartum psychosis, delirium, borderline personality disorder and neurological or organic disorders (such as dementia or Parkinson's disease). Hallucinations in the general population are associated with victimisation experiences, average and below-average IQ and female sex (Chaudhury, 2010).

> Hallucination is considered a core symptom of psychosis.

A multitude of circumstances can trigger hallucinations in normal persons (as well as clinical populations). These include deprivation (food, sensory, sleep), fatigue, sleep-related states, life-threatening states, grief reaction, medications, prolonged perceptual isolation, sexual abuse, religious ritual activities and trance states.

History and Examination

When a person presents with hallucinatory experiences, the first step is to clarify whether these are:

- Illusions. These may be misrepresentations of sensory input or fantasy related, as with imaginary friends. Questions to determine this include: Can you bring them on? Do you see them and hear them as you see and hear me now?
- Intrusive thoughts or inner images. These occur in obsessions, where ego-dystonic experiences are personalised and attributed to an external source. Questions to determine this include: Are they like the voices you normally hear through your ears, or are they more like thoughts as when you are thinking about things?
- Post-traumatic flashbacks. These may be involuntary and intrusive vivid inner images or sounds from past traumatic memories.

Once the presence of hallucinations is established, the second task is to document their complexity. Simple hallucinations, such as occasionally hearing the bleeping of a hand-held radio or fleetingly seeing shadows out of the corner of one's eye, are regarded as non-clinically significant. Complex hallucinations demonstrate the inability to determine experience from reality.

Lastly, the consultation will need to determine whether hallucinations are part of psychotic states and, if not, whether there are any pointers to why this symptom is presenting at this particular time, including possible vulnerabilities and stressors in addition to other psychiatric morbidity. This assessment process is not always straightforward, and it benefits from the input of other clinicians in a multidisciplinary team.

Management

A patient presenting with hallucinations as one of their symptoms needs complete psychiatric and neurological diagnostic evaluations to reach the correct diagnosis. Treatment options typically include CBT, individual development of coping strategies and pharmacological treatment where organic psychosis is considered the main cause.

The Importance of Social Prescribing

Social prescribing and community-based support, which is part of the comprehensive model for personalised care, allows patients to have more control over their care and how it is delivered.

In relation to patients with mental ill health, the care model focuses on shared decision making with targeted and specialist interventions. Social prescribing is considered one of those interventions. After a referral from the clinician to social prescribing services, a link worker will assess the needs of the patient and can, where appropriate, refer onto appropriate services. These services can include pharmacies, multi-disciplinary teams, other allied healthcare professionals, job centres, social care services, community projects, as well as third-sector, community and voluntary organisations. It is worth checking what services are available in the local area, as some areas already have social prescribers working as part of a multi-disciplinary team within primary care practice.

Chapter Summary

In summary, managing patients in primary care that present with mental health conditions is often complex and multi-factorial. This chapter has given an overview of some of the more common presentations and aims to direct the clinician to resources that may aid in their assessment. The principles of the assessment can be applied to most presentations and provide a structured, methodical approach.

Unfortunately, nationwide demand outweighs capacity, and it is very difficult to carry out a full mental health assessment within the limited timeframe found in primary care consultations. Therefore, paramedics may find it beneficial to utilise screening tools in conjunction with available guidance to help navigate their clinical encounters in this territory.

CHAPTER 6   Mental Health Presentations

Case Study 1

You are working in your usual clinic when you see a patient registered to you that you have not met before. She is a 36-year-old female patient presenting with multiple symptoms. She was honourably discharged from the armed forces three months ago.

History

PC: She attended the surgery having booked a double appointment marked 'personal'. She explained that she needed something to 'help her sleep'.

HxPC: On further questioning, she described that for the last three or four months she had been experiencing sleep disturbance, loss of appetite, loss of interest in her hobbies, nightmares and flashbacks. She had become very angry and had been experiencing intrusive thoughts. Further discussion took place around her career in the armed forces and she detailed some of the 'horrors of war' that she had witnessed.

PMHx: Looking at her previous history, there were very few entries as she had been in the armed forces for many years.

DHx: None.

SHx: Lives with partner, no children, smoker, social alcohol drinker.

FHx: Nil of note.

ROS: Alert and orientated.

There were no concerns regarding her physical health.

A – Maintaining own.
B – Normal work of breathing.
C – Good colour, pulse and BP within normal limits.

Examination

- Mental state exam.
- Appearance: Dressed appropriately for weather, well-groomed, slim appearance. Normal posture and gait.
- Behaviour: She was calm throughout the assessment, and made appropriate eye contact. She was co-operative and engaged in the conversation. She was quite fidgety.
- Cognition: Alert; GCS 15/15.
- Speech: Quietly spoken; slow, well-articulated and clear conversation.
- Mood: She appeared blunted and anxious at times, especially when discussing the tours that she was deployed on. She showed sadness throughout.
- Insight and capacity: She has capacity and has emotional awareness of her feelings.
- Thought (form and content): She reports occasional intrusive thoughts, no obvious thought blocking or thought insertion, no references were made of suicidal ideation. She does mention flashbacks and nightmares which continue to occupy her mind.
- Hallucinations and illusions: She denies any auditory or visualisations.

Preferred Diagnosis
- Suspected PTSD.

Management
- She will need a referral for specialist help – consider CBT.
- She may also benefit from medication (the British National Formulary currently recommends paroxetine or SSRIs).
- She will also need a follow-up in one month's time.

Case Study 2

You are working in your usual clinic in general practice and see a patient you have previously managed for her hypertension. She is an 88-year-old female, recently widowed after 60 years with her husband.

History

PC: She explains that she has been crying a lot, feels angry at times and can't believe her husband has died. She says that she still expects him to walk through the door. She doesn't know how to 'feel better' and would like some help.
HxPC: She explained that her husband passed away suddenly two months previously and since then she has been really struggling.
PMHx: Hypertension, hyperlipidemia.
DHx: Amlodipine, simvastatin.
SHx: Lives alone, non-smoker, no alcohol, walks unaided. Has two grown children.
Allergies: Penicillin.
ROS: Alert and orientated.

She has no physical pain.

A – Maintaining own.
B – Normal respiratory effort.
C – Good colour, pulse and BP within normal parameters.

Examination
- Mental state exam.
- Appearance: Very well-dressed, appropriate for weather. Walks unaided, albeit slowly.
- Behaviour: She was calm but very tearful throughout. Appropriate eye contact and engaged with conversation.
- Cognition: Alert; GCS 15/15.
- Speech: Normal tone and speed of speech. Clear and well-articulated.
- Mood: Feels low in mood, sad all the time.
- Insight and capacity: She understands why she feels this way, knows it is grief. She has capacity and there are no concerns regarding this.

CHAPTER 6   Mental Health Presentations

- Thought (form and content): No intrusive thoughts, no indication of suicidal ideation. There was no flight of ideas.
- Hallucinations and illusions: No visual or auditory hallucinations; she does not see anything out of the ordinary.

Preferred Diagnosis
- Grief reaction or bereavement.

Management
- Advise her to speak with her children about how she is feeling.
- Give contact numbers for Cruse Bereavement Support.
- Try and encourage her to meet friends and continue with her hobbies.
- Arrange a follow-up appointment in one month or sooner if necessary.

References

Carvalho, A. and McIntyre, R. (2017) *Mental Disorders in Primary Care: A Guide to Their Evaluation and Management*. Oxford: Oxford University Press.

Chaudhury S. (2010) Hallucinations: Clinical aspects and management. *Industrial Psychiatry Journal* 19(1): 5–12.

Cleary, M. and Raeburn, T. (2019) Personality disorders. In Evans, K., Nizette, D., O'Brien, A. et al. (eds) *Psychiatric and Mental Health Nursing in the UK*. London: Elsevier Health Sciences, pp. 323–336.

Demyttenaere, K., Bruffaerts, R., Posada-Villa, J. et al. (2004) Prevalence, severity, and unmet need for treatment of mental disorders in the World Health Organization World Mental Health Surveys. *Journal of the American Medical Association* 292(21): 2581–2590.

Fineberg, N.A., Haddad, P.M., Carpenter, L. et al. (2013) The size, burden and cost of disorders of the brain in the UK. *Journal of Psychopharmacology* 27(9): 761–770.

Flewett, T. (2010) *Clinical Risk Management: An Introductory Text for Mental Health Clinicians*. London: Elsevier.

Goodwin, F. and Jamison, K. (2007) *Manic-depressive Illness: Disorders and Recurrent Depression*. Oxford: Oxford University Press.

Health and Care Professions Council (HCPC) (2014) *Standards of Proficiency – Paramedics*. London: Health and Care Professions Council.

Lee, R. (2017) Mistrustful and misunderstood: A review of paranoid personality disorder. *Current Behavioural Neuroscience Reports* 4(2): 151–165.

Melhem, N.M. (2011) Grief in children and adolescents bereaved by sudden parental death. *Archives of General Psychiatry* 68(9): 911.

Mental Health Foundation (2016) Fundamental facts about mental health 2016. Available at: https://www.mentalhealth.org.uk/publications/fundamental-facts-about-mental-health-2016 (accessed 10 June 2022).

Mind (2022) Stress. Available at: https://www.mid.ord.uk/information-support/types-of-mentla-health-problems/stress/useful-contacts/ (accessed 10 June 2022).

References

Monroe, S.M., Slavich, G.M. and Gotlib, I.H. (2014) Life stress and family history for depression: The moderating role of past depressive episodes. *Journal of Psychiatric Research* 49: 90–95.

Mughal, A.F. (2014) Understanding and using the Mental Capacity Act. *Nursing Times* 110(21): 16–18.

Murray, R., Hill, P. and McGuffin, P. (eds) (1997) *The Essentials of Postgraduate Psychiatry*. Cambridge: Cambridge University Press.

National Institute for Health and Care Excellence (NICE) (2011a) Alcohol-use disorders: Diagnosis, assessment and management of harmful drinking and alcohol dependence [CG115]. Available at: https://www.nice.org.uk/guidance/cg115 (accessed 28 January 2023).

National Institute for Health and Care Excellence (NICE) (2011b) Common mental health disorders: Identification and pathways to care [CG123]. Available at: https://www.nice.org.uk/guidance/cg123 (accessed 30 January 2023).

National Institute for Health and Care Excellence (NICE) (2016) End of life care for infants, children and young people with life-limiting conditions: Planning and management [NG61]. Available at: https://www.nice.org.uk/guidance/ng61 (accessed 30 January 2023).

National Institute for Health and Care Excellence (NICE) (2017) Healthy workplaces: Improving employee mental and physical health and wellbeing [QS147]. Available at: https://www.nice.org.uk/guidance/qs147/chapter/quality-statement-3-identifying-and-managing-stress (accessed 30 January 2023).

National Institute for Health and Care Excellence (NICE) (2018a) Preventing suicide in community and custodial settings [NG105]. Available at: https://www.nice.org.uk/guidance/ng105 (accessed 30 January 2023).

National Institute for Health and Care Excellence (NICE) (2018b) Post-traumatic stress disorder [NG116]. Available at : https://www.nice.org.uk/guidance/ng116 (accessed 30 January 2023).

National Institute for Health and Care Excellence (NICE) (2020a) Antenatal and postnatal mental health: Clinical management and service guidance [CG192]. Available at: https://www.nice.org.uk/guidance/cg192 (accessed 30 January 2023).

National Institute for Health and Care Excellence (NICE) (2020b) Generalised anxiety disorder and panic disorder in adults: Management [CG113]. Available at: https://www.nice.org.uk/guidance/cg113 (accessed 30 January 2023).

National Institute for Health and Care Excellence (NICE) (2022a) Depressions in adults: treatment and management [NG222]. Available at: https://www.nice.org.uk/guidance/ng222 (accessed 28 January 2023).

National Institute for Health and Care Excellence (NICE) (2022b) Self-harm: assessment, management and preventing recurrent [NG225]. Available at: https://www.nice.org.uk/guidance/ng225 (accessed 22 February 2023).

NHS Digital (2017) Statistics on drugs misuse: England, 2017. Available at: https://digital.nhs.uk/data-and-information/publications/statistical/statistics-on-drug-misuse/2017 (accessed 30 January 2023).

NHS England (2016) The five year forward view for mental health. The Mental Health Taskforce. Available at: https://assets.publishing.service.gov.uk/government/uploads/system/uploads/attachment_data/file/582120/FYFV_mental_health__government_response.pdf (accessed 30 January 2023).

Office of National Statistics (ONS) (2022) Suicides in England and Wales. Available at: https://www.ons.gov.uk/peoplepopulationandcommunity/birthsdeathsandmarriages/deaths/bulletins/suicidesintheunitedkingdom/2021registrations (accessed 30 January 2023).

Patterson, W.M., Dohn, H.H., Bird, J. et al. (1983) Evaluation of suicidal patients: The SAD PERSONS scale. *Psychosomatics* 9(2).

CHAPTER 6 Mental Health Presentations

Porth, C. and Matfin, G (2008) *Pathophysiology: Concepts of Altered Health States*. 8th edn. Philadelphia: Lippincott Williams and Wilkins.

Royal College of Obstetricians and Gynaecologists (2017) Maternal mental health – Women's voices. Available at: https://www.rcog.org.uk/for-the-public/rcog-engagement-listening-to-patients/maternal-mental-health-womens-voices/ (accessed 30 January 2023).

Royal College of Psychiatrists (2018) Postnatal depression. Available at: https://www.rcpsych.ac.uk/mental-health/problems-disorders/post-natal-depression (accessed 30 January 2023).

Runeson, B., Odeberg, J., Pettersson, A. et al. (2017) Instruments for the assessment of suicide risk: A systematic review evaluating the certainty of the evidence. *PloS One* 12(7): e0180292.

Tonkin, L. (1996) Growing around grief – Another way of looking at grief and recovery. *Bereavement Care* 15(1): 10.

Vos, T., Barber, R.M., Bell, B. et al. (2013) Global, regional, and national incidence, prevalence, and years lived with disability for 301 acute and chronic diseases and injuries in 188 countries, 1990–2013: A systematic analysis for the Global Burden of Disease study. *The Lancet* 386(9995): 743–800.

Williams (2013) *Assessment Made Incredibly Easy!* Philadelphia, PA: Wolters Kluwer Health/Lippincott Williams & Wilkins.

Legislation

Adults with Incapacity Act (Scotland) 2000.
Mental Capacity Act (England and Wales) 2005.
Mental Capacity Act (Northern Ireland) 2016.

Eyes, Ears, Nose and Throat Presentations

7

Ajay Bhatt and Georgette Eaton

Within This Chapter

Eyes
- Acute loss of vision
- Disorders of the eyelids
- Eye discharge
- Red eye

Ears
- Earache (otalgia)
  - Otitis externa
  - Otitis media
- Cholesteatoma
- Hearing loss
- Vertigo (dizziness)

Nose
- Epistaxis
- Nasal obstruction
- Rhinitis
- Sinus pain

Throat
- Neck swelling
  - Mumps
  - Sore throat
- Snoring
- Voice changes

Mouth
- Dental abscess
- Mouth pain
- Oral cancer

Introduction

Whilst eye complaints account for 5% of primary care consultations (Kilduff and Lois, 2016), ear, nose and throat problems make up a further 10% (Mohamed et al., 2019), most of which can be managed effectively in primary care, with a small percentage of cases requiring referral to secondary care. A good understanding of the interrelated anatomy of these systems is crucial in the exploration of presenting complaints.

Assessment

> 💡 A systematic approach to eye, ear, nose and throat (EENT) examination will ensure a thorough consultation for the patient presenting with an EENT problem.

CHAPTER 7   Eyes, Ears, Nose and Throat Presentations

Eye

It is essential to adopt a systematic approach for the examination of the eye, and a thorough examination should be undertaken in all people who present with an eye problem. This should include:

- Visual acuity (distance: Snellen chart; near: fine-print reading)
- Visual fields
- Inspection of the external eye
- Pupillary reflexes (direct pupillary reflex; consensual pupillary reflex; swinging light test; accommodation reflex)
- Eye movements
- Fundoscopy.

> Normally, light shone into either eye should constrict both pupils equally (due to the dual efferent pathways). When the afferent limb in one of the optic nerves is damaged, partially or completely, both pupils will constrict less when light is shone into the affected eye, compared to the healthy eye. Therefore, the pupils appear to relatively dilate when swinging the torch from the healthy to the affected eye, and this is called a relative afferent pupillary defect (RAPD).

Ear

The pinna and post-auricular region should be examined for erythema or swelling.

An auroscope is used to examine the external ear canal whilst the pinna is pulled backwards and slightly upwards in order to straighten the ear canal. Inspection of the canal should account for ward, discharge or foreign bodies. The tympanic membrane should always be seen with a light reflex anteroinferiorly, with a milky white appearance.

Rinne Test

Normally, a tuning fork at 512 Hz will be heard as louder if next to the ear (air conduction) than if placed on the mastoid bone (bone conduction). This is Rinne positive. If the tuning fork is perceived as louder when placed on the mastoid (bone conduction), then a defect in the conducting mechanism of the external or middle ear is present. This is Rinne negative.

Weber Test

A tuning fork placed on the forehead should be perceived symmetrically by the patient with normal hearing (or indeed with symmetrical hearing loss). A patient with unilateral conductive hearing loss will hear the sound loudest in the affected ear, whereas a patient with unilateral sensorineural hearing loss will report the sound to be loudest in the unaffected ear.

Neurological Examination

Following a normal neurological examination (as outlined in Chapter 5 – Neurological Presentations in Primary Care, pp. 96–98), a head impulse, nystagmus and test of skew (HINTS) examination will assist in the assessment and diagnosis of patients with a presenting complaint of dizziness.

Head-impulse Test

Gently move the patient's head side to side, making sure the neck muscles are relaxed. Then ask the patient to keep looking at your nose whilst you turn their head left and right. Then turn the patient's head 10–20° to each side rapidly and then back to the midpoint. In a positive test, patients will have difficulty fixating on the clinician's nose. The eyes will move with the head, then saccade rapidly back to the point of fixation on the clinician's nose (a 'corrective saccade').

Nystagmus

To assess nystagmus, observe the patient's primary gaze while they look straight ahead, then ask the patient to look to the left and to the right without fixating on any object. Unidirectional nystagmus will indicate a peripheral cause of dizziness. However, where nystagmus changes direction or is vertical, this is associated with central pathologies. Any bidirectional nystagmus is highly specific for stroke.

Test of Skew

Ask the patient to look at your nose and subsequently cover one of their eyes. Then, quickly, move your hand to cover the patient's other eye. During this process, observe the uncovered eye for any vertical or diagonal corrective movement. Repeat this manoeuvre on the other eye. Any abnormal movement observed here, often associated with vertical diplopia, is highly specific for a central cause of vertigo.

Nose

The anterior part of the nose can be examined using a nasal speculum and light source. Examination of the nasal cavity and postnasal space requires an endoscope, which is traditionally out of the scope of primary care assessment.

Throat

Good illumination of the throat is essential for examination. Inspection should review the teeth, gums, tongue, floor of mouth, tonsils, soft palate and uvula. Inspection of the pharynx and larynx can only be undertaken with a laryngeal mirror or flexible nasendoscope, which are typically not found in general practice.

CHAPTER 7   Eyes, Ears, Nose and Throat Presentations

Examination of the Neck for Lymph Nodes

A systematic examination of the lymph nodes will start under the chin (submental lymph nodes) then move posteriorly, palpating beneath the mandible (submandibular). From here, turn upwards at the angle of the mandible (tonsillar and parotid lymph nodes) and feel in front of (preauricular lymph nodes) and behind the ears (posterior auricular lymph nodes). Moving down the neck, follow the anterior border of the sternocleidomastoid muscle (anterior cervical chain) down to the clavicle, then palpate up behind the posterior border of the sternocleidomastoid (posterior cervical chain) to the mastoid process.

Then, move to the back of the head to palpate over the occipital protuberance (occipital lymph nodes), before moving to palpate behind the posterior border of the clavicle in the supraclavicular fossa (supraclavicular and infraclavicular lymph nodes) with the patient's head tilted with their ear towards their shoulder, moving each side in turn.

> 💡 Avoid playing the lymph nodes like a piano – use the pads of your second, third or fourth fingers to press the lymph node, and roll it over the surrounding tissue.

Presentations in Primary Care

Eyes

Acute Loss of Vision

Aetiology

Every patient with an unexplained sudden loss of vision requires an ophthalmic referral. Loss of vision can be associated with a variety of underlying aetiologies, with the common causes outlined in Table 7.1.

Table 7.1   Causes of Loss of Vision

Painful loss of vision	Painless loss of vision
Acute angle-closure glaucoma	Cataract
Giant cell arteritis	Open angle glaucoma
Optic neuritis	Retinal detachment
Uveitis	Central retinal vein occlusion
Scleritis	Central retinal artery occlusion
Keratitis	Diabetic retinopathy
Shingles	Vitreous haemorrhage
Orbital cellulitis	Posterior uveitis
Trauma	Age-related macular degeneration
	Optic nerve compression
	Cerebral vascular disease

Presentations in Primary Care

In some cases, visual disturbances (such as blurred vision, diplopia, flashing lights, floaters) may precipitate visual loss. It is important to differentiate eye floaters (tiny spots or specks) from other visual disturbances.

Floaters that drift aimlessly around the field of vision are benign and are caused when part of the vitreous gel becomes loose, leaving the tiny piece of debris floating across the eye. These are more pronounced when gazing at a computer screen or light-coloured background, as shadows from these floaters are cast on the retina as light passes through the eye.

However, a shower of floaters, associated with a flash of light, indicates a posterior vitreous detachment (PVD), where the vitreous membrane separates from the retina. Whilst this in isolation does not require treatment, there is a risk of retina tear or detachment associated with PVD and reports of visual disturbances should have a low threshold for specialist ophthalmic review.

History and Examination

An initial history and examination approach for sudden or rapidly progressive visual loss is summarised in Figure 7.1.

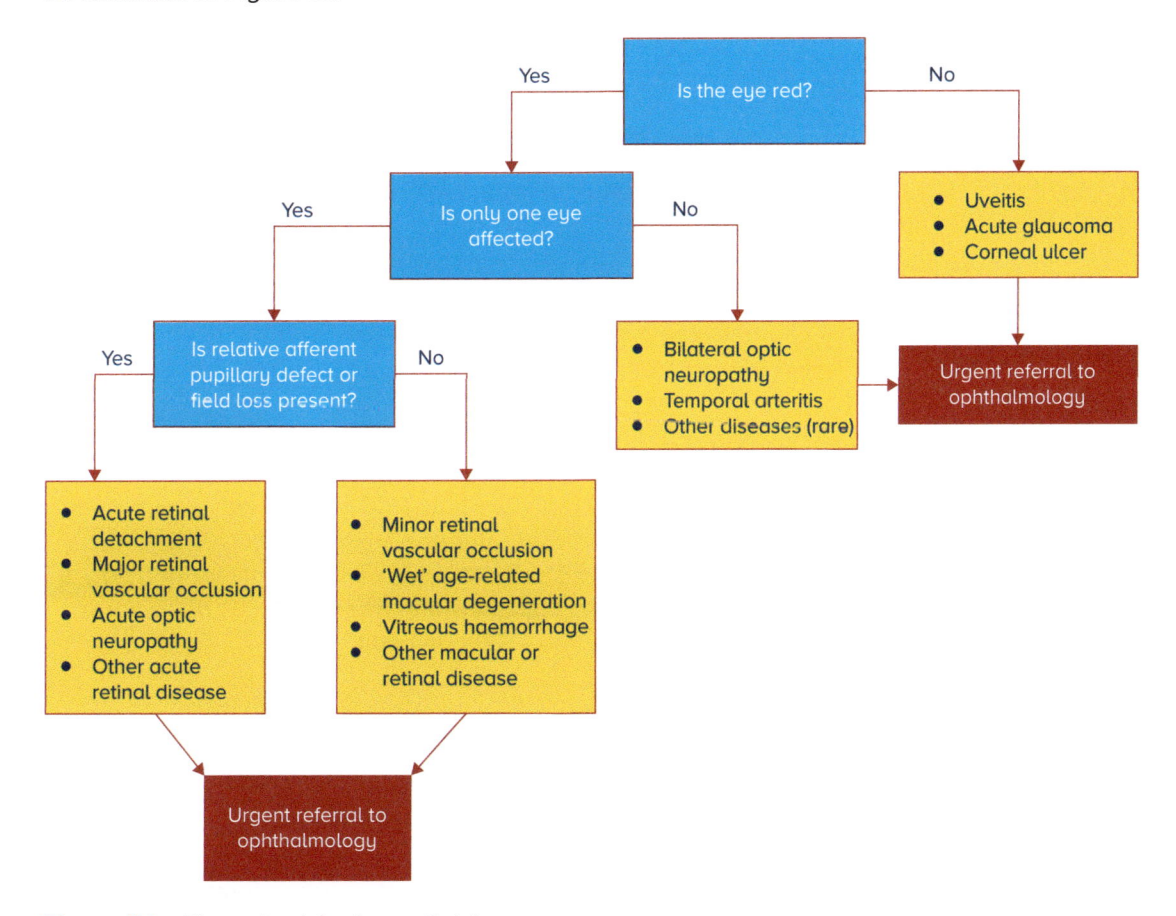

Figure 7.1 Flow chart for loss of vision.
Source: Adapted from Pane and Simcock (2005).

CHAPTER 7 Eyes, Ears, Nose and Throat Presentations

Disorders of the Eyelids

Aetiology

The eyelids provide protection to the eyes and help distribute tear film over the front surface of the globe.

History and Examination

The main disorders of the eyelids are:

- Blepharitis: Inflammation of the lid margins will involve the lashes and lash follicles, which can result in both styes and blockage of the meibomian gland, leading to a chalazion
- Dacryocystitis: Inflammation of the lacrimal sac that results in a painful lump to the side of the nose, adjacent to the lower lid
- Entropion: The lid margin rolling inward, so the lashes are against the globe and effectively act as a foreign body, causing irritation and red eye that can mimic conjunctivitis
- Ectroprion: The lid margin rolling outwards, so it is not opposed to the globe, preventing drainage of tears and resulting in a watery eye
- Trichiasis: Misdirection of the eyelashes towards the cornea.

Management

Symptoms can usually be controlled with self-care measures such as eyelid hygiene and warm compresses, as this prevents bacterial infection and the need for antimicrobials. Topical antibiotics may be considered if eyelid hygiene measures are ineffective. Ectropion can cause keratopathy and entropian and trichiasis can cause corneal irritation and abrasion, and if the paramedic has concern regarding these then routine referral to ophthalmology is required.

Eye Discharge

Aetiology

The most common cause of red eye and eye discharge is inflammation of the conjunctiva, which can arise from a number of viral, bacterial and allergic causes. Of these, bacterial conjunctivitis is the most uncommon, making up 5% of all cases of conjunctivitis, and can be attributed to organisms such as *Haemophilus influenza* and *Streptococcus pneumonia*. Table 7.2 outlines the different clinical features associated with different aetiologies on conjunctivitis (NICE, 2022a; 2022b).

> Urgent opthalmalogical referal is required for conjunctivits that presents with:
> - Reduced visual acuity
> - Marked eye pain, headache or photophobia
> - Copious rapidly progressive discharge
> - Red sticky eye in a neonate
> - Soft contact lens use with corneal symptoms.

Table 7.2 Clinical Features of Conjunctivitis

Types of conjunctivitis	Clinical features
Bacterial conjunctivitis	- Purulent or mucopurulent discharge with crusting of the lids, stuck together on waking - Itching (mild) - Pre-auricular lymphadenopathy
Viral conjunctivitis	- Mild to moderate erythema of the palpebral or bulbar conjunctiva, follicles on eyelid eversion and lid oedema - Petechial subconjunctival haemorrhage - Watery discharge - Itching (mild to moderate) - Pre-auricular lymphadenopathy - Associated respiratory tract infection
Allergic conjunctivitis	- Watery or mucoid discharge - Conjunctival redness - Eyelid oedema - Periorbital oedema in severe cases
Contact lens associated	- Inflammation of the superior conjunctiva
Herpes virus	- Herpes simplex typically presents with unilateral red eye with vesicular lesions visible on the eyelid and watery discharge - Ocular involvement in herpes zoster infection should be assumed if lesions are present at the nose tip (Hutchison's sign)
Sexually transmitted infection	- More severe, and associated with prolonged mucopurulent discharge - Chlamydia presents with a longer (> 2/52) low-grade irritation and mucous discharge in a sexually active person. Pre-auricular lymphadenopathy may be present - Gonorrhoea presents rapidly over 24 hours with copious mucopurulent discharge, eyelid swelling and tender preauricular lymphadenopathy
Ophthalmia neonatorum (ON) (a conjunctival infection within the first 28 days of life)	- Chlamydial ON: Watery or mucopurulent discharge 5–14 days post birth - Gonococcal ON: Copious purulent discharge and eyelid swelling, usually first five days post birth - Viral (usually due to adenovirus or herpes simplex) ON: Petechial or subconjunctival haemorrhages and lymphadenopathy

CHAPTER 7   Eyes, Ears, Nose and Throat Presentations

History and Examination

Common features regardless of the pathological cause include watering and discharge, discomfort described as a 'grittiness' or 'burning' and conjunctival erythema. In general, visual acuity is unaffected, and bacterial conjunctivitis should be suspected when a purulent discharge is present. Chronic conjunctivitis is associated with mild conjunctival injection and a scant purulent discharge.

Management

Most cases of bacterial conjunctivitis resolve within seven days without treatment, and topic antibiotics should be reserved for patients with severe symptoms that require rapid resolution.

Viral conjunctivitis is self-limiting in most cases, and adhering to a regime of regular eye baths, strict hand hygiene and keeping separate towels within the household will be enough to ensure symptoms resolve within one to two weeks. Artificial tears may enable more comfort.

Allergic conjunctivitis is managed in a similar way to viral presentations, plus the avoidance of allergens which may have contributed to the symptoms. If pharmacological measures are required, topical antihistamines can be prescribed.

> 💡 For all types of conjunctivitis, contact lens wearing should be avoided until the symptoms have fully resolved or the treatment (where needed) is completed.

Red Eye

Aetiology

There is a wide differential diagnosis for red eye, each with different underlying aetiological mechanisms.

> 📖 NICE (2021c) Clinical Knowledge Summaries: Management of red eye [online].
> This NICE resource offers a thorough overview of this subject.

History and Examination

The history and examination needs to identify the underlying cause, as well as exclude red flags for any underlying serious conditions. Table 7.3 outlines the common causes of acute red eye, and their corresponding features (NICE, 2021c).

Table 7.3 Common Causes of Acute Red Eye

Cause	Conjunctival injection	Pain	Photophobia	Pupil	Unilateral or bilateral	Vision
Acute glaucoma	Ciliary pattern	Severe	Mild	Mid-dilated	Unilateral	Reduced
Anterior uveitis	Circumcorneal	Moderate	Yes	Constricted	Unilateral	Reduced
Conjunctivitis	Diffuse (conjunctival)	Gritty	No	Normal	Bilateral (unilateral initially)	Normal
Corneal abrasion	Pericorneal	Foreign body sensation	No	Normal	Unilateral	Normal
Corneal ulcer	Mixed	Foreign body sensation	Yes	Normal	Unilateral	Blurred
Episcleritis	Ciliary pattern	Mild	No	Normal	Unilateral or bilateral	Normal
Keratitis	Ciliary pattern	Gritty	Yes	Normal	Unilateral	Reduced
Scleritis	Ciliary pattern	Severe	Yes	Abnormal reactions	Unilateral	Reduced
Subconjunctival haemorrhage	Well-demarcated haemorrhage	None	No	Normal	Unilateral	None

CHAPTER 7 Eyes, Ears, Nose and Throat Presentations

> Indications of a serious and potentially sight-threatening cause of the person's red eye include:
> - Reduced visual acuity
> - Deep pain within the eye
> - Unilateral red eye
> - Contact lens use
> - Photophobia
> - Ciliary injection
> - Unequal or mishappen pupils, abnormal
> - Ophthalmia neonatorum.

Management

For patients with serious and potentially sight-threatening causes of red eye, or if the diagnosis is unclear following clinical assessment, immediate referral to ophthalmology is warranted.

Whilst it appears nasty, subconjunctival haemorrhage will self-resolve in two to three weeks. However, it may be worth undertaking and monitoring blood pressure in these patients, with hypertension being a common cause of this problem.

Ears
Earache

Otalgia, also known as earache or ear pain, can be divided into two areas: primary otalgia, where the pain originates from within the ear; and secondary otalgia, where the pain originates from a different source but is felt in the ear.

Aetiology

Primary otalgia may include:

- Otitis externa (infection of the outer ear)
- Otitis media (infection inside the ear)
- Mastoiditis
- Eustachian tube dysfunction
- Tumours (see section on Cancer)
- Hearing loss (tinnitus)
- Dizziness/vertigo.

Secondary otalgia can be difficult to determine due to the complex nature of the nervous system, and may include:

- Dental pain and dental abscess
- Temporomandibular joint dysfunction (TMJ)

Presentations in Primary Care

- Sinusitis
- Cervical spine arteritis
- Neck and throat problems.

History and Examination

Consider predisposing factors when gathering a history, such as a specific incident that the patient can attribute the current concern to (for example, recent water submersion or blocked ears due to wax). Ascertaining the presence of corresponding elements will guide the examination approach. These may be:

- Pain
- Fever
- Hearing loss
- Discharge from the ear
- Previous auricular history.

Examination includes a visual comparison of both ears:

- The external ear anterior and posterior aspects, pinna, helix, tragus, lobule for erythema and swelling
- Using an otoscope, inspect the canal for inflammation, foreign bodies, discharge and swelling
- Tympanic membrane (TM) – colour, dullness, bulging, retraction, fluid level and perforation (compacted wax may prevent a view of TM).

Followed by a light palpation of the external ear – starting away from the primary focus of pain, feel for temperature, swelling, fluid, lumps and deformity.
Lymph nodes of the head and neck should also be palpated, noting any that are enlarged and tender.

Management

Management of earache should begin with treating the underlying causes. Treating the symptom of earache may involve analgesia or over-the-counter eardrops. If no obvious cause is found, consider reviewing the patient in a few days. If the pain continues and no clear cause can be found, consider rereferral to ear, nose and throat (ENT).

Otitis Externa

Aetiology

Otitis externa is an inflammatory condition of the external ear including the auricle, auditory canal and the outer surface of the ear drum. It can be acute, chronic, diffused or local. Causes range from infection, allergies and irritants to inflammatory conditions (Cross and

CHAPTER 7 Eyes, Ears, Nose and Throat Presentations

Rimmer, 2007). Predisposing factors for the cause include trauma, foreign objects, water submersion, chemicals and eczema.

History, Examination and Management

With different degrees of otitis externa, the history and examination and subsequent management are outlined in Table 7.4.

Table 7.4 Otitis Externa: Clinical Features Present on History and Examination, and Corresponding Management

Otitis externa type	Clinical features	Management
Localised	Usually mild and self-limiting, localised erythema, non-tracking	Oral antibiotics are rarely indicated Pain: simple analgesics, warm compress Consider oral antibiotics when: • Tracking erythema around the ear and face • Systemic signs of infection (NEWS Score > 4) • Immunocompromised patients Consider swab when: • Previous treatment failed • Recurrent or chronic presentation
Acute diffused	• Fever • Tracking erythema • Regional lymphadenopathy • Discharge (serous or purulent) • Conductive hearing loss • Obscured or narrow ear canal preventing topical treatment	🚩 Consider discussion with ENT
Chronic diffused	• Itching and signs of scratches • Fungal infection – *candida* and *aspergillus* • Dermatitis – mild erythema and lichenification • Contact allergies – earplugs or hearing aids	See local guidelines for treatment of candidal dermatitis

Source: NICE (2022e).

Presentations in Primary Care

Otitis Media

Aetiology

Otitis media (OM) is most common in children, and has an incidence of 11.5% among those in their first year of life (Le Saux et al., 2016).

History and Examination

A history of reduced hearing with pain that is relieved suddenly and followed by otorrhoea is suggestive of acute otitis media; examination will reveal a normal external auditory canal, with signs of perforation of the tympanic membrane and discharge. The otorrhoea tends to be mucopurulent, and can also be blood-stained (Dannatt and Jassar, 2013).

Management

Advise that the normal duration for uncomplicated presentations is between three days and one week. Regular analgesia is advised, taking into consideration schedule, age and weight of child.

> Consider immediate referral in:
> - Severe systemic infection
> - Suspected complications, meningitis, mastoiditis, intracranial abscess, facial nerve palsy
> - Children under three months of age with a fever of 38°C.

Cholesteatoma

Aetiology

A build-up of keratin in the middle ear that can subsequently become infected and erodes through neighbouring structures (ossicular chain).

History and Examination

Patients will typically present with a light, foul-smelling discharge and hearing loss. On otoscopy, the appearances can be similar to those of otitis externa. There may be dried discharge in the external auditory canal and crusting over the attic of the tympanic membrane. The appearance of wax deep within the ear, with close proximity to the eardrum, should raise suspicion of cholesteatoma, as wax is not normally seen in this location and so inspection of the attic is crucial.

Cholesteatoma may cause patients to present with facial nerve palsies, nystagmus and/or vertigo. In a patient thought to have otitis externa that is not resolving, cholesteatoma should be considered as an alternative diagnosis (Dannatt and Jassar, 2013).

Management

Suspected cholesteatoma requires urgent assessment and ENT referral for surgical review, with the aim of removing the offending tissue.

CHAPTER 7 Eyes, Ears, Nose and Throat Presentations

Hearing Loss

Aetiology

Hearing loss is a common occurrence and can occur at any age. It can have a rapid or slow onset and can be temporary or permanent. This can be due to conductive or sensory causes, as listed in Table 7.5.

Table 7.5 Aetiology of Hearing Loss

Conductive causes of hearing loss	Aetiology	Sensory causes of hearing loss	Aetiology
Ear wax (cerumen)	Impacted ear wax	Age-related hearing loss	Presbycusis, the most common cause
Foreign body	Hearing aid end piece, cotton bud end. Children: building blocks, beads etc.	Sudden sensorial hearing loss	Sudden onset of hearing loss of 30 dB HL or more which involves three consecutive frequencies and cannot be explained as an outer or inner ear condition (can be temporary or permanent)
TM perforation	Otitis media or cotton bud trauma	Excessive noise	Temporary or permanent
Otitis externa or otitis media	See section on these (pp. 153–155)	Ménière's disease	Generally viewed as abnormal endolymph production and/or absorption causing vertigo and tinnitus
Middle-ear effusion or glue ear	Characterised by a collection of fluid within the middle ear, without signs of acute inflammation	Ototoxic exposure	Examples: gentamycin, furosemide, aspirin, quinine, cisplatin
Neoplasm	Examples: squamos cell carcinoma of the external ear or vascular glomus tumour behind the ear drum	Environmental exposure	Examples: pesticides, cigarette smoke and heavy metals like lead and mercury
Exostoses	Hard bony growths in the ear canal (associated with swimming in cold water)	Labyrinthitis	Labyrinthitis is an inner ear infection. It causes a delicate structure deep inside the ear called the labyrinth to become inflamed, affecting hearing and balance

Conductive causes of hearing loss	Aetiology	Sensory causes of hearing loss	Aetiology
Otosclerosis	Abnormal bone growth affecting the small bones in the ear (stapes)	Ménière's disease	Cause of the disease is unknown. Many factors are thought to be involved, such as increased pressure of the fluid in the endolymphatic sac; allergic factors damaging the inner ear or other unknown factors. Uncommon cause of vertigo
		Vestibular schwannoma (acoustic neuroma)	A slow-growing, benign tumour, which causes hearing loss
		Infection	Meningitis, measles, shingles and mumps

Source: NICE (2019a).

History and Examination

History taking should concentrate on whether the hearing loss is unilateral or bilateral and whether it is has had a sudden onset (over the last 72 hours), is rapidly progressive (within 90 days), slowly progressive (more than 90 days) or fluctuating. Associated features such as dizziness, headache, otorrhoea, otalgia or a sensation of pressure in the ear should be considered.

> 💡 Also consider the occupation of the patient (such as environmental exposure to noise) and the impact of the hearing loss on the ability to communicate at home, in education/work and socially.

Alongside an ear examination, Weber and Rinne tuning fork tests can help distinguish between conductive and sensorineural hearing loss, and a neurological examination can exclude focal neurology contributing to symptoms.

Management

Findings of the examination will depend on whether the patient can be treated in primary care or will need a referral to secondary care.

CHAPTER 7 Eyes, Ears, Nose and Throat Presentations

> 📖 NICE (2019a) Clinical Knowledge Summaries: Hearing loss in adults.
> This outlines when a patient should be referred or managed in primary care.

Vertigo (dizziness)

Aetiology

Dizziness is a common presentation to general practice and emergency departments, affecting 15–35% of the population, with a 12-month incidence of 3% (Neuhauser, 2016). Vertigo is a form of dizziness where there is an illusion of movement, often horizontal and rotary, and a sensation of the environment moving in relation to the patient or vice versa (Kanagalingam et al., 2005). The diagnosis may be uncertain and may have many causes, especially in older patients (Cross and Rimmer, 2007). The symptoms can often be vague, and the causes are hard to pinpoint.

> ⚠️ It is therefore important to exclude more serious causes which may be classified as pre-syncope:
> - Cardiovascular (for example, disorders reducing cerebral perfusion)
> - Neurological (for example, head injury, sudden onset head ache, stroke, TIA, increased ICP, MS)
> - Metabolic (for example, thyroid disease and diabetes)
> - Adverse drug reaction.

The three commonest causes of vertigo are:

1. Central causes of vertigo would present with:
   - Prolonged or severe vertigo
   - New onset headache of head injury
   - Cardiovascular risk factors.
2. Peripheral vertigo would present with:
   - A normal neurological exam
   - Severe nausea and vomiting
   - Hearing loss (can also be present in cerebrovascular accident (CVA) and intercranial tumours).

> 💡 Vestibular neuronitis is a disorder characterised by acute, isolated, spontaneous and prolonged vertigo of peripheral origin. Vestibular neuronitis and labyrinthitis have been used interchangeably; however, it is now acknowledged that these should be differentiated (NICE, 2017).

Presentations in Primary Care

Vestibular neuronitis is thought to be caused by an inflammation of the vestibular nerve. It often occurs after a viral infection, with no hearing loss, whereas labyrinthitis is thought to be caused by inflammation of the labyrinth, with hearing loss (NICE, 2017).

3. Benign paroxysmal positional vertigo (BPPV)

This is thought to be caused by loose calcium carbonate debris in the semi-circular canals, causing motion of the fluid of the inner ear, with causes the symptoms of vertigo (Wippermen, 2014). Symptoms may include vertigo with positional movements of the head and the feeling of being thrown backwards.

History and Examination

Vertigo is best classified by its duration:

- Short < 1 minute
- Medium < 2 hours
- Long > 1 week.

A thorough neurological examination is required to differentiate the cause of dizziness from an acute neurological event. If this is normal, a head impulse, nystagmus and test of skew (HINTS) examination will assist in determining whether vertigo is of peripheral or central origin.

Additionally, the Dix-Hallpike manoeuvre may be used, though it should only be performed by a paramedic competent in its execution.

Management

Depending on the ability to differentiate between the causes of the dizziness, two initial treatment options may be considered:

- A repositioning manoeuvre such as the Epley should be offered and Brandt-Daroff exercises considered
- Pharmacological management is not usually helpful in BPPV but can be useful in peripheral vertigo.

> Referral should be undertaken in a patient with the following (NICE, 2017):
> - Hospital admission if there is severe nausea and vomiting and inability to tolerate fluids
> - ENT referral if:
>   - Repositioning manoeuvre such as the Epley is not available in primary care.
>   - Repositioning manoeuvre such as the Epley has been performed and repeated and symptoms persists
>   - Symptoms have persisted and not resolved in four weeks
> - Neurology referral where there have been three of more episodes in which the patient has experienced symptoms.

CHAPTER 7   Eyes, Ears, Nose and Throat Presentations

Nose

Epistaxis

Aetiology

Nose bleeds are idiopathic in 80–85% of cases (Oxford Medical Education, 2014), frequently originating from Little's area (Kiesselbach's plexus) on the anterior-inferior septum. Secondary causes of epistaxis can be local or systematic, as outlined in Box 7.1.

> **BOX 7.1   Aetiology of Epistaxis**
>
> - Local
>   - Trauma (nose picking, foreign body, fracture)
>   - Iatrogenic (surgery, intranasal steroids)
>   - Neoplasm (malignancy, nasal, paranasal sinus or nasopharyngeal tumours
> - Systemic
>   - Anticoagulants; anti-platelets
>   - Haematological disorders (haemophilia, leukaemia)
>   - Osler-Weber-Rendu syndrome (familial haemorrhagic telangiectasia)
>   - Severe hypertension

History and Examination

A thorough history regarding the presenting complaint of epistaxis should not overlook from which nostril bleeding is from, the onset and duration of the bleed and the presence of a posterior drip down the back of the throat. Social history should consider the potential for cocaine use and any occupational risks of nasopharyngeal carcinoma (exposure to cotton dust, acids and caustics) (Health and Safety Executive, 2012).

Investigation

If the presentation of epistaxis is suspicious, investigation of systematic causes should be undertaken, including full blood count and clotting factors.

Management

> ⚠️ Basic first aid measures should be enough to control a majority of presentations of epistaxis, and the patient may be instructed to sit forward, pinch the soft fleshy part of their nose, apply ice on the forehead or back of the neck and spit blood into a bowl (rather than swallowing). If bleeding continues after 15–20 minutes, admission to ENT is required (NICE, 2022d).

Presentations in Primary Care

Nasal Obstruction

Aetiology

Nasal obstruction is a symptom, rather than a diagnosis. Patients suffering from nasal obstruction often present with a feeling of fullness in the nasal cavity and reduced airflow. Causes can significantly impact a patient's quality of life and can include:

- Nasal polyps (inflammation and oedema of the sinus nasal mucosa that prolapses into the nasal cavity)
- Septal haematoma (a development of a haematoma between the septal cartilage and overlying mucoperichondrium following nasal trauma)
- Foreign body.

History and Examination

A detailed history may be sufficient to obtain a diagnosis, but some examination may aid the process. The nose should be inspected to determine any bony and cartilaginous nasal deformities. Nasal airflow may be assessed in two ways:

- Occlusion of one nostril and assessing the inflow and outflow through the opposite nostril, and the second uses a metal tongue depressor, observing the misting on the metal surface and comparing the two nostrils
- 'Cottle's manoeuvre' (improvement of airflow while holding the patient's cheek, preventing the collapse of the nasal valve) can also be carried out (Mohamed et al., 2019).

Examination should also ascertain the presence of these key discreet symptom sets that relate to common presentations:

- Nasal polyps: Identified as glistening swellings which are insensate on inspection using a nasal speculum
- Septal haematoma: Commonly presents with nasal obstruction, pain, rhinorrhoea and fever, usually in the context of a nasal injury
- Foreign bodies: Usually seen in children who present with a unilateral nasal discharge. Clinical examination of the nose with a light source reveals a foreign body.

Management

Nasal polyps: Intranasal corticosteroids can help reduce the size, though if they are large and unresponsive to steroid use then ENT referral for surgery is necessary.

Septal haematoma: Urgent ENT referral is required for drainage and IV antibiotics to prevent nasal deformity and infective complications (Sanyaolu et al., 2014).

Foreign bodies: Require removal to prevent aspiration. This can be achieved through direct mechanical extraction or positive-pressure expulsion (accomplished by orally applied pressure via a parent's mouth) (Kiger et al., 2008). If removal is not achieved after two attempts, then referral to ENT is warranted.

CHAPTER 7   Eyes, Ears, Nose and Throat Presentations

Rhinitis

Aetiology

Rhinitis is defined clinically as sneezing attacks, nasal discharge or nasal blockage occurring for more than an hour on most days either for a limited time each year (seasonal or intermittent rhinitis) or throughout the whole year (perennial rhinitis) (Kumar and Clark, 2017). Allergic rhinitis is an IgE-mediated inflammatory disorder of the nose, which occurs when the nasal mucosa is exposed to allergens (Scadding et al., 2017) and results in erythema of the nasal mucosa and hypertrophy of the inferior turbinates. Typical allergens include house dust mites; grass, tree and weed pollens; moulds; animal dander (such as cat and dog hair); or occupational exposure involving latex, chlorine, flour, wood dust or laboratory animals (Lipworth et al., 2017).

History and Examination

Diagnosis rests on a history that should assess the type, frequency, persistence and severity of symptoms. Exploration to identify possible causative triggers and allergens, and any associated symptoms such as asthma, eczema or sinusitis (NICE, 2021a). Examination features inspection of the face and nose, for outward signs of congestion, such as:

- Horizontal crease across the dorsum of the nose
- Deviated or perforated nasal septum
- Depressed or widened nasal bridge
- Grey discolouration to the nasal mucosa.

In addition, a nasal intonation of the voice is indicative of congestion.

> 'Allergic shiners' are darkened eye shadows under the lower eyelids due to chronic congestion, and an outward sign of rhinitis.

Management

Allergen avoidance techniques and nasal irrigation with saline are non-pharmacological management options for allergic rhinitis. Allergen avoidance should be tailored to the specific causative agent (if known) for maximum treatment effects.

For mild–moderate intermittent or mild persistent symptoms, intranasal antihistamines are recommended as the first course of action (NICE, 2021a).

For moderate–severe persistent symptoms, a regular intranasal corticosteroid may be added to the treatment regime, with a review within four weeks to determine ongoing management.

Sinus Pain

Aetiology

Sinusitis is defined as symptomatic inflammation of the paranasal sinuses. Sinus mucosa oedema, obstruction of the sinus ostia and reduction in mucociliary action allow secretions to stagnate and give bacteria a suitable environment in which to grow, although only 2% of people with such inflammation will subsequently develop a bacterial infection and acute sinusitis (Gwaltney, 1996). Whilst likely to be a more inflammatory than infective process, chronic sinusitis has more multifactorial aetiology, involving inflammation, infection and obstruction of sinus ventilation (ENT UK and Royal College of Surgeons, 2016).

> The term 'rhinosinusitis' is considered more accurate because inflammation of the nasal cavities almost always accompanies sinusitis.

History and Examination

Acute sinusitis usually follows a respiratory infection, such as the common cold, and is defined as an increase in symptoms after five days, or persistent symptoms beyond ten days (but less than two weeks). There are slightly different presentations between adults and children (Table 7.6).

Table 7.6 Presenting Features for Acute Sinusitis

Children	Adults
- Nasal blockage (obstruction/congestion) - Discoloured nasal discharge - *with* facial pain/pressure - *and/or* cough	- Nasal blockage (obstruction/congestion) - *or* nasal discharge - *with* facial pain/pressure/headache - *and/or* reduction/loss of smell - Tenderness/swelling/redness over cheekbone or periorbital areas - Nasal intonation - Cough

Acute sinusitis refers to sinusitis that completely resolves within 12 weeks. Acute bacterial sinusitis is considered when the following are present:

- Symptoms for more than ten days
- Purulent nasal discharge with unilateral predominance
- Severe local pain with unilateral predominance
- Temperature > 38°C
- A marked deterioration after initial mild fold of the illness.

Recurrent acute sinusitis refers to four or more annual episodes of sinusitis, without persistent symptoms in the intervening periods. Chronic sinusitis refers to sinusitis that causes symptoms that last for more than 12 weeks. Uncomplicated sinusitis refers to sinusitis where inflammation does not extend beyond the paranasal sinuses and nasal cavity (NICE, 2021d).

Examination features inspection of the nasal cavity (using a nasal speculum) to determine the presence of nasal inflammation, mucosal oedema and purulent nasal discharge. The opportunity should also be used to review for other associated pathology

CHAPTER 7 Eyes, Ears, Nose and Throat Presentations

such as nasal polyps or septal deviation. Following this, palpation of the maxillofacial area can elicit swelling and tenderness.

> ⚠️ Arrange hospital admission for people with acute or chronic sinusitis and:
> - Intracranial complications, including swelling over the frontal bone, symptoms or signs of meningitis, severe frontal headache or focal neurological signs
> - Intraorbital or periorbital complications, including periorbital oedema or cellulitis, a displaced eyeball, double vision, ophthalmoplegia or newly reduced visual acuity (NICE, 2021d).

Investigations

Investigations should consider whether the person is systemically well (recording pulse rate, blood pressure and temperature). ESR or CRP can be undertaken to determine the diagnosis of acute bacterial sinusitis, though the practicality of this criterion may be limited in primary care depending on the speed of laboratory reporting.

Management of Acute Sinusitis

The management of sinusitis depends on the duration of symptoms experienced.

Symptoms for Ten Days or Less

Those with symptoms for ten days or less usually require self-care measures such as paracetamol or ibuprofen for pain or fever. There is no evidence to support the use of nasal decongestants, antihistamines, mucolytics, steam inhalation or face packs. Acute sinusitis in this time period usually resolves in two to three weeks, and a majority of patients do not need antibiotics.

Symptoms for Ten Days or More

High-dose nasal corticosteroids are advocated for 14 days for adults and children aged 12 years and over.

Antibiotics should only be considered for patients who are very unwell, with signs of systemic infection but not requiring hospital admission.

> ⚠️ Consider referral for people with acute sinusitis and:
> - A suspected allergic or immunological cause
> - Anatomic defect(s) causing obstruction
> - Comorbidities complicating management such as nasal polyps
> - Frequent recurrent episodes (more than three episodes requiring antibiotics each year)
> - Immunocompromise
> - Treatment failure after extended courses of antibiotics
> - Unusual or resistant bacteria.

Presentations in Primary Care

Management of Chronic Sinusitis

Chronic sinusitis requires a long-term management plan to avoid allergic triggers, smoking cessation and good dental hygiene. Nasal irrigation with saline solution can relieve congestions and nasal discharge.

Intranasal corticosteroids can be used for up to three months when there is an allergic cause but should involve paediatrician support when considered in children.

> Consider referral to an appropriate specialist (for example, ENT specialist or immunologist) if there are:
> - Allergic or immunological risk factors that need investigating
> - Nasal polyps (particularly in children)
> - Persistent symptoms despite compliance with three months of treatment
> - Recurrent episodes of otitis media and pneumonia in a child
> - Symptoms that significantly interfere with functioning and quality of life
> - Unilateral symptoms (consider urgent referral with suspicion of neoplasia)
> - Unusual opportunistic infections.

Throat

Neck Swelling

Aetiology

Neck lumps and bumps are common and have numerous possible causes (Table 7.7). They may arise from the skin or from structures underneath. The tendency on finding a lump is to worry that it might be cancer. Whilst this should be excluded, thankfully the vast majority of neck lumps are not cancer, particularly in children and younger adults.

History

> Important elements of the questioning within the clinical history need to be considered, focusing on:
> - Duration and onset
> - Changes in size and shape
> - Associated symptoms
>   - Hard and fixed lumps
>   - Associated otalgia, dysphagia, stridor or hoarse voice
>   - Epistaxis or unilateral nasal congestion
>   - Unexplained weight loss, night sweats, fever or rigors
>   - Cranial nerve palsies
> - Past medical and social history (smoking, alcohol, radiation exposure).

CHAPTER 7 Eyes, Ears, Nose and Throat Presentations

Table 7.7 Aetiology, Assessment and Management of Lumps in the Neck

Aetiology	Assessment	Management
Trauma: Recent fall or injury	Head, neck and range of movement	Simple analgesia
Infection: May cause lymph nodes in the neck to become inflamed	Full ENT examination. Palpate lymph nodes of the head and neck. Access for systemic infection/sepsis	One or more neck lymph nodes often enlarge in response to an upper respiratory infection, throat infection or dental infection. These nodes are soft, not tender, and typically return to normal shortly after the infection goes away
Salivary glands: They become enlarged if blocked with stones and can become infected	Inspect the mouth and look under the tongue; they are not always visible. Palpate lymph nodes of head and neck	Self-management – gentle massage, drinking plenty of water. Painful and infected glands may need to be referred to ENT if the patient is unwell
Thyroid glands: Can become enlarged, most common type is 'Goiter' (benign)	ENT assessment to rule out other causes. Thyroid function test/blood test	Depending on how big the swelling is and other symptoms, consider specialist referral

Source: NICE (2020).

Mumps

Aetiology

Mumps is an acute infectious disease caused by the paramyxovirus. It has an incubation period of 16–18 days and is most infections around one to two days before the onset of symptoms and then up to nine days after (NICE, 2018). Fifteen to twenty per cent of cases will be asymptomatic. This is particularly common in children, with over 90% of cases found in people aged 15 years or over. Nearly all people will develop lifelong immunity after being infected.

> One in three males who get mumps after puberty will experience orchitis. Just under half of those with mumps-related orchitis notice some shrinkage of their testicles, and an estimated one in ten men experience a drop in their sperm count. However, this is very rarely large enough to cause infertility.

Presentations in Primary Care

History and Examination

Questions regarding exposure to other known cases should be asked. A full ENT assessment and observations should be undertaken, and it is expected that parotitis (swollen parotid glands) will be found in 95% of symptomatic cases.

Other non-specific symptoms for mumps include:

- Fever
- Headache
- Malaise
- Muscle aches
- Loss of appetite
- Epididymo-orchtis – in patients with testes.

> During history and examination, it is crucial that the presence of mumps encephalitis (which presents with altered level of consciousness and focal neurology) and mumps meningitis (parotitis alongside symptoms of meningitis) is excluded.

Management

Mumps is self-limiting and should resolve in one to two weeks; antibiotics are not required. Children should remain off school for five days after the initial presentation of parotitis.

Advice to give the patient and parents for the management of mumps includes:

- Rest
- Drink adequate fluids
- Take paracetamol and ibuprofen for symptom relief
- Warm or cold compress can be applied to the parotoid gland
- NB: Aspirin should be avoided in children under 16.

> Mumps is a notifiable disease and in any suspicion of infection, the local Health Protection Unit (HPU) should be notified. They will arrange testing kits and surveillance.

Sore Throat

Aetiology

The causes of sore throat can be bacteria, virus, fungi, coughing, acid reflux, smoking, medication, shouting, snoring, hay fever or the environment.

History and Examination

The term 'sore throat' describes the symptom of pain at the back of the throat. They are common and usually nothing to worry about. They normally get better by themselves within a week. Most sore throats can be self-treated by gargling warm salty water (not for children), drinking plenty of water and taking simple analgesia. The aetiology, assessment and management of sore throats is outlined in Table 7.8.

CHAPTER 7 Eyes, Ears, Nose and Throat Presentations

Table 7.8 Aetiology, Assessment and Management of Sore Throats

Aetiology	Assessment	Management
Laryngitis: Inflammation of the vocal cords	Full ENT examination Palpate lymph nodes of the head and neck Assess for systemic infection and sepsis	Simple analgesia, NSAIDS and paracetamol
Viral infections: Common colds and flu	Full ENT examination Palpate lymph nodes of the head and neck Assess for systemic infection and sepsis	Keep hydrated, take paracetamol to manage symptoms. Consider OTC medication
Acute pharyngitis: Inflammation of the part of the throat behind the soft palate; it can be associated with pharyngeal exudate and cervical lymphadenopathy	Full ENT examination Palpate lymph nodes of the head and neck Assess for systemic infection and sepsis Swab	Consider antibiotics as per local guidelines for patients that have FEVER pain score (4–5) and/or CENTOR score (3–4)
Tonsilitis: Inflammation of the tonsils; can be associated with tonsillar exudate, erythema and swelling	Full ENT examination Palpate lymph nodes of the head and neck Assess for systemic infection and sepsis Swab	Consider antibiotics as per local guidelines for patients that have FEVER pain score (4–5) and/or CENTOR score (3–4)
Epiglottitis: Inflammation and swelling of the epiglottis, potential for airway compromise	Full ENT examination Palpate lymph nodes of the head and neck Assess for systemic infection and sepsis Swab	Patients with stridor, dyspnoea and respiratory distress should be treated as a medical emergency

Source: NICE (2022f).

Assessment:

- Ask about ability to swallow own saliva
- Inspect back of throat using a tongue depressor and pen torch
- Examine head and neck for raised lymph nodes
- Look for signs of acute infection
- Use FeverPAIN and CENTOR criteria.

Management

Signs of systemic infection should be considered for hospital. Antibiotics should be considered for patients with severe symptoms and if there is concern about clinical condition.

Snoring

Aetiology

Snoring occurs when there is an obstruction to the free flow of air through the passages at the back of the mouth and nose. More specifically, the area where the tongue and upper throat meet the soft palate and uvula. Snoring occurs when these come into contact with each other during breathing (General Practice Notebook, 2020).

Management

Excessive snoring may be secondary to conditions causing an encroachment on the pharynx or conditions causing nasal obstruction. Excessive snoring may be associated with sleep apnoea.

> General Practice Notebook (2020) Snoring.
> Further reading on the management of conditions associated with excessive snoring and sleep apnoea.

Voice Changes

Aetiology

Voice problems are often multifactorial. Sound is produced in the larynx by vibration of the vocal cords. Resonance occurs in the pharynx, nose and mouth; articulation uses the mouth and tongue. The vocal cords are subject to high forces and so are vulnerable to voice overuse or misuse (Knott, 2021). Whilst most voice changes can be attributed to voice overuse, serious pathology (such as cancers) must be excluded.

History and Examination

A systematic approach to assessment includes:

- Symptoms, duration and onset patterns
- Precipitating factors – recent upper respiratory tract infection, change in voice use – for example, shouting or singing
- Past medical history, especially chest, head, neck and neurological symptoms
- Social history (occupation, smoking and alcohol use)
- Associated ENT symptoms
- Presence of acid reflux.

> To assist with smoking cessation, alcohol abuse or social needs affecting health and well-being, consider engagement with a local health and well-being group or input from a social prescribing link worker.

CHAPTER 7   Eyes, Ears, Nose and Throat Presentations

Examination should assess laryngeal function, head and neck for swelling and lumps. If any signs of systemic infection are found, conduct a chest and neurological exam.

> Patients who report persistent and progressive change in voice for more than three weeks, especially in smokers and with a unilateral persistent sore throat, should be referred under 2WW criteria.

Management

Management depends on the specific cause. The first-line treatment for non-serious pathology will be:

- Voice hygiene advice
- Adequate hydration
- Avoidance of vocal strain
- Smoking cessation and alcohol reduction
- Reduction in caffeine
- Treatment of any acid reflux with a PPI.

Mouth

Dental Abscess

Aetiology

A dental abscess is a localised collection of pus in the teeth, periodontal ligament, alveolar bones or gums. This occurs as a result of bacterial infection affecting the structure around and in the tooth. There are two main types of dental abscess:

- Periapical abscess: Caused by an infection of the root canal
- Periodontal abscess: Originates in the deep periodontal pocket between the tooth and gum.

In the primary care setting, these are treated the same (Siqueira and Rocas, 2013).

History and Examination

Enquire about recent dental treatment or trauma and the presence of:

- Pain
- Facial swelling
- Fever
- Erythema
- Drooling.

Management

Within the UK, treatment is typically overseen by a dentist. However, antibiotics may be provided in systemically unwell patients or those who are immunocompromised (NICE, 2022c), though this should still have dental follow-up or involvement.

Presentations in Primary Care

Mouth Pain

Aetiology

A painful mouth can manifest in many different ways. The health of the mouth is dependent on intact oral mucosa, normal saliva production, balanced bacterial floral and intact immune system. Trauma, medication and disease can cause disruption to this delicately balanced system.

History and Examination

Enquire about dry mouth, oral pain, halitosis, change in taste, excessive salivation, difficulty chewing, difficulty swallowing, difficulty speaking and any bleeding. Be particularly vigilant in those patients with a compromised immune system and on medication that causes dry mouth.

Two common presentations associated with mouth pain are oral candida (presenting with painful mouth and a creamy white curd like plaques on mucosal surface) and mouth ulcers (round or oval white, red, yellow or grey sores in the mouth on the cheeks, lips and tongue). Inspection of the mouth should determine the presence of these.

Management

For oral thrush, topical nystatin or miconazole is the first-line treatment (NICE, 2021b).

For mouth ulcers, most are treated using mouthwash, analgesia and lozenges. Mouth ulcers lasting three weeks or more should be investigated (NHS Scotland, 2020).

Oral Cancer

Aetiology

Head and neck squamous cell carcinomas are the sixth most common cancers worldwide. They account for 2.5% of all new cancer cases and 1.9% of all cancer deaths annually. More than 90% of oral cancers (occurring in the mouth, lip and tongue) are oral squamous cell carcinoma. The incidence rate of oral cancer varies widely throughout the world, with an evident prevalence in South Asian countries. This high incidence occurs in correlation with oral cancer-associated behaviours such as alcohol and tobacco use (Ali et al., 2017). Different types of oral cancer are outlined in Table 7.9.

History and Examination

Regardless of the aetiology, common features of oral cancer which will be picked up within the history and examination are (Cancer Treatment Centers of America, 2021):

- A lump or thickening in the inside of the mouth
- A lump or thickening on the lip
- A neck mass
- A sore on the lip that does not heal
- A white or red patch on the gums, palate, tonsil or lining of the mouth
- A white or red patch on the lip
- Difficulty moving the jaw or tongue

CHAPTER 7 Eyes, Ears, Nose and Throat Presentations

- Difficulty swallowing or chewing
- Persistent lip pain or numbness
- Persistent tongue or jaw pain.

Table 7.9 Different Types of Oral Cancer

Type of cancer	Description
Squamous cell carcinoma	Accounts for 90% of oral cancer. The throat and mouth are lined with 'squamous cells', which are flat and look like fish scales on a microscopic level. Squamous cell carcinoma develops when some squamous cells mutate and become abnormal
Verrucous carcinoma	About 5% of all oral cavity tumours are verrucous carcinoma, a type of very slow-growing cancer made up of squamous cells. This type of oral cancer rarely spreads to other parts of the body, but it may invade nearby tissue
Minor salivary gland carcinomas	This disease includes several types of oral cancer that may develop on the minor salivary glands, which are located throughout the lining of the mouth and throat
Lymphoma	Oral cancers that develop in lymph tissue, which is part of the immune system, are known as lymphomas. The tonsils and base of the tongue both contain lymphoid tissue
Benign oral cavity tumours	Several types of non-cancerous tumours and tumour-like conditions may develop in the oral cavity and oropharynx. Sometimes, these conditions may develop into cancer. For this reason, benign tumours are often surgically removed

Source: Cancer Treatment Centers of America (2021).

Management

Any concern regarding the possibility of oral cancer should be managed with a two-week referral within local pathways, and appropriate support networks as required.

Chapter Summary

Problems relating to the eyes, ears, nose and throat are commonly seen as acute presentations in primary care. A good understanding of the interrelated anatomy of these systems is crucial in the exploration of presenting complaints. The key to paramedics managing EENT conditions confidently is to recognise the red flag symptoms, use contemporaneous clinical guidelines (such as NICE Clinical Knowledge Summaries) to guide treatment and be aware of limitations, and to seek referral when required.

Case Study 1

You are working in a GP surgery and a 58-year-old male patient presents to you complaining of sudden onset of blurred vision in his left eye that began yesterday morning and has become gradually worse.

History

PC: Blurred vision.
HxPC: Blurred vision began in his left eye yesterday morning and has become gradually worse, with moving dark shadows and flashes of light that are affecting his ability to see clearly. He noticed a sudden increase in floaters seven days ago but put it down to a recent medication review.
PMHx/SHx: Hypertension; cataract surgery to the L eye three weeks ago.
DHx: Lisinopril.
SHx: Non-smoker.
FHx: No ocular history.
ROS: Denies recent illness or any new CNS, heart, lung, GI, skin or joint symptoms.

Examination

- Visual acuity: R 6/7.5; L counting fingers at 3 feet.
- Pupils: Equal, round and reactive to light.
- Swinging light test: RAPD present L eye.
- Red light reflex: Asymmetric.
- Extraocular movements: Full. No nystagmus.
- Confrontational visual fields: R full to finger counting; central, inferior and nasal field deficits L eye.
- Lids and lashes: Normal.
- Conjunctiva/sclera: Normal.
- Cornea: Clear.
- Anterior chamber: Normal.
- Retina: Wrinkled retinal folds.

Preferred Diagnosis

Retinal detachment should be suspected if there is one or more of:

- New onset of floaters
- New onset of flashes
- Sudden-onset painless and usually progressive visual field loss
- A reduction in visual acuity, blurred or distorted vision, causing persistent and progressive visual loss.

The clinical examination indicates that there is a vision loss, with fundoscopic findings of retinal detachment.

CHAPTER 7 Eyes, Ears, Nose and Throat Presentations

Differential Diagnoses
- This retinal break is likely due to vitreous traction on the periphery and may have been precipitated by the recent cataract surgery. Cataract surgery creates more space in the vitreous chamber (the new lens is thinner than the extracted cataract) and allows the vitreous jelly to shift. As the vitreous jelly moves to fill this new space, it can tug on the retina and cause a retinal break.

Management
- Immediate referral to an ophthalmologist on the same day is required for patients with sight-threatening disease, such as visual field loss (or changes in visual acuity) or fundoscopic signs of retinal detachment or vitreous haemorrhage (NICE, 2019b).

Case Study 2

Within your role at the GP surgery, you see a 45-year-old male who presents with a history of ear pain for two weeks.

History
PC: Ear pain.
HxPC: The patient had pain in his left ear for the past three days, which became much worse yesterday. He has taken paracetamol and ibuprofen irregularly since onset. This morning, he awoke to blood on his pillow, loss of hearing and little or no pain.
PMHx/SHx: None.
DHx: None.
SHx: Professional drummer.
FHx: None.
ROS: Denies recent illness.

Examination
- Inspection: Right ear – nothing abnormal identified. Left ear – no external swelling, erythema, bruising or deformity. Visual inspection of the ear canal shows dried blood and view of TM shows a perforation.

Preferred Diagnosis
- Perforation of the TM secondary to otitis media.

Differential Diagnosis
- Cholesteatoma.

Management
NHS self-care (NHS UK, 2020) advice is suitable for this patient, and should include:
- Avoid putting anything in the ear, such as cotton buds or eardrops, and be careful when showering to avoid water entering the ear.

- Avoid blowing your nose too hard, as this can damage your eardrum as it heals.
- Warm flannels against the ear can help reduce any pain.
- Take regular paracetamol and ibuprofen as needed.

Case Study 3

You are working the Saturday out-of-hours surgery and an 18-year-old male patient presents to you concerned that he has fractured his nose following a football injury.

History

PC: Swollen nose.
HxPC: The patient was involved in an altercation during a poor tackle, resulting in his face hitting the pitch. He has noted a blocked nose and pain since injury, with no focal neurological signs.
PMHx/SHx: None.
DHx: None.
SHx: Smokes socially; works in retail.
FHx: None.
ROS: Denies recent illness or any new CNS, heart or MSK symptoms.

Examination
- Inspection: Swollen nose with some associated bruising to the bridge and obvious nasal deviation to the right. Nasal speculum identifies a bilateral cherry red swelling arising from the nasal septum.

Preferred Diagnosis
- Septal haematoma.

Differential Diagnoses
- Fractured nose
- Soft tissue injury.

Management
- Immediate referral to ENT for emergency review.

Case Study 4

You are working at a walk-in-centre and see a 22-year-old female with a sore throat.

History

PC: Sore throat.
HxPC: The patient reports an increasing sore throat over the past four days. Over the last two days she has developed a fever and is now finding it difficult swallow.

CHAPTER 7 Eyes, Ears, Nose and Throat Presentations

PMHx/SHx: None.
DHx: None.
SHx: Smokes ten a day. Nurse.
FHx: None.
ROS: Denies recent illness.

Examination
- Inspection: Lymph nodes, left tonsillar and cervical chain are inflamed and tender. On visual inspection of the throat, you see bilaterally swollen tonsils, which are red and inflamed. With no white exudate.

Preferred Diagnosis
- Viral tonsillitis.

Differential Diagnoses
- Bacterial tonsillitis
- Pharyngitis.

Management
- NHS self-care advice is suitable for this patient and should include conservative measures such as over-the-counter analgesia (paracetamol and ibuprofen) as needed and ensure adequate rehydration. Clear worsening advice should be given for the patient to monitor their ability to swallow fluids and the presence of voice changes, dribbling or neck swelling that could indicate a worsening infection.

References

Ali, J., Sabiha, B., Jan, H.U. et al. (2017) Genetic etiology of oral cancer. *Oral Oncology* 70: 23–28.

Cancer Treatment Centers of America (2021) Types of oral cancer: Common, rare and more varieties. Available at: https://www.cancercenter.com/cancer-types/oral-cancer/types (accessed 6 April 2021).

Cross, S. and Rimmer, M. (2007) *Nurse Practitioner Manual of Clinical Skills*. 2nd edn. London: Elsevier.

Dannatt, P. and Jassar, P. (2013) Management of patients presenting with otorrhoea: Diagnostic and treatment factors. *British Journal of General Practice* 63(607): e168–e170.

ENT UK and Royal College of Surgeons (2016) Commissioning guide: Chronic rhinosinusitis. Available at: https://www.entuk.org/resources/114/commissioning_guide_for_rhinosinusitis/ (accessed 28 January 2023).

General Practice Notebook (2020) Snoring. Available at: https://gpnotebook.com/simplepage.cfm?ID=1369047114 (accessed 6 April 2021).

Gwaltney, J.M. (1996) Acute community-acquired sinusitis. *Clinical Infectious Diseases* 23(6): 1209–1223.

Health and Safety Executive (2012) The burden of occupational cancer in Great Britain: Nasopharynex/pharynx. Available at: https://www.hse.gov.uk/research/rrpdf/rr863.pdf (accessed 30 January 2023).

References

Kanagalingam, J., Hajioff, D. and Bennett, S. (2005) Vertigo. *British Medical Journal* 330(7490): 523.

Kiger, J., Brenkert, T. and Losek, J.D. (2008) Nasal foreign body removal in children. *Pediatric Emergency Care* 24(11): 785–792.

Kilduff, C. and Lois, C. (2016) Red eyes and red-flags: Improving ophthalmic assessment and referral in primary care. *BMJ Quality Improvement Reports* 5(1): u211608.w4680.

Knott, D. (2021) Voice hoarseness. Available at: https://patient.info/doctor/hoarseness-pro#ref-5 (accessed 9 March 2021).

Kumar, P. and Clark, L. (2017) *Clinical Medicine*. 9th edn. New York: WB Saunders Company.

Le Saux, N., Robinson, J.L. and Canadian Paediatric Society, Infectious Diseases and Immunization Committee (2016) Management of acute otitis media in children six months of age and older. *Paediatrics and Child Health* 21(1): 39–50.

Lipworth, B., Newton, J., Ram, B. et al. (2017) An algorithm recommendation for the pharmacological management of allergic rhinitis in the UK: A consensus statement from an expert panel. *NPJ Primary Care Respiratory Medicine* 27(3): 1–8.

Mohamed, S., Emmanuel, N. and Foden, N. (2019) Nasal obstruction: A common presentation in primary care. *British Journal of General Practice* 69(689): 628–629.

National Institute for Health and Care Excellence (NICE) (2017) Clinical Knowledge Summaries: Vestibular neuronitis. Available at: https://cks.nice.org.uk/topics/vestibular-neuronitis/ (accessed 30 January 2023).

National Institute for Health and Care Excellence (NICE) (2018) Clinical Knowledge Summaries: Mumps. Available at: https://cks.nice.org.uk/topics/mumps/ (accessed 30 January 2023).

National Institute for Health and Care Excellence (NICE) (2019a) Clinical Knowledge Summaries: Hearing loss in adults. Available at: https://cks.nice.org.uk/topics/hearing-loss-in-adults/ (accessed 30 January 2023).

National Institute for Health and Care Excellence (NICE) (2019b) Clinical Knowledge Summaries: Management of suspected retinal detachment. Available at: https://cks.nice.org.uk/topics/retinal-detachment/management/management-of-suspected-retinal-detachment/ (accessed 30 January 2023).

National Institute for Health and Care Excellence (NICE) (2020) Assessment and diagnosis of neck lumps. Available at: https://cks.nice.org.uk/topics/neck-lump/diagnosis/assessment/ (accessed 28 January 2023).

National Institute for Health and Care Excellence (NICE) (2021a) Clinical Knowledge Summaries: Allergic rhinitis. Available at: https://cks.nice.org.uk/topics/allergic-rhinitis/diagnosis/assessment/ (accessed 28 January 2023).

National Institute for Health and Care Excellence (NICE) (2021b) Clinical Knowledge Summaries: Oral. Available at: https://cks.nice.org.uk/topics/palliative-care-oral/management/oral-candida-infection/ (accessed 28 January 2023).

National Institute for Health and Care Excellence (NICE) (2021c) Clinical Knowledge Summaries: Management of red eye. Available at: https://cks.nice.org.uk/topics/red-eye/management/management-of-red-eye/ (accessed 30 January 2023).

National Institute for Health and Care Excellence (NICE) (2021d) Clinical Knowledge Summaries: Sinusitis. Available at: https://cks.nice.org.uk/topics/sinusitis/background-information/ (accessed 28 January 2023).

National Institute for Health and Care Excellence (NICE) (2022a) Clinical Knowledge Summaries: Conjunctivitis infective. Available at: https://cks.nice.org.uk/topics/conjunctivitis-infective/ (accessed 28 January 2023).

CHAPTER 7 Eyes, Ears, Nose and Throat Presentations

National Institute for Health and Care Excellence (NICE) (2022b) Clinical Knowledge Summaries: Conjunctivitis allergic. Available at: https://cks.nice.org.uk/topics/conjunctivitis-allergic/ (accessed 28 January 2023).

National Institute for Health and Care Excellence (NICE) (2022c) Clinical Knowledge Summaries: Dental abscess. Available at: https://cks.nice.org.uk/topics/dental-abscess/management/management/ (accessed 28 January 2023).

National Institute for Health and Care Excellence (NICE) (2022d) Clinical Knowledge Summaries: Epistaxis. Available at: https://cks.nice.org.uk/topics/epistaxis-nosebleeds/management/recurrent-epistaxis/ (accessed 28 January 2023).

National Institute for Health and Care Excellence (NICE) (2022e) Clinical Knowledge Summaries: Otitis externa. Available at: https://cks.nice.org.uk/topics/otitis-externa/ (accessed 28 January 2023).

National Institute for Health and Care Excellence (NICE) (2022f) Clinical Knowledge Summaries: Sore throat – acute. Available at: https://cks.nice.org.uk/topics/sore-throat-acute/ (accessed 28 January 2023).

Neuhauser, H. (2016) Chapter 5: The epidemiology of dizziness and vertigo. In Furman, J. and Lempert, T. (eds) *Handbook of Clinical Neurology*. Amsterdam: Elsevier, pp. 67–82.

NHS Scotland (2020) Mouth ulcer symptoms and treatments. Available at: https://www.nhsinform.scot/illnesses-and-conditions/mouth/mouth-ulcer (accessed 9 March 2021).

NHS UK (2020) Cholesteatoma. Available at: https://www.nhs.uk/conditions/cholesteatoma/ (accessed 28 January 2023).

Oxford Medical Education (2014) Epistaxis. Available at: https://www.oxfordmedicaleducation.com/wp-content/uploads/2014/07/ENT-Epistaxis.pdf (accessed 30 January 2023).

Pane, A. and Simcock, P. (2005) *Practical Ophthalmology: A Survival Guide for Doctors and Optometrists*. London: Churchill Livingstone.

Sanyaolu, L.N., Farmer, S.E.J., and Cuddihy, P.J. (2014) Nasal septal haematoma. *British Medical Journal* 349: g6075.

Scadding, G., Kariyawasam, H., Scadding, G. et al. (2017) BSACI guideline for the diagnosis and management of allergic and non-allergic rhinitis. *Clinical & Experimental Allergy* 47(7): 856–889.

Siqueira, J. and Rocas, I. (2013) Scottish dental clinical effectiveness programme. *SDCEP*. Available at: https://www.sdcep.org.uk/in-development/prevention-and-treatment-of-periodontal-diseases-in-primary-care/ (accessed 9 March 2021).

Wipperman, J. (2014) Dizziness and vertigo. *Primary Care: Clinics in Office Practice* 41(1): 115–131.

Respiratory Presentations

8

Marc Gildas Thomas

> **Within This Chapter**
> - Acute cough/bronchitis
> - Allergy
> - Asthma
> - Bronchiectasis
> - Bronchiolitis in children
> - Chronic obstructive pulmonary disease (COPD)
> - Lung cancer
> - Obstructive sleep apnoea
> - Suspected infection – pneumonia
>   - Aspirational pneumonia
>   - Atypical pneumonia
>   - Community-acquired pneumonia (CAP)
>   - COVID-19 (coronavirus)
>   - Hospital-acquired pneumonia (HAP)
>   - Viral pneumonia

Introduction

The management of patients with respiratory presentations within primary care can be very different from what is required when managing patients who present with emergency respiratory symptoms to the ambulance service. A bonus within primary care is that paramedics have greater ability to review previous test results, request further tests, actively monitor and refer patients to specialities for more enhanced diagnostic investigations and treatments.

> 💡 Do not consider shortness of breath in isolation. Consideration should also be given to other system assessments, such as cardiovascular, to confirm the diagnosis.

CHAPTER 8   Respiratory Presentations

Assessment

As autonomous clinicians working in primary care, the main function of a respiratory assessment is to identify any red flags and to increase or decrease clinical suspicions identified during the initial history taking. Is it important to note signs such as dyspnoea, pallor or cyanosis which may be detectable at the very start of the consultation. Examination then starts with determining the patient's respiratory rate, rhythm and pattern of breathing – looking to determine the degree of any shortness of breath.

> - Can they speak to you in a full sentence?
> - Do they look cyanosed?
> - Are they out of breath from walking down the corridor to your room? Or on answering the phone to you?
> - Are they tripoding, diaphragmatic breathing or do they have any chest recession with increased accessory muscle use?
> - In infants and children, is there any nasal flaring, pursed lip breathing or head bobbing?
> - Are they confused?
>
> If any patient presents with red flag symptoms, treat as an emergency and contact 999.

The Medical Research Council dyspnoea scale should be used to assess the severity of breathlessness (Table 8.1).

If no red flags are present, then continue with the respiratory assessment. This starts with inspection of the patient's hands (Thomas and Monaghan, 2015):

- Determine the presence of peripheral cyanosis to the nails, fingers and hands.
- Inspect the nails for finger clubbing, which occurs as a result of low oxygen in the blood and is a sign of various lung diseases including bronchiectasis, cancer, cystic fibrosis, empyema, fibroma, mesothelioma and pulmonary fibrosis.
- Look for nicotine staining to the fingers, indicating the presence of cigarette smoking.

Table 8.1   Medical Research Council Dyspnoea Scale

Grade	Level of activity
1	Not troubled by breathlessness except during strenuous exercise
2	Short of breath when hurrying or walking up a slight hill
3	Walks slower than contemporaries on the level because of breathlessness, or has to stop for breath when walking at own pace
4	Stops for breath after walking about 100 yds or after a few minutes on the level
5	Too breathless to leave the house, or breathless when dressing or undressing

Source: Adapted from Fletcher (1952). Used with the permission of the Medical Research Council.

Assessment

- Ask the patient to extend their arms and abduct their fingers, assessing for fine finger tremor associated with salbutamol use.
- In suspected carbon dioxide retention, ask the patient to hold hands outstretched with wrists dorsiflexed for 30 seconds to assess for asterixis (though noting that this can also have hepatic pathology).

Move upwards to the patient's face, head and neck (Douglas et al., 2013), firstly inspecting the eyes to determine the presence of:

- Iritis, which can be found in tuberculosis (TB)
- Conjunctivitis, which can again be found in TB or sarcoidosis

Then inspect the nose and mouth for:

- Candidiasis, which is common with inhaled steroid or immunosuppressant use
- Central cyanosis – even just slightly, this is an indication of low oxygen saturations and hypoxia
- Dry mucous membranes, demonstrating dehydration
- A hoarse voice, and whether this is normal or has been a rapid onset (and if associated with a bovine (non-explosive) cough and unilateral pain/weakness to the arm and hand, consider Pancoast tumour)
- Nasal flaring, seen particularly in acute shortness of breath

Before moving down the neck to:

- Inspect the trachea, to determine if it is in a midline position without deviation (such as in plural effusion or pneuomothorax)
- Ensure that the jugular venous pressure (JVP) is not raised over 3 cm, which is indicative of cor pulmonale (right ventricular hypertrophy which occurs in response to increased pressure caused by respiratory distress, severe chronic obstructive pulmonary disease (COPD), emphysema).
- Inspect and palpate lymph nodes – if a node is enlarged or tender, look for a cause. Tender nodes may indicate inflammation or infection, whereas hard painless nodes are more suggestive of malignancy.

> When conducting a respiratory assessment on paediatric patients, it is important to add in the Paediatric Assessment Triangle (PAT) as it considers their appearance, work of breathing and circulation to the skin (Fuchs and Klein, 2019).

Now, start the chest examination. Inspect the anterior chest wall for:

- Shape: Asymmetry of shape, deformity
- Barrel deformities: Rounded thorax with increased anterior posterior (AP) diameter – hyperinflation (marker of chronic obstructive lung disease)
- Bruising/swelling: Signifies possible history of trauma
- Pectus carinatum (pigeon chest): Prominent sternum and costal cartilages which protrude from the chest, which can be caused by an increased respiratory effort when the bones are still malleable in childhood (asthma, rickets)

CHAPTER 8   Respiratory Presentations

- Pectus excavatum (funnel chest): This is where the sternum and costal cartilages appear to be depressed into the chest
- Scars: Possibly caused by operative procedures or radiotherapy, which can provide important clues to the underlying pathology.

> 💡 This may be a good time to assess the patient's posture, looking for any signs of lordosis, kyphosis or scoliosis which can restrict breathing (Rawles et al., 2015).

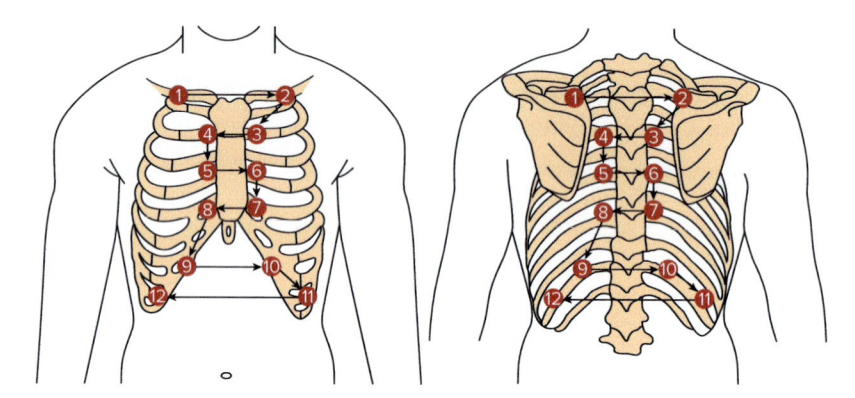

Figure 8.1   Sites for auscultation of the chest.

Undertake auscultation as outlined in Figure 8.1, looking for:

- Normal sounds (vesicular): This is the normal passage of air through large and small airways until it reaches the stethoscope
- Decreased/reduced sounds: Can be localised (pneumonia, tumour, pleural effusion, pneumothorax, collapsed lung) or widespread (asthma, COPD)
- Bronchial breathing: Loud, hollow sounds similar to those of trachea, heard on both inspiration and expiration; signifies increased thickness of substance within lung(s)
- Crackles: Also referred to as rales or crepitations. Can be course (affecting larger airways) or fine (affecting smaller airways). Caused by infection or fluid in the airways
- Pleural rub: This is caused by the parietal and visceral pleura layers rubbing against each other as they are inflamed; can be caused by a pulmonary embolism or infection (pneumonia)
- Wheeze: Sometimes known as rhonchi – polyphonic (narrowing of multiple airways) linked with asthma and exacerbations of COPD. Monophonic (narrowing of a single airway) which can signify a carcinoma or even a foreign body obstruction. Inspiratory wheeze is associated with the upper airway and expiratory wheeze is linked with the lower airways
- Silent chest: A sign of life-threatening asthma.

Then look to undertake egophony. Egophony is an auscultatory finding due to a change in the quality (timbre) of the voice. A solid (consolidated), fluid-filled or compressed lung decreases the amplitude and only allows select frequencies to pass through. This changes the sound of the vowel 'E' to 'A'. This is typically undertaken in the posterior bases:

- Vocal resonance: Ask patient to say 'blue balloon'. The sound will be louder over consolidated or collapsed areas of lung as sound is conveyed somewhat better through a solid lung compared to an air-filled lung
- Whispering pectoriloquy: Ask the patient to whisper. A whisper is clearly heard over areas of consolidation or collapse.

Move on to percussion of the chest wall, following the same locations as in Figure 8.1 for auscultation. Look for:

- Resonant sound: A normal lung
- Hyperresonant sound: Indicative of pneumothorax
- Dull sound: Indicative of pulmonary consolidation, pulmonary collapse, severe pulmonary fibrosis
- Stoney dull sound: Indicative of pleural effusion, haemothorax.

Lastly, palpate the chest wall:

- Assess chest expansion: Less than 2 cm of chest expansion in an adult signifies a pathological cause. Asymmetrical expansion can indicate a pleural effusion, pneumothorax or consolidation of fibrosis. Reduced expansion bilaterally indicates a diffuse abnormality such as a chronic airways disease or fibrosing alveolitis.
- Tenderness over chest wall: This will suggest musculoskeletal problems, for example, fractured rib or costochondritis (inflammation of the cartilages in the ribcage).
- Tactile vocal fremitus: Palpable for a vibration which is felt over the chest wall during low frequency vocalisation when asking the patient to say '99'. This vibration is increased over areas of consolidation and is decreased or absent over a pneumothorax (Douglas et al., 2013).

> For children under the age of five, the National Institute for Health and Care Excellence (NICE) traffic light system for detecting serious illness is an excellent clinical tool (NICE, 2019a).

Presentations in Primary Care

Acute Cough/Bronchitis
Aetiology

An acute cough associated with an upper respiratory infection is defined as a cough that has developed within the last three weeks (Simon et al., 2016). It is most frequently caused by a viral infection such as a cold or the flu which irritates the area anywhere between the pharynx and the lungs (BMJ, 2022). Acute bronchitis is a temporary inflammation of the trachea and bronchi, causing mucous production and a cough but with no evidence of pneumonia (Kinkade and Long, 2016). It can be bacterial or viral in aetiology, with common

CHAPTER 8   Respiratory Presentations

viruses including rhinovirus, enterovirus, influenza A and B, parainfluenza, coronavirus, human metapneumovirus, respiratory syncytial virus (RSV) and adenovirus (BMJ, 2022; Kinkade and Long, 2016). The approximate annual incidence of acute bronchitis within the adult population of the United Kingdom (UK) is 44 per 1,000, with most cases occurring during the autumn and winter months (NICE, 2019b).

> There are other infective causes of an acute cough, such as bronchiectasis, bronchiolitis, pneumonia and croup (NICE, 2019b). Non-infective causes could be attributed to exacerbations of asthma or COPD, heart failure, interstitial lung disease, lung cancer, pulmonary embolisms (PEs), pneumothorax or even gastro-oesophageal reflux disease (GORD) (NICE, 2019b).

History and Examination

Important things to ascertain during the history taking are whether the cough is productive or dry, the duration of symptoms and if there are any additional symptoms such as fever, pleuritic pain, wheeze and shortness of breath. Smoking status is also important to establish.

> Consider the presence of red flags during the history taking, which may indicate that the presentation is not a simple acute cough or acute bronchitis:
>
> - Confusion
> - Haemoptysis
> - Hypotension
> - Lethargy
> - Low oxygen saturations
> - Night sweats
> - Persistent cough (< 3 weeks)
> - Pleuritic pain
> - Recent foreign travel
> - Shortness of breath
> - Tachycardia
> - Weight loss.

On examination, although patients are not normally systemically unwell with acute bronchitis, they may also have a raised temperature which is not normally above 38°C. Crackles and wheezes may be present on auscultation, which normally improve when the patient coughs (with some production of sputum) (NICE, 2019b, 2020a).

> A chest X-ray is not indicated for an acute cough but may be warranted in a chronic or persistent cough (cough that lasts over three weeks) (NICE, 2021c).

Management

Acute cough and acute bronchitis are normally mild and self-limiting, resolving within three to four weeks (NICE, 2019b, 2020a). Antibiotics should not be routinely offered for patients who are systemically not unwell.

Self-care such as honey and lemon drinks (in patients over one year old) and over-the-counter cough expectorants or cough suppressants may be considered, although there is limited evidence for the benefits of the latter (NICE, 2019b).

Some groups of patients are more at risk of complications, and so antibiotics are indicated (NICE, 2020a). These are: premature children; patients with existing respiratory, heart, liver, renal, diabetes or neuromuscular disease; those who are immunosuppressed; those who use oral steroids; and those over 65 years old who have two or more of these criteria, or over 80 years old who have one these criteria.

Antimicrobial prescribing, should it be required, would typically follow:

Adults
- Doxycycline (first choice); alternative first choices are amoxicillin, clarithromycin or erythromycin.

Children
- Amoxicillin (first choice); alternative first choices are clarithromycin or erythromycin
- Doxycycline (over 12 years old) (BMJ, 2022).

However, refer to your local guidelines for which treatment is indicated first or second line, as these may differ.

> 💡 Be mindful that pneumonia can be a complication of acute bronchitis, which is particularly prevalent in the elderly and more vulnerable patients (BMJ, 2022).

Allergy
Aetiology

An allergic reaction normally does not occur on first exposure to the allergen, as it is repeated exposure that sensitises the patient to it which leads to histamine release. This histamine release becomes more significant as it increases with repeated exposure to the allergen (Phipps and Lugg, 2016), and it is this that can result in the rapid systemic hypersensitivity reaction that can lead to anaphylaxis and circulatory collapse within seconds (Resuscitation Council UK, 2021).

> ❗ Whilst most allergies do not become anaphylactic reactions, the potential for deterioration should be considered during the consultation.

CHAPTER 8 Respiratory Presentations

Some common allergen triggers are:

- Dust and pollen
- Food (nuts, cow's milk, eggs)
- Insect stings (wasp, bee, spiders) and animals (horse fur, cat fur)
- Medications (antibiotics, non-steroidal anti-inflammatory drugs (NSAID), chemotherapy).

> 💡 It should also be noted that an anaphylactic reaction can be idiopathic, with no known cause being identified in many cases (Resuscitation Council UK, 2021).

History and Examination

The history should focus on the onset of symptoms (whether sudden or progressive), the duration of symptoms (whether this is worsening each time exposure occurs) and the symptoms that are experienced. Identification of a potential trigger may also be useful, though this is not always present. Table 8.2 outlines some of the common symptoms experienced with different allergen types.

Table 8.2 Symptoms of Allergies

Allergen	Symptoms
Dust and pollen	- Blocked or congested nose - Cough - Itchy eyes or nose - Runny nose - Swollen/watery eyes
Food	- Abdominal pain - Diarrhoea - Swelling of the lips - Tingling in the mouth - Vomiting
Insect stings and animals	- Cough - Itchy skin - Restlessness - Significant swelling at the site of the sting/bite - Urticaria
Medication	- Abdominal pain - Diarrhoea - Lethargy - Peritus - Rashes (notably urticaria or purpura)

Presentations in Primary Care

> ⚠️ Beware of symptoms that pre-empt systemic failure and circulatory shutdown, including airway, breathing and circulatory problems and a general sense of 'impending doom'. In such situations, emergency anaphylactic protocols should be followed (Resuscitation Council UK, 2021).

Management

Treatment will depend on the symptoms present and the regularity of exposure. In allergies that are mild and related to particular contact such as animal fur or certain food types (such as fruit), then avoidance may be the best treatment option.

If contact cannot be avoided and for seasonal allergies, over-the-counter antihistamines may be considered the first-line treatment option.

> ⚠️ Consider 'watchful waiting' of mild allergies, but with specific worsening care advice to monitor for allergy progression and deterioration.

Where the allergen is not clear, and symptoms are increasing or becoming more regular, consider referral to a specifical allergy clinic for patch testing and blood tests. These clinics can also offer advice for diet adjustments.

Asthma

Aetiology

Asthma is a chronic inflammatory condition of the airways in the lungs (GINA, 2020). Asthma can occur at any age, and is associated with genetic, atopic and environmental factors. It is more common in urbanised areas of developed countries, particularly in the UK (Ashelford et al., 2019; Kumar and Clark, 2017).

Physiologically, there are three key features of asthma:

- Airflow limitation
- Bronchiole inflammation and excess mucus production
- Hyperresponsiveness causing bronchospasm of the airways.

These physiological changes can be elicited by exposure to atopic and environmental factors such as (Ashelford et al., 2019; Kumar and Clark, 2017):

- Cigarette smoke
- Cold air
- Exercise
- House dust mites
- Industrial irritants
- Non-steroidal anti-inflammatory medication (NSAID)
- Pollen
- Viral infections.

CHAPTER 8   Respiratory Presentations

History and Examination

Symptoms present in the history, indicative of asthma, include an intermittent cough, wheeze (predominantly bilateral and expiratory) and chest tightness or breathlessness which is worse in the early morning or during the night. Exploration of environmental factors (as above) may also guide the history and should include a family history of asthma or childhood asthma, or any related atopy or rhinitis (Kumar and Clark, 2017; NICE, 2020a).

> 💡 Look for recurrent episodes of symptoms, presence of wheezes on auscultation, personal history of atopy and absence of symptoms of alternative diagnosis (SIGN, 2019).

Investigations

Investigating for asthma can be difficult as there is no specific test for diagnosis. However, spirometry, bronchodilator reversibility (BDR), fractional exhaled nitric oxide (FeNO) testing and peak expiratory flow rate (PEFR) readings or diary (taken over a two- to four-week period) can support the diagnosis of asthma (ICST, 2020a; NICE, 2020a). However, these tests should not be performed in children < 5 years old as they cannot carry them out reliably.

> 💡 Laughter and emotion can cause asthma symptoms in young children (Sugand et al., 2019).

> ❗ Consider the differential diagnosis of asthma (ICST, 2020a):
> - Hyperventilation syndrome
> - COPD
> - Low level of physical fitness or obesity
> - GORD
> - Heart failure
> - Bronchiectasis.

Management

The goals of asthma treatment are to minimise asthma symptoms; maintain normal lung function; not limit activity or exercise; reduce the need for rescue medication; and prevent exacerbations or attacks.

This can be achieved through both pharmacological and non-pharmacological treatment.

Presentations in Primary Care

Pharmacological Treatment

The basic premise of pharmacological treatment is to assess symptoms, measure lung function, check inhaler technique and adherence, adjust dose and implement and review a self-management plan (SIGN, 2019). Treatment of asthma, therefore, should be considered on a sliding scale, best outlined in Figure 8.2 from the Scottish Intercollegiate Guidelines Network (SIGN). Figure 8.3 demonstrates pharmacological treatment in children.

> ⚠️ It is important to note that there are many different clinical guidelines for asthma, including those by NICE, the British Thoracic Society (BTS), SIGN, the Global Initiative for Asthma (GINA) and the All Wales Guidance; application will depend on the country within which you are employed.

Asthma – suspected	Adult asthma – diagnosed
Diagnosis and Assessment	Evaluation: • Assess symptoms, measure lung function, check inhaler technique and adherence • Adjust dose • Update self-management plan • Move up and down as appropriate

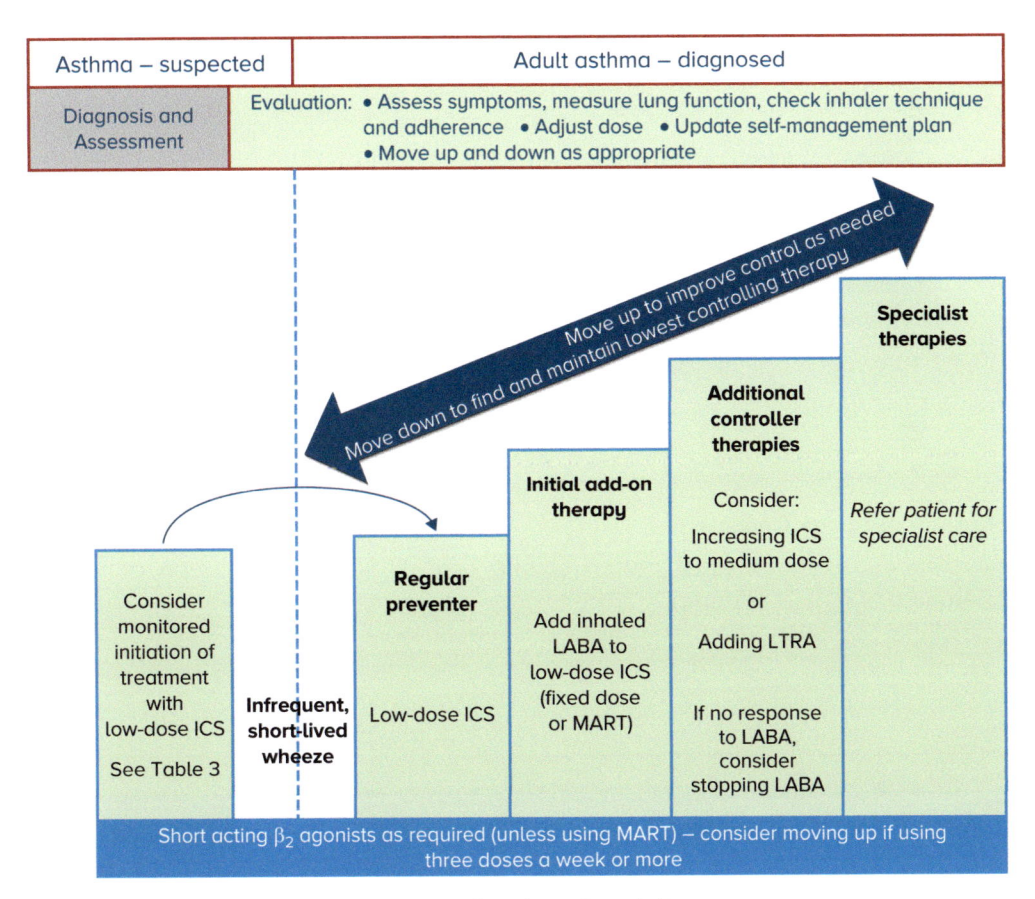

Move up to improve control as needed
Move down to find and maintain lowest controlling therapy

- **Consider monitored initiation of treatment with low-dose ICS** See Table 3
- **Infrequent, short-lived wheeze**
- **Regular preventer** — Low-dose ICS
- **Initial add-on therapy** — Add inhaled LABA to low-dose ICS (fixed dose or MART)
- **Additional controller therapies** — Consider: Increasing ICS to medium dose or Adding LTRA. If no response to LABA, consider stopping LABA
- **Specialist therapies** — Refer patient for specialist care

Short acting β₂ agonists as required (unless using MART) – consider moving up if using three doses a week or more

Figure 8.2 Pharmacological treatment of asthma in adults.
Source: SIGN (2019). Reproduced with permission.

CHAPTER 8 Respiratory Presentations

Asthma – suspected	Paediatric asthma – diagnosed
Diagnosis and Assessment	Evaluation: • Assess symptoms, measure lung function, check inhaler technique and adherence • Adjust dose • Update self-management plan • Move up and down as appropriate

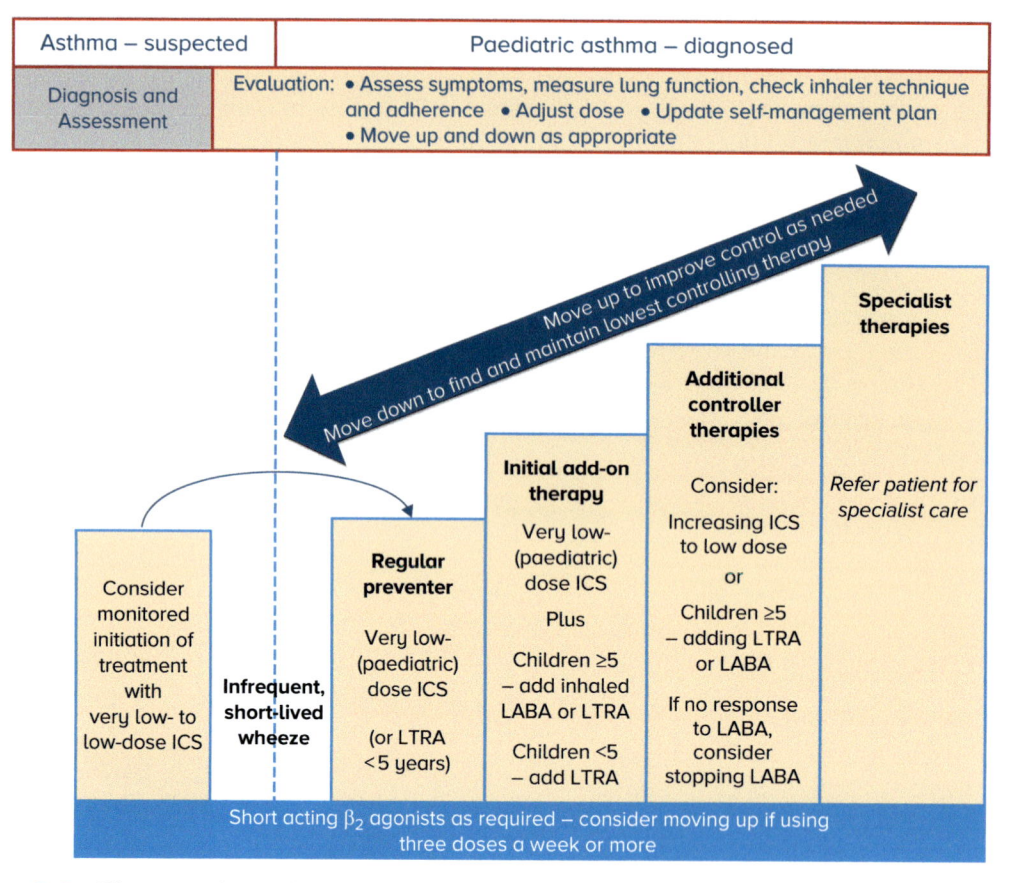

Move up to improve control as needed
Move down to find and maintain lowest controlling therapy

Specialist therapies
Refer patient for specialist care

Additional controller therapies
Consider:
Increasing ICS to low dose
or
Children ≥5 – adding LTRA or LABA
If no response to LABA, consider stopping LABA

Initial add-on therapy
Very low-(paediatric) dose ICS
Plus
Children ≥5 – add inhaled LABA or LTRA
Children <5 – add LTRA

Regular preventer
Very low-(paediatric) dose ICS
(or LTRA <5 years)

Consider monitored initiation of treatment with very low- to low-dose ICS

Infrequent, short-lived wheeze

Short acting β₂ agonists as required – consider moving up if using three doses a week or more

Figure 8.3 Pharmacological treatment of asthma in children.
Source: SIGN (2019). Reproduced with permission.

Non-pharmacological Treatment
- Avoidance of triggers (dust, pollen, smoke, cold air, NSAID medication, *et cetera*)
- Removal of mould or damp
- Smoking cessation
- Weight loss (NICE, 2020a).

> To assist patients with weight loss and smoking cessation, consider engagement with a local health and well-being group or input from a social prescribing link worker.

Presentations in Primary Care

Regular Asthma Reviews

All patients with asthma should receive a review, at least annually. This will need to be more frequent if poor asthma control is identified and will need to be face to face. All patients should be reviewed after emergency admission or exacerbation (ICST, 2020a).

Bronchiectasis

Aetiology

Categorised as a persistent or progressive chronic debilitating disease characterised by permanent dilation of the bronchi due to irreversible damage to the elastic and muscular components of the bronchial wall. The most common cause is severe lower respiratory tract infection, and in UK studies the most frequent pathogen found in bronchiectasis is *Haemophilus influenzae* (20–40%), followed by Pseudomonas aeruginosa (10–30%), *Moraxella catarrhalis*, *Streptococcus pneumoniae*, *Staphylococcus aureus* and *Enterobacteriaceae*. Non-tuberculous mycobacteria (NTM) accounts for 1–10% of cases (Quint and Smith, 2019). Non-infective causes include aspiration or inhalation injury or mucociliary clearance disorders. Two-thirds of people who experience it have comorbidities, with 43% of these being asthma and 36% COPD.

History and Examination

Bronchiectasis should be suspected in adults who present with:

- Purulent sputum
- Dyspnoea
- Fever
- Reduced exercise tolerance or exertional breathlessness
- Rhinosinusitis
- Non-pleuritic chest pain
- An absence of cigarette smoking.

Symptoms are similar in children, with the addition of:

- Asthma that does not respond to treatment
- Previous or recurrent episodes of pneumonia
- A recurrent or persistent wet cough.

On respiratory examination, there might be wheezes, coarse crackles in the lower lungs, high inspiratory squeak or rhonchi. Finger clubbing is much more common in children than adults (NICE, 2022).

Investigations should consist of chest X-ray, sputum culture, spirometry and full blood count.

Management

Referral to respiratory teams is required to confirm the diagnosis, and this may also include a CT scan (Sugand et al., 2019).

191

CHAPTER 8   Respiratory Presentations

> Patients diagnosed with bronchiectasis require annual review within primary care. This may also be a good opportunity for input with a social prescribing link worker, to support understanding of the condition, smoking cessation and compliance with airway clearing techniques and yearly vaccinations.

Bronchiolitis in Children

Aetiology

Bronchiolitis is a viral lower respiratory tract infection, which affects infants and children under two years old (Fuchs and Klein, 2019). It most frequently occurs during the first year of life, with approximately one in three infants developing bronchiolitis during this time, and 2–3% requiring hospital treatment (NICE, 2021a). It occurs during the winter months, being generally caused by the highly infectious RSV, although it can also be caused by influenza, parainfluenza and adenovirus (Miall et al., 2016).

> Risk factors for bronchiolitis:
> - < 3 months old
> - chronic lung disease
> - congenital heart disease
> - immunodeficiency
> - neuromuscular disorders
> - premature birth (NICE, 2021a; Simon et al., 2016).

History and Examination

Suspect bronchiolitis if a there is a one- to three-day history of coryzal symptoms accompanied with:

- Chest recession
- Crackles or wheeze on chest auscultation
- History of poor feeding
- Mild fever
- Persistent cough
- Tachypnoea.

> Focal crackles on auscultation and a pyrexia of > 39°C are indicative of pneumonia, not bronchiolitis (NICE, 2021a).

Management

If symptoms are mild with no respiratory distress or recession and the patient is feeding well, children can be monitored closely at home, with thorough safety-netting advice given to parents or carers.

Presentations in Primary Care

> ⚠️ When giving such safety-netting advice, consider the ability for the parents or carers to look after the infant or child with bronchiolitis and whether they have the knowledge and confidence to recognise deterioration and act on it promptly (contacting 999, or presenting to the emergency department). Additional time may be needed to clearly explain the symptoms of worsening condition to the parents or carers and to ensure this is understood.

Specific worsening care advice should include monitoring the child for:

- Apnoea (observed or reported)
- Central cyanosis
- Oral intake not sufficient or difficulty breastfeeding
- Persistent oxygen saturations of < 92%, when breathing air for babies under 6 weeks or children of any age with underlying health conditions (if measurable)
- Increased respiratory rate of > 60 breaths per minute.

It should be emphasised that if this occurs, admission to hospital is required (NICE, 2021a; Simon et al., 2016).

Chronic Obstructive Pulmonary Disease (COPD)
Aetiology

COPD is defined as a progressive obstructive airway disorder characterised by airway limitation with little or no reversibility, which encompasses two chronic conditions: chronic bronchitis and emphysema (Kumar and Clark, 2017; Wilkinson et al., 2017).

- Chronic bronchitis: Three-month history of increased sputum production and cough which occurs over two successive years (Sugand et al., 2019)
- Emphysema: Defined as destruction to the walls of the alveolar, accompanied with enlargement of the airspaces beyond the terminal bronchioles, resulting in the loss of elasticity and the narrowing or collapse of the airways (Ashelford et al., 2019).

Long-term exposure to toxic gases and particles from cigarette smoking or occupational or environmental exposure are causes of COPD (NICE, 2020a). Although, COPD can also be caused by alpha1-antitrypsin deficiency, a genetic bronchial hyperresponsiveness disorder (Simon et al., 2016), this rare hereditary deficiency accounts for approximately 2% of all cases of emphysema within the UK (Kumar and Clark, 2017).

> ⚠️ Patients with severe advanced COPD may develop pulmonary hypertension, which can lead to the enlargement of the right ventricle, with right ventricular failure ensuing (cor pulmonale) (see Chapter 9 – Cardiovascular Presentations) (Kumar and Clark, 2017).

COPD patients can experience exacerbations due to lung infections. These infections reduce gas exchange, by increased airway inflammation which can lead to severe respiratory failure and even death (Ashelford et al., 2019).

CHAPTER 8 Respiratory Presentations

History and Examination
- Signs of progressive symptoms (NICE, 2019c).

And exposure to risk factors:

- Environmental or occupational exposure
- Smoking – how long for? How many smoked daily? Pack years (number of cigarette packs smoked daily multiplied by number of years smoked).

> 💡 Remember that COPD can have a significant impact on the psychological well-being of an individual affected by it, and consider asking around the past medical history of symptoms of anxiety or depression.

Patients presenting with COPD may appear to be cachexic, with hyperinflation to their chest and pursed lip breathing. A general examination should be carried out, including respiratory rate, heart rate, blood pressure, temperature and oxygen saturations. This should be followed by a respiratory examination, which may find:

- On auscultation, crackles or wheeze present
- Peripheral oedema or raised JVP (consider cor pulmonale).

Investigations
Investigations will include:

- ECG
- Body mass index (BMI)
- Spirometry: Used for diagnosis and prognosis as it assesses the severity of airflow obstruction. Can also be used for monitoring disease progression
- Chest X-ray: COPD might not show until severe. Also useful for exclusion of other causes such as heart failure, tuberculosis, lung cancer and bronchiectasis
- Bloods: Full blood count to identify polycythaemia or anaemia and serum natriuretic peptides if cardiac disease or pulmonary hypertension are suspected
- Sputum culture: To identify infective organism
- Echocardiogram (follow local guidelines)
- Computed tomography (CT) thorax: If abnormality of chest X-ray or another diagnosis such as bronchiectasis is suspected
- Serum alpha-1 antitrypsin: If early onset or young age, with minimal history of smoking or risk factors; may also have a positive family history (NICE, 2020a).

> ❗ Differential diagnosis will include asthma, congestive cardiac failure, bronchiectasis and tuberculosis (GOLD, 2020), and it is important that these are considered during the decision-making process.

Management

When a diagnosis of COPD has been confirmed, for smokers the initial management is smoking cessation, and this is the most significant and important factor in preventing the development of COPD. All COPD patients should be encouraged to stop smoking regardless of age or years of smoking (Walker and Whittlesea, 2012), and should be referred for smoking cessation therapy (ICST, 2020b).

For non-smokers, patients should be managed with non-pharmacological treatments first, including offering pneumococcal and influenza vaccinations, as well as pulmonary rehabilitation as needed. Inhaled therapies should only be offered if clinically indicated to relieve breathlessness and once patients have been trained in their use (ICST, 2020b; NICE, 2019c).

> 💡 Respiratory nurse input is vital for managing patients with COPD, and opportunities for referral and engagement should be sought.

Management can then be split into the following phenotypes:
Patient phenotype 1 (Figure 8.4)

- COPD with predominant breathlessness
- Dyspnoea with fewer than two exacerbations per year.

Patient phenotype 2 (Figure 8.5)

- COPD with exacerbation or breathlessness
- Two or more exacerbations per year.

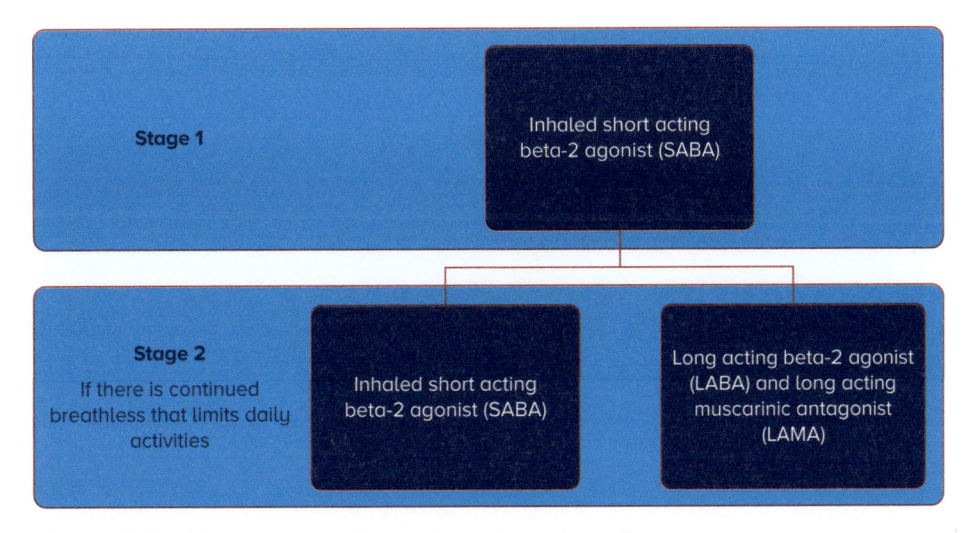

Figure 8.4 Management for patient phenotype 1.

CHAPTER 8 Respiratory Presentations

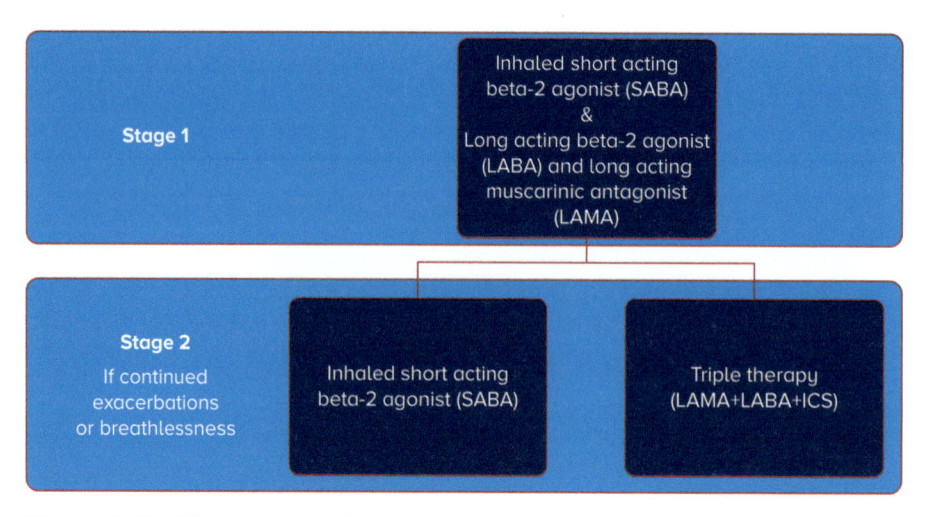

Stage 1: Inhaled short acting beta-2 agonist (SABA) & Long acting beta-2 agonist (LABA) and long acting muscarinic antagonist (LAMA)

Stage 2: If continued exacerbations or breathlessness → Inhaled short acting beta-2 agonist (SABA) | Triple therapy (LAMA+LABA+ICS)

Figure 8.5 Management for patient phenotype 2.

Patient phenotype 3 (Figure 8.6)

- COPD with asthma overlap
- Evidence of significant symptomatic or lung function response to steroids (oral or inhaled)
- Raised blood eosinophil count.

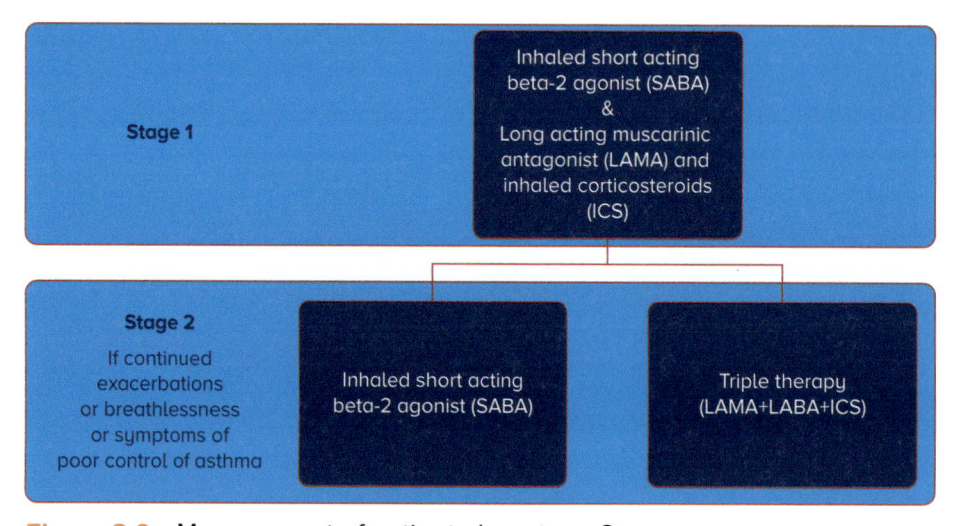

Stage 1: Inhaled short acting beta-2 agonist (SABA) & Long acting muscarinic antagonist (LAMA) and inhaled corticosteroids (ICS)

Stage 2: If continued exacerbations or breathlessness or symptoms of poor control of asthma → Inhaled short acting beta-2 agonist (SABA) | Triple therapy (LAMA+LABA+ICS)

Figure 8.6 Management of patient phenotype 3.
Source: ICST (2020b); NICE (2019a).

Acute Infective Exacerbations

As the paramedic in primary care, it is highly likely you will see acute exacerbations of COPD. These can be spontaneous but are commonly caused by respiratory tract infections, pollutants and smoking (NICE, 2019c).

Presentations in Primary Care

Following the same examination skills, and if there is no need for emergency admission, the treatment for acute infective exacerbations of COPD include:

- Short-acting inhaled bronchodilators
- Antibiotics (doxycycline, or if doxycycline unsuitable clarithromycin or amoxicillin. Co-amoxiclav can be considered if the patient has been exposed to antibiotics within the last three months)
- Corticosteroids (for example, prednisolone).

Local guidelines should be followed for the exact treatment summaries (NICE, 2019c, 2020a; Walker and Whittlesea, 2012).

> To assist patients with managing this condition, consider engagement with a local health and well-being group or input from a social prescriber or link worker.

Lung Cancer

Aetiology

Approximately 43,000 new cases of lung cancer are diagnosed annually in the UK (NICE, 2021d). Lung cancers are the commonest cause of cancer death in males, accounting for around 15% of all cancer diagnosis in the UK (Sugand et al., 2019). Histologically, lung cancers can be classed into two different types: small cell and non-small cell (Simon et al., 2016; Sugand et al., 2019).

Smoking (including passive smoking) is the most significant modifiable risk factor; other risk factors include exposure to asbestos or to products of coal combustion (Kumar and Clark, 2017).

History and Examination

> Patients are likely to present with (Kumar and Clark, 2017; Simon et al., 2016; Sugand et al., 2019):
>
> - Cervical or supraclavicular lymphadenopathy
> - Cough (persistent > 3 weeks, especially in a smoker)
> - Decreased appetite
> - Dyspnoea
> - Fatigue
> - Finger clubbing
> - General malaise or fatigue
> - Haemoptysis
> - Hoarseness
> - Recurrent chest infections
> - Stridor
> - Unexplained chest pain
> - Unintentional weight loss.

CHAPTER 8   Respiratory Presentations

Investigations and Management

Patients over 40 years of age with two or more of these symptoms (or one symptom if they are a smoker) should be offered an urgent chest X-ray, to be performed within two weeks (NICE, 2021d).

Once the decision to refer has been made, make sure it is carried out within one working day.

> 💡 Explain to people who are being referred with suspected cancer that they are being referred to a cancer service. Reassure them, as appropriate, and discuss alternative diagnoses with them.

Obstructive Sleep Apnoea

Aetiology

Apnoeic episodes (characterised by cessation of breathing > 10 seconds) occur during sleep as the pharyngeal airway completely closes, provoking transient arousal as increased inspiratory effort is sensed by the brain. This can also present as choking episodes during sleep (Simon et al., 2016).

Causes of obstructive sleep apnoea include:

- Alcohol (especially consumed in the evening)
- Enlarged tonsils
- Hypothyroidism
- Increased BMI
- Nasal congestion
- Smoking.

> 💡 Children may present with symptoms of obstructive sleep apnoea due to enlarged tonsils during an upper respiratory tract infection (URTI) (Simon et al., 2016).

History and Examination

As sleep apnoea affects sleep, it is likely that patients will present with daytime lethargy, irritability and decreased libido and concentration (Kumar and Clark, 2017). A careful history is needed to determine the presence of sleep apnoea against other differentials.

One way to assess excessive sleepiness is using the Epworth Sleepiness Scale.

Management

Management focuses on lifestyle changes, which can tackle the causes (especially if due to high BMI, consuming alcohol in the evening or smoking).

Presentations in Primary Care

> To assist patients with managing this condition, consider engagement with a local health and well-being group or input from a social prescriber or link worker.

Patients may also be advised to change sleeping position or to elevate the head of the bed and to treat nasal congestion with over-the-counter remedies.

Referral to respiratory physiology may be considered for sleep assessment, with possible treatment with continuous positive airway pressure (CPAP) therapy at night.

> ! If a positive diagnosis is made of obstructive sleep apnoea, the patient must inform the Driver and Vehicle Licensing Agency (DVLA).

Pneumonia

Aetiology

Pneumonia can be described as an acute infection of the bronchioles and alveoli within the lung tissue, often with associated pleural inflammation resulting in consolidation (Lim et al., 2009). This infection can be either located in one or more lobes (lobar pneumonia) or spread over both lung fields including the bronchi and bronchioles (bronchopneumonia) (Campbell, 2011). There are many types of pneumonia; they can have a bacterial, viral or dual aetiology, and can be contracted within the community or in hospital (Gibson and Waters, 2017).

Aspirational Pneumonia

Acutely aspirated gastric acid into the lungs can be particularly serious due to the destructive nature of gastric acid (Kumar and Clark, 2017). Aspirational pneumonia tends to be most prevalent in the right middle and lower lobes, due to the lower angle of the right primary main bronchus to the trachea making it much more likely that any aspirated contents end up in the right bronchus (Williams, 2020). Impaired glottal closure, dysphasia and inadequate cough are contributary factors in aspirational pneumonia which should be suspected in patients who are elderly or have a history of dementia or stroke which impairs their ability to swallow or cough effectively. If aspirational pneumonia is suspected and the patient is not severely ill, then a prompt swallow assessment should be arranged (BMJ, 2021).

Atypical Pneumonia

Atypical pneumonia presents differently from community-acquired pneumonia's (CAP) cough, fever and dyspnoea (Wilkinson et al., 2017). It is usually characterised by symptoms such as general malaise, headache, low-grade fever and cough, with the constitutional findings prevailing over respiratory ones initially. Most cases are mild; however, be aware that severe pneumonia can occur, including hospitalisation. Patients admitted to hospital with atypical pneumonia tend to be young (less than two years old), so suspicions of atypical pneumonia must be factored into any acutely unwell child (BMJ, 2021).

CHAPTER 8 Respiratory Presentations

Community-acquired Pneumonia (CAP)

CAP is described as a pneumonia which is acquired outside of hospital, in the community setting. It can occur in any age; however, it is more common at the extremities of age (Kumar and Clark, 2017). Most CAP infections are caused by the *Streptococcus pneumonia* and *Haemophilus influenzae* organisms, with patients typically presenting with signs of a lower respiratory tract infection, such as cough, fever, productive cough or pleuritic chest pain) (Wilkinson et al., 2017).

Risk factors include:

- Comorbidities (diabetes mellitus, chronic kidney disease, HIV or chronic respiratory conditions such as COPD, cystic fibrosis and bronchiectasis)
- Recent viral respiratory illness
- Extremities of age (< 16 or > 65 years old)
- Lifestyle (smoking, excessive alcohol consumption)
- Medication (prolonged corticosteroid use, immunosuppressant therapy such as methotrexate) (Kumar and Clark, 2017).

> 💡 It is important to note that a common cause of CAP is influenza, which is a highly infectious disease that mutates every two to three years between type A, B and C, annually occurring between the months of October to May (Gibson and Waters, 2017).

COVID-19 (Coronavirus Disease)

The first case of COVID-19 was identified in Wuhan City, China in 2019. It is an acute respiratory infection which is caused by severe acute respiratory syndrome coronavirus 2 (SARS-CoV-2) (BMJ, 2021). It has since spread worldwide, causing a global pandemic in 2020 as it is highly contagious and spreads and evolves rapidly within the human population (Liu et al., 2020). Coronaviruses previously have caused mild upper respiratory conditions in humans, but two coronaviruses within the last 20 years (SARS-CoV and MERS-CoV) have been linked to severe cases of pneumonia, leading to death in humans (Stewart et al., 2020). COVID-19 is a respiratory virus which is spread mainly by droplets from a cough or sneeze. The droplets are either directly inhaled or are picked up on hands from surfaces and transferred when someone touches their face, mouth or eyes (Liu et al., 2020). COVID-19 causes severe respiratory symptoms in people who are older or immunocompromised, including those who have comorbidities such as chronic lung disease, cancer and diabetes mellitus (Liu et al., 2020; Stewart et al., 2020).

Hospital-acquired Pneumonia (HAP)

HAP is defined as an acute respiratory tract infection which develops following at least 48 hours of hospital admission. It is more likely to be caused by an antibiotic-resistant pathogen, so therefore can increase hospital stay and mortality (particularly in the elderly and those with risk factors and comorbidities) (BMJ, 2021; Gibson and Waters, 2017). The risk factors for HAP are like those of CAP, although the organisms that cause HAP are most commonly aerobic Gram-negative bacteria such as *P. aeruginosa*, *Escherichia coli* and *K. pneumoniae* (Kumar and Clark, 2017).

Viral Pneumonia

Patients who are immunosuppressed or at the extremes of age are at increased risk of viral pneumonia. Both CAP and HAP can be due to a viral aetiology and are often caused by RSV, parainfluenza virus and influenza virus (Gibson and Waters, 2017). These can be further complicated by pathogens such as *Staphylococcus aureus* and *Streptococcus pneumonaie*, as co-infection between a viral and bacterial pathogen can increase bacterial virulence, thereby increasing morbidity and mortality (BMJ, 2021).

History and Examination

Regardless of the aetiology, there are common features of pneumonia. Whilst it is categorised by a productive cough and fever, patients may present with some subtle signs such as abdominal pain, lethargy and general malaise (AMLSC NAEMT, 2019).

Other clinical features include:

- Dyspnoea
- Haemoptysis
- Pleuritic pain
- Purulent sputum.

Examination findings may include:

- Confusion
- Cyanosis
- Hypotension
- Hypothermia
- Pyrexia
- Tachycardia
- Tachypnoea.

On chest examination, signs of consolidation within the lungs may be present:

- Bronchial breathing
- Crackles auscultated over area(s) of consolidation
- Decreased chest expansion
- Hyporesonance on percussion over area(s) of consolidation
- Increased vocal resonance over area(s) of consolidation (Wilkinson et al., 2017).

> ⚠ Caution must be taken when assessing for pneumonia, especially in the old or very young, who can present with atypical symptoms such as confusion or headache (Simon et al., 2016).

CHAPTER 8 Respiratory Presentations

A bacterial cause of pneumonia may be more likely if the patient:
- Becomes acutely unwell within a few days
- Has pleuritic pain
- Has a productive cough with purulent sputum
- Has no history of COVID-19 symptoms or exposure (NICE, 2021b).

> The CURB65 score can be useful alongside clinical judgement to assist with decision making (NICE, 2019c).

Investigations

As well as respiratory examination, investigations may include physiological observations, bloods (FBC, U&E, LFT, CRP) and chest X-ray (NICE, 2020b).

> If available, point-of-care CRP can determine the severity of the illness and the potential for deterioration due to sepsis (Wilkinson et al., 2017).

Management

An essential part of the management of pneumonia is assessing whether the patient is suitable to be treated at home or admitted to hospital.

> Treat all children who have a clear clinical diagnosis of pneumonia with antibiotics, as it is difficult and unreliable to distinguish between bacterial and viral pneumonia in children (AWMSG, 2022; BTS, 2011).

Amoxicillin is the antibiotic of choice, as it is a broad-spectrum beta-lactam antibiotic that is effective whilst safeguarding against high levels of antibiotic resistance, specifically to co-amoxiclav, and reducing the Clostridium difficile risk (ICST, 2019; Thomas, 2020).

Antibiotic Treatment for Adults

All antibiotic treatments should be adopted with the current local antimicrobial guidance.
- CRB65 score of 0: First choice = amoxicillin
    - Alternative = doxycycline or clarithromycin
- CRB65 score of 1 (at home): First choice = amoxycillin plus clarithromycin
    - Alternative = doxycycline (AWMSG, 2022; BTS, 2015).

Antibiotic Treatment for Children
- Recommended: amoxicillin
- Penicillin allergy: clarithromycin
- Pneumonia associated with influenza: co-amoxiclav (AWMSG, 2022; BTS, 2011).

> ⚠ Ensure that patients are clinically reviewed and assessed for severity in the community setting within 48 hours, or sooner if clinically indicated. If there is no improvement within this period, hospital admission or a chest X-ray should be considered (AWMSG, 2022; BTS, 2011).

Chapter Summary

Paramedics may be very au fait with assessing respiratory presentations as they enter work in primary care, and the ability to recognise and assess severity of respiratory symptoms is paramount to the safe investigation and management of these patients. It is important that paramedics review and comply with local antimicrobial treatment guidelines in the management of their patients, and have a low threshold for involvement of other teams, such as review by respiratory nurses or involvement of respiratory specialists where necessary.

Case Study 1

You are working in a general practice and a 60-year-old male presents with a one-week history of a productive cough.

History

PC:	Productive cough and shortness of breath on exertion (SOB).
HxPC:	No haemoptysis, no chest or pleuritic pain. Patient complaining of increased shortness of breath on exertion, also states that for the last few years he has been having a similar presentation at this time of year.
PMHx:	Hypertension.
DHx:	Ramipril, no illicit drugs.
Allergies:	None.
SHx:	Self-employed builder, married, two adult children, social weekend alcohol consumption, lifelong cigarette smoker (> 40 years, 20 cigarettes daily), no recent foreign travel.
FHx:	Mother (hypertension, type 2 diabetes) and father (bronchiectasis, hypertension) both deceased, two siblings (brother and sister) both with hypertension.
ROS:	Alert, orientated, no confusion, slight shortness of breath following walking down the corridor which eased at rest during the consultation, speaking in full complete sentences, no cyanosis.

CHAPTER 8   Respiratory Presentations

Examination
- Vital signs: BP 118/74 mmHg; HR 98 bpm (regular); RR 20–24/min; SpO_2 94% on air; temperature 38.1°C.
- Blood sugar: 6.4 mmol/L.
- Auscultation: Bilateral widespread course crackles with a slight expiratory wheeze present, equal chest expansion, no deformities, resonant on percussion, good bilateral air entry throughout, no peripheral or sacral oedema.
- CRB65 = 0.
- ECG = normal sinus rhythm (NSR).

Preferred Diagnosis
- Acute infective exacerbation of undiagnosed COPD.

Differential Diagnoses
- Acute cough
- CAP
- Bronchiectasis.

Management
Initial management of the acute infective exacerbation:

- Short-acting inhaled bronchodilators
- Antibiotics
- Corticosteroids
- Sputum sample to identify infective organism
- Chest X-ray and blood test if no improvement
- Smoking cessation (counselling, support and assistance to achieve this)
- Close monitoring and follow-up assessments.

Local guidelines should be followed for the exact treatment summaries.
Management following full recovery of the episode of this acute infective exacerbation:

- Spirometry
- Chest X-ray (if not already carried out previously)
- Flu vaccination
- Consider referral for exercise and pulmonary rehabilitation.

Case Study 2
A 64-year-old male presenting with a four-month history of a non-productive cough.

History
PC: Cough.
HxPC: The patient states he has been feeling lethargic recently and has also lost some weight which has been unplanned.

PMHx: Normally fit and well.
DHx: Over-the-counter paracetamol taken occasionally.
SHx: Divorced with one child who is 36 years old, employed as a car sales executive, has been smoking 10 cigarettes daily for the last 40 years, no recent foreign travel
FHx: Father 78 years old (myocardial infarction (MI), hypertension), mother 74 years old (breast cancer).
ROS: Alert, orientated, good colour, no shortness of breath, speaking in full complete sentences.

Examination
- Vital signs: BP 130/84 mmHg; HR 88 bpm (regular); RR 18/min; SpO$_2$ 95% on air; temperature 36.8°C.
- BM: 5.4 mmol/L.
- Auscultation: Fine scattered crackles noted right lung, good bilateral air entry, equal chest expansion, resonant on percussion, no deformities, no peripheral or sacral oedema.
- ECG = NSR.

Preferred Diagnosis
- Lung cancer.

Differential Diagnoses
- GORD
- Infection.

Management
- Urgent chest X-ray (on the day or the next day) to assess for lung cancer, then referral under the two-week wait pathway depending on results.

References

Advanced Medical Life Support Committee of the National Association of Emergency Medical Technicians (AMLSC NAEMT) (2019) *AMLS Advanced Medical Life Support: An Assessment-based Approach.* 2nd edn. Burlington, MA: Jones and Bartlett Learning.

All Wales Medicines Strategy Group (AWMSG) (2022) Primary care antimicrobial guidelines. Available at: https://awttc.nhs.wales/medicines-optimisation-and-safety/medicines-optimisation-guidance-resources-and-data/prescribing-guidance/primary-care-antimicrobial-guidelines/ (accessed 31 January 2023).

Ashelford, S., Raynsford, J. and Taylor, V. (2019) *Pathophysiology and Pharmacology in Nursing.* 2nd edn. London: Sage.

British Medical Journal (BMJ) (2021) Best Practice Guideline: Overview of pneumonia. Available at: https://bestpractice.bmj.com/topics/en-gb/1113 (accessed 31 January 2023).

CHAPTER 8   Respiratory Presentations

British Medical Journal (BMJ) (2022) Best Practice Guideline: Acute bronchitis. Available at: http://bestpractice.bmj.com (accessed 31 January 2023).

British Thoracic Society (BTS) (2011) Guidelines for the management of community acquired pneumonia in children: Update 2011. *Thorax BMJ* 66(2): 1–23.

British Thoracic Society (BTS) (2015) Annotated BTS Guideline for the management of CAP in adults: Update 2009. Available at: https://www.brit-thoracic.org.uk/quality-improvement/guidelines/pneumonia-adults/ (accessed 30 January 2023).

Campbell, J. (2011) *Campbell's Physiology Notes.* Carlisle: Lorimer Publications.

Douglas, G., Nicol, F. and Robertson, C. (2013) *Macleod's Clinical Examination.* 13th edn. London: Churchill Livingstone.

Fletcher, C.M. (1952) The clinical diagnosis of pulmonary emphysema – An experimental study. *Proceedings of the Royal Society of Medicine* 45(9): 577–584.

Fuchs, S. and Klein, B. (2019) *Paediatric Education for Prehospital Professionals.* 3rd edn. Burlington, MA: Jones and Bartlett.

Gibson, V. and Waters, D. (2017) *Respiratory Care.* London: CRC Press.

Global Initiative for Asthma (GINA) (2020) Global strategy for asthma management and prevention (2020 update). Available at: https://ginasthma.org/wp-content/uploads/2020/06/GINA-2020-report_20_06_04-1-wms.pdf (accessed 30 January 2023).

Global Initiative for Chronic Obstructive Lung Disease (GOLD) (2020) GOLD teaching slide set. Available at: https://goldcopd.org/gold-teaching-slide-set/ (accessed 18 January 2021).

Institute of Clinical Science and Technology (ICST) (2019) The All Wales secondary care community acquired pneumonia guideline. Available at: https://allwales.icst.org.uk/wp-content/uploads/2021/01/GUIDELINE-All-Wales-Secondary-Care-Community-Acquired-Pneumonia-Guideline.pdf (accessed 31 January 2023).

Institute of Clinical Science and Technology (ICST) (2020a) The All Wales asthma diagnosis guideline. Available at: https://www.clinicalscience.org.uk/assets/all-wales-asthma-diagnosis-guideline.pdf.

Institute of Clinical Science and Technology (ICST) (2020b) The All Wales COPD and management prescribing guideline. Available at: https://allwales.icst.org.uk/wp-content/uploads/2020/07/The-All-Wales-COPD-Management-and-Prescribing-Guideline.pdf (accessed 30 January 2023).

Kinkade, S. and Long, N. (2016) Acute bronchitis. *American Family Physician* 94(7): 560–565.

Kumar, P. and Clark, M. (2017) *Kumar and Clark's Clinical Medicine.* 9th edn. London: Elsevier.

Lim, W., Baudouin, S., George, R. et al. (2009) British Thoracic Society guidelines for the management of community acquired pneumonia in adults: Update 2009. *Thorax BMJ* 64(3): 55.

Liu, Y., Kuo, R. and Shih, S. (2020) COVID-19: The first documented coronavirus pandemic in history. *Biomedical Journal* 43(4): 328–333.

Miall, L., Rudolf, M. and Leven, M. (2016) *Paediatrics at a Glance.* 4th edn. Oxford: Blackwell.

National Institute for Health and Care Excellence (NICE) (2019a) Traffic light system for identifying risk of serious illness in under 5s. Available at: https://www.nice.org.uk/guidance/ng143/resources/support-for-education-and-learning-educational-resource-traffic-light-table-pdf-6960664333 (accessed 31 January 2023).

National Institute for Health and Care Excellence (NICE) (2019b) Cough (acute): Antimicrobial prescribing [NG120]. Available at: https://www.nice.org.uk/guidance/ng120/chapter/Recommendations (accessed 22 December 2020).

References

National Institute for Health and Care Excellence Guideline (NICE) (2019c) Chronic obstructive pulmonary disease in over 16s: Diagnosis and management [NG115]. Available at: https://www.nice.org.uk/guidance/ng115 (accessed 31 January 2023).

National Institute for Health and Care Excellence (NICE) (2020a) Clinical Knowledge Summaries: Asthma. Available at: https://cks.nice.org.uk/topics/asthma/ (accessed 29 April 2021).

National Institute for Health and Care Excellence (NICE) (2020b) COVID-19 rapid guideline: Managing suspected or confirmed pneumonia in adults in the community. Available at: https://www.nice.org.uk/guidance/ng165/chapter/3-Diagnosis-and-assessment (accessed 22 December 2020).

National Institute for Health and Care Excellence (NICE) (2021a) Bronchiolitis in children diagnosis and management [NG9]. Available at: https://www.nice.org.uk/guidance/ng9/ (accessed 7 February 2023).

National Institute for Health and Care Excellence (NICE) (2021b) Clinical Knowledge Summaries: Chest infections. Available at: https://cks.nice.org.uk/topics/chest-infections-adult/background-information/prevalence/ (accessed 31 January 2023).

National Institute for Health and Care Excellence (NICE) (2021c) Clinical Knowledge Summaries: Chronic obstructive pulmonary disease. Available at: https://cks.nice.org.uk/topics/chronic-obstructive-pulmonary-disease/ (accessed 31 January 2023).

National Institute for Health and Care Excellence (NICE) (2021d) Clinical Knowledge Summaries: Lung and pleural cancers – recognition and referral. Available at: https://cks.nice.org.uk/topics/lung-pleural-cancers-recognition-referral/ (accessed 30 March 2021).

National Institute for Health and Care Excellence (NICE) (2022) Clinical Knowledge Summaries: Bronchiectasis. Available at: https://cks.nice.org.uk/topics/bronchiectasis/ (accessed 31 January 2023).

Phipps, O. and Lugg, O. (2016) *RAPID Emergency and Unscheduled Care.* Chichester: Wiley Blackwell.

Quint, J.K. and Smith, M.P. (2019) Paediatric and adult bronchiectasis: Diagnosis, disease burden and prognosis. *Respirology* 24(5): 413–422.

Rawles, Z., Griffiths, B. and Alexander, T. (2015) *Physical Examination Procedures for Advanced Practitioners and Non-Medical Prescribers Evidence and Rationale.* 2nd edn. London: CRC Press.

Resuscitation Council UK (2021) Emergency treatment of anaphylactic reactions guidelines for healthcare providers. Available at: https://www.resus.org.uk/library/additional-guidance/guidance-anaphylaxis/emergency-treatment (accessed 31 January 2023).

Scottish Intercollegiate Guidelines Network (SIGN) (2019) British guideline on the management of asthma. Available at: https://www.sign.ac.uk/our-guidelines/british-guideline-on-the-management-of-asthma/ (accessed 31 January 2023).

Simon, C., Everitt, H., van Dorp, F. et al. (2016) *Oxford Handbook of General Practice.* 4th edn. Oxford: Oxford University Press.

Stewart, K., Connelly, D. and Robinson, J. (2020) Everything you should know about the coronavirus outbreak. *The Pharmaceutical Journal*, 4 May. Available at: https://www.pharmaceutical-journal.com/news-and-analysis/features/everything-you-should-know-about-the-coronavirus-outbreak/20207629.article?firstPass=false (accessed 31 January 2023).

Sugand, K., Berry, M., Yusuf, I. et al. (2019) *Oxford Handbook for Medical School.* Oxford: Oxford University Press.

CHAPTER 8 Respiratory Presentations

Thomas, J. and Monaghan, T. (2015) *Oxford Handbook of Clinical Examination and Practical Skills.* 2nd edn. Oxford: Oxford University Press.

Thomas, M.G. (2020) Use of co-amoxiclav for the treatment of dog bites. *Journal of Paramedic Practice* 12(5): 1–7.

Walker, R. and Whittlesea, C. (2012) *Clinical Pharmacy and Therapeutics.* 5th edn. Oxford: Churchill Livingstone.

Wilkinson, I., Raine, T., Wiles, K. et al. (2017) *Oxford Handbook of Clinical Medicine.* 10th edn. Oxford: Oxford University Press.

Williams, N. (2020) The respiratory system. In Knight, J., Nigam, Y. and Cutter, J. (eds) *Understanding Anatomy and Physiology in Nursing.* London: Sage, pp. 82–106.

Cardiovascular Presentations

9

Jessica Willetts

Within This Chapter

- Angina
- Atrial fibrillation
- Chest pain
    - Acute coronary syndrome
    - Bornholm disease
    - Costochondritis
    - Endocarditis
    - Musculoskeletal (including costochondritis)
    - Myocarditis
    - Pericarditis
- Deep vein thrombosis
- Fits, faints and funny turns
- Heart failure
- Hyperlipidaemia
- Hypertension
- Peripheral vascular disease
- Pulmonary embolism

Introduction

Cardiovascular complaints are common reasons for attendance in primary care (Brown, 2022), forming 6% of all presentations (Salisbury et al., 2013). The primary care presentations of cardiac disease can be highly varied and challenging. Primary care cardiovascular work comprises both prevention (for example, management of hypertension) and same-day urgent presentations (for example, cardiac sounding chest pain). Therefore, the primary care paramedic needs to be skilled in both chronic and emergency assessment and management of cardiovascular complaints.

    This chapter will provide the reader with a comprehensive, practical guide of the assessment and management of cardiovascular presenting complaints that are commonly seen by paramedics working in a primary care setting.

CHAPTER 9   Cardiovascular Presentations

Assessment

A systematic approach to a cardiovascular examination will ensure a thorough consultation for the patient presenting with a cardiovascular problem. This starts with a general inspection of the patient, looking at visible clues indicating cardiovascular insufficiency:

- Corneal arcus (a white ring around the iris) is associated with high cholesterol levels. There appears to be a clear association between arcus and age, and its presence in younger people is more strongly suggestive of cardiovascular disease (Chambless et al., 1990)
- Cyanosis
- Finger clubbing
- Frank's sign (a bilateral diagonal crease in the ear lobe) is suggestive of cardiovascular disease – although it is poorly specific, especially in older men, where it is also a sign of ageing (Mallinson and Brooke, 2017)
- Janeway lesions (rare – red swellings on the palms indicative of endocarditis)
- Osler's nodes (red nodules on the fingers, indicative of endocarditis)
- Splinter haemorrhage (sometimes seen in endocarditis, though more commonly due to trauma)
- Xanthomas in other body areas, especially tuberous xanthoma (areas such as elbows and knees) or tendinous xanthoma (usually hands, feet or Achilles tendon) are more strongly associated with hyperlipidaemia (Ngan and Stanway, 2005).

> 💡 Xanthelasma (fatty deposits around the eyelids) is frequently taught as a sign of hyperlipidaemia, although there is some debate about this. Kavoussi et al. (2016) showed a linkage between low-density lipoprotein (LDL) ('bad' cholesterol) and xanthelasma, but overall lipid levels were similar to control.

Auscultation

The most important examination undertaken in primary care is auscultation of heart sounds to identify heart murmurs, which can be heard best in the locations shown in Figure 9.1. The mnemonic 'Ambulance Paramedic Tea Makers' can be a fun way to remember the valves best heard at each site (aorta, pulmonary, tricuspid, mitral).

Palpation

Palpating for the apex beat is also useful (it may move in cardiomegaly). Heaves and thrills are rarely felt but it is useful to check for them (though care should be taken not to tell the patient you are feeling their chest for thrills!). Heaves are felt when your hand is lifted by the force of contraction and usually indicated hypertrophy. Thrills are vibrations created by a murmur and may be felt through your hand (Douglas et al., 2009).

Presentations in Primary Care

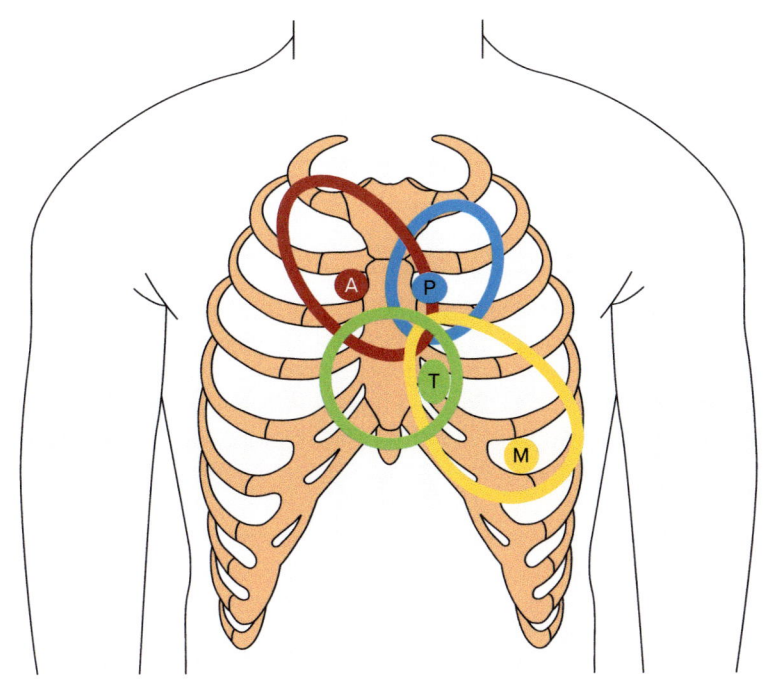

Figure 9.1   Sites for cardiac auscultation.

Presentations in Primary Care

Angina

Aetiology

A mismatch between the heart's oxygen demand and supply will cause chest pain. Normally, the coronary arteries will vasodilate to supply more oxygen but if there is damage from atherosclerosis, or spasm (Prinzmetal's angina), this is harder to achieve. Where there is significant atherosclerosis, a small increase in oxygen demand from exertion can be enough to exceed the heart's ability to supply more oxygen, resulting in pain (Van Meter and Hubert, 2014).

Stable angina occurs in about 8% of men and 3% of women and increases with age (Simon et al., 2014), as with other cardiac disease. Annual mortality is between 0.5% and 4%, normally after an acute cardiac event such as myocardial infarction (MI) (Simon et al., 2014).

> Angina can also occur in severe anaemia (reduced oxygen supply), in tachycardia due to uncontrolled hyperthyroidism or where uncontrolled hypertension increases the force of cardiac contraction (Van Meter and Hubert, 2014).

CHAPTER 9   Cardiovascular Presentations

Unstable angina-type chest pain may occur at rest or with less-than-usual exertion. It should be treated as a type of acute coronary syndrome (ACS) – emergency admission to hospital is required.

History and Examination

Angina is primarily a clinical diagnosis, and a comprehensive history is vital. In particular, a full history of the pain is required, including provoking and relieving factors. Anginal pain is usually brought on by exertion (though may be due to cold, emotion or other factors) and goes after a few minutes of rest (or use of glyceryl trinitrate (GTN)). It is typically cardiac in nature, with central chest pain described as 'crushing' or 'like a band', which may radiate to the jaw or neck. There may be accompanying pallor, diaphoresis or breathlessness.

Assess for cardiac risk factors such as hyperlipidaemia, smoking, hypertension, vascular disease and stroke or transient ischaemic attack (TIA) history. History of previous cardiac disease (MI, angioplasty) and relevant family history are also essential.

Measure pulse, blood pressure and body mass index (BMI), and examine for carotid bruits. Assess for signs of aortic stenosis (an ejection systolic murmur) and cardiomyopathy, which are both causes of anginal pain unrelated to the coronary arteries (NICE, 2016a). In addition, assess for other signs of chest pain (see section on Chest Pain).

NICE discuss 'typicality' in assessing possible angina by using three key symptoms:

- Constricting pain in the chest, neck, shoulders, jaw or arm
- Brought on by exertion
- Relieved by rest or GTN within five minutes.

'Typical' angina has all three symptoms, 'atypical' angina two. Non-anginal chest pain has one or none of these (NICE, 2016b). Factors that make stable angina less likely include:

- Continuous, or prolonged, chest pain
- Pain unrelated to activity
- Pleuritic pain (brought on by inspiration or expiration)
- Symptoms such as palpitations, dizziness, tingling or problems swallowing.

However, these factors do not in themselves exclude a cardiac cause; it just may not be angina. The National Institute for Health and Care Excellence (NICE) notes that an angina diagnosis should only be excluded if there are no other aspects of the history suggestive of angina.

> NICE comments that chest pain and angina symptoms should be assessed the same way regardless of sex or ethnicity. However, there is evidence that women are less likely to exhibit the 'normal' chest pain symptoms – and more likely to have their symptoms attributed to a non-cardiac cause than men (Canto et al., 2012; Lichtman et al., 2018).

Investigations

- Arrange initial blood tests, including a full blood count to exclude anaemia and thyroid function if hyperthyroidism is a possible cause. Lipids and HbA1C should be measured to assess for cardiac risk factors and underlying diabetes.
- ECG.

Management

If stable angina is suspected, refer the person to a rapid-access chest pain clinic, arranging initial investigations including ECG, full blood count, lipids, HbA1C and thyroid function.

Follow your local rapid-access chest pain clinic guidelines for treatment prior to the patient being seen in clinic.

Hospital investigations may include:

- CT coronary angiography
- Non-invasive functional testing (such as myocardial perfusion scan, stress echo or MRI)
- Invasive angiography (you will be familiar with this from STEMI management).

NICE no longer recommends exercise ECGs (treadmill) for diagnosis of stable angina.

Once the diagnosis is confirmed, management may include:

- Patient education in regard to the nature of the disease
- Symptom management
- Risk reduction (lifestyle advice such as weight loss and smoking cessation)

> To assist with smoking cessation and weight loss, consider engagement with a local health and well-being group or input from a social prescribing link worker.

- Short-acting nitrate (GTN spray or tablet) to relieve symptoms and education of how and when to use

> Patients may faint after GTN usage if not used correctly. Educate your patient on when to use the spray, how to use it and what side effects may occur (headache, dizziness). In particular, ensure they are clear about when to call an ambulance.

- Secondary prevention
  - Aspirin 75 mg daily
  - Statin
  - Hypertension management (consider ACE inhibitors in diabetes with angina)
- A beta blocker or calcium channel blocker
- Further treatments as indicated to relieve symptoms, including long-acting nitrates, ivabradine, nicorandil or ranolazine. These are likely to be outside the scope of a paramedic in primary care but you may encounter patients on them
- Possibly bypass (coronary artery bypass graft) or angioplasty to relieve symptoms.

Other Variants

Prinzmetal's angina is caused by vasospasm and causes ST elevation on an ECG. It is rapidly relieved by nitrates. Refer to hospital as an emergency to exclude ACS. If confirmed, management is with calcium channel blockers.

CHAPTER 9   Cardiovascular Presentations

Cardiac syndrome X should be considered where anginal chest pain occurs but angiography shows normal coronary arteries. It is poorly understood but can be managed similarly to stable angina in most cases. Take cardiology advice.

Atrial Fibrillation

Aetiology

Atrial fibrillation (AF) is a very common cardiac dysrhythmia, affecting 2.5% of the population of England (PHE, 2020). It is commonly undiagnosed, with around 250,000 people unaware they have AF (NICE, 2021). The risk of developing AF roughly doubles with each decade of life, with approximately 9% of 80–90-year-olds affected (Barra and Fynn, 2015). AF contributes to approximately 20% of strokes (Barra and Fynn, 2015), and thus early detection and treatment can be significantly beneficial. AF increases the overall risk of adverse cardiac events, with an increase in all-cause mortality of 46% and a 96% increase in risk of a major cardiac event (Odutayo et al., 2016). Whilst stroke is most commonly associated with AF, there are other health risks, in particular increased rates of heart failure and chronic kidney disease. There are also significant effects on quality of life, with patients experiencing reduced exercise tolerance (Odutayo et al., 2016).

History and Examination

The patient may present with breathlessness, palpitations, dizziness or syncope, chest discomfort or stroke or TIA, or they could be completely asymptomatic and AF is an incidental finding.

> 💡 NICE (2021) recommend manually palpating a pulse, as a patient with AF may be asymptomatic. Auscultate heart sounds for murmurs and check the patient's blood pressure.

Investigations

An irregular pulse should trigger an ECG. AF will show on an ECG as an irregularly irregular rhythm in the absence of P waves (Figure 9.2). If this confirms AF, then further treatment should be considered. Paroxysmal AF should be considered as a cause of the patient's symptoms, and if this is not detected on an ECG, a 24-hour ambulatory monitor may be arranged. If a high suspicion of AF continues, an implantable loop recorder might be considered; however, this would be arranged in secondary care.

> 💡 Consider arranging an echocardiogram (echo) if your examination leads you to suspect heart failure or valve dysfunction (for example, a murmur). It may also be arranged by cardiology if they are considering rhythm control.

Presentations in Primary Care

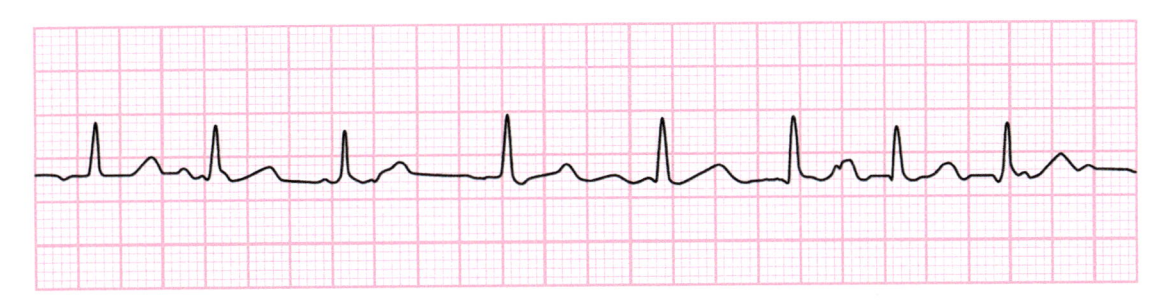

Figure 9.2 ECG of atrial fibrillation.

Management

Most patients with AF are managed in primary care with rate control and anticoagulation. There may be local treatment pathways to assist you in when to refer to secondary care. Some presentations of new AF may be acutely unwell with very fast heart rates (fast AF) and haemodynamic compromise. These should be managed via 999, with supportive care given in the primary care setting prior to ambulance arrival.

Patients with a clear new onset of AF in the last 48 hours should be offered cardioversion (NICE, 2021), which in practical terms will mean via a cardiology admission.

Rate Control

Rate control is important in managing symptoms, especially palpitations or dizziness where the ventricular rate is often high. Beta blockers (commonly bisoprolol as it is relatively cardio-selective) are commonly used, and doses should be titrated to achieve an acceptable rate. Other options include rate-limiting calcium channel blockers such as verapamil. Digoxin can also be considered if the patient is primarily sedentary. Drug choice, however, depends on patient comorbidities (NICE, 2021).

Anticoagulation

Anticoagulation is a mainstay of AF management which aims to reduce the threat of stroke. However, it comes with risks, in particular of major bleeding, such as intracranial haemorrhage or gastrointestinal bleeding. Patients were traditionally anticoagulated with warfarin; however, the difficulty in dosing and the need for regular checks of the international normalised ratio (INR) of clotting means that a newer group of drugs, known originally as novel oral anti-coagulants (NOACs) but more commonly now called direct oral anti-coagulants (DOACs), has become popular. These only require annual monitoring of renal function. Two of the most popular drugs in this class are rivaroxaban and apixaban (NICE, 2022a). Many studies have shown these drugs to be as good as warfarin for stroke prevention in AF, but research suggests that rivaroxaban is probably as likely, or more likely, than warfarin to have adverse bleeding effects. Apixaban has lower incidents of major bleeding than warfarin (Vinogradova et al., 2018).

NICE (2021) recommends that patients have an individual assessment of the risk of stroke using the CHA_2DS_2-VASc score (Table 9.1). Men with a score of 1 or more, and women with a score of 2 or more, should be offered anti-coagulation. The ORBIT (Table 9.2) score is now

CHAPTER 9   Cardiovascular Presentations

the preferred tool to assess bleeding risk (NICE, 2021), but the HAS-BLED (Table 9.3) is still in widespread use and it will likely take some time for clinicians, clinical systems and local guidance to catch up. The risk of bleeding should be assessed when making decisions about anti-coagulation therapy. These scores can be calculated by primary care clinical systems or websites such as the MDCalc website.

Table 9.1 CHA_2DS_2-VASc

Factor	Score
Age	< 65: 0; 65–74: 1; ≥ 75: 2
Sex	Female: 1
Congestive heart failure	1
Hypertension	1
Stroke/TIA/thromboembolism	2 (for any, do not score one for each)
Vascular disease (prior MI, peripheral arterial disease, aortic plaque)	1
Diabetes	1

Source: MDCalc, 2023a. Reproduced with kind permission.

Table 9.2   ORBIT

Haemoglobin (levels depend on sex)	2 if below normal
Age > 74	1
History of GI/intercranial bleeding or haemorrhagic stroke	2
GFR < 60 mL/min/1.73 m²	1
Treatment with antiplatelets	1

Source: MDCalc, 2023c. Reproduced with kind permission.

Table 9.3   HAS-BLED

Hypertension (uncontrolled, > 160 mmHg systolic)	1
Abnormal liver or renal function (dialysis, transplant; creatinine > 200 µmol/L; cirrhosis or bilirubin > 2 x normal with AST/ALT/ALP > 3 x normal)	1 or 2
Stroke history	1
Bleeding history or predisposition	1
Labile INR	1
Elderly > 65	1
Drugs (aspirin, non-steroidal anti-inflammatory drugs (NSAIDs)) alcohol	1 or 2

Source: MDCalc, 2023b. Reproduced with kind permission.

Presentations in Primary Care

> 📖 Patients should have their individual risk assessment discussed with them and should be supported to make a decision about whether to commence anti-coagulation. NICE produces a useful decision aid, and the SPARC Tool website (https://www.sparctool.com) can be very helpful to illustrate an individual's risk of stroke and bleeding with various treatment options.

Patient concordance should also be considered, as various studies show that around one-third of patients will stop taking their DOAC within three months (Jackevicius et al., 2017), and around 26% of warfarin patients stopped within a year (Fang et al., 2010). It might be expected that warfarin, with regular checks of INR and hence contact with health professionals, would have higher concordance, but this is not borne out in the studies. Similarly, it might be expected that rivaroxaban would have higher concordance due to the once-daily dosing, but in fact similar concordance rates are found across the DOACs.

Prescribers should note that DOACs have specific dosing changes in patients with reduced renal function and that this should use creatinine clearance rather than estimated glomerular filtration rate (eGFR). Creatinine clearance using the Cockcroft-Gault formula takes into account weight as well as age and sex to give a more refined measure of renal function.

Rhythm Control

Rhythm control is usually achieved by electrical cardioversion, and rhythm may be maintained by a variety of medications – primarily beta blockers, but also drugs such as dronedarone or amiodarone. Some studies, such as Wyse et al. (2002), recommend anti-coagulation be continued in rhythm-controlled patients, due to the difficulty in maintaining the patient in sinus rhythm (Van Gelder et al., 2002).

Rhythm control may be considered by secondary care in situations such as:

- AF with a reversible cause (for example, infection)
- Heart failure caused by AF
- Atrial flutter
- New onset (within 48 hours) of AF, or life-threatening haemodynamic instability
- Unsuccessful rate control or ongoing symptoms.

Some patients with infrequent paroxysmal AF, or where a trigger is known, may use 'pill in the pocket' medication approaches. Others may undergo cardiac ablation, possibly with a pacemaker, especially where drug treatment has failed or AF is causing heart failure. This will be managed in secondary care.

> 📖 NICE (2021) Atrial fibrillation: Diagnosis and management [online].
> AF is a huge topic and there are a considerable number of variables in considering both the underlying cause and the treatment options. This section presents a brief overview. This NICE guideline should be considered during investigation and treatment.

CHAPTER 9 Cardiovascular Presentations

Chest Pain

Aetiology

Chest pain represents about 1.5% of primary care presentations (Harskamp et al., 2019). Paramedics in primary care will need to be confident in diagnosing and differentiating the emergency presentations from the more minor presentations. It is not possible to rule out ACS on history and clinical examination alone, and a low threshold must be adopted for referral into hospital. Harskamp et al. (2019) report a sensitivity of 69% and a specificity of 89% for ACS by GPs. The emergency experience and 'spidey sense' or 'clinical gestalt' that paramedics bring to this area is invaluable. If there is any concern that the patient is presenting with ACS or that something 'just isn't right', then refer the patient to the emergency department (ED).

History and Examination

History is key to the assessment of chest pain. Main points to cover include:

- Onset
- Radiation
- Character (pleuritic, dull, ache, heavy, stabbing)
- Severity
- Palpitations
- Pallor, diaphoresis
- Breathlessness
- Nausea or vomiting
- Past medical history (especially cardiovascular risk factors such as hypertension, hyperlipidaemia or smoking)
- Family history of heart disease
- Palliating or provoking factors (such as on movement, leaning forwards)
- Tender chest wall
- Cough (including haemoptysis)
- Calf pain or swelling
- Recent chest wall injury or lifted something heavy.

Examination should consider:

- 'End-of-bed assessment' – do they look well or unwell? Colour, distress, diaphoresis
- Basic observations (pulse, blood pressure, respiratory rate, oxygen saturations, temperature)
- Jugular venous pressure
- Heart sounds and apex beat
- Lung sounds
- Any local tenderness to the chest wall
- Rashes (shingles)
- Pain on movement
- Calves for signs of deep vein thrombosis (DVT) – swelling, tenderness.

Presentations in Primary Care

Investigations

Obtain an ECG (remember that a normal ECG alone does not rule out ACS). Look for ECG changes suggestive of ACS (ST elevation, new left bundle branch block, STEMI mimics such as Wellens) but also of PE (sinus tachycardia, S1Q3T3 right heart strain), pericarditis, arrhythmia or signs of ischaemia. Blood tests may be indicated if there is an unclear cause for the pain; however, this depends on the diagnosis. Chest X-ray may be indicated.

Management

ACS or STEMI

In a primary care setting, this is likely to include aspirin, GTN and possibly morphine. Collate notes and an ECG for the ambulance crew, organise emergency admission.

Bornholm Disease

A viral illness (usually Coxsackie B) causing fever, headache and myalgia. It causes pain in the lower chest or upper abdomen which is usually pleuritic. There is usually localised tenderness. Treatment is supportive. Note: Coxsackie virus can also cause pericarditis and myocarditis, which may present similarly (Simon et al., 2014).

Costochondritis and Tietze's Syndrome

Inflammation of the costochondral or costo-sternal junctions of the ribs (where the ribs join the sternum with cartilage). There is usually a history of recent illness with lots of coughing, or of strenuous exercise. Examination will show a well-localised tenderness in this area. In Tietze's Syndrome there will also be a swelling – usually over the second or third ribs. Both usually self-resolve with simple analgesia such as NSAIDs, providing there are no contraindications.

Endocarditis

This is an infection of the endocardium. It is easy to miss and can present with a wide variety of clinical features (Gould et al., 2011). The disease will be managed in hospital. Diagnosis is complicated and should be made in hospital by a cardiologist and infection specialist working together. An echocardiogram is the key diagnostic test, and diagnosis may also be made based on blood cultures. The role of the primary care clinician is to retain a high index of suspicion and refer appropriately.

Patients at higher risk are those with valvular heart disease (for example, aortic stenosis), a history of valve replacement or congenital heart disease (other than repaired atrial septal defect, ventricular septal defect or patent ductus arteriosus), previous infective endocarditis and hypertrophic cardiomyopathy.

Guidelines recommend consideration of endocarditis in the following situations (from Gould et al., 2011: 271):

- Febrile illness and new regurgitation murmur
- Febrile illness, a pre-existing at-risk cardiac lesion without clinically obvious site of infection

CHAPTER 9 Cardiovascular Presentations

- Febrile illness with any of:
  - Predisposition and recent intervention with associated bacteraemia
  - Evidence of congestive heart failure
  - New conduction disturbance
  - Vascular or immunological symptoms: embolic event, Roth spots, splinter haemorrhage, Janeway lesions, Osler's nodes
  - New stroke
  - Peripheral abscesses (renal, splenic, cerebral, vertebral) of unknown origin
- Protracted history of sweats, weight loss, anorexia or malaise and an at-risk lesion
- New unexplained embolic event (cerebral or limb ischaemia)
- Unexplained, persistently positive blood cultures
- Intravascular catheter-related blood stream infection with persistently positive cultures 72 hours after catheter removal.

Musculoskeletal Chest Pain

A common primary care presentation, often with a preceding history of trauma or following an upper respiratory tract infection causing lots of coughing. The pain should be localised, tender and reproducible on palpation. Be cautious in excluding more sinister causes of chest pain. Treatment is with simple analgesia. Consider the use of oral non-steroidal such as ibuprofen or naproxen in suitable patients, as these will also help inflammation. However, many people are unable to take these. Topical non-steroidal anti-inflammatory drugs (NSAIDs) may be helpful in these patients.

Myocarditis

Inflammation of the myocardium. It can present with a variety of symptoms including fatigue, dyspnoea, chest pain, fever or palpitations. There may be a variety of ECG changes (including ST elevation or depression, or AV block). Causes are varied; 50% are idiopathic, others include infection and drugs. Suspected cases should be referred to cardiology as they will need further investigation and management. There is a risk of progression to heart failure (Longmore et al., 2014).

Pericarditis

Inflammation of the pericardium. It classically causes sharp sternal pain which is relieved by leaning forwards (reducing the pressure on the pericardium from the chest wall). Causes include infection, MI, malignancy, trauma, hypothyroidism and others. It has a distinctive ECG pattern of global concave ST elevation. Management should be referral to cardiology, pain relief (usually NSAIDs) and treatment of the underlying cause. Pericardial effusion can occur (Simon et al., 2014).

Deep Vein Thrombosis (DVT)

Aetiology

DVT is the formation of a clot in the deep venous system. Most commonly, it occurs in the calves, but it can also occur in the arms, the mesentery and the central sinus – which

Presentations in Primary Care

has come to prominence as a rare side effect of some COVID-19 vaccines (Lee and Lee, 2021).

History and Examination

A history of risk factors associated with DVT will raise clinical suspicion. These include (Simon et al., 2014: 290):

- Age over 40
- Smoking
- Obesity
- Recent long-distance travel
- Pregnancy or post-partum period
- Hormone usage (combined pill, HRT)
- Recent surgery or trauma
- Malignancy
- Heart failure
- Nephrotic syndrome
- Previous DVT
- Inflammatory bowel disease
- Inherited clotting disorders
- Chronic illness.

In the leg, it will present with unilateral leg swelling, pain and tenderness. There may also be warmth, pitting oedema and distended superficial veins.

> Consider differential diagnoses, which include:
>
> - Cellulitis
> - Baker's cyst
> - Thrombophlebitis
> - Lymphoedema
> - Other causes of leg swelling (venous obstruction, hypoproteinaemia)
> - Arthritis
> - Injury (muscle or ligamental tear, or fracture).

Investigations

Use the DVT Wells score (Table 9.4) to assess the probability of DVT. Note that the Wells score does not rule out DVT; it merely assesses the risk and guides further management (Wells et al., 1995). If you clinically suspect DVT, you need to follow the onward management steps to exclude it.

CHAPTER 9   Cardiovascular Presentations

Table 9.4   DVT Wells Score

Clinical feature	Points
Active cancer (current treatment or treatment within six months, or palliative)	1
Paralysis, paresis or recent plaster cast	1
Recently bedridden for > 3 days, or major surgery requiring general or reginal anaesthesia in the last 12 weeks	1
Localised tenderness along distribution of the deep venous system	1
Entire leg swollen	1
Calf swelling at least 3 cm larger than the other side	1
Pitting oedema on the affected leg only	1
Collateral superficial veins (non-varicose)	1
Previous DVT	1
Alternative diagnosis at least as likely as DVT	−2

A score of 2 points or more makes DVT likely; a score of 1 or less makes it unlikely.
Source: Reproduced from NICE, adapted from Wells et al. (1995).

Management

Local procedures will vary. If you have access, this will somewhat simplify the management of the 'unlikely' group of possible DVTs. Otherwise, you may need to send a blood sample for the laboratory to test d-dimer. Alternatively, you will likely have access to a DVT clinic where you can refer suspected DVTs and they will perform d-dimer and ultrasound testing. Note that d-dimer can be elevated for many reasons and definitive diagnosis is via ultrasound.

Your local pathway may require initiation of interim anti-coagulation (recommended by NICE when d-dimer or ultrasound is not available within four hours). This has traditionally been via low molecular weight heparin (LMWH) such as clexane, but off-label use of DOACs such as rivaroxaban or apixaban is becoming more common as this is significantly more convenient.

Fits, Faints and Funny Turns
Aetiology

Fits, faints and funny turns, including dizziness, is a presentation, along with headache, which often produces an internal sigh in primary care clinicians due to the complexity of these presentations. The differentials are enormous and include many benign but also many serious pathologies. Obtaining a history can be difficult, as patients may use 'dizzy' to describe several different symptoms, and if there was a loss of consciousness they may not be able to tell you a complete history.

This section focuses on cardiovascular causes of fits, faints and funny turns, including dizziness and syncope, which affects about 6% of the UK population (Simon et al., 2014).

Presentations in Primary Care

Other chapters will cover the other causes of these presentations, which might be neurological (Chapter 5 – Neurological Presentations in Primary Care), endocrine (Chapter 16 – Endocrine Presentations) or ENT (Chapter 7 – Eyes, Ears, Nose and Throat Presentations) in origin.

History and Examination

An excellent history is pivotal to these presentations. Key questions include:

- What were they doing immediately prior – in detail? Had they just finished urinating (micturition syncope), had they stood up too fast (postural hypotension), had they just had a shock (vasovagal syncope)?
- Where were they, when did it happen?
- How were they feeling? Was there an aura (epilepsy)? Did they feel lightheaded, clammy or nauseated (syncope). Did they have palpitations or chest pain?
- If they were 'dizzy', how did it feel – 'on a boat', 'like everything spinning', 'lightheaded' – distinguish rotational vertigo from light headedness or pre-syncope.
- What happened during the event? Did their vision blur, or do they seem to have passed out (everything went white, or black)? Did they lose consciousness? Can they remember everything?
- Is there any collateral history – did the patient jerk? How long for (remember myoclonic jerks can occur briefly in syncope)? What did the jerks look like? Did they lose consciousness?
- Did they bite their tongue or lose bowel or bladder control (more common in epilepsy, but absence does not rule out a seizure).
- What happened afterwards? If they were lying down, did they rapidly recover (more suggestive of syncope) or did it take some time (post-ictal). Were they confused or amnesic afterwards (usually very brief in syncope, longer in a post-ictal phase)?

Then consider general medical history, in particular:

- Previous similar events
- Cardiovascular and neurological history (including meningitis, encephalitis)
- Psychiatric history (anxiety, panic attacks)
- Family history of epilepsy or cardiac problems (Brugada, hypertrophic obstructive cardiomyopathy)
- Family history of sudden cardiac, or unexplained, death, especially in the young (suggestive of structural or electrical abnormality in the heart)
- Previous head injury
- Drug history – including recreational drug and alcohol usage.

A cardiovascular examination should be comprehensive, including:

- Pulse (rate, rhythm, strength)
- Respiratory rate
- Temperature
- ECG
- Heart sounds and apex beat

CHAPTER 9 Cardiovascular Presentations

- Carotid bruits
- Blood pressure (BP) (consider lying or standing BPs if postural hypotension is suspected).

Investigations

Investigations should always include an ECG. In the context of transient loss of consciousness (TLOC), NICE (2014) recommends that any of the following is a red flag if reported on an automated ECG interpretation:

- Complete left or right bundle branch block
- Any degree of heart block
- Long or short QT interval
- Any ST segment or T wave abnormalities.

The full list of abnormalities (if competent to interpret them) are:

- Inappropriate bradycardia
- Any ventricular arrhythmia (including ventricular ectopic beats)
- Long QT (corrected > 450 ms) and short QT (< 350 ms)
- Brugada syndrome
- Ventricular pre-excitation (a part of Wolff-Parkinson-White)
- Left or right ventricular hypertrophy
- Abnormal T wave inversion
- Pathological Q waves
- Atrial arrhythmia.

Consider blood tests, such as blood glucose levels, HbA1c and full blood count.

Management

> If there was a TLOC, then assess for red flags:
>
> - Any ECG abnormality (see above)
> - Heart failure history or signs on examination
> - TLOC on exertion
> - Family history of sudden cardiac death in people under 40.
>
> Any red flags should be referred for specialist assessment within 24 hours – local pathways will vary as to how this referral should be made. This might be via the cardiologist on call or same day emergency care (SDEC) or another pathway. Efforts should be made to make a formal referral rather than just sending the patient to the ED – the patient will receive care in a more appropriate timeframe, and pressure will be taken from our ED colleagues. Advice and Guidance (A&G) services are becoming increasingly common for obtaining assistance from secondary care consultants; however, they should be used with caution in this instance given NICE guidance for specialist assessment within 24 hours.

If the history is suggestive of a cardiac event but there is no diagnosis from above, or events are recurring, then consider a Holter monitor (a 24-hour, or longer, ECG). A cardiology referral may be required. In secondary care, sometimes an implantable loop recorder is used to capture infrequent events.

Remember that other serious pathology, such as pulmonary embolism, can also present with syncope.

A diagnosis of uncomplicated vasovagal syncope (simple faint) can be made when there is nothing to suggest an alternative diagnosis and the 'three Ps' suggest simple faint:

- Provoking factors (such as pain, medical procedure)
- Prodrome (sweating, pallor, feeling warm or hot)
- Posture (prolonged standing, similar events prevented by lying down).

Consider situational syncope when TLOC is consistently related to straining during urination, coughing or swallowing. Discuss possible triggers and how to avoid them (for example, urination whilst seated) and encourage the patient to keep a diary to record possible triggers.

Orthostatic hypotension occurs when blood pressure falls on change in position (often lying to standing). The person may present as having fallen, with dizziness or TLOC. It is defined as a systolic drop of 20 mmHg or diastolic drop of 10 mmHg within three minutes of standing. It occurs as a result of fluid shift on position change, where there is a failure of the baroreflex system (compensatory vasoconstriction and tachycardia), end-organ dysfunction or volume depletion.

Neurogenic causes include Parkinson's disease or other causes of central lesions – it can be an early sign of Parkinson's disease. Neuropathy (for example, from diabetes) can also cause orthostatic hypotension. Other non-neurogenic causes include cardiac problems (for example, from MI or valve disorders), adrenal insufficiency, volume depletion or vasodilation (for example, in infection). However, probably the most common causes are iatrogenic. Common drugs include:

- Diuretics
- Alpha-adrenoceptor blockers for hypertension or prostate disease (for example, doxazosin)
- Anti-hypertensives (such as ACE inhibitors or thiazide-like diuretics)
- Calcium channel blockers
- Insulin and levodopa can also cause a drop in some patients.

Medication-induced orthostatic hypotension can often be resolved with a thorough medication review; however, if other causes are suspected, or the situation cannot be managed with simple measures (such as drinking more, getting up slowly), referral to a falls clinic should be considered for a full multi-factorial assessment. Treatment options can include fludrocortisone or midodrine which help reduce the postural drop, as well as an overall assessment of reducing falls risk.

Refer for specialist assessment if no apparent cause can be identified or more serious disease such as arrhythmia or structural heart disease is suspected. Depending on the local situation, it may be appropriate to request additional investigations such as an echocardiogram or ambulatory ECG (also known as a '24-hour tape' or 'Holter monitor') at the same time as referral.

CHAPTER 9   Cardiovascular Presentations

Heart Failure

Aetiology

Heart failure can be defined as the inability of the heart to provide sufficient cardiac output to meet the demands from the body (Simon et al., 2014). Heart failure is the end-stage disease process for all cardiac disease, affecting 900,000 UK adults. It can be caused by many conditions, such as valve disease, chronic respiratory disease or congenital defects, but the major cause is coronary artery disease (Van Meter and Hubert, 2014).

Heart failure carries a high risk of mortality; 25–50% of patients will die within five years of diagnosis, reaching 75% if admission is needed. Death can also be sudden; 54% of people dying in the next 72 hours had been expected to live for at least six months (Longmore et al., 2014).

Heart failure is better described as 'pump failure'. The ventricles of the heart can no longer supply the body with enough blood. The body responds pathologically in several ways:

- Vasoconstriction and increased heart rate from sympathetic nervous system activation leads to:
  - Reduced ventricular filling (less time to fill between beats)
  - Renin-angiotensin-aldosterone system activation, which:
    o Increases blood pressure
    o Inhibits sodium and water diuresis, causing increased blood volume.

All this places greater strain on the heart muscle, which responds by enlarging (hypertrophy) like any muscle. This enlargement of the heart makes it harder for the heart to pump blood from the ventricles. This causes 'forward' effects (Van Meter and Hubert, 2014) of reduced blood flow to the organs, causing fatigue and shortness of breath on exertion.

Heart failure is usually divided into left- and right-sided failure:

- Left sided – because the left ventricle is not emptying as expected, blood backs up into the lungs causing pulmonary oedema
- Right sided – blood backs up into the systemic circulation, causing peripheral oedema.

It can also be classified as systolic failure, where the ventricle cannot pump with sufficient force to push blood into the circulation, and diastolic failure, where the ventricle cannot properly relax as it has become stiff, causing the ventricle to not properly fill during diastole.

History and Examination

Patients will likely present with the following symptoms:

- Cold intolerance
- Confusion
- Cough – may be nocturnal, or with white or pink frothy sputum (due to lung irritation from oedema)
- Dizziness
- Fatigue or lethargy

- History of cardiovascular disease (poorly controlled hypertension, MI, AF)
- History of severe respiratory disease (for example, advanced COPD)
- Orthopnoea (needing to sleep more upright due to pulmonary oedema) – ask if they have needed more pillows recently
- Paroxysmal nocturnal dyspnoea (seen more in acute failure but can occur in chronic disease) – waking suddenly in the night feeling very short of breath. Classically, patients will describe having to rush to the window or back door to get fresh air
- Peripheral oedema
- Shortness of breath on exertion
- Weight gain or loss, muscle wasting.

On examination, there may be:

- Bibasal crepitations
- Changes to heart sounds or presence of heaves
- Organomegaly
- Pallor
- Pitting peripheral oedema (ankle swelling)
- Raised jugular venous pressure
- Signs of enlarged heart such as a displaced apex beat
- Tachycardia.

Investigations

The key investigation is brain naturetic peptide (BNP) (most labs now measure the precursor peptide NT-pro-BNP), which is produced in the heart by myocytes in response to increased stretching of the ventricles. A rise in BNP levels is strongly predictive of heart failure, although like any laboratory value there are other reasons for a rise in BNP. It is worth noting that various drugs (especially ACE inhibitors, beta blockers and diuretics) can falsely lower the BNP value, as can obesity (Simon et al., 2014).

An NT-pro-BNP value of > 2000 ng/l is highly suggestive of heart failure and the patient should be referred urgently for an echocardiogram and specialist assessment. Intermediate values (400-2000 ng/l) should be referred to be seen within six weeks. If the NT-pro-BNP value is below 400 ng/l, heart failure is very unlikely and the diagnosis should be reconsidered (NICE, 2018). AF can raise NT-pro-BNP levels (Richards et al., 2013); NICE recognise this but do not advise using different cut-offs for heart failure investigation.

> BNP is a relatively expensive laboratory investigation, and labs may restrict access to it or require a clear clinical justification for performing it. Check with your local lab.

Also arrange:

- 12-lead ECG (look especially for signs of AF, hypertrophy or previous MI)
- Chest X-ray, which may show classic signs of heart failure or cardiomegaly but also helps exclude other causes of the symptoms

CHAPTER 9 Cardiovascular Presentations

- Laboratory investigations should include:
  - a full blood count (may see anaemia of chronic disease, or secondary polycythaemia)
  - urea and electrolytes (essential if diuretic treatment is being considered)
  - thyroid function as hypothyroidism can cause leg swelling (as reflected in the older name, myxoedema)
  - Lipid profile
  - HbA1C
  - Liver function.

You may also want to consider urinalysis, peak flow and spirometry (to assess for other causes of symptoms) (NICE, 2018).

An echocardiogram will assess for valve disease and also assess the systolic and diastolic function of the heart.

Management

Heart failure is usually classified using the New York Heart Association criteria (Simon et al., 2014).

If there is a rapid onset or worsening of symptoms (increasing breathlessness, fatigue, ankle or abdominal swelling and rapid weight gain), then consider emergency admission or same-day discussion with on-call cardiology.

All patients with heart failure should have a holistic assessment, including education about their disease (and the prognosis) and lifestyle advice. There is no need to routinely advise fluid, although it may be needed where patients drink large amounts of fluid resulting in dilutional hyponatraemia. Patients also do not need to specifically reduce their salt intake, although normal healthy living advice on salt content should be followed.

Most areas will have specialist heart failure nurses, who can provide this holistic assessment, ongoing support and monitoring. They will develop a self-management plan with the patient to promote maximal independence. They are often able to offer advice to other health professionals and will be a useful contact point.

The mainstay of drug treatment for heart failure is diuretic therapy, usually with a loop diuretic such as furosemide or bumetanide as the first line treatment.

> 💡 40 mg of furosemide is equivalent to 1 mg of bumetanide. Both work similarly, although if one is not working it can be worth trying the other. Always measure electrolytes carefully when changing diuretics or dose. Hyponatraemia is common, hypokalaemia less so. If hypokalaemia occurs but diuresis is succeeding, consider adding adjunctive mineralocorticoid receptor antagonists (such as spironolactone). Similarly, this can be useful if higher doses of furosemide alone are resulting in hyponatraemia. Close monitoring is required – see the British National Formulary (BNF).

Presentations in Primary Care

Diuretic therapy should be titrated to symptoms and may need to be altered up and down. Some patients manage this titration well themselves. Patients should monitor their weight daily and report significant changes to their GP practice as this will show if diuretic dosage is too high or low.

> The diuretic effects can be difficult for people to manage as they can be very pronounced. For this reason, diuretics are often advised to be taken in the morning (to avoid nocturia). Explain to patients that they can alter the timings to suit their lifestyles – for example, some patients give up activities they enjoy because they are in the morning and do not know they could safely take furosemide at lunchtime.

For patients with reduced ejection fraction, additional drugs should be used. The aim is to minimise the body's pathophysiological response explained above. ACE inhibitors should usually be started and titrated to the maximum tolerated dose (symptomatic of hypotension or postural hypotension indicate this). Monitor urea and electrolytes (U&Es) after each dose change, and check BP monthly for the first three months after the maximal dose has been reached, then six-monthly (NICE, 2018). Angiotensin receptor blockers can be used if Angiotensin-converting enzyme inhibitors (ACEIs) are not tolerated (see Hypertension section).

Beta blockers will reduce the effects of the sympathetic nervous system activation and should be started in a 'start low, go slow' manner with careful monitoring of heart rate and blood pressure.

Consider mineralocorticoid receptor antagonists (for example, spironolactone, eplerenone) in patients whose heart failure remains symptomatic. Carefully measure blood pressure and closely monitor electrolytes when initiating or changing dosage.

Specialist treatments include:

- Ivabradine – reduces heart rate by reducing the current in the sinoatrial node
- Sacubitril valsartan (brand name Entresto) – combination drug. Valsartan is an angiotensin receptor blocker and sacubitril acts to cause blood vessel dilation and reduced blood volume (by increasing sodium excretion)
- Hydralazine with nitrate – specialist option if ACE inhibitors not tolerated
- Digoxin – used for rate control where heart failure is worsening despite first line treatments.

All these treatments should only be started by heart failure specialists; however, you are likely to encounter patients on them.

Hyperlipidaemia

Aetiology

Approximately half the UK population have cholesterol levels above the recommended amount (BHF, 2023). This increases the risk of cardiovascular events through atherosclerosis. Except in very high levels of cholesterol, which are usually due to genetic factors in familial hyperlipidaemia, there is no specific acceptable value for cholesterol, but risk will depend on

CHAPTER 9 Cardiovascular Presentations

a multitude of other factors. However, a total cholesterol below 5.0 mmol/L is recommended (McGhee, 2009).

There are three main types of cholesterol (McGhee, 2009):

- HDL – high-density lipoprotein. This is 'good' cholesterol as it helps remove 'bad' cholesterol from the body.
- Non-HDL – 'bad' cholesterol. This used to be seen in lab reports as LDL but now includes all non-HDL cholesterol as it is all felt to be harmful.
- Triglycerides are stored in fat cells. Higher levels are associated with high-fat diets and obesity. They are also associated with atherosclerosis and with pancreatitis in very high levels.

Management of hyperlipidaemia falls into two main categories:

- Primary prevention – preventing a person having a cardiovascular event through lifestyle modification and drug therapy where appropriate
- Secondary prevention – where a cardiovascular event has already occurred, to reduce the risk of recurrence.

History and Examination

Most hyperlipidaemia is diagnosed by laboratory testing, but there may be indications in the history and examination that give clues. A history of smoking or diabetes increases risk, as does male sex and South Asian ethnic origin (BHF, 2023). A family history of both heart disease and hyperlipidaemia should always be assessed.

Clinical examination can be of limited value, but some clinical signs can lead to a suspicion of hyperlipidaemia (see the overall Assessment section at the start of the chapter).

Diagnosis is usually on the basis of laboratory testing. The test does not need to be a fasting sample. If you think statin therapy may be indicated, it is worth also checking liver function, thyroid function and renal function at the same time, as these should be checked prior to initiating treatment. This helps exclude secondary causes of hyperlipidaemia such as liver disease, hypothyroidism or uncontrolled diabetes (NICE, 2023).

The QRISK2 scoring tool should be used to calculate a person's overall cardiovascular risk. The result is given as a percentage, which represents the person's overall risk of having a cardiovascular event over the next ten years. People with possible familial hypercholesterolemia (total cholesterol above 9 mmol/L, non-HDL above 7.5 mmol/L) should be referred to specialist care. Triglycerides over 20 mmol/L should be urgently referred (where not due to poor diabetic control or alcohol). Values of 10–20 mmol/L should be repeated after 5–14 days and specialist advice obtained if persistently high.

QRISK2 can be calculated using primary care systems, or online at qrisk.org. Show the patient how it is calculated and show them the effect that lifestyle modification can have on their risk. This can be an effective way of supporting patients to make lifestyle modifications.

For primary prevention, lifestyle modification should be encouraged, and support offered by referrals into appropriate local services (such as stop-smoking clinics, weight loss, *et cetera*). If lifestyle modification is ineffective when lipids are rechecked after a few months, a lipid-lowering drug should be considered. Where secondary prevention is the concern, statins should be commenced straight away.

> Lipid modification therapy is likely to be lifelong or very long term and so a shared informed decision with the patient is important for concordance – there is a patient decision aid from NICE which can help with these discussions.

Management

Where a person has a 10% or greater QRISK2 score, they should be offered a high-intensity statin, usually atorvastatin 20 mg. The BNF gives a helpful list of statin dosages and intensities. Exceptions to this are people with chronic kidney disease or type 1 diabetics (refer to NICE guidance). Cholesterol should be checked again after three months, and if a 40% reduction is not achieved (and the patient is concordant), consider a dose increase. For secondary prevention, 80 mg is the normal starting dose.

Monitoring requirements are quite simple – ALT/AST liver enzymes should be measured after three months and again at 12 months but there is no need for ongoing monitoring (NICE, 2023).

> To assist patients with multiple long-term conditions, consider engagement with a local health and well-being group or input from a social prescribing link worker.

Hypertension

Aetiology

Hypertension affects more than 25% of the adult UK population, with a slightly higher prevalence in men. Hypertension plays a part in over half of all heart attacks and is a significant risk factor for kidney disease, stroke and dementia.

> Social determinants of health are important to consider as hypertension is significantly more common in deprived areas, and is a leading cause of premature death, behind smoking and poor diet which are also associated with deprivation (PHE, 2017).

Management of hypertension is hugely improved with good understanding of the renin-angiotensin-aldosterone system. This explains how the body maintains blood pressure normally, and aids understanding of how the various anti-hypertensive medications work.

Hypertension guidelines use various terms which it is useful to be familiar with, as outlined in Table 9.5.

Table 9.5 Terminology Associated with Hypertension

Stage	Clinic BP range	Home/ambulatory range
One	140/90–159/99	135/85–149/94
Two	160/100–179/119	Above 150/95
Three	Systolic over 180 mmHg or diastolic over 120 mmHg	

Source: NICE (2022b).

> 'White coat hypertension' is a well-known phenomenon where blood pressures in clinic are significantly higher than home readings. It is defined as a difference between clinic and home/ambulatory BPs of more than 20/10 mmHg.

History and Examination

History in a new diagnosis of hypertension can be difficult as it is only rarely symptomatic. One of the key issues in hypertension management is patient concordance with treatment – many patients will understandably not want to take a tablet when they feel well, especially one they will have to remain on for the rest of their lives. A new diagnosis of hypertension may also come alongside diagnosis of other disease processes such as hypocholesteraemia or diabetes, meaning more tablets.

Some patients will present feeling non-specifically unwell and are unable to characterise it. They may be getting low-level mild headaches. On examination, they may be found to be hypertensive.

> Red flags for hypertensive emergency include (Boffa et al., 2019):
> - Retinal haemorrhage
> - Papilloedema
> - New confusion
> - Chest pain
> - Heart failure
> - Acute kidney injury.

Possibly the more common scenario in primary care is a patient with a diagnosis of hypertension referred by the practice nurse or other professional as their blood pressure is found to be high during an annual check or opportunistically. The primary care paramedic thus needs to be able to manage both the initial diagnosis of hypertension and onward management in established hypertension, or at least be aware of the pharmaceutical treatments and their relation to the severity of the hypertension (a prescribing paramedic may not feel this is within their remit).

> ⚠ Be aware of the possibility of phaeochromocytoma (a rare tumour of adrenal gland tissue resulting in the release of too much epinephrine and norepinephrine) presenting with severe hypertension. This may be accompanied by postural hypotension, palpitations, tachycardia, abdominal pain, sweating or pallor.

Measurement

Given the lifelong consequences in terms of medication burden of a hypertension diagnosis, it is important that the initial diagnosis is correct. NICE recommends the following approach (NICE, 2022b):

- Measure blood pressure in both arms. If there is a difference of 15 mmHg, repeat. If on the second reading the difference remains, use the arm with the higher reading from then onwards.
- If blood pressure is 140/90 mmHg or higher, take a second reading. If this is significantly different from the first, take a third. Use the lower reading as the clinic blood pressure.
- If clinic blood pressure is between 140/90 mmHg and 180/120 mmHg, then ambulatory blood pressure monitoring should be arranged. Where this is not possible or the patient cannot tolerate it, encourage patients to do home blood pressure monitoring.

> 💡 It was once commonly taught that significant difference in bilateral blood pressures indicated an aneurysm. This is incorrect and physiologically implausible (unless a dissection occurred between the two subclavian artery branches on the aortic arch – at which point the patient is likely to be seriously ill).

Diagnosis of hypertension requires a clinic blood pressure of 140/90 mmHg or above and a daytime ambulatory pressure or home blood pressure average of 135/85 mmHg or above.

Home blood pressure monitoring should be twice a day, for four to seven days, with two readings morning and evening whilst seated and relaxed.

Investigations

New diagnoses should be assessed for end organ damage and cardiovascular risk. Most clinical systems will be able to calculate a risk score using systems such as QRISK. It is usually best to arrange these investigations whilst waiting for the results of ambulatory or home blood pressure monitoring.

Blood tests should include urea and electrolytes, eGFR, total and HDL cholesterol and HbA1C (to check for diabetes). Patients should have their urine dipped for haematuria and sent to the lab for an albumin creatinine ratio (ACR) to assess for renal damage.

CHAPTER 9 Cardiovascular Presentations

> 💡 Ensure you are familiar with your practice processes for handling urine samples and make clear in your notes that the sample is for an ACR. It can be frustrating for the clinician and the patient if the sample is mistakenly dipped and sent for microscopy. Urine for ACR needs to remain in a normal urine sample bottle, not one with boric acid preservative (as used for urinary tract infection).

Arrange an ECG, and examine, or refer for examination, for retinopathy – often it is best to recommend the patient has a sight test.

Management

Explain what hypertension is to patients – it can be useful to use analogies such as hard water furring up the pipes (and that happening faster at higher pressure). The analogy can then be extended to explain the risks of heart attack or stroke (if a bit of the limescale breaks off and blocks the pipe). With really high blood pressure, explain that blood vessels can burst (causing things like epistaxis).

Give patients lifestyle advice – in particular, stopping smoking (recall that nicotine is a vasoconstrictor), diet, exercise, dietary salt reduction and weight loss. Where possible, refer to local support services to increase the chances of success.

For patients with Stage 2 hypertension, NICE advises *offering* drug treatment (taking into account frailty). For patients under 80 with any of the below, *discuss* drug treatment:

- End organ damage
- Cardiovascular disease
- Renal disease
- Diabetes
- Risk score of 10% of more.

In Stage 3 hypertension, immediately start drug therapy whilst awaiting further investigation.

For patients over 80, or who are frail, careful assessment is needed of the risks and benefits. Some literature suggests that use of hypertensive and lower systolic blood pressure in the frail increases all-cause mortality (Streit et al., 2018).

Evidence suggests that anti-hypertensives may be more effective taken at bedtime, with a reduction in cardiovascular events of 45% (Hermida et al., 2019). This may also avoid an initial hypotensive effect. The evidence is still emerging, and the mechanism is unclear, but this is a low-risk intervention with a possible large benefit. Patients taking diuretics should usually take them in the morning to avoid excessive nocturia. When initiating anti-hypertensive therapy, also consider the need to optimise or initiate other cardiovascular risk prevention medication. Ensure diabetes is well controlled and re-emphasise the need for good glycaemic control. Consider starting a statin where appropriate.

Presentations in Primary Care

> Drug therapy should always follow current local and national guidelines, especially for specific patient groups (renal disease, type 1 diabetes or women with hypertension who are planning to become, or are, pregnant). Refer to the BNF or NICE guidelines for the most current treatment algorithm.

Drug Side Effects

> There are some common problems associated with hypertension management and it is well worth counselling patients on possible side effects. Calcium channel blockers may well cause ankle swelling which is dose dependent so may only be seen when the dose is increased. Warn the patient this may occur, and what to do, otherwise patients will panic and may seek urgent or even emergency advice.
>
> With ACE inhibitors, the most common side effect is a dry, persistent cough. The usual solution is to change to an angiotensin receptor blocker (ARB) medication such as losartan. The cough should slowly resolve (but may take some months).
>
> Diuretic therapy will make the patient urinate more often and this may be inconvenient or bothersome. Discuss this with patients before starting therapy as it may not be suitable for a number of reasons.

Peripheral Vascular Disease

Aetiology

Peripheral vascular disease (PVD) is a disease where there is abnormality of the veins or arteries outside of the heart; atheroma formation occurs, which may restrict or occlude the vessel. The most common cause of disease is atherosclerosis, which may result in pain, sensory problems or motor problems in the lower limbs in particular. Just as in the heart, partial and complete occlusions occur.

> A complete occlusion may result in loss of blood supply to a part of the body which can result in ulcers, necrosis, gangrene and ultimately possibly amputation.

History and Examination

There may be a history of circulatory disease, or cardiovascular risk factors. The patient may report a sensation of weakness in the limbs on exertion, sensory problems (numbness, pins and needles, burning) or skin problems such as ulcers.

> The Edinburgh Claudication Questionnaire (ECQ) is a validated questionnaire to diagnose intermittent claudication in epidemiological surveys of peripheral arterial disease (Leng and Fowkes, 1992).

235

CHAPTER 9 Cardiovascular Presentations

Examine in particular skin condition, peripheral pulses, reflexes and temperature. Patients with PVD may have thinner, shinier skin with hair loss. They may also have dependent rubor (redness) with elevation pallor; that is, their legs are red hanging down but go pale when lifted up (Simon et al., 2014; Van Meter and Hubert, 2014).

Investigations

The primary additional investigation is ankle-brachial pressure index, which compares the blood pressure in the brachial artery to that at the ankle. This can often be performed in primary care (Simon et al., 2014). Values ≤ 0.9 indicate PVD, although note that in some patients values may be falsely elevated – especially in diabetes or renal failure due to calcification (Morley et al., 2018).

Other tests should include blood tests: FBC, U&E, creatinine, eGFR, HbA1C, lipids (Simon et al., 2014).

Acute Limb Ischaemia

> Recall the '6 Ps' (Brearley, 2013) – there will be a sudden onset:
> - Pain
> - Pulseless
> - Pallor
> - Power loss
> - Paraesthesia
> - Perishing cold.

> ❗ These patients should be referred urgently to the vascular team as the condition is limb threatening.

Intermittent Claudication

This is pain reproducible after a period of exertion, often feeling like cramp. ABPI ≤ 0.9 in the affected limb supports the diagnosis. Pain may be in the calf, thigh or buttock depending on the location of the atheroma.

Management includes graduated exercise (trying to walk a bit further each day to the point of maximal pain), anti-platelets and management of lipids and other cardiovascular risk factors.

Critical Limb Ischaemia

This is defined as a history of peripheral artery disease and one or more of:
- Ulceration
- Gangrene
- Rest pain in the foot for over two weeks.

Patients may report relief by hanging the leg out of bed at night (Morley et al., 2018).

ABPI ≤ 0.5 is indicative of critical limb ischaemia. This should be referred urgently to the vascular team.

Presentations in Primary Care

Pulmonary Embolism (PE)

Aetiology

Pulmonary embolism (PE) is a clot within the pulmonary system. They usually arise as the result of a clot elsewhere (DVT) breaking off and travelling to the lungs, although other causes such as sepsis, neoplasm or MI exist (Longmore et al., 2014). The rate of PE is approximately 60–70 per 100,000 people (approximately half the rate of DVT), although this is thought to be an underestimate (Bělohlávek et al., 2013). Untreated PE carries a mortality rate of 30%, but with treatment this falls to 8% (Bělohlávek et al., 2013).

History and Examination

PE is one of the most difficult diagnoses on clinical grounds alone. The most common symptoms include dyspnoea, cough and tachypnoea occurring in around 60% of patients, whilst pleuritic pain and haemoptysis occur in 8% and 12% respectively. Even symptoms that might be regarded as making a PE less likely, such as fever, occur in 22% of patients (Ji et al., 2017), although other studies put this much lower, at 7% (Miniati et al., 1999). The latter study is more reliable as it required angiographic confirmation of all PEs – Ji et al. used the presence of DVT with PE symptoms in some patients. Tachycardia is the most common abnormality, seen in 44% of patients. Sudden-onset dyspnoea, chest pain and fainting (on their own or in combination) were present in 96% of patients with PE (Miniati et al., 1999). COVID-19 increases the risk of thromboembolism; you should have a low threshold for referring these patients for investigation for PE. The risk can continue after hospital discharge and apparent recovery (Kanso et al., 2020).

A general clinical examination should be performed to include a complete set of clinical observations and a respiratory examination.

Investigations

ECG changes can be very varied and are relatively rare – the classic sign of S1Q3T3 is seen in 19% of patients, whilst other signs such as T wave inversion in the precordial leads are somewhat more common at 23% (Ji et al., 2017). S1Q3T3 refers to a specific ECG pattern with a large S wave in lead 1 and a Q wave and inverted T wave in lead 3.

> C. Till (2021) *Clinical ECGs in Paramedic Practice*. Bridgwater: Class Professional Publishing.
> Check out this book for an example of a PE shown on an ECG.

Point-of-care d-dimer tests, if available, may assist with diagnosis in the 'unlikely' group (although there are many reasons for an elevated d-dimer, such as infection).

Management

In patients with a low clinical possibility of PE, estimated by the clinician to be below 15% considering medical history and examination, the PE rule-out criteria (PERC) score can be used to help make decisions on whether further investigations are needed (NICE, 2020). Only if all factors are absent can PE safely be ruled out clinically.

- Age ≥ 50
- Heart rate ≥ 100
- Oxygen saturations < 95%
- Unilateral leg swelling
- Haemotypsis
- Recent surgery or trauma (within four weeks, requiring general anaesthetic)
- Prior PE or DVT
- Hormone use (oral contraceptive use, hormone replacement therapy or oestrogenic hormone use). Note some therapies for prostate cancer can be oestrogenic.

If PE is suspected, then use the two-level PE Wells score (note this is different to the Wells score for DVT) (Table 9.6).

Patients in the 'PE likely' category should be referred to hospital using your local procedures. This may be via the ED or an ambulatory care or SDEC) process. They are likely to require imaging, usually a computerised tomography pulmonary angiogram (CTPA).

Management of patients in the 'PE unlikely' category should have a d-dimer test – again this may be in hospital or more locally depending on local referral pathways. It is likely there will be a delay obtaining blood tests and their results in the community – note that NICE recommend a d-dimer within four hours (with interim anticoagulation if this is not possible).

Table 9.6 Two-Level PE Wells Score

Clinical feature	Points
Clinical signs and symptoms of DVT (minimum of leg swelling and pain with palpation of the deep veins)	3
An alternative diagnosis is less likely than PE	3
Heart rate more than 100 beats per minute	1.5
Immobilisation for more than three days or surgery in the previous four weeks	1.5
Previous DVT/PE	1.5
Haemoptysis	1
Malignancy (on treatment, treated in the last six months or palliative)	1
Clinical probability simplified score	Points
PE likely	More than 4 points
PE unlikely	4 points or less

Source: Reproduced from NICE (2020).

> Clinical rules such as PERC and Wells can help assess the likelihood of a PE but remember that they are intended to be used alongside d-dimer testing and clinical intuition and judgement.

Chapter Summary

This chapter has covered a broad range of cardiovascular topics which commonly occur in primary care. History is the key for cardiovascular presentations, as for all medical problems. You have less immediate access to tests and investigations in primary care and must decide which ones to undertake based on your history. Develop your abilities to take a really good history – in the words of Osler, 'listen to the patient, he [sic] is telling you the diagnosis' (Pitkin, 1998).

Chronic disease management such as hypertension and hyperlipidaemia are core primary care work, and likely your colleagues will have significant expertise in their management. Draw on the expert knowledge of the practice nurses, GPs and practice pharmacists in these areas.

Whilst this may be the bread-and-butter clinical presentation for ambulance paramedics, chest pain is a minefield with a very broad range of differential diagnoses, some of which you may not have seen in an ambulance service context. If in doubt, consult senior colleagues. Most chest pain presenting to primary care is not ACS – but some will be, and you should maintain a high index of suspicion.

Faints, fits and funny turns can be very difficult to diagnose and can confuse the most expert of practitioners. Take a careful history, then if in doubt, ask.

Case Study 1

You are asked to see a 56-year-old man who came in for his annual diabetes review and has been asked for your review following the results.

History

PC: Abnormal blood pressure.
HxPC: The practice nurse noted his blood pressure was somewhat high at 158/88. He arranged an ambulatory blood pressure monitor for him, which showed an average blood pressure of 150/76. He has come to see you to discuss management of his blood pressure.
PMHx/SHx: Type 2 diabetes, hyperlipidaemia.
DHx: Metformin 500 mg BD, atorvastatin 20 mg. Concordant with both medications. No known drug or food allergies.
SHx: Senior manager, lives with his partner and their two children. Drinks socially at weekends. Never smoked tobacco. Recreational drug usage (cocaine) in his 20s.
FHx: Mother had hypertension and type 2 diabetes. Father had hypertension and died from lung cancer (smoker). No siblings.
ROS: Unremarkable, clinical observations normal apart from an elevated blood pressure of 148/82.

CHAPTER 9 Cardiovascular Presentations

Examination
- He has recently had routine monitoring bloods for his diabetes, showing good renal function, no proteinuria and good diabetic control (HbA1c 50). His cholesterol is elevated, and his QRISK score is 11%.

Preferred Diagnosis
- Essential hypertension.

Management
- He is at higher risk of complications of hypertension due to his diabetes and poor cholesterol levels. He is offered ramipril at an initial dose of 5 mg (an ACE inhibitor is preferred despite his age due to his diabetes). Having explained the QRISK score to him, his statin is up-titrated to 40 mg. His blood pressure and renal function is checked after two weeks and he is found to have a blood pressure of 126/70.

Case Study 2

You see an urgent appointment for a 72-year-old woman who has been experiencing palpitations for the last two weeks.

History

PC: Palpitations.
HxPC: Palpitations do not make her dizzy, but she finds she needs to sit down whilst they occur. They last for 10–20 minutes at a time. She does not become short of breath and does not have any chest pain. She describes the palpitations as feeling like her heart is racing. She is worried she may have something wrong with her heart.
PMHx/SHx: Anxiety, hypertension.
DHx: Sertraline 100 mg, amlodipine 5 mg.
SHx: Recently lost her wife to cancer. She describes her as 'her rock'. They had been together for 40 years. Social drinker and has been drinking a bit more recently 'to help me sleep'. Smoked until 20 years ago – 30 pack years. She has not used recreational drugs since smoking 'some special cigarettes' in the 1960s.
FHx: She was adopted and doesn't know her family history.
ROS: She appears anxious and nervous. She is well dressed. There is no evidence of shortness of breath, she has a normal skin colour and she appears to have a normal BMI.

Examination
- Vital signs: BP 132/75 mmHg; HR 116 bpm (irregularly irregular); RR 14/min; SpO_2 98%.

Case Study 2

- Auscultation: Chest is clear, normal heart sounds.
- ECG shows an irregularly irregular rhythm at a rate of 116 bpm with no visible P waves.

Preferred Diagnosis
- AF. Although there is a history of anxiety and presents as anxious, which may have worsened due to her bereavement, her examination and ECG are suggestive of AF.

Differential Diagnoses
- Anxiety (possibly due to bereavement).

Management
- Explain the diagnosis.
- Assess her risk of serious bleeding or stroke due to AF:
  - ORBIT score of 0
  - HAS-BLED of 2 (due to her increased alcohol consumption)
  - CHA_2DS_2-VASc of 3.
- She feels able to cut down on her drinking and decides to start anticoagulation.
- Start apixaban 5 mg bd and bisoprolol 2.5 mg od.
- Bloods to exclude other causes (thyroid function, full blood count, liver function, renal function, electrolytes).
- Review in a week to check heart rate is controlled. She feels much better and the palpitations have stopped.
- Signpost to counselling support about bereavement.

> Careful consideration needs to be given to starting a DOAC whilst on an SSRI (such as sertraline). SSRIs can increase the risk of bleeding. The patient did not feel able to cope without her sertraline at present, but is very worried about having a stroke, so you agree to start apixaban with a proton-pump inhibitor (lansoprazole 15 mg od) to try to reduce this risk. Once her mental health has improved, consideration could be given to changing to an alternative medication such as mirtazapine, which does not have this interaction.

> To assist with those who need support with their mental health, are lonely or isolated or have complex social needs which affect their well-being, consider engagement with a local health and well-being group or input from a social prescriber or link worker.

CHAPTER 9 Cardiovascular Presentations

Case Study 3

A 25-year-old patient walks into reception with chest pain, and you are alerted to his presence by the emergency bell from reception.

History

PC: Dry cough and chest pain.
HxPC: 3/7 history of an ongoing dry cough and chest pain. He recently had a cold (with a negative COVID-19 PCR). The pain is mainly in his lower chest and is worse on deep inspiration but is alleviated by leaning forwards.
PMHx/SHx: None. No surgical history.
DHX: He has been taking paracetamol and ibuprofen for the pain. Fully vaccinated against COVID-19.
SHx: Social drinker, drinks somewhat to excess on the weekend. Occasionally smokes cannabis.
FHx: Nil of note. Both parents still alive, no medications. One sibling who is well.
ROS: Looks well but is uncomfortable when seated.

Examination

- Vital signs: BP 122/74 mmHg; HR 65 bpm (regular); RR 13/min; SpO$_2$ 100% on air; temperature 36.8°C.
- Auscultation: Chest is clear. He has some mild chest wall tenderness over the right side and sternal area. Heart sounds are normal (I+II+0).
- An ECG shows concave ST elevation in all leads.
- There is no calf swelling or tenderness.

Preferred Diagnosis

- Pericarditis. The patient's history of recent illness, pain location and nature and ECG are typical of this. Costochondritis or Bornholm disease would be consistent with the finding of chest wall tenderness and recent illness but could also be consistent with frequent coughing.
- Pulmonary embolism is less likely given the presentation, lack of dyspnoea and lack of risk factors. The PERC score is 0, which means PE can be safely ruled out.

Differential Diagnoses

- Pericarditis (based on ECG)
- Costochondritis
- Bornholm disease
- Pulmonary embolism.

Management

- Refer to cardiology.
- Management of pain and symptoms with NSAIDs.

References

Barra, S. and Fynn, S. (2015) Untreated atrial fibrillation in the United Kingdom: Understanding the barriers and treatment options. *Journal of the Saudi Heart Association* 27(1): 31–43.

Bělohlávek, J., Dytrych, V. and Linhart, A. (2013) Pulmonary embolism, part I: Epidemiology, risk factors and risk stratification, pathophysiology, clinical presentation, diagnosis and nonthrombotic pulmonary embolism. *Experimental and Clinical Cardiology* 18(2): 129–138.

Boffa, R., Constanti, M., Floyd, C. et al. (2019) Hypertension in adults: Summary of updated NICE guidance. *British Medical Journal* 21(367): l5310.

Brearley, S. (2013) Acute leg ischaemia. *British Medical Journal* 346: f2681.

British Heart Foundation (BHF) (2023) BHF statistics factsheet – UK. Available at: https://www.bhf.org.uk/-/media/files/research/heart-statistics/bhf-cvd-statistics-uk-factsheet.pdf?la=en (accessed 1 February 2023).

Brown, H. (2022) Ten most common conditions seen by GPs. *British Journal of Family Medicine*. Available at: https://www.bjfm.co.uk/ten-most-common-conditions-seen-by-gps (accessed 1 February 2023).

Canto, J., Rogers, W., Goldberg, R. et al. (2012) Association of age and sex with myocardial infarction symptom presentation and in-hospital mortality. *Journal of the American Medical Association* 307(8): 318–322.

Chambless, L., Fuchs, F., Linn, S. (1990) The association of corneal arcus with coronary heart disease and cardiovascular disease mortality in the Lipid Research Clinics Mortality Follow-up Study. *American Journal of Public Health* 80(10): 1200–1204.

Douglas, G., Nicol, E. and Robertson, C. (2009) *Macleod's Clinical Examination*. 12th edn. Edinburgh: Elsevier Churchill Livingstone.

Fang, M.C., Go, A.S., Chang, Y. et al. (2010) Warfarin discontinuation after starting warfarin for atrial fibrillation. *Circulation: Cardiovascular Quality and Outcomes* 3(6): 624–631.

Gould, F., Denning, D., Elliott, T. et al. (2011) Guidelines for the diagnosis and antibiotic treatment of endocarditis in adults: A report of the Working Party of the British Society for Antimicrobial Chemotherapy. *Journal of Antimicrobial Chemotherapy* 67(2): 269–289.

Harskamp, R.E., Laeven, S.C., Himmelreich, J.C. et al. (2019) Chest pain in general practice: A systematic review of prediction rules. *BMJ Open* 9(2): e027081.

Hermida, R., Crespo, J., Domínguez-Sardiña, M. et al. (2019) Bedtime hypertension treatment improves cardiovascular risk reduction: The Hygia Chronotherapy Trial. *European Heart Journal* 41(48): 4565–4576.

Jackevicius, C.A., Tsadok, M.A., Essebag, V. et al. (2017) Early non-persistence with dabigatran and rivaroxaban in patients with atrial fibrillation. *Heart* 103(17): 1331–1338.

Ji, Q., Wang, M., Su, C. et al. (2017) Clinical symptoms and related risk factors in pulmonary embolism patients and cluster analysis based on these symptoms. *Nature – Scientific Reports* 7(1): 14887.

Kanso, M., Cardi, T., Marzak, H. et al. (2020) Delayed pulmonary embolism after COVID-19 pneumonia: A case report. *European Heart Journal – Case Reports* 4(6): 1–4.

Kavoussi, H., Ebrahimi, A., Rezaei, M. et al. (2016) Serum lipid profile and clinical characteristics of patients with xanthelasma palpebrarum. *Anais Brasileiros de Dermatologia* 91(4): 468–471.

Lee, E.-J. and Lee, A.I. (2021) Cerebral venous sinus thrombosis after vaccination: The UK experience. *The Lancet* 398(10306): 1107–1109.

CHAPTER 9 Cardiovascular Presentations

Leng, G.C. and Fowkes, F.G. (1992) The Edinburgh Claudication Questionnaire: An improved version of the WHO/Rose Questionnaire for use in epidemiological surveys. *Journal of Clinical Epidemiology* 45(10): 1101–1109.

Lichtman, J., Leifheit, E., Safdar, B. et al. (2018) Sex differences in the presentation and perception of symptoms among young patients with myocardial infarction. *Circulation* 137(8): 781–790.

Longmore, M., Wilkinson, I., Baldwin, A. et al. (2014) *Oxford Handbook of Clinical Medicine*. 9th edn. Oxford: Oxford University Press.

Mallinson, T. and Brooke, D. (2017) Frank's Sign as a clinical marker of cardiovascular disease. *Journal of Paramedic Practice* 9(1): 8–10.

McGhee, M. (2009) *A Guide to Laboratory Investigations*. Oxford: Radcliffe.

MDCalc (2023) CHA_2DS_2-VASc Score for Atrial Fibrillation Stroke Risk. Available at: https://www.mdcalc.com/calc/801/cha2ds2-vasc-score-atrial-fibrillation-stroke-risk (accessed 14 April 2023).

MDCalc (2023) HAS-BLED Score for Major Bleeding Risk. Available at: https://www.mdcalc.com/calc/807/has-bled-score-major-bleeding-risk (accessed 14 April 2023).

MDCalc (2023) ORBIT Bleeding Risk Score for Atrial Fibrillation. Available at: https://www.mdcalc.com/calc/10227/orbit-bleeding-risk-score-atrial-fibrillation (accessed 14 April 2023).

Miniati, M., Prediletto, R., Formichi, B. et al. (1999) Accuracy of clinical assessment in the diagnosis of pulmonary embolism. *American Journal of Respiratory and Critical Care Medicine* 159(3): 864–871.

Morley, R., Sharma, A., Horsch, A. et al. (2018) Peripheral artery disease. *British Medical Journal* 360: j5842.

National Institute for Health and Care Excellence (NICE) (2014) Transient loss of consciousness ('blackouts') in over 16s [CG109]. Available at: https://www.nice.org.uk/guidance/cg109/ (accessed 1 February 2023).

National Institute for Health and Care Excellence (NICE) (2016a) Recent-onset chest pain of suspected cardiac origin: Assessment and diagnosis [CG95]. Available at: https://www.nice.org.uk/Guidance/CG95 (accessed 1 February 2023].

National Institute of Health and Care Excellence (NICE) (2016b) Stable angina: Management [CG126]. Available at: https://www.nice.org.uk/guidance/cg126/ (accessed 1 February 2023).

National Institute for Health and Care Excellence (NICE) (2018) Chronic heart failure in adults: Diagnosis and management. Available at: https://www.nice.org.uk/guidance/ng106 (accessed 1 February 2023).

National Institute for Health and Care Excellence (NICE) (2020) Venous thromboembolic diseases: diagnosis, management and thrombophilia testing [NG158]. Available at: https://www.nice.org.uk/guidance/NG158 (accessed 1 February 2023).

National Institute for Health and Care Excellence (NICE) (2021) Atrial fibrillation: Diagnosis and management [NG196]. Available at: https://www.nice.org.uk/guidance/ng196 (accessed 1 February 2023).

National Institute for Health and Care Excellence (NICE) (2022a) Clinical Knowledge Summaries: Anticoagulation – Oral: Management. Available at: https://cks.nice.org.uk/topics/anticoagulation-oral/management/ (accessed 1 February 2023).

National Institute for Health and Care Excellence (NICE) (2022b) Hypertension in adults: Diagnosis and management [NG136]. Available at: https://www.nice.org.uk/guidance/ng136/ (accessed 1 February 2023).

References

National Institute for Health and Care Excellence (NICE) (2023) Cardiovascular disease: Risk assessment and reduction, including lipid modification [CG181]. Available at: https://www.nice.org.uk/guidance/cg181/ (accessed 21 February 2023).

Ngan, V. and Stanway, A. (2005) Xanthoma. *Dermnet NZ*. Available at: https://dermnetnz.org/topics/xanthoma/ (accessed 1 February 2023).

Odutayo, A., Wong, C., Hsiao, A. et al. (2016) Atrial fibrillation and risks of cardiovascular disease, renal disease, and death: Systematic review and meta-analysis. *British Medical Journal* 354: i4482.

Pitkin, R.M. (1998) Listen to the patient. *British Medical Journal* 316(7139): 1252.

Public Health England (PHE) (2017) Health matters: Combating high blood pressure. Available at: https://www.gov.uk/government/publications/health-matters-combating-high-blood-pressure/health-matters-combating-high-blood-pressure#:~:text=High%20blood%20pressure%20affects%20more,over%20the%20last%20few%20years (accessed 1 February 2023).

Public Health England (PHE) (2020) Atrial fibrillation prevalence estimates for local populations. Available at: https://www.gov.uk/government/publications/atrial-fibrillation-prevalence-estimates-for-local-populations (accessed 1 February 2023).

Richards, M., Somma, S.D., Mueller, C. et al. (2013) Atrial fibrillation impairs the diagnostic performance of cardiac natriuretic peptides in dyspneic patients results from the BACH study (Biomarkers in ACute Heart Failure). *JACC: Heart Failure* 1(3): 192–199.

Salisbury, C., Procter, S., Stewart, K. et al. (2013) The content of general practice consultations: Cross-sectional study based on video recordings. *British Journal of General Practice* 63(616): e751–e759.

Simon, C., Dorp, F. and Everitt, H. (2014) *Oxford Handbook of General Practice*. 4th edn. Oxford: Oxford University Press.

Streit, S., Poortvliet, R. and Gussekloo, J. (2018) Lower blood pressure during antihypertensive treatment is associated with higher all-cause mortality and accelerated cognitive decline in the oldest-old. Data from the Leiden 85-plus Study. *Age and Ageing* 47(4): 545–550.

Till, C. (2021) *Clinical ECGs in Paramedic Practice*. Bridgwater: Class Professional Publishing.

Van Gelder, I.C., Hagens, V.F., Bosker, H.A. et al. (2002) A comparison of rate control and rhythm control in patients with recurrent persistent atrial fibrillation. *New England Journal of Medicine* 347(23): 1834–1840.

Van Meter, K. and Hubert, R. (2014) *Gould's Pathophysiology for the Health Professions*. 5th edn. St. Louis, WA: Elsevier.

Vinogradova, Y. Coupland, C., Hill, T. et al. (2018) Risks and benefits of direct oral anticoagulants versus warfarin in a real world setting: Cohort study in primary care. *British Medical Journal (Clinical Research ed.)* 362: k2505.

Wells, P.S., Hirsh, J., Anderson, D.R. et al. (1995) Accuracy of clinical assessment of deep-vein thrombosis. *Lancet* 345(8961): 1326–1330.

Wyse, D.G., Waldo, A.L., DiMarco, J.P. et al. (2002) A comparison of rate control and rhythm control in patients with atrial fibrillation. *New England Journal of Medicine* 347(23): 1825–1833.

Gastrointestinal and Hepatic Presentations

Ant Kitchener

10

Within This Chapter

Alimentary-related common presentations
- Change in bowel habit – blood in stools, mucus in stools
- Coeliac disease
- Constipation
- Diarrhoea
- Inflammatory bowel disease (IBD)
- Irritable bowel syndrome (IBS)
- Peptic ulcers
- Poor appetite
- Rectal bleeding
- Stoma issues

Hepatic-related common presentations
- Alcohol use disorder (alcohol dependency syndrome)
- Alpha-1 antitrypsin deficiency (A1AD)
- Cholecystitis
- Haemochromatosis
- Hepatitis
- Non-alcoholic fatty liver disease (NAFLD)
- Pancreatitis
- Primary biliary cirrhosis (PBC)
- Primary sclerosing cholangitis (PSC)
- Wilson's disease

Introduction

Abdominal complaints are a frequent consultation within primary care and form part of a common, yet complex, spectrum from trivial to sinister pathologies. Pain, bloating, reflux, distension and bleeding are among the leading reasons for abdominal-related consults (Hunt et al., 2013). Routine screening of seemingly well patients may also present abnormalities, which may have a gastrointestinal (GI) origin and may warrant further investigations, for example deranged liver or renal blood tests. Detection of hepatic disease is commonly difficult due to its insidious and often asymptomatic development. Nevertheless, groups of symptoms such as jaundice, dark urine, pale stools, generalised itching and hepatitis-related abdominal pain can alert the paramedic to potential hepatic involvement.

CHAPTER 10 Gastrointestinal and Hepatic Presentations

Assessment

It is likely that the paramedic in primary care will have vast experience of abdominal examination, and this short section serves as a refresher to those skills. As autonomous clinicians working in primary care, the main function of an abdominal assessment is to identify any red flags and to increase or decrease clinical suspicions identified during the initial history taking.

Blood Tests

Liver function tests (LFTs) are a common set of primary care investigations for abdominal complaints (Table 10.1) and may in many cases be the first sign of abdominal pathology. However, it is worth noting that their results are non-specific. Second-line liver investigations should be made where the origin of the LFT abnormality is unclear (Table 10.2), as well as correlating with broader blood tests, imaging and stool samples.

Table 10.1 Common Primary Care Investigations: Liver Function Tests

Chemical	Use	Common pathology	Notes
Alanine transaminase (ALT)	Is used by the body to metabolise protein. If there is hepatic damage or poor liver function, ALT may be released into the blood and detected on serum blood testing	A high result could be a sign of liver stress (such as in alcohol binge) and very high levels may indicate viral hepatitis, ischaemic hepatitis or injury from drugs or other chemicals, amongst other pathologies	
Aspartate aminotranferase (AST)	Is an enzyme found in several parts of the body (heart, brain, pancreas, liver and muscles). When there is hepatic damage, a high result may indicate a liver damage pathology. As this is non-specific, viewing in combination with ALT is more helpful	Liver or muscle disease, in the absence of a raised ALT and/or bilirubin, is less likely to be hepatic disease in origin	

Chemical	Use	Common pathology	Notes
Alkaline phosphatase (Alk Phos)	Is an enzyme found in the bones, bile ducts and liver. This may indicate liver disease, an outflow blockage or bone destruction	May be liver inflammation or an obstruction such as gallstones or pancreatic carcinoma, amongst other pathologies. If the other liver chemicals are normal, also consider destructive bony pathology	If raised, repeat with a fasting sample including a gamma-glutamyl transferase (GGT) screen, AST and full blood count. If normal GGT, consider vitamin D deficiency or Paget's disease. If raised GGT, consider second-line investigations to assess for fatty liver, viral hepatitis, alcoholic liver disease fibrosis, primary sclerosing cholangitis, primary biliary cholangitis, autoimmune hepatitis, gallstone disease, hepatic vascular disorders and hepatic metabolic disorders
Albumin	Is the main protein made by the liver. Albumin nourishes tissue and transport hormones, vitamins and other processes. It is also important in osmotic balance	Low albumin may be present in malnourished patients (including chronic alcohol use disorders, chronic respiratory disease, etc.), or may be a sign of liver cirrhosis or cancer	
Bilirubin	Is a waste product from the breakdown of red cells. Normally this would be broken down by the liver. In liver disease, there may be excess bilirubin due to poor breakdown. Destruction of red cells may also cause bilirubin release (haemolysis). It is responsible for jaundice, stool and urine coloration and globalised itch seen in liver disease	Consider pre-hepatic, intrahepatic and post-hepatic causes	If raised bilirubin **and** raised ALP or AST or ALT and jaundice: immediate referral to acute medical assessment is required. If no jaundice, then urgent referral to hepatology/gastroenterology is required. If asymptomatic, consider if the patient is anaemic and consider haemolysis screen

CHAPTER 10   Gastrointestinal and Hepatic Presentations

Table 10.2   Second-line Tests for Abnormal LFTs

Test	Pathology
Serology for hepatitis B and C	Hepatitis B virus, hepatitis C virus
Serum iron and total iron binding capacity	Increased iron load suggests haemochromatosis
Serum caeruloplasmin levels	Decreased levels suggest Wilson's disease
Serum protein electrophoresis	Increased polyclonal immunoglobulin suggests autoimmune hepatitis; decreased alpha-globulin suggests alpha-1 antitrypsin deficiency
Liver autoimmune serology	Especially in females. Autoimmune hepatitis
Full blood count	Anaemia
Thyroid function tests	Thyroid disease
HBa1c	Diabetes screen
Anti-TTG	Coeliac screen

GI Presentations in Primary Care

Change in Bowel Habit: Blood in Stools, Mucus in Stools
Aetiology

A change in bowel habit can be caused by a range of psychosocial as well as pathological causes. Conditions such as irritable bowel syndrome (IBS) may have an unknown cause but often have triggers that can lead to constipation, bloating or diarrhoea presentations, or fluctuations of this range (Chey et al., 2015). Where a change of bowel habit persists for longer than six months and is associated with abdominal pain or bloating, a diagnosis of IBS should be considered once other pathologies are excluded. Change in bowel habit can be a sign of cancer, and exploration of this area may be an important aspect if described by the patient. Colorectal cancer guidance from the National Institute for Health and Care Excellence (NICE) identifies that any (unexplained) change in bowel habit in those aged over 60, or in younger adults where there is coexisting rectal bleeding, should warrant rapid investigation (NICE, 2020). Having a small amount of mucus in the stool may be normal and can result from both dehydration and constipated states. Mucus in stools can be associated with inflammatory bowel disease, some food intolerances, gastroenteritis and bowel obstructions.

> 🚩 Stools with blood or pus and abdominal distension where bowel obstruction cannot be excluded are a red-flag presentation.

History and Examination

Asking about any change in bowel habit, including patterns and triggers, may help identify possible causes. Asking about systemic history may indicate underlying or background pathologies, so ask about anorexia, weight loss, nausea, fatigue, fever, pruitis and confusion. Asking about lower GI symptoms may help localise pathology, so ask about abdominal pain, distension, constipation, diarrhoea, steatorrhoea, melaena and haematochezia. A general abdominal assessment including digital rectal examination may help inform the clinical picture. Consider GI risk factors, including pre-existing GI disease (gastro-oesophageal reflux disease (GORD), IBD) and familial history, recreational drug and alcohol use, smoking and diet. Travel history is useful in considering risk of malaria, campylobacter, shigella or contaminated waters, such as hepatitis A infection. Drug history is useful, noting some drugs alter gut transit (such as laxatives, proton pump inhibitors, non-steroidal anti-inflammatory drugs (NSAIDs), antibiotics and immunosuppressants).

Management

- Refer urgently under a two-week cancer pathway for those aged over 60 who have had altered bowel habits for over three weeks, or for younger adults with prolonged altered bowel habit associated with bleeding.
- In cases that do not self-limit, consider investigation for underlying infection or pathology.

Coeliac Disease

Aetiology

This is an autoimmune disease when exposure to gluten causes an immune reaction that leads to inflammation in the small bowel. This is more than just an intolerance presentation, as inflammatory pathology occurs of epithelial cells in the gut (NICE, 2016b). The jejunum, known as the small bowel, is most affected and it causes atrophy of intestinal villi, which is the absorption area, so therefore the patient becomes malabsorbed and this can present as a failure to thrive in young children.

History and Examination

Diarrhoea, fatigue, weight loss and anaemia (from deficiency of iron, B12 and folate) can occur, so a B12 and folate blood test should be done to exclude pernicious anaemia (NICE, 2015a). There is an abdominal rash called dermatitis hepitiformis that occurs in coeliac disease and it is itchy and blistering. It can also present with neurological disease, and all diabetes patients should be screened for coeliac disease.

Investigations

As well as B12 and folate, there are two IgA antibodies which may be present: anti-tissue transglutaminase (anti-TTG) and IgA anti-endomysial antibodies are found in 90% of coeliac patients. An IgA antibody—total IgA should be checked for deficiency (Ciacci and Zingone, 2021).

CHAPTER 10 Gastrointestinal and Hepatic Presentations

Management
Definitive diagnosis is via endoscopy whilst still having a gluten-containing diet, and a referral to the relevant team is warranted.

> ❗ Lymphoma is linked with coeliac disease, so cautious observations of lymph nodes are warranted.

Constipation

Aetiology
Constipation is a symptom-based disorder which describes defecation that is unsatisfactory because infrequent, difficulty passing stools or the sensation of incomplete emptying (Rao et al., 2021). Constipation is a common primary care presentation and can present with significant abdominal pain or discomfort. Some of the common causes include poor hydration, use of opiate medication or other drugs which slow gut transit or bind stools, such as metformin or oral iron supplements. Differential should explore whether the patient has a congested state of constipation, whether stools are impacted or whether there is a bowel obstruction. Bowel obstruction can lead to bowel perforation, peritonitis and sepsis. Therefore, any presentation of potential bowel obstruction must be excluded, or at least monitored that intervention such as laxatives has decongested the colon. Functional constipation is a common presentation in paediatrics, including reluctance to stool during toilet training or when defecation is painful (Barberio et al., 2021). Environmental factors, including attending school or unfamiliar environments, may contribute to functional constipation. Assessment of constipation will require a digital rectal examination to check that stool has progressed through the terminal colon and is not proximally obstructed. Chronic constipation is typically applied to cases in excess of a three-month duration. Constipation is more common in children, the elderly and those who are pregnant. Poor urinary voiding or urinary retention can commonly be caused by a constipated state, so should be considered in these presentations (Kuronen et al., 2021).

History and Examination
A thorough symptom history is important, including assessing longevity of symptoms. Assessing hydration status can be helpful. The use of a stool chart to identify the type of stool is sometimes supportive, or using an assessment tool such as the Rome IV tool (Dimidi et al., 2019). A history of drug use, including over-the-counter and prescribed medicines, can be helpful, including looking for drugs that commonly induce constipation, such as analgesics. An abdominal assessment, including assessment of abdominal distension, will be needed. Digital rectal examination is required to assess for bowel obstruction (Sayuk, 2022).

Management
Where bowel obstruction is suspected, this is a common surgical emergency and should be acutely admitted to hospital (Lee et al., 2019). Where constipation is drug induced,

you should perform a medication review and consider stopping causative drugs or reducing the dosing. Addressing the hydration status of the patient and increasing oral fluids may be helpful. Provide advice on diet, including fibre content, and exercise that can support regular stooling. Laxative choices are either osmotic or stimulant in nature but ensuring adequate hydration of osmotic laxatives will support their work. Coaching on titration of laxative, in response to effect, should be given. Bulk-forming laxatives such as ispaghula are good first-line agents, switching to osmotic laxatives if symptoms are unresponsive. Lactulose is an effective second-line agent. There may be other factors that affect the choice of laxative, and prescribing guidelines should be consulted accordingly. Occasionally enemas such as glycerine suppositories can be helpful. Where constipation is chronic and non-refectory, further clinical workup including assessing for other conditions is warranted. Non-pharmacological treatments should also be explored (Wegh et al., 2022).

Diarrhoea

Aetiology

Diarrhoea is the passage of three or more loose stools per day, or more frequently than normal for the patient. Acute diarrhoea is loose stools for less than two weeks, whereas persistent diarrhoea lasts for more than two weeks and chronic diarrhoea lasts for more than four weeks. It is often helpful to define with the patient what they mean by diarrhoea and consider describing in terms that they would understand, such as asking if the stool is the consistency of water or toothpaste, lumpy or solid. Acute diarrhoea tends to be either infectious in nature or the result of food poisoning, although consideration around common drugs such as selective serotonin reuptake inhibitors (SSRIs) should be considered. Anxiety can contribute to increased stooling, and inflammatory bowel conditions may have flares where diarrhoea may present. Tenesmus associated with acute appendicitis should also be a consideration, with appropriate clinical correlation.

History and Examination

Asking about any change in bowel habit, including patterns and triggers, may help identify possible causes. Asking about systemic history may indicate underlying or background pathologies, so ask about anorexia, weight loss, nausea, fatigue, fever, pruitis and confusion. Asking about lower GI symptoms may help localise pathology, so ask about abdominal pain, distension, constipation, diarrhoea, steatorrhoea, melaena and haematochezia. Ask about potential food poisoning (around 72 hours prior to presentation of diarrhoea). A general abdominal assessment including digital rectal examination may help inform the clinical picture. Consider GI risk factors, including pre-existing GI disease (GORD, IBD), familial history, recreational drug and alcohol use, smoking and diet. Travel history is useful in considering risk of malaria, campylobacter, shigella or contaminated waters, such as hepatitis A infection. Assess for clinical features of dehydration, which can result from diarrhoea (Table 10.3).

CHAPTER 10   Gastrointestinal and Hepatic Presentations

Table 10.3   Stages of Dehydration

Stage of dehydration	Clinical features
Mild	- Lassitude - Anorexia - Nausea - Light-headedness - Postural hypotension - Usually no signs
Moderate	- Apathy/tiredness - Dizziness - Nausea/headaches - Muscle cramps - Dry tongue or sunken eyes - Reduced skin elasticity - Postural hypotension - Tachycardia - Oliguria
Severe	- Profound apathy - Weakness - Confusion, leading to coma - Shock - Tachycardia - Peripheral vasoconstriction - Systolic BP < 90 mmHg - Oliguria or anuria

Source: Farthing et al. (2013).

Drug history is useful, noting some drugs alter gut transit (such as laxatives, proton pump inhibitors, NSAIDs, antibiotics and immunosuppressants).

> Blood in stool, recent antibiotic treatment, weight loss, evidence of dehydration and nocturnal symptoms are red-flag presentations.

Management

Management can be split into two approaches, according to whether it is acute (duration of less than four weeks) or chronic diarrhoea (duration of more than four weeks).

Acute Management
- Send a faecal specimen for microbiology assessment (Box 10.1), especially if systemically unwell, pus or blood in the stool, immunocompromised, diarrhoea after travel or need to exclude infectious disease.

- Consider if a public health referral is required (people in high-risk groups such as food handlers, elderly residents in care homes and healthcare workers, or if suspected food-poisoning outbreak).
- Admit to hospital if the person is vomiting and unable to retain oral fluids, has features of severe dehydration (see Table 10.3) or is in a high-risk group (such as over 60, with coexisting medical conditions or immunosuppressed).

Chronic Management
- Assess for underlying contributing pathology (such as cancers or inflammatory diseases).
- Look for features suggestive of other underlying causes (such as infectious agents, laxative abuse, adverse drug reactions, abdominal surgery, family history, diet, alcohol intake).
- Assess for features of IBS.
- Perform an abdominal examination looking for distension and abdominal mass, organomegaly or tenderness.
- Perform a digital rectal examination for local lesion, prostate hypertrophy or impaction.

> **BOX 10.1** Guidance for Sending a Faecal Specimen
> - Send a specimen in the appropriate stool pot; the sample will typically not be assessed if in a formed state.
> - For an exotic travel history, or prolonged diarrhoea, request ova cysts and parasites (with detail of travel area on the request).
> - Detail clinical history on the request, such as bloody stools, pain, suspected food causes, travel, antibiotic history, untreated water exposure, contact with any other outbreak, to help guide the microbiologist.

Inflammatory Bowel Disease (IBD)

This is an umbrella term for the two main GI tract inflammation diseases of Crohn's disease and ulcerative colitis (UC). Both conditions flare and remit over time and can be exacerbated. Crohn's disease can affect the entire GI tract and in patches, from mouth to anus. However, the terminal ilium is the most affected area and is often transmural. UC is typically limited to the colon and rectum and it only affects the superficial mucosa (Gomollon et al., 2016).

History and Examination

A common presentation is frequent and recurring diarrhoea and abdominal pain as well as lower GI bleeding. Blood and stool mucus is much less common in Crohn's disease compared with UC (Mowat et al., 2011). There is a strong link between UC and primary sclerosing cholangitis (PSC). Crohn's disease is more associated with weight loss, strictures and fistulas. UC has more continuous inflammation compared to Crohn's disease, so endoscopy findings will be different.

Investigations

Testing includes blood tests to check anaemia, thyroid function, kidney function and liver function. A c-reactive protein (CRP) blood test would indicate active infection or disease. Undertaking a faecal calprotectin stool test or erythrocyte sedimentation rate (ESR) blood test could indicate chronic inflammation in the body (Dignass et al., 2015). Definitive assessment is with endoscopy and biopsy.

Management

NICE (2015b) guidelines for Crohn's disease management describe inducing remission, known as settle and maintain remission, by keeping gut health. Recommendations for inducing remission include oral or parental steroids. If steroids do not work alone, other immune-suppressive medication can be used under the direction of a consultant (NICE, 2019c). Maintenance therapy should be under the guidance of a consultant, so the patient will need referral to the IBD clinic, and often have access to an IBD nurse specialist for specific advice.

For UC, there are NICE guidelines that describe the same settle/maintain approach. The first-line treatment in mild to moderate UC is aminosalicylates, such as mesalazine, either orally or as a foam rectal enema. Second-line treatment includes steroid treatment or more aggressive biological agents (NICE, 2019e). Surgery may be an option in both conditions.

Irritable Bowel Syndrome (IBS)

Aetiology

This is a functional bowel disorder with no underlying organic disease (Drossman, 2016). The NICE (2017) guidelines therefore suggest that it is a condition of exclusion of other pathologies first.

History and Examination

Symptoms are that of the function of an otherwise healthy bowel. It is common in the young and female. The three aspects of the syndrome are bowel frequency changes, such as diarrhoea or constipation, including fluctuation between the two. Abdominal pain and bloating are common. Post-prandial irritation and post-defecation relief are also characteristic (El-Serag et al., 2004).

> **!** Abdominal examination may be unremarkable.

Investigations

Initial investigations should include a full blood count for anaemia and inflammatory markers (ESR/CRP). If these are normal, this makes IBS more probable when clinically linked to the described symptoms. Coeliac disease antibodies should be checked via an anti-TTG blood test, and a faecal calprotectin stool test will help exclude IBD-related pathologies. The two-week wait criteria for cancer should also be excluded.

Management

Reassurance and an information prescription are useful in this condition. Limiting alcohol and caffeine intake may also be helpful in this group of patients. A fermentable oligosaccharides, disaccharides, monosaccharides and polyols (FODMAP) diet is a recognised diet used to help manage the symptoms of IBS and again this may be helpful to present as an information prescription; a dietetics referral can support this (Ford and Vandvik, 2015). Symptomatic relief of symptoms, such as loperamide for diarrhoea and laxatives (but avoid lactulose) for constipation. Anti-spasmodic, tricyclic antidepressants and SSRI anti-depressants may be used (Halland and Saito, 2015).

> Referral for social prescribing initiatives and psychological interventions such as cognitive behavioural therapy (CBT) may be helpful.

Peptic Ulcers

Aetiology

Peptic ulcers involve ulceration of the protective mucosal layer of the stomach lining. Ulceration of the stomach is termed a gastric ulcer and ulceration of the duodenum is termed a duodenal ulcer, with duodenal ulcers being more common (Ford and Moayyedi, 2013). The stomach mucosa secretes bicarbonate to act as a pH neutraliser, but with the destruction of the mucosal layer this is inhibited.

History and Examination

The presentation is often with localised epigastric discomfort or pain, which may be tender on palpation. Indigestion-type symptoms may be prevalent and if bleeding occurs this will present as haematemesis (coffee ground vomit) or melaena (black tar-like stools). Prolonged bleeding, even a low level, can lead to an iron deficiency anaemia and this may present as a 'tired all the time' presentation.

> Iron deficiency anaemia associated with the abdomen should be presumed to be cancerous until excluded.

Eating will typically worsen the pain of a gastric ulcer but conversely may ease the pain of a duodenal ulcer. If you have a patient with suspected ulceration, this can be confirmed with upper GI endoscopy which allows for cancer biopsy of ulcers. Medical management would typically include the use of proton pump inhibitors (PPIs) and lifestyle advice (Lanas and Chan, 2017).

CHAPTER 10 Gastrointestinal and Hepatic Presentations

> 💡 The most common drug causes are steroid and NSAID use and, if dyspepsia or upper GI bleeding presentations, these medicines should be stopped.

Investigations
Helicobacter pylori (HP/H. pylori) is the most common pathogenic cause and can be easily diagnosed through an antigen breath test or stool sample (PHE, 2016).

Management
H. pylori infection can be eradicated by using a triple-therapy approach, such as two antibiotics and an acid reduction medication. Too much stomach acid can also lead to peptic ulcers, so lifestyle factors which may contribute should be checked and advised against accordingly, including increased stress, smoking, too much caffeine use and spicy foods (NICE, 2019d).

> 🚩 Peritonitis is also possible if the ulceration is to such depth that it perforates, and this may present as generalised infection or sepsis and warrants emergency surgical admission.

Poor Appetite
Aetiology
Poor appetite is a non-specific presentation but could indicate underlying pathology or psychosomatic presentation. Body mass index is a common measurement of weight and height to assess body habitus, with visceral fat around the abdomen being associated with increased cardiovascular risk (Omura-Ohata et al., 2019). Thenar eminence atrophy may be an early sign of weight loss.

> 🚩 Rapid unplanned weight loss is a red-flag presentation.

Poor appetite can be associated with local presentations related to the mouth; for example, poor dentition, stomatitis, peritonsillar abscess or tonsilitis. It may also be associated with a nauseated state, such as in early pregnancy, or a feeling of satiety, such as with gastric banding.

History and Examination
A change in eating behaviours may be associated with dieting or restrictive eating processes, such as in religious fasting. Some GI conditions such as coeliac or uncontrolled diabetes may also present with poor appetite. Altered behaviours such as laxative overuse, induced vomiting or excessive exercise may be contributory and should be assessed. Alcohol use disorders, chronic respiratory disease and thyroid conditions can present with cachexia.

GI Presentations in Primary Care

Physical signs of poor nutrition include:

- Poor circulation
- Dizziness
- Palpitations
- Fainting
- Pallor.

> Unexplained appetite loss may be a symptom suggestive of cancer. Possible cancers include lung cancer, oesophageal cancer, stomach cancer, colorectal cancer, pancreatic cancer, bladder cancer and renal cancer. Referral under the appropriate two-week wait cancer referral pathway may be appropriate in these cases.

You should have an awareness that eating disorders can affect anyone but have the highest prevalence in females aged 13–17. Eating disorders are also associated with certain professions, such as sports, dancing and fashion modelling (Galmiche et al., 2019). Faltering growth and delayed puberty can be associated with poor nutrition. Faltering growth in the newborn should prompt screening for genetic conditions and thyroid disease.

Management

As a generic presentation, management would depend on the underlying pathology.

> NICE (2019b) Clinical Knowledge Summaries: Eating disorders: When should I suspect an eating disorder? [online].
> Refer to this NICE resource for the clinical features of anorexia nervosa, bulimia nervosa, binge eating disorders and atypical eating disorders.

For dental presentations, assessment by a dental surgeon is warranted. Localised non-dental oral presentations may benefit from soothing gels or local preparations. For infectious states of the oropharynx, reference to local antibiotic prescribing formulary should be used.

Rectal Bleeding

Aetiology

Rectal bleeding is a common primary care presentation and can include both trivial and sinister pathology. Bright red, painless rectal bleeding is the most common symptom of haemorrhoids and is typically associated with defecation (Lohsiriwat, 2012). Occult rectal bleeding (haematochezia) may be associated with lower colon disease, such as inflammatory states of UC, Crohn's disease or proctitis. Localised trauma is sometimes seen post anal penetration or injury. Local tears around the anus may present (fissures) as well as localised dermatological presentations. In children, excoriation is sometimes seen from

CHAPTER 10 Gastrointestinal and Hepatic Presentations

helminth (parasitic worm) infestation. Pruitis ani (itch) is a dermatological presentation that causes persistent itch, and associated scratching and can sometimes present as bleeding.

History and Examination

Checking the origin of bleeding is helpful, as this is sometimes confused with vaginal, urological or skin origins. Ask if the bleeding is bright red and painless, is associated with defecation or with streaks seen on the toilet paper or toilet bowl or is coated on the outside of stools (but not mixed within it). Check if there is any associated anal itch, which is common in haemorrhoids but also in other localised dermatological conditions. A feeling of rectal fullness or a feeling of incomplete defecation may be present where there is local pressure from haemorrhoids. Is there any soiling (thinking about conditions of the sphincter/neurological presentations) and is the soiling blood stained? Is there associated pain with the bleeding, which is less typical of haemorrhoids (unless prolapsed)? Awareness that localised haemorrhoids may be symptomatic of other pathologies, such as portal hypertension, or cancerous pathology so should be clinically correlated through history taking.

Management

External inspection of the anal area is important to assess for localised dermatology and external lesions. Where the origin of the bleeding is unclear, it may be warranted to progress to an internal examination via a digital rectal examination or proctoscopy. Where there is active bleeding of unknown cause, with future possibility of haemodynamic compromise, acute admission should be considered.

Stoma Issues

Aetiology

Several diseases and operations may necessitate stoma and the patient may have concerns about how this affects their activities of daily living. A stoma is an artificial opening on the abdomen to divert the flow of faeces or urine into an external pouch located outside of the body (Hill, 2020). This procedure may be temporary or permanent. Colostomy and ileostomy are the most common forms of stoma but a gastrostomy, jejunostomy, duodenostomy or caecostomy may also be performed.

History and Examination

Look for signs of bowel obstruction, including a non-producing stoma if digestive waste becomes blocked. Consider B12 deficiency caused by poor absorption due to stoma bypass. Monitor for local infection, irritation or stoma shape change which may make it difficult to attach an external collection bag.

Management

Consider involvement of the local stoma nurse specialist or liaison with the supplies company which will often have adaptations or support offers available.

Hepatic Presentations in Primary Care

Hepatic disease can be split into pre-hepatic, intra-hepatic and post-hepatic presentations. This section focuses on intra-hepatic and post-hepatic pathology.

Alcohol Use Disorder (Alcohol Dependency Syndrome)

Aetiology

Commensal background flora enable the gut to work efficiently. Such bacteria are usually prevented from being absorbed into the gut due to the barrier effect of the gut wall and covering mucus. However, recurring and excessive use of alcohol weakens that protective barrier. If bacteria progress through this weakened wall, they can enter the bloodstream into the portal hepatic vein, which is where the liver changes can occur.

The bacteria activate cells which release inflammatory markers, known as interleukin 1, 6, 12 and TNF-alpha, and this starts a process of inflammatory changes in the liver, such as hepatitis. Further insult causes other cells to lose their ability to store vitamin A and then release further inflammatory markers, like interleukin 8, which adds to inflammatory changes and prompts the development of collagen fibres, starting the journey of fibrous tissue. These are known as fibrous liver changes. As these progress, these fibres prevent nutrients getting to hepatocytes (liver cells), causing them to die off, which leads to liver cirrhosis. This scarring is an irreparable state for the liver.

As well as the infiltration of bacteria, there is a chemical pathway breakdown that uses enzymes known as alcohol dehydrogenase. The body is chronically overwhelmed in long-term alcohol use and may be forced to use alternative breakdown pathways, which have acidotic side effects, and this could make the patient prone to a metabolic acidosis. In addition, there are nutritional insults, as often the source of nutritional intake may be just the alcohol, meaning that the patient becomes vitamin deficient. Deficiency of vitamin B1, known as thiamine, places the patient at risk of an encephalopathy (Babor et al., 2001) and this may present as an acute confusion or psychosis such as Wernicke's encephalopathy. This would require an acute emergency admission.

History and Examination

The history may support recurring and excessive alcohol use (Day et al., 2015) and inflammatory changes may present as painful hepatitis.

The inflamed liver may be palpable as hepatomegaly and the inflammatory or cirrhotic changes may be visible on ultrasonography, so organising this via a community pathway may help support a liver damage diagnosis.

Management

Management will depend on the resulting effects of alcohol use. Raised pressures in the hepatic portal vein as a result of changes to the liver also cause backpressure to the spleen and this can cause the spleen to enlarge and may be palpated as splenomegaly. The spleen cannot move cells out, so the patient can become anaemic, thrombocytopenic and immunocompromised. The backpressure in the veins around the oesophagus also places the patient at risk of bleeding. Backpressure into the veins

CHAPTER 10   Gastrointestinal and Hepatic Presentations

around the anus can cause haemorrhoids, with again an increased non-clotting risk and the veins around the oesophagus can lead to profuse and often fatal bleeding, known as oesophageal varices.

> Paramedics working within primary care will need to consider both the biological changes and the psychosocial support required to address alcohol use disorders. Treatment priorities include taking advantage of social prescribing initiatives and arranging psychosocial support through the local alcohol cessation service, with self-referral being the best option to support self-actualisation (NICE, 2010).

Thiamine should be prescribed to provide cover against Wernicke-Korsakoff syndrome.

> Monitoring should be made for acute alcohol withdrawal, including the red-flag symptoms of seizures, fever and delirium tremens.

> A dementia presentation called Korsakoff syndrome may also be present with chronic alcohol use disorders and often requires extensive and intensive therapy, which may include supported living arrangements.

Alpha-1 Antitrypsin Deficiency (A1AD)

Aetiology
Alpha-1 antitrypsin (A1A) is a protease inhibitor and is a genetic condition of deficiency of this inhibitor. A deficiency of A1A protease inhibitor leads to an excess of protease enzymes and these enzymes attack liver and lung tissue. This can result in liver cirrhosis or early onset chronic obstructive pulmonary disease (COPD)-like presentation (NICE, 2019a).

History and Examination
Alpha-1 antitrypsin deficiency (A1AD) may present in a hepatitis abdominal pain or with respiratory issues similar to those of COPD. The blood test serum A1A can be ordered in primary care and it may be low in a deficiency.

Management
There is no clear treatment for the condition, although smoking cessation is recommended to minimise disease progression in the lungs. Long-term treatment of A1AD will depend on how severe the condition is and any related conditions that develop. Patients with A1AD should have their lung and liver functions monitored.

Cholecystitis
Aetiology
A blockage may be caused by a stone (lithiasis) in, or inflammation in or around, the gall bladder. Gall bladder-related presentations are one of the most common causes of right upper quadrant pain. The obstruction typically occurs around the gall bladder neck or within the cystic duct. Acalculous cholecystitis is seen in under 15% of acute cholecystitis presentations but has a much higher mortality (up to 50% mortality), so this presentation should be taken seriously (Kimura et al., 2013). Bile stasis or thickening is thought to contribute to obstruction, and bacterial colonisation is thought to contribute to the risk. Occasionally, these can self-settle but progressive obstruction on infection can lead to necrosis of the gallbladder, perforation of the gall bladder, biliary peritonitis, pericholecystic abscess, fistula, jaundice or sepsis.

> Risk factors for stones includes being female, over 40, obese, having liver disease and using certain drugs. Parathyroid disease, high cholesterol and dehydration can also contribute to stone formation (Srivastav et al., 2017).

History and Examination
Gallstones can be a painful presentation. New onset of acute right upper quadrant pain with a positive Murphy's sign, particularly if associated with fever or vomiting, should be admitted for same-day surgical opinion (RCS, 2016). As there is a 10% mortality rate with this condition (Kimura et al., 2013), a low threshold for admission should be considered. Non-specific or chronic presentations may be investigated with an LFT panel looking for an obstructive picture, and community ultrasonography can be helpful in sub-acute or chronic presentations.

Management

> Where acute cholecystitis is suspected, the person should be referred to hospital for abdominal ultrasound and blood tests. Treatment may include intravenous fluids, antibiotics and analgesia (NICE, 2021a).

Ongoing management of cholecystitis includes lifestyle changes, such as diet change and exercise, as well as an analgesia regime to manage pain.

Haemochromatosis
Aetiology
Haemochromatosis is a genetic condition of high iron levels and is an iron-storage disorder. The gene that is mutated is responsible for iron breakdown, and so fails to metabolise iron. As a result, iron is deposited in excessive levels in tissues where it should not be and so exhibits a pathological effect.

CHAPTER 10   Gastrointestinal and Hepatic Presentations

History and Examination
Patients can present with 'tired all the time' symptoms, arthralgia, pigmentation (known as bronze discolouration of skin), alopecia, erectile dysfunction, amenorrhoea as well as memory and mood changes (Neghina and Anghel, 2011).

> Patients with iron levels significant enough to cause symptoms typically present in their late 40s, although this may be later in females as menstruation acts as a bloodletting mechanism.

Diagnosis is made by the blood test serum ferritin. Ferritin can rise for several reasons, including infection and inflammation, so a transferrin saturation level is needed to confirm haemochromatosis. As well as ferritin and transferrin levels, iron deposition in the pancreas can cause diabetes (Raju and Venkataramappa, 2018) and so a HbA1c screen should be considered. Deposition in the liver can cause cirrhosis, and deposition in pituitary gland or gonads can result in endocrine or sexual dysfunction, so it is important to consider prolactin and testosterone screening in these cases. Deposition in the heart can cause cardiomyopathy and heart failure, so an electrocardiogram (ECG) and B-type natriuretic peptide (pro-BNP) screening would be appropriate. Deposition in the thyroid can lead to hypothyroidism, so you should consider a thyroid function test (TFT) in addition.

Management
Referral to a hepatology service will be required when haemochromatosis is diagnosed. Management is through regular removal of iron via venesection. Regular ferritin levels will be needed as monitoring (BSH, 2018).

Hepatitis
Aetiology
Inflammation of the liver, also termed hepatitis, is most commonly caused by viral or autoimmune disease. Despite this, secondary causes such as alcoholic hepatitis, hepatitis secondary to non-alcoholic fatty liver disease (NAFLD) and drug-induced hepatitis (for example, due to paracetamol overdose) may also occur. There is a spectrum of inflammatory changes associated with hepatitis, from local spots to widespread inflammation which can lead to the formation of necrosed areas of the liver. It is important to note that the disease course of hepatitis can differ quite significantly with regards to mode of transmission, incubation period, liver damage and chronicity, depending on its aetiology.

History and Examination
There is a spectrum of presentation types for hepatitis, ranging from the asymptomatic patient to those in acute fulminant hepatic failure. Whilst specific considerations for the most prevalent forms of hepatitis are considered below, history taking may elicit non-specific signs and symptoms such as malaise, myalgia, anorexia, pruritus (itching) and jaundice. Nausea, vomiting and diarrhoea with or without fever may also occur,

and abdominal pain, if present, may locate to the right, specifically the right upper quadrant. The more generic symptoms of hepatitis are:

- Fever
- Vomiting
- Pale-coloured stools
- Extreme fatigue
- Unexplained weight loss
- Headache
- Yellow skin and eyes
- Loss of appetite
- Dark urine.

Findings on physical examination relate to the presence of an acute infection or liver disease. They are often non-specific, however reproducible abdominal pain, specifically in the right upper quadrant, may increase your suspicion for hepatitis.

In addition, an LFT screen may show abnormal results, including raised transaminases (AST/ALT), with a raise in alkaline phosphate (ALP) also being possible, all of which indicate an inflammatory process in the liver. Bilirubin and urobilinogen measurements may be present on dipstick urinalysis, the presence of which may be an early indicator of liver disease.

> Whilst findings such as hepatomegaly, palmar erythema, spider naevi, caput medusa and asterixis are commonly cited in physical examination literature, they are more common in advanced disease and so are rare observations.

Management

There are slightly different treatment approaches for each type of hepatitis, and early referral to a hepatologist, or to a gastroenterologist or infectious disease specialist with an interest in hepatology, is required (NICE, 2017). All categories of hepatitis are notifiable diseases to Public Health England (HPA, 2010).

> As well as referral to counselling, psychotherapy and/or psychiatry, ongoing support such as referral to hepatitis support groups and referral to support for benefits advice is a vital component of the treatment plan.

Hepatitis A

The faecal-oral-transmitted virus hepatitis A is the most common across the world (Payne and Coulombier, 2009), but is relatively rare in the UK. Nausea, vomiting, anorexia and jaundice can be the presenting problems (Wasley et al., 2009). Slowing of bile through the exit tubes from the liver, known as cholestasis, can also occur and this presents with dark urine and pale stools. This occurs as bilirubin starts to be excreted through the urine but

CHAPTER 10   Gastrointestinal and Hepatic Presentations

cannot exit to the gut to colour the stools, so the stool is pale in colour. On palpation, the liver may be enlarged, known as hepatomegaly, and tender. The virus is often self-limiting in one to three months.

> NICE (2021a) Clinical Knowledge Summaries: Hepatitis A [online].
> Read further regarding the diagnosis and management of hepatitis A in the NICE Clinical Knowledge Summaries.

> Those undertaking foreign travel should consult fit-for-travel guidelines for hepatitis A vaccination (https://www.fitfortravel.nhs.uk/destinations).

Hepatitis B

Hepatitis B virus (HBV) is a blood-borne disease and those who have unprotected sexual intercourse (UPSI) and intravenous drug users (IVDUs) are at a significantly increased risk. Contact through open lesions such as cuts or sharing of toothbrushes also provides a risk of transmission. It can also be transmitted to an unborn foetus (Aspinall et al., 2011). Most infected patients recover from hepatitis B within two months without treatment, but one in ten patients will go on to become chronic HBV carriers: it becomes replicated within DNA. A confirmed case should be referred to the local hepatology service. Table 10.4 details blood tests for different types of hepatitis.

When screening for HBV, testing for HBV surface antigen will show active infection. HBV core antibody will also show a previous infection. If these results are positive, it indicates that the patient could have a current infection. At this stage, further testing using the HBV-E antigen and HBV DNA viral load can be used to evaluate levels of the infection, although this could be done in a specialist clinic (Department of Health, 2013). HBV vaccination is part of the child vaccination programme in the UK.

> Screening for HBV should be done in those with risk, and those with positive results should be referred to a sexual health screening for broader disease screening.

Table 10.4   Blood Tests for Hepatitis B

Blood test	Meaning
HBV surface antigen	Indicates an active infection
HBV-E antigen	A marker of viral replication (high infection rate)
HBV core anti-body	Indicates current or past infection
HBV surface antibody	Previous exposure or vaccination
HBV DNA	Direct count of the viral load in circulation

Hepatitis C

Hepatitis C virus (HCV) is spread by blood and bodily fluid. There is no HCV vaccine. HCV is curable with direct-acting anti-viral medication (SIGN, 2013). A quarter of infected patients will self-limit and recover, with the rest progressing to become chronic HCV patients. Complications, including liver cirrhosis, can occur and these patients are at increased risk for hepato-cellular carcinoma.

> HCV screening is with the HCV antibody test and, if positive, further HCV RNA testing will confirm the infection (PHE, 2015). Once confirmed, the patient should be referred to hepatology services and a notifiable disease form should be completed. HCV treatment resolves about 90% of cases within three months (NICE, 2013).

Autoimmune Hepatitis

The cause is unknown but there may be genetic factors. If clinical detection of hepatitis is found, the patient should be referred to the local rheumatology or hepatology service. These patients may have high immunoglobulin G (IgG) levels, LFTs will be deranged and auto-immune anti-bodies will be positive.

Treatment involves high-dose steroids which are tapered as immuno-suppressants. Immune suppression is typically lifelong to prevent return of the disease. Post-transplant recurrence may also occur in these patients.

Non-alcoholic Fatty Liver Disease (NAFLD)

Aetiology

NAFLD is a common condition that is quickly becoming one of the leading causes of cirrhosis and end-stage liver disease. An estimated 30% of adults have some degree of NAFLD detectable on ultrasound (NICE, 2016a). NAFLD encompasses a number of conditions that demonstrate build-up of fat in liver cells, with these 'fatty deposits' causing interreference with normal liver functioning. In the early stages, NAFLD may not cause issues and is mostly asymptomatic; however, progression of the disease can lead to hepatitis and cirrhosis in a similar fashion to alcohol use disorder.
A raised GGT blood test may indicate a fatty liver presentation.

In addition to its direct impact on liver functioning, a consensus of evidence demonstrates the strong association between NAFLD and metabolic syndromes – an accumulation of pathologies leading to greatly increased risk of diabetes, heart disease and stroke (Preuss et al., 2018). These associations hint to the underlying aetiology which, whilst complex, is likely to result from a combination of obesity, dyslipidaemia, insulin resistance and resulting hyperinsulinaemia. There are four stages to NAFLD:

1. Non-alcoholic fatty liver
2. Non-alcoholic steatohepatitis (NASH), which is hepatitis that is secondary to the fatty liver
3. Fibrosis
4. Irreparable liver cirrhosis and liver failure.

CHAPTER 10 Gastrointestinal and Hepatic Presentations

History and Examination

NAFLD is often asymptomatic, and diagnosis is, in most cases, incidental. History taking should focus on ascertaining risk factors for NAFLD and metabolic syndromes, such as age, poor diet, obesity, lack of exercise and smoking. In the latter stages of disease, NAFLD may present as a hepatitis-like abdominal pain; however, the more likely situation is finding abnormalities on routine investigations, such as raised liver enzymes or lowered platelets or albumin.

> Two common situations where NAFLD may be diagnosed are:
> - By ultrasound when investigating another suspected pathology, such as gallstones
> - By ultrasound when investigating raised liver enzymes of unknown cause.

Investigation can be achieved through community ultrasound to confirm hepatosteatosis (fatty liver). This, however, does not identify severity of disease or whether there is fibrotic progression. For confirmation and further investigation, a routine referral to hepatology services should be made for an enhanced liver fibrosis (ELD) screen and specialised ultrasound.

Management

> Lifestyle changes should be recommended as part of the treatment regime, which can be supported through effective signposting to social prescribing initiatives in your area.

Pharmacotherapy management is aimed at targeting elements of metabolic syndrome as the mainstay of treatment, including optimising management of hypertension, diabetes and raised cholesterol where present.

Pancreatitis

Aetiology

Pancreatic disease can be both acute and chronic and is a serious condition with a potential mortality rate of 10–25% (Hines and Pandol, 2019). The condition is associated with alcohol use disorder. Acute pancreatitis can affect local tissue, and the organ is partly in the abdominal cavity, as well as the retroperitoneal cavity, giving differing characteristics of pain (anterior-posterior pain presentation). The severity can be categorised into mild, moderate or severe (see Table 10.5).

History and Examination

Anterior abdominal pain is typically generalised where the head of the pancreas is involved, but with the latter two-thirds of the pancreas being in the retroperitoneal cavity, a more localised feeling of radiation towards the back may occur. The patient may present as a post-hepatic jaundice. Initial investigations are likely to include lipase or amylase blood tests and diagnostic imaging.

Hepatic Presentations in Primary Care

Table 10.5 Severity of Pancreatitis

Mild	Moderate	Severe
No local or systemic complications or organ failure Uneventful recovery and resolves within the first week Most common form	Local complications or transient organ failure which resolves within 48 hours	Persistence of single multi-organ failures for > 48 hours

Management

An urgent admission is likely needed to manage pain (Tenner et al., 2013) and complications of the disease. Referral for management of underlying causes, such as alcohol use, may be warranted beyond the acute flare.

Primary Biliary Cirrhosis (PBC)

Aetiology

Primary biliary cirrhosis (PBC) is autoimmune disease where the exit ducts from the liver become enlarged and blocked. Bile cannot exit the liver and cholestasis occurs (Selmi et al., 2011). The build-up and backpressures from this obstruction can lead to liver fibrosis and cirrhosis. Bile build-up causes widespread itching, known as pruritis. Bilirubin build-up causes jaundice. Cholesterol build-up presents as xanthelasma. Xanthoma causes cholesterol in tendons and ligaments and atheroma is a build-up in blood vessels which increases vascular risk. As bile cannot enter the duodenum to breakdown fat, fatty stools, known as steatorrhoea, occur. As bilirubin cannot exit into the duodenum, stools are not coloured and become pale.

History and Examination

Patients may present with 'tired all the time symptoms', generalised gastrointestinal disturbance and abdominal pain. LFTs may show a raised ALP, as this is an exit block presentation, although raised ALP may be from bony destruction so be cautious in the interpretation. There are two antibodies which are associated with this condition. The first is anti-mitochondrial antibodies and these are most specific to PBC (Hirschfield et al., 2019). The second is anti-nuclear antibodies (ANAs), which are less specific to PBC but are common across auto-immune disorders. Erythrocyte sedimentation rate (ESR) may be raised, but again it is non-specific. IgM immunoglobulins may also be raised. Diagnosis is by liver biopsy, and thus if suspected should be referred to hepatology services. Later stages may present with ascites.

> Pruritis is a common symptom with a wide differential diagnosis spanning from dermatological conditions (such as eczema) to renal conditions (such as chronic kidney disease) through to liver disease. Cast a broad net when observing these patients and ensure consideration of red-flag diagnoses.

269

CHAPTER 10   Gastrointestinal and Hepatic Presentations

> NICE (2021b) Clinical Knowledge Summaries: Itch – widespread. Guidance in this area can be helpful.

Management

Ursodeoxycholic acid (UDCA) reduces intestinal absorption of cholesterol. Another medication which reduces cholesterol is cholestyramine and this binds to bile acids in the gut and prevents their absorption. This can help with pruritis symptoms.

Immuno-suppression may help slow the disease but it raises the risk of infection.

Primary Sclerosing Cholangitis (PSC)

Aetiology

PSC is an autoimmune condition that causes a stiff and inflamed bile duct, both inside and outside the liver. The narrowing (known as strictures) and hardening (known as fibrosis) of the bile duct causes an obstruction to the outflow of bile from the liver into the intestine (Chapman et al., 2019). The long-term backflow of bile pressure into the liver causes inflammation and eventually cirrhosis. Whilst the cause is unclear, there is believed to be a genetic and local bacterial environment set of factors associated with this condition.

History and Examination

Hepatomegaly may be palpable and tender on examination. LFTs will show a cholestatic picture, which is a slowing of bile duct flow, and ALP will be the most deranged LFT and may be the only initial abnormality.

As the disease progresses, bilirubin may rise and finally the transaminases may rise. There are no specific auto-immune antibodies, but 35% of PSC patients produce anti-endothelial-cell antibodies (AECAs) and 75% perinuclear antineutrophil cytoplasmic antibodies (pANCAs).

> PSC and UC have a strong link. UC is seen in approximately 70% of PSC cases, and whichever one presents, the other must be a consideration. This patient presents with a hepatitis-like picture.

Management

A definitive diagnosis will be via a magnetic resonance cholangiopancreatography (MRCP) (Hirschfield et al., 2019), which can be achieved through a hepatology service referral.

Wilson's Disease

Aetiology

Wilson's disease is a genetic condition of excessive accumulation of copper.

History and Examination

Patients may present with liver disease, neurological problems or psychiatric presentation, so this is not exclusive to the liver. Copper deposition in the liver leads to hepatitis, which can lead to liver cirrhosis.

The initial investigation is a cerulopasmin blood test. Be aware that false positives occur in cancer and inflammation (EASL, 2012). Kayser Fleischer, which are brown rings, may occur around the eyes.

Management

Referral to the hepatology service is required. Treatment is with copper chelation, which can be arranged by the consultant teams (Walshe et al., 2003).

Chapter Summary

Differentiating the acute abdomen, which requires urgent surgical intervention, from less immediate presentations is a cornerstone of general practice clinical risk management. Presentations should be considered in the context of their clinical risk, and paramedics should use the tools at their disposal (such as examination and investigations) to work to correctly assess, investigate and diagnose presentations relating to the GI and hepatic systems.

Case Study 1

You are working in primary care when a 24-year-old presents with abdominal pain, nausea and low-grade fever.

History

PC:	Abdominal pain.
HxPC:	Pain started in the mid-abdominal region six hours ago and is now in the right lower quadrant of the abdomen. The pain was steady in nature and aggravated when defecating or tensing their abdominal muscles.
PMHx/SHx:	None.
DHx:	None.
FHx:	None.
ROS:	Denies recent illness.

Examination

- Physiological observations reveal a fever of 38°C, a tachycardia of 110bp, a slightly raised respiratory rate and a normal blood pressure.
- Inspection: Clear discomfort, no other peripheral stigmata of chronic disease.
- Palpation: Pain on palpation at right lower quadrant (McBurney's sign), as well as pain on raising the right, for example against resistance (psoas sign).
- Movement: Localised pain with any movement or walking.

CHAPTER 10   Gastrointestinal and Hepatic Presentations

Preferred Diagnosis
- Possible appendicitis.

Differential Diagnoses
- Mesenteric adenitis is a common alternative diagnosis of appendicitis.
- Other conditions that mimic appendicitis may include Crohn's disease, cholecystitis, diverticulitis, ectopy of pregnancy, endometriosis, colitis, gastric or duodenal ulcer disease, hepatitis, kidney disease and live abscess (and numerous others).

Management
- Due to the mortality risk, anyone with any one of the four clinical examination signs for appendicitis (McBurney's, Rovsing's, psoas or obturator) should be admitted under the surgeons as a same-day urgent admission.

Case Study 2

You are working in out-of-hours when a 40-year-old woman presents with sudden new right upper quadrant pain.

History

PC: New right upper quadrant pain.
HxPC: Onset of pain post-prandial (after eating a four-cheese pizza). Pain is generalised across the right upper abdomen and is associated with vomiting. The patient is writhing in pain which comes in spasmodic waves.
PMHx/SHx: Three-month history of reflux presentation treated with proton pump inhibitors. Depression and anxiety presentations.
DHx: Omperazole 20 mg; sertraline 50 mg.
SHx: Works as a schoolteacher, smoker, no recreational drug use. Social drinker only.
FHx: None.
ROS: Denies recent illness.

Examination
- Physiological observations: No fever but slightly tachycardic at 114 bpm and visibly unsettled. BP 125/80 mmHg.
- Inspection: Clear discomfort, no other peripheral stigmata of chronic disease.
- Palpation: Pain on palpation at right upper quadrant (Murphy's sign).
- Movement: Not exacerbated by movement, but generally writhing in pain.

Preferred Diagnosis
- Cholecystitis.

Differential Diagnoses
- Biliary colic, empyema of the gall bladder, mucocoele, perforation, biliary obstruction, acute cholangitis, acute pancreatitis, bowel obstruction (amongst many others).

Management
- Right upper quadrant pain associated with fever or vomiting should be admitted for surgical opinion as a same-day urgent admission.

References

Aspinall, E.J., Hawkins, G. and Fraser, A. (2011) Hepatitis B prevention, diagnosis, treatment and care: A review. *Occupational Medicine* 61(8): 531–540.

Babor, T.F., Higgins-Biddle, J.C., Saunders, J.B. et al. (2001) *The Alcohol Use Disorders Identification Test: Guidelines for Use in Primary Care.* New York: World Health Organization.

Barberio, B., Judge, C., Savarino, E. et al. (2021) Global prevalence of functional constipation according to the Rome criteria: A systematic review and meta-analysis. *Lancet* 6(8): 638–648.

British Society for Haematology (BSH) (2018) *Clinical Guidelines from the British Society for Haematology on the Management of Haemachromatosis.* London: British Society for Haematology.

Chapman, M.H., Thorburn, D., Hirschfield, G.M. et al. (2019) *British Society of Gastroenterology and UK-PSC Guidelines for the Diagnosis and Management of Primary Sclerosis Cholangitis.* London: British Society of Gastroenterology.

Chey, W.D., Kurlander, J. and Eswaran, S. (2015) Irritable bowel syndrome: A clinical review. *Journal of the American Medical Association* 313(9): 949–958.

Ciacci, C. and Zingone, F. (2021) New perspectives on the diagnosis of adulthood coeliac disease. In A. Schieptti and D. Sanders (eds) *Coeliac Disease and Gluten Related Disorders.* London: Academic Press, Elsevier, pp. 201–211.

Day, E., Copello, A. and Hull, W.D. (2015) Assessment and management of alcohol use disorders. *British Medical Journal* 350: 715–715.

Department of Health (2013) Immunisation procedures. In *The Green Book.* London: Department of Health, pp. 25–34.

Dignass, A.U., Gasche, C. and Bettenworth, D. (2015) European consensus on the diagnosis and management of iron deficiency and anaemia in inflammatory bowel diseases. *Journal of Crohn's and Colitis* 9(3): 211–222.

Dimidi, E., Cox, C., Grant, M. et al. (2019) Perceptions of constipation among the general public and people with constipation differ strikingly from those of general and specialist doctors and the Rome IV criteria. *American Journal of Gastroenterology* 114(7): 1116–1129.

Drossman, D.A. (2016) Functional gastrointestinal disorders: History, pathophysiology, clinical features. *Gasroenterology* 150: 1262–1279.

El-Serag, H.B., Pilgrim, P. and Schoenfeld, P. (2004) Systematic review: Natural history of irritable bowel syndrome. *Alimentary Pharmacology & Therapeutics* 19(8): 861–870.

European Association for the Study of the Liver (EASL) (2012) Management of Wilson's disease. *Journal of Hepatology* 56(3): 671–685.

Farthing, M., Salam, M., Lindberg, G. et al. (2013) WGO Guideline: Acute diarrhea in adults and children: A global perspective. *Journal of Clinical Gastroenterology* 47(1): 12–20.

Ford, A.C. and Moayyedi, P. (2013) Dyspepsia. *British Medical Journal* 347: 1–5.

Ford, A.C. and Vandvik, P.O. (2015) Irritable bowel syndrome: Dietary interventions. *BMJ Clincial Evidence* 30: 1–13.

CHAPTER 10   Gastrointestinal and Hepatic Presentations

Galmiche, M., Dechelotte, P., Lambert, G. et al. (2019) Prevalence of eating disorders over the 2000–2018 period: A systematic literature review. *The American Journal of Clinical Nutrition* 109(5): 1402–1413.

Gomollon, F., Dignass, A. and Annese, V. (2016) 3rd European evidence-based consensus on the diagnosis and management of Crohn's disease. *Journal of Crohn's and Colitis* 11(1): 3–25.

Halland, M. and Saito, Y.A. (2015) Irritable bowel syndrome: New and emerging treatments. *British Medical Journal* 350: 1–14.

Health Protection Agency (HPA) (2010) *Guidance on Infection Control in Schools and Other Child Care Settings*. London: Health Protection Agency.

Hill, B. (2020) Stoma care: Procedures, appliances and nursing considerations. *British Nursing Journal* 29(22): S14–S19.

Hines, O.J. and Pandol, S.J. (2019) Management of severe acute pancreatitis. *British Medical Journal* 367: i6227.

Hirschfield, G.M., Dyson, J.K., Alexander, G.J.M. et al. (2019) The British Society of Gastroenterology/UK-PBC primary biliary cholangitis treatment and management guidelines. *Gut British Medical Journals* 67(9): 1568–1594.

Hunt, R., Quigley, E. and Zaigham, A. (2013) Coping with common gastrointestinal symptoms in the community. *Clinical Gastroentrology* 48(7): 567–578.

Kimura, Y., Takada, T. and Strasberg, S.M. (2013) TG13 current terminology, etiology, and epidemiology of acute cholangitis and cholecystitis. *Journal of Hepato-Biliary-Pancreatic Sciences* 20(1): 8–23.

Kuronen, M., Hantunen, S., Alanne, L. et al. (2021) Pregnancy, puerperium and perinatal constipation – An observational hybrid survey on pregnant and postpartum women and their age-matched non-pregnant controls. *International Journal of Obstetrics and Gynaecology* 128(6): 1057–1064.

Lanas, A. and Chan, F.K. (2017) Peptic ulcer disease. *Lancet* 3736(16): 1–12.

Lee, M.J., Sayers, A.E., Drake, T.M. et al. (2019) National prospective cohort study of the burden of acute small bowel obstruction. *British Journal of Surgery Open* 3(3): 354–366.

Lohsiriwat, V. (2012) Hemorrhoids: From basic pathophysiology to clinical management. *World Journal of Gastroenterology* 18(17): 2009–2017.

Mowat, C., Cole, A. and Windsor, A. (2011) Guidelines for the management of inflammatory bowel disease in adults. *Gut* 60(5): 571–607.

National Institute for Health and Care Excellence (NICE) (2010) Alcohol-use disorders: Prevention [PH24]. Available at: https://www.nice.org.uk/guidance/ph24 (accessed 31 January 2023).

National Institute for Health and Care Excellence (NICE) (2013) Hepatitis B and C testing: People at risk of infection [PH43]. Available at: https://www.nice.org.uk/guidance/ph43 (accessed 31 January 2023).

National Institute for Health and Care Excellence (NICE) (2015a) Coeliac disease: Recognition, assessment and management [NG20]. Available at: https://www.nice.org.uk/guidance/ng20 (accessed 31 January 2023).

National Institute for Health and Care Excellence (NICE) (2015b) Inflammatory bowel disease [QS81]. Available at: https://www.nice.org.uk/guidance/qs81 (accessed 31 January 2023).

National Institute for Health and Care Excellence (NICE) (2016a) Non-alcoholic fatty liver disease (NAFLD): Assessment and management [NG49]. Available at: https://www.nice.org.uk/guidance/ng49 (accessed 31 January 2023).

References

National Institute for Health and Care Excellence (NICE) (2016b) Coeliac disease [QS134]. Available at: https://www.nice.org.uk/guidance/qs134 (accessed 31 January 2023).

National Institute for Health and Care Excellence (NICE) (2017) Irritable bowel syndrome in adults: Diagnosis and management [CG61]. Available at: https://www.nice.org.uk/guidance/cg61 (accessed 31 January 2023).

National Institute for Health and Care Excellence (NICE) (2019a) Chronic obstructive pulmonary disease update [NG115]. Available at: https://www.nice.org.uk/guidance/ng115 (accessed 31 January 2023).

National Institute for Health and Care Excellence (NICE) (2019b) Clinical Knowledge Summaries: Eating disorders: When should I suspect an eating disorder? Available at: https://cks.nice.org.uk/topics/eating-disorders/diagnosis/clinical-features/ (accessed 31 January 2023).

National Institute for Health and Care Excellence (NICE) (2019c) Crohn's disease: Management [NG129]. Available at: https://www.nice.org.uk/guidance/ng129 (accessed 31 January 2023).

National Institute for Health and Care Excellence (NICE) (2019d) Gastro-oesophageal reflux disease and dyspepsia in adults: Investigation and management [CG184]. Available at: https://www.nice.org.uk/guidance/cg184 (accessed 31 January 2023).

National Institute for Health and Care Excellence (NICE) (2019e) Ulcerative colitis: Management [NG130]. Available at: https://www.nice.org.uk/guidance/ng130 (accessed 31 January 2023).

National Institute for Health and Care Excellence (NICE) (2020) Colorectal cancer [NG151]. Available at: https://www.nice.org.uk/guidance/ng151 (accessed 31 January 2023).

National Institute for Health and Care Excellence (NICE) (2021a) Clinical Knowledge Summaries: Cholecystitis – acute. Available at: https://cks.nice.org.uk/topics/cholecystitis-acute/ (accessed 31 January 2023).

National Institute for Health and Care Excellence (NICE) (2021b) Itch – widespread. Available at: https://cks.nice.org.uk/topics/itch-widespread/ (accessed 31 January 2023).

Neghina, A.M. and Anghel, A. (2011) Hemochromatosis genotypes and risk of iron overload — a meta-analysis. *Annals of Epidemiology* 2(1): 1–14.

Omura-Ohata, Y., Son, C., Makino, H. et al. (2019) Efficacy of visceral fat estimation by dual bioelectrical impedance analysis in detecting cardiovascular risk factors in patients with type 2 diabetes. *Cardiovascular Diabetology* 18(137).

Payne, L. and Coulombier, D. (2009) Hepatitis A in the European Union: Responding to challenges related to new epidemiological patterns. *Eurosurveillance* 14(3): 19101.

Preuss, H.G., Kaats, G.R., Mrvichin, N. et al. (2018) Examining the relationship between nonalcoholic fatty liver disease and the metabolic syndrome in nondiabetic subjects. *Journal of the College of Nutrition* 37(6): 457–465.

Public Health England (PHE) (2015) *Hepatitis C in the UK*. London: Public Health England.

Public Health England (PHE) (2016) *Test and Treat for Helicobacter Pylori (HP) in Dyspepsia. Quick Reference Guide for Primary Care: For Consultation and Local Adaptation*. London: Public Health England.

Raju, K. and Venkataramappa, S.M. (2018) Primary hemochromatosis presenting as type 2 diabetes mellitus: A case report with review of literature. *International Journal of Appied Basic Medical Research* 8(1): 57–60.

Rao, S.S., Kearns, K., Orleck, K.D. et al. (2021) Diagnosis, management and patient perspectives of the spectrum of constipation disorders. *Alimentary Pharmacology and Therapeutics* 53(12): 1250–1267.

CHAPTER 10 Gastrointestinal and Hepatic Presentations

Royal College of Surgeons (RCS) (2016) *Commissioning Guide: Gallstone Disease.* London: Royal College of Surgeons.

Sayuk, G.S. (2022) The digital rectal examination. *Gastroenterology Clinics* 51(1): 25–37.

Scottish Intercollegiate Guidelines Network (SIGN) (2013) *Management of Hepatitis C.* Ediburgh: Scottish Intercollegiate Guidelines Network.

Selmi, C., Bowlus, C.L. and Gershwin, M.E. (2011) Primary biliary cirrhosis. *The Lancet* 377(9777): 1600–1609.

Srivastav, A., Srivastava, M. and Paswan, R. (2017) Spectrum of clinico-pathological presentations of gall bladder. *International Journal of Contemporary Medicine Surgery and Radiology* 4(1): A18–A24.

Tenner, S., Baillie, J., De Witt, J. et al. (2013) Management of acute pancreatitis. *American Journal of Gastroenterology* 108(9): 1400–1415.

Walshe, J.M., Vinken, P.J. and Lawans, H.L. (2003) Wilson's disease. *Diagnosis and Phenotypic Classification of Wilson Disease* 23(3): 139–142.

Wasley, A.M., Feinstone, S.M. and Bell, B.P. (2009) *Hepatitis A Virus.* London: Churchill Livingstone.

Wegh, C.A., Baaleman, D.F., Tabbers, M.M. et al. (2022) Nonpharmacologic treatment for children with functional constipation: A systematic review and meta-analysis. *The Journal of Paediatrics* 240(5): 136–149.

Genitourinary and Gynaecological Presentations

Sarah Brown and Elizabeth Steer

11

Within This Chapter

- Urinary symptoms
- Urinary tract infection (UTI)
- Urinary retention
- Penile pain and discharge
  - Balanoposthitis
  - Frenulum tears
  - Paraphimosis
- Testicle pain and swelling
- Breast pain
  - Cyclical breast pain
  - Mastitis
- Early pregnancy
  - Confirmation of pregnancy
  - Termination of pregnancy (TOP)
  - Miscarriage, pregnancy loss, and ectopic pregnancy
- Pelvic pain and masses
  - Fibroids
  - Pelvic inflammatory disease (PID)
- Vaginal bleeding
  - Dysmenorrhoea
  - Menorrhagia
  - Post-coital bleeding
  - Postmenopausal bleeding
  - Sexual assault
  - Female genital mutilation (FGM)
- Vaginal discharge
  - Bacterial vaginosis (BV)
  - Vulvovaginal candidiasis

Introduction

Paramedics working within primary care will frequently encounter patients presenting with genitourinary or gynaecological symptoms. Patients are often hesitant to discuss symptoms related to 'down there', so paramedics must approach this topic with sensitivity. A detailed history, including sexual history, is vital to establishing an accurate diagnosis, so it is important to explain that any information shared will be confidential. There are many different over-the-counter options sold with an aim to treat odour, itch and discomfort, so it is also important to establish if a patient has been self-treating, with what product and for how long. Many conditions are simple to treat but the paramedic must be alert for red flags and be prepared to consult senior colleagues and escalate care or refer if they have any concerns.

Gynaecological History Taking

Undertaking a gynaecological history is pertinent to several of the presentations within this chapter. Taking a detailed gynaecological history can help you form a clinical opinion.

CHAPTER 11   Genitourinary and Gynaecological Presentations

It is important to optimise the environment in which the history is taken; some people may wish to be alone, others may feel more comfortable with a chaperone. Some elements of history to consider are:

- Menstrual history, including last menstrual period (LMP), age to start menstruating, cycle lengths and changes, painful cramping
- Presence of bleeding: heavy bleeding, out-of-cycle bleeding
- History of fertility problems
- Cervical screening history
- Gastrointestinal symptoms
- Unexplained weight loss
- Pelvic pain
- Weight loss
- Discharge: colour, smell, rashes
- Pregnancy and obstetric history
- Sexual history
- Contraception
- Pain and discomfort: type of pain, duration, radiation and aggravating factors.

Assessment

Abdominal Assessment

A structured assessment of the abdomen, as outlined in Chapter 10 – Gastrointestinal and Hepatic Presentations (pp. 248–250), will be important when assessing patients with genitourinary or gynaecological symptoms, as they may also be experiencing abdominal pain. Additional to this is examination of genitalia.

Examination of Hernias

The process is the same for either sex. Inspect for any asymmetry or bulging area. Ask the patient to cough or bear down, which will increase intra-abdominal pressure, making any hernia more visible. Palpate left and right groin for presence of any inguinal hernia.

> It is important to consider that patients may not identify with the sex they were assigned at birth. In this situation, patients may have delayed presentation of symptoms and may find discussion and assessment of genitals they do not associate with distressing. The paramedic must always therefore be mindful of this and adapt their assessment as required.

Examination of the genitals should be performed if appropriate to aid the paramedic to establish a diagnosis. It is important to explain the procedure to the patient before gaining consent and to offer a chaperone (Bickley et al., 2020).

Male Genitalia

Examination of the penis and scrotum should if possible be completed whilst the patient is standing.

Assessment

The Penis

Inspection: Examine for any ulceration, erythema, scars or discharge. If the foreskin is present, then ask the patient to retract this so that the glans can be fully examined. Ensure the foreskin is replaced after inspection. Check the urethral meatus for sign of discharge. If the patient reports discharge, then they may be able to milk the penis in order for discharge to be produced and a swab taken for testing (Bickley et al., 2020).

Palpation: Note any tenderness or induration to the length of the penis.

Scrotum

Inspection: Examine for any swellings, erythema, pustules, lice or abrasions. Ensure to lift the scrotum to examine the posterior surface.

Palpation: Examine for shape, size, tenderness and any abnormal lumps. Both testes, the epididymis and the spermatic cords should be examined (Bickley et al., 2020).

Female Genitalia

Breast and Axillae

Inspection: This should be completed with the patient sitting, leaning forwards and then semi-recumbent. Examine for breast size and symmetry, colour and any dimples, masses or rashes. Examine the nipples for ulceration, inversion and change in colour or position.

Palpation: This is best completed with the patient supine or semi-recumbent. Examine the breast tissue for tenderness, masses or change in skin texture. Palpate the axilla for any swollen lymph nodes, masses or tenderness (Bickley et al., 2020).

Vulva

Inspection: This is best completed with the patient semi-recumbent with heels raised to the buttocks and knees allowed to fall out to the side. Many women may be familiar with this position from cervical screening or previous gynaecological examination. Examine for any rash, ulceration, pustules, lice, laceration or excoriation. Also examine for signs of discharge. You may also note the presence and formation of the labia.

Palpation: This will only be appropriate in specific circumstances such as abnormal swelling or mass in order to establish the characteristics of this (Bickley et al., 2020).

Internal Examination of Vagina and Cervix

This should only be completed by a paramedic who has received appropriate training and education. If internal examination is required, then consider who is appropriate to complete this procedure; this may require a referral to a sexual health clinic, a senior colleague or the gynaecological team (Bickley et al., 2020).

Urinalysis

Urinalysis is initially completed using dipstick testing and the results are used to aid diagnosis. It is a quick and simple test that can be completed whilst with the patient.

CHAPTER 11   Genitourinary and Gynaecological Presentations

When to Use
Urinalysis should be completed in:

- Any patient experiencing urinary symptoms but where diagnosis is uncertain based on the history alone
- Pregnant women with abdominal pain or urinary symptoms
- Children – where UTI is suspected
- Patients over 65 years of age – where UTI is suspected.

How to Complete
The sample should be 'mid-stream' to reduce risk of contamination. Acquiring a 'clean-catch' sample from children, the elderly or those with limited mobility may prove difficult if using a white-topped universal sterile container, due to the small opening. Gallipots are useful in this situation, and urine can then be transferred to other containers as needed. Urinalysis strips are not sterile and best practice is not to place strips into a sample if this is to be sent to the lab for microscopy (Johnson et al., 2019). Instead, a sterile pipette can be used to place urine onto the strip and excess urine can be blotted from the strip to avoid bleeding of colour. Urine samples in red pots containing boric acid are not suitable for use with urinalysis strips as they may give false results.

Interpretation of Results
Read the instructions of the urinalysis strips carefully, as each test on the strip will need to be read after a set length of time. The instructions will also give guidance on after how long results become invalid.

Each urinalysis kit will contain several different tests on each strip. Examples are:

- pH: A measure of the amount of acid in the urine. Normal pH of urine is 4.5–8. A pH that is above normal may be a sign of kidney stones, urinary infections, kidney problems or other disorders. A pH below normal may be a sign of severe gout, dehydration or starvation.
- Protein: Can be a sign of strenuous exercise, fever, UTI, vaginal discharge, pre-eclampsia, renal disease, diabetes mellitus or hypertension.
- Glucose: Normally because of diabetes mellitus. Can be as a result of contamination if patient has used a non-sterile container such as a jam jar.
- Ketones: Can be a sign of starvation, persistent vomiting or diabetic ketosis.
- Microscopic haematuria: Can be due to menstruation, UTI, urethral trauma, kidney stones, renal cancer or kidney infection.
- Leukocyte esterase: Detects intact and lysed leucocytes produced in inflammation, and is a sign of UTI or can be due to vaginal discharge or contamination.
- Nitrate: Indicates high probability of UTI. Nitrate is produced by the action of bacterial nitrate reductase in urine. Contact time between the bacteria and urine is needed for this to form. Patients who drink large volumes of water may have a false negative result due to flushing urine out of the bladder before the reaction has occurred. Early morning samples are more accurate.
- Bilirubin: May be a sign of liver disease.

Presentations in Primary Care

Urinary Symptoms

Urinary symptoms include:

- Dysuria: Discomfort, pain, burning, tingling or stinging associated with urination
- Frequency: Passing urine more often than usual
- Urgency: A strong desire to empty the bladder, which may lead to urinary incontinence
- Nocturia: Passing urine more frequently at night
- Suprapubic discomfort
- Changes in urine appearance or consistency
- Urine may appear cloudy or change colour
- Change in odour
- Haematuria may present as red or brown discolouration of urine or as frank blood.

Patients may present with one or more urinary symptoms, so accurate history taking and physical assessment is crucial to developing a diagnosis, as many conditions have similar symptoms (NICE, 2022f).

Urinary Tract Infection (UTI)

Aetiology

UTI is one of the most common conditions presenting in primary care, and up to 50% of women experience a UTI (NICE, 2022f). UTIs are predominantly caused by bacteria from the gastrointestinal tract entering the urinary tract, with *Escherichia coli* being the most common cause (NICE, 2022f). Less commonly identified organisms include *Staphylococcus saprophyticus* (approximately 5–10%), *Proteus mirabilis* (more common in males, associated with renal tract abnormalities or calculi) and *Klebsiella* species (NICE, 2022f).

History and Examination

Urine colour should be examined, and if the urine is cloudy there is a 97% chance of UTI (SIGN, 2012). Any non-pregnant woman less than 65 years of age presenting with two or more symptoms of new nocturia, cloudy urine or dysuria, in the absence of vaginal discharge or irritation, should be considered to have a UTI and should be treated without need for urine dipstick (PHE, 2020).

Urine dip should be completed for all children, men, pregnant women, recurrent infections or if treatment has failed. Sample should be sent to lab if any abnormality noted.

> Three days after the antibiotic course has been completed, a repeat urine dip should be conducted:
>
> - For pregnant women, to check for incomplete treatment, or
> - If haematuria or microhaematuria is present on urinalysis, as persistence is a sign of bladder or renal cancer.

CHAPTER 11   Genitourinary and Gynaecological Presentations

It is important to consider acute prostatitis in men who present with urinary symptoms and discomfort in the back passage or fever or irritative voiding symptoms. Prostatitis is an infection of the prostate gland and is often secondary to UTI and may require prolonged treatment with antibiotics. Also ask male patients about hesitancy, dribbling or poor urinary stream, which if prolonged are red flags for enlarged prostate and possible prostate cancer and require further investigation.

It is important to check for uraemic symptoms, which could be signs of systemic disease. These include nausea, vomiting, tachycardia, fever, malaise, poor appetite, muscle cramps, pruritis and confusion. The paramedic should consider referral to the emergency department (ED) for any signs of sepsis or pyelonephritis in pregnant women or children.

> UTI in children under three months or urine retention with palpable bladder or persistent unexplained haematuria are all red flags that require escalation of care.

Management

Follow local guidelines for prescribing based on local sensitivities. Simple UTI in women and children can be treated with a three-day course of antibiotics. Pregnant women, men and those with recurrent symptoms should receive an initial seven-day course of antibiotics (NICE, 2022f). The patient should be encouraged to return if there is any worsening of symptoms or if symptoms do not resolve after the course of treatment has been completed.

> SIGN (2012) Management of suspected bacterial urinary tract infection in adults: A national clinical guideline 88 [online].
> This gives a particularly good background to the research base for the current guidelines regarding UTI.

Urinary Retention

Aetiology

This is most common in male patients and can be a result of prostatic hyperplasia, cancer, urethral stricture, multiple sclerosis (MS), infection or post-operative complication.

History and Examination

Patient reports inability to pass urine, as well as pain over the bladder. Examination will show a tender enlarged bladder with dullness on percussion.

Management

The bladder needs to be drained using a catheter and the volume of drained urine noted. This is normally completed in an ED as they can also investigate the underlying cause.

Presentations in Primary Care

> Check for signs of sepsis in any patient that presents with having not passed urine in the preceding 12 hours.

Penile Pain and Discharge

Aetiology

Penile pain can have several causes and may or may not be associated with discharge. The onset of pain and lifestyle factors are important to establish in order to develop a diagnosis.

The most common causes of penile pain and discharge are paraphimosis, minor tears to the frenulum and balanoposthitis (NICE, 2022e).

Balanoposthitis

This is a common cause of penile pain and describes inflammation of the glans penis (balantis) and foreskin (posthitis). This can have several causes, as outlined in Table 11.1, and a detailed history taking alongside physical assessment is crucial to establish an accurate diagnosis (NICE, 2022a).

Frenulum Tears

Minor tears of the frenulum are common and often occur because of masturbation or vigorous intercourse. These do not need treatment unless bleeding is excessive, in which case these will need to be managed in an ED.

Paraphimosis

Paraphimosis occurs in uncircumcised patients when the retracted foreskin cannot be replaced and becomes trapped behind the corona. This can occur because of intercourse, masturbation or erection. It can lead to strangulation of the glans, painful vascular compromises and (worst case) necrosis.

> During inspection, check for objects such as rings, hair or rubber bands that could be restricting the blood supply, which can imitate foreskin trapping.

Management

Any physical object causing restriction needs to be carefully cut and removed. Attempts to reduce the swelling should be made by running cool water over the glans penis. If attempts to reduce the swelling are unsuccessful and the foreskin cannot be replaced, then emergency referral to urology will be required.

CHAPTER 11 Genitourinary and Gynaecological Presentations

Table 11.1 Aetiology of Balanoposthitis

Symptom	Aetiology	History and examination	Management
Genital thrush	Candida	Symptoms develop over days or weeks. Redness on the under-surface of the glans penis. There may be small, eroded itchy papules on the glans, shaft of the penis and scrotal skin. A white curd-like discharge is often present	Treat with topical antifungal or oral if symptoms severe. With or without topical steroid depending on severity of inflammation ⚑ If symptoms of thrush are severe or do not improve after treatment, consider underlying immunosuppression, such as undiagnosed diabetes mellitus, and arrange for further investigation.
Cellulitis	Organisms such as group *A beta-haemolytic streptococci* and *Staphylococcus aureus*	Symptoms develop over days and increasing pain without treatment. Erythema and oedema of the foreskin or shaft of the penis. Often without discharge	Consider antibiotics as per local guidelines
Symptoms associated with sexually transmitted infections	*Chlamydia, herpes simplex, trichomonas, syphilis* or anaerobes such as *Gardnerella*	Considered based on the history or if any ulceration, blisters or inguinal lymphadenopathy are present	Referral or self-presentation to the sexual health clinic
Trauma	History of foreskin 'fiddling' common in young boys. Trauma during intercourse or vigorous cleaning	Will present with redness but no associated rash or discharge	Advise the person to clean under the foreskin daily with lukewarm water and to dry it gently. Do not use soap or bubble bath, which may irritate the area

Presentations in Primary Care

Symptom	Aetiology	History and examination	Management
Allergic reaction	Exposure to potential irritants or allergens, such as soaps, creams, latex condoms or lubricants	Red rash, itchy, possible hives	Advice on avoidance of triggers and application of topical steroid if needed

Testicle Pain and Swelling
Aetiology
Testicular swelling can be unilateral or bilateral and can develop suddenly or over several weeks. Most patients are concerned about cancer and may have delayed presentation due to embarrassment.

History and Examination
A history of sudden severe pain and swelling should be considered testicular torsion until proven otherwise and as such patients should have urgent referral to urology. Physical examination of the scrotum is important to establish the position of the pain and swelling in relation to the testes.
   Other conditions associated with testicle pain and swelling include:

- Hydrocele or groin hernia (characterised by swelling without pain)
- Epididymo-orchitis (which is more common in older men, and concurrent symptoms of UTI on dipstick testing are often seen).

> Severe pain, scrotal mass, lymphadenopathy or an abdominal mass are red-flag symptoms as they can be signs of cancer.

Management
Ultrasound should be arranged for any unexplained scrotal swelling or if there is a history of trauma and scrotal pain, or persistent testicular symptoms.
   Epididymo-orchitis can be treated with antibiotics as per local guidelines and consider referral to sexual health clinic if there is any suspicion that epididymo-orchitis is caused by a sexually transmitted infection (STI).

Breast Pain
Aetiology
Patients can develop breast pain for a variety of reasons. They may present with a new episode or ongoing history of breast pain. Patients may also have noticed changes to the breast, including a lump, nipple discharge, skin changes or change in size or shape.

CHAPTER 11 Genitourinary and Gynaecological Presentations

Patients may have delayed presentation due to concerns about being examined or fear of cancer diagnosis.

> Refer all patients for two-week wait to breast clinic if:
> - They are aged 30 years or over and have an unexplained breast lump with or without pain. They are aged 50 years or over with discharge, retraction or other changes of concern in one nipple only.
> - They present with skin changes to the breast such as tethering or *peau d'orange*.
> - They are aged 30 years or over with an unexplained lump in the axilla.

Consider non-urgent referral in people aged under 30 years with an unexplained breast lump with or without pain (NICE, 2020).

Cyclical Breast Pain

Aetiology

Breast pain associated with the menstrual cycle is common and affects up to two-thirds of women. One in ten females report moderate to severe pain.

History and Examination

Patients usually report pain that starts within two weeks before their period, increasing until menstruation begins and improving after menses. Pain is dull, heavy or aching in nature and is usually bilateral. It may extend to the axilla and be poorly localised.

> ! Physical assessment is crucial to rule out symptoms of malignancy or infection.

Management

Ask the patient to record a breast pain diary, including dates of menstrual cycle, to aid diagnosis.

Advise the patient to ensure they wear a well-fitting bra during the day as well as a soft-support bra at night. Simple over the counter analgesics such as paracetamol or ibuprofen may be helpful, and patients should be advised to take as per the packet instructions. Referral to a specialist may be required if the pain is severe and affecting quality of life and does not respond to initial treatment after three months.

Mastitis

Aetiology

Mastitis is a painful inflammation of the breast which may be accompanied by infection. It usually occurs in lactating females due to statis of milk. The accumulated milk causes an inflammatory response which may or may not progress to infection. Infective mastitis is most commonly caused by *Staphylococcus aureus* (NICE, 2023).

History and Examination
Patient reports unilateral breast pain and swelling.
Examination shows a tender, red, swollen and hard area of the breast, often in a wedge-shaped distribution.

> Mastitis can develop into a breast abscess and will require urgent referral for consideration of surgery. Symptoms include a painful, swollen lump in the breast, with redness, heat and swelling of the overlying skin and fever or general malaise.

Management
Advise to use simple analgesics and to apply a warm compress to the breast to help with pain. Encourage breastfeeding women to continue feeding if possible, including from the affected breast, as this will help to reduce stasis of milk. Prescribe oral antibiotics as per local guidelines if indicated.

Early Pregnancy
Confirmation of Pregnancy
Women may present to primary care for confirmation of pregnancy. This may be following a positive home pregnancy test or due to missed periods and a suspicion of pregnancy. A simple urine dip can confirm pregnancy. At this point, the patient can be booked for antenatal care, or encouraged to self-refer to maternity services as per local guidelines.

Patient Information
Patients can be directed to the NHS website (NHS, 2022) for further advice on their pregnancy.

Termination of Pregnancy (TOP)
When discussing termination of pregnancy (TOP) with patients, it is important to be non-judgemental or critical of their decisions. Patients may have anxiety about being perceived negatively by healthcare professionals and others. TOP is a complex decision that is undertaken for a variety of reasons. Undertaking a gynaecological history will enable you to roughly estimate the gestation of the pregnancy.

In most cases, these patients should be referred to the termination of pregnancy clinic as per local guidance. Timely access to these services is important, as these clinics have specific gestations up to which they will accept referrals. As a paramedic, it is important that you are aware of the requirement to raise any safeguarding concerns (NICE, 2019a). For more information on patients who do not wish to continue their pregnancy, see p. 342 in Chapter 13 – Obstetric Presentations.

CHAPTER 11 Genitourinary and Gynaecological Presentations

Early Pregnancy Bleeding, Miscarriage and Early Pregnancy Loss (Including Ectopic)

Aetiology

A miscarriage is the loss of a pregnancy during the first 23 weeks. Miscarriage is common and affects approximately one in eight pregnancies. The reason for miscarriage is rarely known, but it is thought that most miscarriages are in relation to chromosomal abnormality.

History and Examination

The most common symptoms associated with early pregnancy loss are bleeding and lower abdominal pain and cramping. It is important that a gynaecological history is taken and an abdominal or pelvic examination is conducted.

Ectopic pregnancy can present with a variety of signs and symptoms (NICE, 2021a). Most commonly:

- Pelvic tenderness
- Abdominal tenderness
- Adnexal tenderness.

Other signs and symptoms:

- Rebound tenderness or peritoneal signs
- Abdominal distention
- Pallor
- Tachycardia, hypotension or clinical signs of shock
- Cervical motion tenderness
- Enlarged uterus
- Orthostatic hypotension
- Gastrointestinal and urinary symptoms
- Nausea and vomiting.

> It is important to rule out an ectopic pregnancy. Ectopic pregnancy requires immediate referral to hospital and, in cases of a rupture, requires emergency surgery.

Management (NICE, 2021a)

Immediate referral is required in patients with pain and abdominal tenderness, pelvic tenderness or cervical motion tenderness.

Refer patients to an early pregnancy service or out-of-hours gynaecological service if they report bleeding and other symptoms (such as pain) and show signs of early pregnancy, are over six weeks' gestation or a pregnancy of an unknown gestation. The urgency of these types of referrals is in relation to the clinical situation.

Patients with pregnancies of less than six weeks' gestation who are bleeding but not in pain, with no risk factors and no previous history of ectopic pregnancy, can be sent home with appropriate safety netting. Advise the patient to return if bleeding continues or worsens or if they develop pain. Advise them to repeat a pregnancy test in seven to ten days' time and return to primary care if it is positive. A negative pregnancy test result would mean the patient miscarried.

Presentations in Primary Care

Patient Support and Referral

> There are many organisations and charities available to help support patients and families through this difficult time. Signposting to these organisations and charities can help people find support and process what has happened to them. Examples of these include the Miscarriage Association and Tommy's. Patients may require ongoing psychological support depending upon the individual circumstances.

Pelvic Pain and Masses

Pelvic pain or masses can have several possible causes. The most common causes are fibroids and pelvic inflammatory disease (PID), but if there is any doubt about diagnosis then refer to a senior colleague for further assessment.

Fibroids

Aetiology

Fibroids develop at reproductive age and in females uterine fibroids are the most common benign tumour. Fibroids can be single or multiple and vary in size. Fibroids may be an incidental finding during investigations for gynaecological problems as they commonly cause no symptoms (NICE, 2022c).

Risk factors (NICE, 2022c):

- Increasing age
- Obesity
- Early puberty
- Black or Asian ethnicity – incidences are higher in Black and Asian women than in white women; they also may occur at a younger age and are more likely to be symptomatic
- Family history of fibroids in first-degree relatives.

History Taking and Examination

Undertake a gynaecological and medical history. Establish cervical screening history, history of fertility problems and any risk factors.

Symptoms

Patients are commonly asymptomatic; however, symptoms can include:

- Pelvic pain, pressure or discomfort
- Abdominal distention or distortion
- Heavy menstrual bleeding
- Urinary and bowel symptoms
- Fertility issues.

289

CHAPTER 11 Genitourinary and Gynaecological Presentations

Examination

On palpation, an enlarged firm irregularly shaped non-tender uterus is characteristic of uterine fibroids. This should be able to be moved slightly side to side (NICE, 2022c).

Management

In people who present with ascites and masses, an urgent referral should be undertaken. A routine referral for an ultrasound scan should be undertaken in patients who present with typical features of uterine fibroids but no cancerous features (NICE, 2022c).

> In people who present with pelvic masses associated with any other cancer feature (such as weight loss or unexplained bleeding), the suspected cancer pathway referral should be undertaken (two-week wait referral).

Pelvic Inflammatory Disease (PID)

Aetiology

PID is a general term for infection of the upper-genital tract. It is commonly due to STI, such as *Chlamydia trachomatis* (14–35%) (NICE, 2022d).

The infection travels upwards from the endocervix, causing one or more of the following (BASHH, 2018):

- Endometritis
- Salpingitis
- Parametritis
- Oophoritis
- Tubo-ovarian abscess
- Pelvic peritonitis.

> For more information on sexual health presentations, refer to Chapter 12 – Contraception and Sexual Health.

History Taking and Assessment

Undertake a gynaecological history. Establish if any recent procedures have involved instrumentation of the uterus or interruption of the cervical barrier, as this increases the risk of PID. Examples include placement of an intrauterine device or a termination-of-pregnancy procedure.

Signs and symptoms include:

- Pelvic pain and lower abdominal pain (usually bilateral)
- Vaginal discharge

- Abnormal bleeding (post coital, intermenstrual or heavy)
- Dysmenorrhoea
- Fever (> 38°C in moderate to severe cases)
- Adnexal tenderness of bimanual vaginal examination (which should only be undertaken by paramedics who have been trained and are competent to do so in primary care).

Management

Patients with suspected PID should ideally be managed in a genito-urinary medicine (GUM) clinic or sexual health service. A high vaginal swab should be taken, alongside a pregnancy test. Prescription of antibiotics should be in line with local policy (BASHH, 2018), and may also be required for sexual partners.

> Urgent admission to hospital is required in cases where there are signs of significant infection, where other emergency presentations cannot be ruled out such as ectopic pregnancy, acute appendicitis or pelvic peritonitis or where a woman is pregnant (NICE, 2019b).

> Remember, if the patient is unwell and there is diagnostic doubt, refer to hospital.

> BASHH (2018) 2018 United Kingdom national guideline for the management of pelvic inflammatory disease [online].

Vaginal Bleeding

Dysmenorrhoea

Aetiology

Dysmenorrhea is painful cramping before or during menstruation, or both. It is extremely common. There are two types of dysmenorrhoea:

- Primary dysmenorrhoea: Occurs in the young female in the absence of any underlying pelvic pathology. This presents usually 6–12 months after the first menstrual cycle (BMJ, 2022).
- Secondary dysmenorrhoea: Occurs in females with pelvic pathology. This often presents several years after the first menstrual cycle. The pain is not consistent with menstruation alone and may occur through other phases of the menstrual cycle. The most common causes are endometriosis, chronic PID, adenomyosis, presence of an intrauterine device (IUD), fibroids and polyps. Less common causes include congenital uterine abnormalities, ovarian pathology and cervical stenosis (BMJ, 2022).

CHAPTER 11   Genitourinary and Gynaecological Presentations

History and Examination

Undertake a gynaecological history. It is important to rule out secondary dysmenorrhoea prior to diagnosing primary dysmenorrhoea. Establish when the symptoms started in relation to the first menstrual period. Perform an abdominal assessment to identify any clinical pathologies such as masses or large fibroids. Perform or arrange for a pelvic examination, including speculum examination of the cervix, unless the symptoms present in a young non-sexually active woman and so primary dysmenorrhoea is the most likely diagnosis. Undertake a pregnancy test to exclude an ectopic pregnancy, and consider arranging an ultrasound scan, high vaginal swab and endocervical swab.

Management

Primary dysmenorrhoea: Offer non-steroidal anti-inflammatory drugs (NSAIDs) unless contraindicated. If NSAIDs are contraindicated, not tolerated or not providing adequate pain relief, offer paracetamol in line with local guidelines (NICE, 2018b). If a patient does not wish to conceive, consider prescribing three to six months of a hormonal contraceptive in line with local policy and guidelines (NICE, 2018b). Self-care can include local application of heat (heat patch or hot water bottle) or a transcutaneous electrical nerve stimulation (TENS) machine.

Secondary dysmenorrhoea: This will depend on the underlying cause.

> Refer under the suspected cancer pathway if:
> - Ascites or pelvic or abdominal masses are present and not thought to be uterine fibroids.
> - There is an abnormal cervix on examination.
> - There is persistent intermenstrual or post-coital bleeding.

In other cases, consider other causes of dysmenorrhoea and manage symptoms such as PID and fibroids if pain newly presents after several years of painless periods (NICE, 2018b).

Menorrhagia: Heavy Menstrual Bleeding (HMB)

Aetiology

Most women will lose 80 mL of blood during a period. Heavy menstrual bleeding (HMB) is defined as losing more than 80 mL in a period or having a period lasting more than seven days, or both (NHS, 2021). HMB can have a range of causes. The most common are:

- Fibroids
- Endometriosis or adenomyosis
- Polyps.

HMB may have no underlying pathology, but it can have a major impact on the quality of a person's life and the interventions undertaken are to look at improving quality of life, not necessarily reducing the total blood loss (NICE, 2021b).

Presentations in Primary Care

History and Examination
The patient may report a long history of HMB. Most patients know what is normal for them, so will be able to report out-of-character bleeding. Unexplained changes in bleeding characteristics should be investigated. Abdominal assessment and pelvic assessment may show signs of underlying pathology, but findings may be normal.

Management
Undertake a full blood count and test for coagulation disorders. Consider thyroid function in patients showing evidence of thyroid disease. If the patient does not wish to conceive, consider prescribing three to six months of a hormonal contraceptive in line with local policy and guidelines (NICE, 2018b). If HMB is presenting with pain, consider the management of dysmenorrhoea below.

> 🚩 If presence of cancer symptoms, refer into the suspected cancer pathway for a two-week wait appointment (NICE, 2021b).

> ⚠️ Insertion of foreign body objects into the vagina can cause pain or bleeding. If the object is still in situ, this will require referral to hospital. If no longer in situ, consider the infection risk and significance of the trauma as to whether the patient requires onward referral or exam.

Post-coital Bleeding

Aetiology
The most common cause of post-coital bleeding is cervical ectropion, but it can also present because of cervical polyps or cervical cancer.

History and Examination
Normally disclosed by the patient due to concerns about the cause. Speculum examination by an appropriately trained clinician may show the presence of polyps or cervical ectropion but the clinician should not be falsely reassured by this.

Management
Patients should be referred as per local guidelines, to rule out cervical cancer or STI. Recent normal cervical screening is not a suitable alternative to assessment by a gynaecological department.

Postmenopausal Bleeding

Aetiology
Menopause itself is usually diagnosed in women over 45 years old who have not had a period for more than a year. Postmenopausal bleeding is not usually serious, but it can be a sign of cancer. Causes of postmenopausal bleeding are highlighted in Table 11.2.

293

CHAPTER 11   Genitourinary and Gynaecological Presentations

Table 11.2   Causes of Postmenopausal Bleeding

Cause	Treatment
Cervical polyps	May need to be removed by a specialist
Endometrial hyperplasia	Varied treatment options available, from no treatment, hormone medications or a total hysterectomy
Ovarian cancer	Often a total hysterectomy
Womb cancer	Often a total hysterectomy
Side effect of hormone replacement treatment (HRT)	Change or stop in medication
Endometrial atrophy	No treatment, or oestrogen cream or pessaries

Source: NHS (2021b).

Management

Referral under the suspected cancer pathway or postmenopausal bleeding pathway for a two-week wait appointment.

> It may be useful to direct patients to the NHS website for some background information (NHS, 2020).

Sexual Assault

A patient who presents disclosing that they have experienced sexual assault needs to be carefully supported in all aspects of their onward care journey. Where possible, these patients should be encouraged to report these incidences to the police. As healthcare professionals, we have a responsibility to safeguard as per local policy, taking into consideration the individual circumstances.

Management

These patients require onward referral to a specialist centre, such as a sexual assault referral centre (SARC) or the Havens, depending on your local pathways.

> Not all disclosures of sexual assault are recent. In cases of non-recent sexual assault, the management of these types of cases may differ, so follow local policies and guidelines.

> BASHH (2012) UK national guidelines on the management of adult and adolescent complainants of sexual assault 2011 [online].

Presentations in Primary Care

Female Genital Mutilation (FGM)

Female genital mutilation (FGM) refers to all acts of cutting or mutilation of the external female genitalia or genital organs for non-medical purposes. FGM is practised for a variety of reasons, usually in the incorrect belief that it is beneficial for vaginal hygiene, but it has no health benefits and is illegal in the United Kingdom (RCOG, 2015). It is important to follow the local guidelines for safeguarding these patients.

The immediate symptoms of FGM can include bleeding, severe pain, infection, urinary symptoms, tissue injury and damage to organs such as the urethra and bowel. Long-term effects of FGM are extensive, but can include recurrent infections, blood-borne viruses, urinary symptoms, painful or abnormal periods, fertility issues, complications in pregnancy and psychological distress.

> RCOG (2015) Female genital mutilation and its management (Green-top Guideline No. 53) [online].
> Female Genital Mutilation Act (England and Wales) 2003.

Vaginal Discharge

Aetiology

Vaginal discharge is common and is not normally pathological (NICE, 2019b). Bacterial vaginosis (BV) is the most common cause of abnormal vaginal discharge in women of child-bearing age, with vulvovaginal candidiasis (genital thrush) estimated to be the second most common cause (Lopez, 2015). It is also important to consider STI.

> Consider STI in patients who are younger than 25 years of age or have had a new sexual partner or more than one sexual partner in the last 12 months or have had a previous STI. This is covered in more detail in Chapter 12 – Contraception and Sexual Health.

History and Examination

The symptoms, aetiology and likely diagnosis of instances of abnormal vaginal discharge are shown in Table 11.3.

> Post-coital bleeding or unusual per vaginum (PV) bleeding, pelvic pain and recent gynaecological procedure are all red flags that would prompt referral to gynaecology.

> In children with itchy genitals but no discharge, consider the possibility of threadworms.

CHAPTER 11   Genitourinary and Gynaecological Presentations

Table 11.3   Discharge Symptoms

Symptom	Aetiology	Diagnosis
White, 'cheese-like' and non-malodorous discharge, with itch	*Candida* is most common causative organism, although other yeasts can occasionally be implicated	Vulvovaginal candidiasis
Fishy-smelling, thin, grey or white discharge without itching or soreness	Caused by an overgrowth of anaerobic organisms (such as *Gardnerella vaginalis*, *Prevotella* species, *Mycoplasma hominis* and *Mobiluncus* species) and a loss of lactobacilli. The vagina loses its normal acidity, increasing to a PH of greater than 4.5	Bacterial vaginosis

Source: NICE (2018a).

Management

Non-pregnant women with asymptomatic BV do not usually require treatment. Patients with symptoms characteristic of BV can be treated without need for empirical testing if they are not pregnant or post termination or gynaecological procedure and if symptoms are not recurrent. Thrush can also be treated without the need for empirical testing; however, if recurrent, it should be confirmed with genital swab. Treatments should be prescribed as per local guidelines. Treatment for both BV and genital thrush can be purchased over the counter, so do check what the patient has already tried, before considering treatment. Most presentations can be managed with self-care and many clinical commissioning groups will have guidance on when patients should be encouraged to treat with over-the-counter medications. If there is any indication of STI, then referral or self-presentation to a sexual health clinic is recommended (NICE, 2022b; 2018a). Neither BV or thrush are sexually transmitted and there is no need to test sexual partners.

Self-care

Wash vulva only once daily with no soaps or wipes. If bathing, do not use products in the water and avoid hot baths. Avoid tight-fitting underwear made of synthetic fibres.

Chapter Summary

Many patients may be apprehensive about disclosing genitourinary and gynaecological symptoms to a clinician, which can make history taking more difficult. If a paramedic has effective communication skills and can notice patient cues, then diagnosis is easier and more accurate. Often conditions are simple to treat, and the patient may have been self-treating for some time before seeking help. Paramedics must therefore be very alert to red-flag symptoms and be willing to seek early senior support if necessary.

Case Study 1

You are working in a GP surgery and a 30-year-old female presents to you complaining of vaginal discharge.

History

PC:	Vaginal discharge.
HxPC:	Seven days of thick, white, odourless vaginal discharge. Vulva feeling increasingly itchy and sore.
PMHx/SHx:	Same sexual partner for two years, with recent negative STI check.
DHx:	Completed course of antibiotics ten days ago for paronychia.
SHx:	None.
FHx:	None.
ROS:	No other symptoms.

Examination
- Inspection not indicated unless diagnosis unclear or patient requests for reassurance.

Preferred Diagnosis
- Genital thrush (vulvovaginal candidiasis).

Differential Diagnoses
- Bacterial vaginosis
- UTI.

Management
- Treat with OTC clotrimazole 1% cream with intravaginal cream or pessary depending on patient preference.
- Return if symptoms not resolved after 10–14 days of treatment.
- Return if develops bleeding PV or new urinary symptoms.

Case Study 2

You are working in a GP surgery and 26-year-old female presents with new PV bleeding and abdominal pain.

History

PC:	Minimal bleeding PV and lower abdominal pain.
HxPC:	Patient is thought to be eight weeks pregnant and last night noticed frank blood in her underwear. Since then, the patient reports cramping abdominal pain.
PMHx/SHx:	One male sexual partner for last four years; denies chance of STI.
DHx:	Taken paracetamol within last four hours with no relief.
SHx:	None.
FHx:	None.
ROS:	No other symptoms.

CHAPTER 11 Genitourinary and Gynaecological Presentations

Examination
- Abdominal assessment: No abnormality found, no tenderness.
- Pelvic assessment: No masses or tenderness.

Preferred Diagnosis
- Miscarriage.

Differential Diagnosis
- Ectopic pregnancy.

Management
- Referral to the early pregnancy unit or out-of-hours gynaecological service, dependent upon local service provision.

References

Bickley, L., Szilagyi, P., Hoffman, R. et al. (2020) *Bates' Guide to Physical Examination and History Taking*. 13th edn. Philadelphia, PA: Lippincott Williams and Wilkins.

British Association for Sexual Health and HIV (BASHH) (2012) UK national guidelines on the management of adult and adolescent complainants of sexual assault 2011. Available at: https://www.bashhguidelines.org/media/1079/4450.pdf (accessed 28 January 2023).

British Association for Sexual Health and HIV (BASHH) (2018) 2018 United Kingdom national guideline for the management of pelvic inflammatory disease. Available at: https://www.bashhguidelines.org/media/1170/pid-2018.pdf (accessed 28 January 2023).

British Medical Journal (BMJ) (2022) Best practice guideline: Dysmenorrhoea. Available at: https://bestpractice.bmj.com/topics/en-gb/420 (accessed 1 February 2023).

Female Genital Mutilation Act (England and Wales) 2003. Available at: https://www.legislation.gov.uk/ukpga/2003/31/contents (accessed 21 February 2023).

Johnson, G., Hill-Smith, I. and Bakhai, A. (2019) *The Minor Illness Manual*. Boca Raton, FL: Taylor and Francis.

Lopez, J. (2015) Candidiasis (vulvovaginal). *BMJ Clinical Evidence*: 0815.

National Health Service (NHS) (2020) Postmenopausal bleeding. Available at: https://www.nhs.uk/conditions/post-menopausal-bleeding/ (accessed 1 February 2023).

National Health Service (NHS) (2021) Heavy periods. Available at: https://www.nhs.uk/conditions/heavy-periods/ (accessed 28 February 2023).

National Health Service (NHS) (2022) Your NHS pregnancy journey. Available at: https://www.nhs.uk/pregnancy/finding-out/your-nhs-pregnancy-journey/ (accessed 1 February 2023).

National Institute for Health and Care Excellence (NICE) (2018a) Clinical Knowledge Summary: Bacterial vaginosis. Available at: https://cks.nice.org.uk/topics/bacterial-vaginosis/ (accessed 28 February 2023).

National Institute for Health and Care Excellence (NICE) (2018b) Clinical Knowledge Summary: Dysmenorrhoea. Available at: https://cks.nice.org.uk/topics/dysmenorrhoea/ (accessed 1 February 2023).

References

National Institute for Health and Care Excellence (NICE) (2019a) Abortion care [NG140]. Available at: https://www.nice.org.uk/guidance/ng140/ (accessed 28 February 2023).

National Institute for Health and Care Excellence (NICE) (2019b) Clinical Knowledge Summary: Vaginal discharge. Available at: https://cks.nice.org.uk/topics/vaginal-discharge/ (accessed 28 February 2023).

National Institute for Health and Care Excellence (NICE) (2020) Clinical Knowledge Summary: Breast cancer – recognition and referral. Available at: https://cks.nice.org.uk/topics/breast-cancer-recognition-referral/ (accessed 28 February 2023).

National Institute for Health and Care Excellence (NICE) (2021a) Ectopic pregnancy and miscarriage: Diagnosis and initial management [NG126]. Available at: https://www.nice.org.uk/guidance/ng126 (accessed 1 February 2023).

National Institute for Health and Care Excellence (NICE) (2021b) Heavy menstrual bleeding: Assessment and management [NG88] . Available at: https://www.nice.org.uk/guidance/ng88/ (accessed 1 February 2023).

National Institute for Health and Care Excellence (NICE) (2022a) Clinical Knowledge Summary: Balanitis. Available at: https://cks.nice.org.uk/topics/balanitis/ (accessed 1 February 2023).

National Institute for Health and Care Excellence (NICE) (2022b) Clinical Knowledge Summary: Candida – female genital. Available at: https://cks.nice.org.uk/topics/candida-female-genital/ (accessed 1 February 2023).

National Institute for Health and Care Excellence (NICE) (2022c) Clinical Knowledge Summary: Fibroids. Available at: https://cks.nice.org.uk/topics/fibroids/ (accessed 1 February 2023).

National Institute for Health and Care Excellence (NICE) (2022d) Clinical Knowledge Summary: Pelvic inflammatory disease. Available at: https://cks.nice.org.uk/topics/pelvic-inflammatory-disease/ (accessed 1 February 2023).

National Institute for Health and Care Excellence (NICE) (2022e) Clinical Knowledge Summary: Scrotal pain and swelling. Available at: https://cks.nice.org.uk/topics/scrotal-pain-swelling/ (accessed 1 February 2023).

National Institute for Health and Care Excellence (NICE) (2022f) Clinical Knowledge Summary: Urinary tract infection (lower) – women. Available at: https://cks.nice.org.uk/topics/urinary-tract-infection-lower-women (accessed 1 February 2023).

National Institute for Health and Care Excellence (NICE) (2023) Clinical Knowledge Summary: Mastitis and breast abscess. Available at: https://cks.nice.org.uk/topics/mastitis-breast-abscess (accessed 1 February 2023).

Public Health England (PHE) (2020) Diagnosis of urinary tract infections: Quick reference tool for primary care for consultation and local adaptation. Available at: https://www.gov.uk/government/organisations/public-health-england (accessed 28 January 2023).

Royal College of Obstetricians and Gynaecologists (RCOG) (2015) Female genital mutilation and its management (green-top guideline no. 53). Available at: https://www.rcog.org.uk/globalassets/documents/guidelines/gtg-53-fgm.pdf (accessed 28 January 2023).

Scottish Intercollegiate Guidelines Network (SIGN) (2012) Management of suspected bacterial urinary tract infection in adults: A national clinical guideline 88. Available at: https://www.sign.ac.uk/our-guidelines/management-of-suspected-bacterial-urinary-tract-infection-in-adults/ (accessed 28 January 2023).

Contraception and Sexual Health

Alyesha Proctor

12

Within This Chapter

This chapter will follow the current Faculty of Sexual and Reproductive Healthcare UK Medical Eligibility Criteria (FSRH, 2016), the British Association for Sexual Health and HIV guidance (BASHH, 2021) and relevant National Institute for Health and Care Excellence (NICE) guidance throughout. Current local guidelines should also be followed in line with these guidelines. This chapter specifically covers contraception and sexual health queries, as outlined below.

Contraception

- The contraceptive injection
- The intrauterine device (IUD) (copper coil) and intrauterine system (IUS) (Mirena coil)
- The contraceptive implant
- The progesterone-only pill (POP)
- The combined oral contraceptive pill (COCP)
- The combined transdermal patch
- The combined vaginal ring
- Condom and diaphragm use
- Vasectomy and female sterilisation
- Approaches to health promotion
- Legal and ethical requirements concerning contraception

Emergency Contraception

This section will include options for emergency contraception, indications and contraindications for use, instructions for use and important considerations such as pregnancy testing and STI screening.

- The copper coil (Cu-IUD)
- Levonorgestrel
- Ulipristal

CHAPTER 12   Contraception and Sexual Health

> **Sexually Transmitted Infections (STIs)**
> - Chlamydia
> - Genital herpes
> - Genital warts
> - Gonorrhoea
> - Hepatitis B
> - Human immunodeficiency virus (HIV)
> - Syphilis
> - Trichomoniasis

Introduction

Good sexual health is a vital aspect of overall public health and well-being (BASHH, 2021). Most adults are sexually active, and poor sexual health can lead to unintended pregnancies and sexually transmitted infections (STIs) (NICE, 2019b). In England, conceptions in women aged 18 and under have been reducing over time. While this reduction cannot be credited to any one factor, it is thought that 86% of the decline in the teenage pregnancy rate is due to enhanced contraceptive use (ONS, 2018). The number of newly diagnosed STIs has stabilised over the last two years; however, trends such as an increase in antimicrobial resistant infections are concerning. Most diagnoses of STIs are in younger people (aged 15–24). Other disproportionally affected groups include men who have sex with men (MSM) and Black and minority ethnic (BME) groups (NICE, 2019b).

Paramedic practitioners working in primary care are expected to have generalist knowledge on a range of issues, including sexual health and contraception. The requirement for contraception is a common occurrence in general practice, and this is something that was traditionally managed by sexual health nurses, practice nurses or GPs. Paramedics working in primary care may have very little experience of managing sexual health and contraceptive issues. This chapter presents current up-to-date guidance to provide you with the knowledge to manage patients presenting with sexual health complaints and contraceptive queries.

Contraception

Building the knowledge, skills, resilience and ambitions of young people, as well as providing easy access to welcoming services, helps them to delay sex until they are ready to enjoy healthy, consensual relationships and to use contraception effectively to prevent unplanned pregnancy (PHE, 2018). Helping women to choose the method of contraception that suits them will help to reduce unplanned pregnancies (NICE, 2019b). To prevent unwanted pregnancies, contraception needs to be used up until the menopause. The menopause is typically determined as two years after last having a period if the patient is under the age of 50 and one year if the patient is over the age of 50 (FPA, 2020).

Contraception

Options for contraception:

- Long-acting reversible contraception (LARC), which includes the contraceptive injection, the contraceptive implant and intrauterine contraception devices (copper intrauterine devices (Cu-IUDs)) and levonorgestrel intrauterine systems (LNG-IUS)
- The progesterone-only pill (POP)
- The combined contraceptive pill (COCP)
- The combined contraceptive patch
- The combined vaginal ring
- Condoms.

The FSRH UK Medical Eligibility Criteria

When offering contraception in your clinic, it is important to refer to the FSRH UK Medical Eligibility Criteria (UKMEC), which offers guidance on who can use contraceptive methods safely. These are evidence-based recommendations that allow for consideration of the possible methods that can be used safely by women with certain health conditions (for example, hypertension) or characteristics (for example, smoker, obesity), to prevent unintended pregnancy (FSRH, 2016).

> To assist with weight loss and smoking cessation, consider engagement with a local health and well-being group or input from a social prescribing link worker.

Certain medical conditions are associated with potential or theoretical increased health risks with certain contraceptive methods. For each of the personal characteristics or medical conditions considered by the UKMEC, a category (1, 2, 3 or 4) is given, as outlined in Table 12.1.

Table 12.1 Definition of UKMEC Categories

UKMEC	Definition of category
Category 1	A condition for which there is no restriction on the use of the method
Category 2	A condition where the advantages of using the method generally outweigh the theoretical or proven risks
Category 3	A condition where the theoretical or proven risks usually outweigh the advantages of using the method. The provision of a method requires expert clinical judgement or referral to a specialist contraceptive provider, since use of the method is not usually recommended unless other more appropriate methods are not available or not acceptable
Category 4	A condition which represents an unacceptable health risk if the method is used

Source: FSRH (2016).

CHAPTER 12   Contraception and Sexual Health

> It is important to note that you do not add scores together. You simply take the highest score. For example, if a woman wants the COCP, she smokes and is over the age of 35, this scores her a UKMEC of 3. If her body mass index (BMI) is over 30 then this scores a UKMEC of 2. Her score is still 3 (not 5), as you take the highest score and do not add any scores together.

The initiation or continuation of a method of contraception can be classified differently. At times it may be appropriate to start a contraceptive method; for example, starting the POP if the patient has a history of a stroke gives a UKMEC score of 2, but if the individual had a stroke *while* taking the POP the continuation of the pill is not recommended as this gives a UKMEC score of 3.

Along with the UKMEC, and determining what is a safe contraceptive method for the patient to use, as the consulting practitioner you must also have a discussion with the patient detailing all the available options of contraception and what might work best for them. For example, it may not be ideal for a cabin crew worker to commence the COCP, as they will work in shifts across different time zones, making it very difficult to know when to take their next pill. In this case a LARC would be more suitable. On the other hand, the patient and her partner may be considering starting a family within the next year and therefore a LARC, such as the coil, may not be suitable for them. Written information is often a good idea for patients to read and take their time when considering their choice – you can point them in the direction of the Sex Wise website (Sex Wise, 2021) where this information is freely available. Whichever contraception the patient chooses, it needs to fit her lifestyle.

History Taking

There are many different aspects which should be considered when taking a patient's history concerning contraception and sexual health, such as contraceptive and sexual history, medical history, menstrual history, obstetric history, drug history, family history and social history. Some things to consider within these categories when taking the patient's history are outlined below.

Contraception and sexual history:

- Is the patient already on a method of contraception?
- Any contraception failure such as missed pills or a damaged condom that could increase pregnancy risk? If so, discuss and offer emergency contraception.
- Establish the reason for the patient wanting to start or switch contraception. Is there a new sexual partner? Is it due to menstrual-related issues? Are there any side effects with the current contraception, for example, mood changes?
- If this is a new partner, offer STI screening. If appropriate (if the patient is under the age of 18), ask what age her partner is.
- Ask if the sex is consensual, free from coercion and if the patient is happy in their sexual relationship (you should consult with the patient alone to ask this).
- If the patient is asking for a repeat prescription of a pill, check that she is remembering to take the pill. It can be helpful to ask the patient in an open way,

Contraception

such as 'how many pills have you missed this month?'. Discuss ways of remembering, such as setting an alarm or putting the pill pack by their toothbrush.
- Does the patient have a preference of which contraceptive method they would like to use? Patients often read online about the different methods before contacting you, so this can be a useful starting point. A discussion of the advantages and disadvantages of each method in relation to the patient's personal circumstances should take place.
- Ask questions in relation to specific contraceptive method and the UKMEC to ensure the method the patient wishes to start is safe for them to have.
- If the patient is over the age of 25, it is important that you check during the consultation whether their smear is up to date.
- When starting a new method, always give the individual an NHS patient information leaflet or refer to the appropriate website regarding their contraceptive method, as there is a great deal of information to absorb in the consultation. This will include details on what to do if there is a missed pill or adverse effects, and can serve as a good reminder for patients.

Medical history:
- Does the patient have any medical conditions?
- Are they taking any regular medicines?
- Do they have any drug allergies?

Menstrual history:
- Ask about the patient's last menstrual period, her cycle length, whether there is a pattern, heavy or painful periods, *et cetera*.

Obstetric history:
- Does the patient have any children?
- Were the births normal vaginal delivery or other?

Drug history:
- Ask about any current prescription, non-prescription or illicit drugs.

Family history:
- Any relevant family history.

Social history:
- Alcohol and smoking
- Occupation.

Examination

Depending on each individual's situation and which contraceptive method they are opting for, you may need to take their blood pressure, a BMI (record height and weight) and an up-to-date pregnancy test. A routine annual review at least is recommended by the FSRH;

CHAPTER 12   Contraception and Sexual Health

however, this can be reduced to six monthly if the clinician is concerned (for example, due to age, safeguarding, weight).

> ⚠️ Ensure you are aware of the local policies regarding how to escalate encounters where patients disclose problems with sexual relationships, such as non-consensual sex or sexual violence.

Types of Contraception

Long-acting Reversible Contraception (LARC)

In 2005, NICE published its guideline on the use of LARC, with an aim to increase the use of LARCs because their effectiveness does not depend on the woman remembering to take or use them. In addition, NICE's guideline and quality standard on contraception recommend that women asking for contraception are given information about, and offered a choice of, all methods of contraception including LARC (NHS Digital, 2018). Since this publication, use of user-dependent contraceptives, such as the oral contraceptive pill, has gradually decreased over time from 77% in 2007 to 59% in 2018. During the same time, use of LARCs has increased from 23% to 41% (NICE, 2019b).

The Contraceptive Injection (Depo and Sayana Press)

With careful use, the contraceptive injection is over 99% effective; however, typical use results in around 94% effectiveness, as women sometimes attend late for their injection (FPA, 2020). Women now have the option of both Depo-provera and Sayana Press. Sayana Press is a self-injection that patients are able to give themselves at home, once they have been shown how to do it by a clinician. This suits many women because of their busy lifestyle and being able to inject at home is very convenient; however, others do not like the idea of self-injecting and prefer to opt for the Depo-provera. Make sure that you discuss both options with your patient, so that they can make an informed choice.

The contraceptive injection is a progesterone-only contraceptive, which works by releasing progesterone to stop ovulation, thickening cervical mucus to prevent sperm reaching an egg and thinning the lining of the uterus to prevent a fertilised egg implanting. It lasts for 13 weeks and can be very effective at reducing heavy periods (often bleeding completely stops). Disadvantages of the contraceptive injection include some women suffering with unpredictable and irregular bleeding, and some women gaining weight. Additionally, it is vital to inform your patient that periods and fertility can take a year to return after stopping the injection, which is important if your patient wants to conceive in the near future. Moreover, as the injection is in the body, it cannot be removed, so any side effects may continue until it is out of the patient's system. Women need to receive the injection every 13 weeks for it to be fully effective.

The contraceptive injection can increase the risk of developing osteoporosis and fractures; several studies have shown that bone density decreases by a small amount in women who use this as a contraceptive method (Dennerstein et al., 2018). Therefore, it is essential that women are asked about any family history of osteoporosis and whether they smoke; if the answer is 'yes' to both, it would be worth discussing an alternative option. The injection can be given at any time during the cycle as long as the woman is not pregnant. If the injection is given in the first seven days of a cycle, the patient will be protected against pregnancy straight away. If it is given at any other time, it is vital to inform the patient to use additional contraception, such as condoms, for seven days afterwards or to abstain from sex.

Intrauterine Contraceptive Devices (IUCDs)

Intrauterine contraception is highly effective and long acting, making it a very cost-effective option (FPA, 2020). There are two main types – LNG-IUS and Cu-IUD.

The LNG-IUS

The LNG-IUS is over 99% effective. Once it is fitted it works as a contraceptive for three to six years, depending on the type (Mirena: six years), and therefore is not reliant on remembering to take a pill (FRSH, 2023; FPA, 2020). If the LNG-IUS is fitted under the age of 45 years, it works as a contraceptive for up to six years. If it is inserted at age over 45 years it can be used as a contraceptive until the age of 55 years. It is important to note that the LNG-IUS can only be used for five years as endometrial protection as part of hormone replacement therapy (HRT) (FSRH, 2023).

It involves a small flexible T-shaped plastic device that is inserted into the uterus where it releases progesterone. Many GP surgeries have trained practitioners who can fit IUCDs within the practice, or it may be commissioned outside of primary care within local sexual health clinics. Both IUC methods have a very small chance of an infection occurring within the first 20 days after insertion, and insertion can be uncomfortable (FPA, 2020).

The intrauterine system (IUS) works by thinning the lining of the uterus to stop a fertilised egg implanting, and thickens the cervical mucus so that it is difficult for sperm to reach the egg. In some women it also supresses ovarian function. The effect the LNG-IUS has on bleeding varies from woman to woman; bleeding usually becomes lighter and less painful, and it may completely stop. However, many women do suffer with unpredictable and irregular bleeding in the first six months. When the IUS is removed, the patient's fertility will return to normal instantly. The LNG-IUS can be fitted at any time in the menstrual cycle as long as the patient is not pregnant or at recent risk of pregnancy. If it is fitted in the first seven days of a cycle, the patient will be protected against pregnancy straight away. If it is fitted at any other time, it is vital to inform the patient to use additional contraception, such as condoms, or to abstain from sex for seven days afterwards (FSRH, 2016).

Copper IUD

The copper IUD is over 99% effective and once is it fitted it works as a contraceptive for five to ten years, depending on the type (usually ten years). It involves a small, flexible plastic and copper device being inserted into the uterus. The copper impairs the viability of sperm and eggs and changes cervical mucus to stop sperm from being able to reach the egg. It starts working as soon as it has been inserted (no need to use extra precautions for seven days afterwards) and the patient's fertility will return to normal as soon as the Cu-IUD is removed. An obvious advantage of the Cu-IUD for many women is that it does not use any hormones, which is brilliant for women who want to be protected from pregnancy but do

CHAPTER 12   Contraception and Sexual Health

not want any additional hormones. A disadvantage is that it can make periods heavier and more painful (the patient will still have regular monthly bleeds), making it an unsuitable method if the patient already suffers with dysmenorrhoea and menorrhagia.

The Contraceptive Implant

The implant is highly effective at preventing pregnancy, with over 99% efficacy (FPA, 2020). It is a progesterone-only method and once it is fitted it works for three years, although it can be removed sooner if a patient is getting unwanted side effects or wishes to conceive. According to the UKMEC, it is viewed as one of the safest contraceptives and most GP practices fit contraceptive implants. It involves a small flexible rod that is put under the skin of the upper arm. This releases the progesterone hormone, which stops ovulation, thickens cervical mucus to prevent sperm from reaching an egg and thins the lining of the uterus to prevent an egg implanting. Advantages of the implant include not needing to remember a pill or patch, and that once it is removed fertility returns to normal instantly. Disadvantages of the implant include irregular and unpredictable bleeding patterns and the requirement of a small procedure to fit and remove it (inserted using a local anaesthetic, no stitches required). The patient may be left with a small scar and the implant can cause or worsen acne in some women (Ramdhan et al., 2018). The patient should be advised that they should be able to feel the implant but not see it.

The Progesterone-only Pill (POP)

The POP can also be referred to as the 'mini pill'. It is 99% effective if taken correctly, but with typical use it is around 91% effective. It is a progesterone-only method of contraception. POPs with the progesterone Desogestrel work by stopping ovulation, thickening cervical mucus and thinning the lining of the uterus (FPA, 2020). Other POPs thicken cervical mucus and may stop ovulation. The POP is brilliant for women who want to take a pill as a method, but the combined pill is contraindicated. This is because it comes with fewer risks for certain conditions such as blood clots and breast cancer. For example, women are still able to take the POP if they are overweight, smoke or suffer with migraines. A disadvantage of the POP is that it commonly causes irregular bleeding, particularly in the first three to six months, and may continue to cause bleeding issues after this time (although often bleeding stops altogether). Additionally, if the patient has diarrhoea and vomiting, then the POP may not be fully effective. Often women report side effects of acne and breast pain, therefore this particular method may not be suitable for women who already suffer with spots. The POP can be taken up until the age of 55 (FSRH, 2019a).

How to Take the POP

The main difference between the POP and the COCP is that the POP is taken continuously, without a stop for a withdrawal bleed. There are two different types of POP; the most commonly used is Desogestrel, which must be taken within 12 hours of the same time each day. There is also the 'traditional' POP, such as Northisterone, which should be taken within three hours of the same time each day. There are 28 pills in a POP pack, when a patient finishes a pack, they simply start the next pack. If the patient starts the POP on day one to five of their menstrual cycle, it will work straight away and they will be protected against pregnancy. If they start the progestogen-only pill on any other day of their cycle, they will not be protected from pregnancy straight away and will need additional contraception until they

Types of Contraception

have taken the pill for two days (48 hours). If the patient has just had a baby, she can start the progestogen-only pill on day 21 after the birth and will be protected against pregnancy straight away. If she starts the progestogen-only pill more than 21 days after giving birth, she will need to use additional contraception until she has taken the pill for two days (NHS, 2021c).

> NHS (2021c) The progesterone-only pill [online].
> Specific advice is required for patients who miss taking their pill.

The Combined Oral Contraceptive Pill (COCP)

The COCP is 99% effective if used correctly, but with typical use it is around 91% effective (FPA, 2020). It is a combined method and therefore includes two hormones (oestrogen and progesterone). It works by stopping ovulation, thickening cervical mucus to prevent sperm reaching an egg and thinning the lining of the uterus to prevent an egg implanting.

> The COCP can interact with enzyme inducers. These speed up the breakdown of hormones by the liver, reducing the effectiveness of the pill. Examples include Carbamazepine, Phenytoin and St John's wort.

Use of the COCP may be associated with non-contraceptive health benefits, particularly reducing heavy bleeding, improving painful periods and improving acne. Additionally, the use of the COCP is associated with a significant reduction in the risk of endometrial and ovarian cancer (FPA, 2020). Fertility returns to normal once the combined pill is stopped. Missing pills, vomiting or severe diarrhoea can make the COCP less effective. A clear advantage of the COCP is that a woman can have more control over her monthly bleeds.

> Due to the COCP being a combined method of contraception, it is vital to ask the patient questions in relation to the UKMEC. Combined methods of contraception can be associated with blood clots and breast cancer (still a relatively low risk), and the patient should be made aware of these risks (FSRH, 2020a).

Combined hormonal contraception is associated with a very small increased risk of myocardial infarction (MI) and ischaemic stroke that appears to be greater with higher doses of oestrogen. Due to these risks, the COCP is not suitable for women who:

- Smoke and are over the age of 35
- Are over the age of 50
- Suffer from migraines with aura
- Are obese (BMI over 35)
- Suffer with hypertension

CHAPTER 12 Contraception and Sexual Health

- Have a history of venous thromboembolism (VTE) or a first-degree relative under the age of 45 with a history of VTE
- Have a history of breast cancer.

> 📖 FSRH (2016) UK medical eligibility criteria [online].
> Refer to the UKMEC for a full list of personal characteristics and medical conditions.

There are several different brands of COCP available on the market, each with different doses of oestrogen and type of progesterone. It can be trial and error finding out which COCP works best for each woman in relation to her mood, skin and bleeding patterns. When considering which brand to prescribe, this is constantly changing and you should follow both the FSRH and local guidance.

How to Take the COCP

Traditionally, women on the combined contraceptive pill take a seven-day break at the end of each 21-pill packet. During this monthly break from pill-taking, there is usually a bleed and some women have symptoms like period pain, headache and mood change. However, a new NICE-accredited clinical guideline from the Faculty of Sexual and Reproductive Healthcare (FSRH, 2020a) highlights that there is no health benefit from having this hormone-free interval. Women can avoid monthly bleeding and any associated symptoms by running pill packets together so that they take fewer, or no, breaks. If a hormone-free interval is taken, shortening it to four days could potentially reduce the risk of pregnancy if pills are missed (FSRH, 2020a). However, by not having the seven-day break, women may report 'spotting' or irregular and unpredictable bleeding. Women should be given information about both standard and tailored regimens to broaden contraceptive choice. However, women should be advised that use of tailored regimens is outside the manufacturer's licence but is supported by the Faculty of Sexual and Reproductive Healthcare (FSRH).

> 📖 FSRH (2020a) Combined hormonal contraception [online].
> FSRH summarise the different ways of taking the COCP.

The COCP needs to be taken at around the same time every day. If the patient starts their combined pill on the first day of their period, and up to and including the fifth day of their period, they will be protected from pregnancy straight away and will not need additional contraception. However, if the pill is commenced after this date, then the patient will not be protected from pregnancy straight away and will need additional contraception until they have taken the pill for seven days, or to abstain from sex for that time.

> ❗ The antibiotics rifampicin and rifabutin (which can be used to treat tuberculosis and meningitis) can reduce the effectiveness of the combined pill. Other antibiotics do not have this effect.

If the patients vomits within three hours of taking the COCP, it may not have been fully absorbed; you should advise your patient to take another pill straight away and the next pill at their usual time. If they continue to vomit, they should use another form of contraception until they have taken the pill again for seven days without vomiting or severe diarrhoea. If your patient has just had a baby, is not breastfeeding and does not have any other risk factors, she can most likely start the pill on day 21 after the birth. She will be protected against pregnancy straight away. If she starts the COCP later than 21 days after giving birth, she will need additional contraception for the next seven days. If the woman is breastfeeding, it is not advised to take the COCP until six weeks after the birth (FSRH, 2016).

> NHS (2019) What should I do if I miss a pill? [online].
> Specific advice is required for patients who miss taking their COCP.

The Combined Transdermal Patch

The contraceptive patch is 99% effective if used correctly; however, with typical use it is around 91% effective (FPA, 2020a). It is a small patch that sticks to the skin and releases both oestrogen and progesterone, which stops ovulation, thickens cervical mucus to prevent sperm reaching an egg and thins the lining of the uterus to prevent an egg implanting. The patch can be worn in the bath, when swimming and while playing sports and can be applied to most areas of the skin apart from the breasts. Advantages of the combined patch include not needing to remember a pill every day but still offering the benefits of a combined method. Additionally, it is not affected if the patient has diarrhoea or vomiting, and the patient can determine their monthly bleeds by running patches together. It often makes periods less painful and lighter. A disadvantage of the patch is that it can sometimes be seen. Limited evidence suggests a possible reduction in patch effectiveness in women ≥ 90 kg, and therefore alternatives should be used if the patient is over 90 kg (FSRH, 2019b). In the UK, the patch brand name is Evra.

> Due to the contraceptive patch being a combined method of contraception, it is vital to ask the patient questions in relation to the UKMEC.

How to Use the Combined Transdermal Patch

See the COCP section for different ways of using the contraceptive patch (table to regimens). However, the traditional way of taking the patch involves applying the first patch and wearing it for seven days. On day eight, the patient will need to change the patch to a new one. They will need to change it like this every week for three weeks, and then have a patch-free week. During the patch-free week they will get a withdrawal bleed, although this may not always happen. After seven patch-free days, the patient should apply a new patch and start the four-week cycle again. If the patient starts using the patch on the first day of their period,

CHAPTER 12   Contraception and Sexual Health

and up to and including the fifth day of their period, they will be protected from pregnancy straight away. If they start using it on any other day, they need to use an additional form of contraception for the first seven days, or to abstain from sex for this time (NHS, 2021a).

> NHS (2021a) Contraceptive patch [online].
> Specific advice is required for patients who forget to take their patch off or to put a new one on after the patch-free week.

The Combined Vaginal Ring

The contraceptive vaginal ring is 99% effective if always used according to instructions; however, with typical use it is 91% effective (FPA, 2020). It involves the woman inserting a small, flexible plastic ring into their vagina, where it releases both oestrogen and progesterone (the vaginal ring is a combined method of contraception). It works by stopping ovulation, thickening the cervical mucus to stop sperm reaching the egg and thinning the lining of the uterus to stop an egg implanting. One ring provides contraception for a month. The patient can continue to have sex as usual when the ring is in place; a partner may feel it, but this is not harmful. Unlike the pill, the ring still works even if the patient has vomiting and diarrhoea. For most women, the ring lightens bleeding and makes periods less painful. For women who suffer with acne, the vaginal ring may improve their skin. Occasionally, the ring can come out on its own, but it can be rinsed with warm water and re-inserted within three hours without the need to use additional contraception.

How to Use the Vaginal Ring

The patient can start using the vaginal ring at any time during their menstrual cycle as long as they are not pregnant. Traditionally, the patient needs to leave the ring in for 21 days, then remove it and have a seven-day ring-free break. They are protected against pregnancy during the ring-free break. A new ring is then inserted for another 21 days. The patient will be protected against pregnancy straight away if the ring is inserted on the first day of their period. If the patient starts using the ring at any other time in their menstrual cycle, they will need to use additional contraception, or to abstain from sex, for the first seven days of using it. To insert the ring, the patient will need to clean their hands, squeeze the ring between their thumb and finger and gently insert the tip into the vagina, gently pushing the ring up until it feels comfortable. To remove the ring, the patient will need to clean their hands, put a finger into their vagina and hook it around the edge of the ring, gently pulling the ring out. It can then be put in the special bag provided and thrown in the bin; advise them not to flush it down the toilet. Removing the ring should be painless (NHS, 2021d).

> ! Due to the vaginal ring being a combined method of contraception, it is vital to ask the patient questions in relation to the UKMEC.

Types of Contraception

> NHS (2021d) The vaginal ring, your contraceptive guide [online].
> Specific advice is required for patients who forget to take the ring out or to insert a new ring.

Condoms

The methods of contraception previously discussed do not protect patients from STIs. However, condoms do, if used correctly and consistently (98% effective) (FPA, 2020). With typical use, around 18 in 100 women will become pregnant every year when using condoms as the only form of contraception (FPA, 2020). A condom is made from very thin rubber and it simply covers an erect penis to prevent sperm from entering the vagina. It is important to offer condoms to your patients when they come to see you for any kind of sexual health or contraceptive issue (particularly if they are under the age of 25). Condoms are available in all different shapes and sizes and do not come with any serious side effects. The biggest issue with condoms is that they can sometimes split or slip off if the incorrect size is used, which results in women requiring emergency contraception.

Female (internal) condoms are also available (not as widely available as male (external) condoms) and are made from soft, thin synthetic latex or polyurethane. They are worn inside the vagina to prevent semen getting to the womb and are 95% effective (NHS, 2021b). Diaphragms are non-hormonal barrier methods of contraception that protect women against pregnancy by preventing sperm reaching the cervix. The 'Caya' is the most common and comes in one size (it will accommodate 80% of women).

> If possible, avoid using spermicidal lubricated condoms because they commonly contain a chemical called nonoxinol-9, which may increase the risk of HIV and other infections (FPA, 2020).

Vasectomy

A vasectomy is more than 99% effective. It involves a surgical procedure to seal the tubes that carry sperm, permanently preventing pregnancy. Sperm is prevented from entering the semen; therefore when ejaculation occurs the semen has no sperm to fertilise an egg. It is considered permanent and is very difficult to reverse; therefore it is important to ensure it is the right choice for your patient.

The patient will need to use contraception for at least 8–12 weeks after the operation because sperm will still be in the tubes leading to the penis.

> It is recommended that both patient and partner agree with the vasectomy, but it is not a legal requirement to have partner permission.

CHAPTER 12   Contraception and Sexual Health

Female Sterilisation

Female sterilisation is an operation to permanently prevent pregnancy. The fallopian tubes are blocked or sealed to prevent the eggs reaching the sperm and becoming fertilised. Eggs will still be released from the ovaries as normal, but they will be absorbed naturally into the woman's body. It is very difficult to reverse, and therefore counselling is recommended to ensure the right choice for the patient.

> It does not affect hormone levels and the patient will still have periods.

> FSRH (2016) UK medical eligibility criteria [online].
> Further reading regarding ensuring the method of contraception is safe can be found within the UKMEC guidelines.

Health Promotion When Considering Contraception

Contraception After Childbirth

Fertility may return very quickly and therefore it is important for post-partum women to be offered contraception at the earliest point possible, as supporting women to make an informed choice about contraception will reduce unwanted pregnancies. Moreover, providing advice about contraception after childbirth helps avoid the risk of complications associated with an inter-pregnancy interval of less than 12 months (NICE, 2019b).

Breastfeeding

Breastfeeding can be 98% effective at preventing pregnancy up to six months after giving birth if the woman is exclusively breastfeeding (day and night), their baby is up to six months old and they have not yet had a period (NICE, 2019b).

Opportunities for Health Promotion

More than one in five pregnant young women under the age of 25 reported being a smoker at their first booking appointment, and 25% of young women aged 18–24 are overweight or obese in early pregnancy (AYPH, 2019). Discussing contraceptives with patients can be an excellent opportunity for health promotion, particularly when initiating any combined method of contraception.

> Side effects are an important consideration. There is no evidence of weight gain for any of the contraceptive methods apart from the Depo injection. Hormonal contraception may be associated with mood changes but there is no evidence that hormonal contraceptives cause depression.

Emergency Contraception (EC)

Contraception in Patients Under 18 Years

In 2017, rates of conceptions in the under-18 age group were at their lowest level since 1969, but the UK still has a relatively high rate of births among 15–19-year-olds compared with other similar high-income countries (NICE, 2019b). Understanding the law relating to conversations with patients less than 18 years of age is important.

Legal and Ethical Requirements for Contraception

The most notorious aspect of law concerning contraceptives within England, Wales and Northern Ireland is associated with Gillick and Fraser. It is important to note that these are related, but not interchangeable, terms. Gillick competence refers to the assessment that could be made regarding whether a child under the age of 16 has the capacity to consent to treatment without parental or guardian consent (Griffith, 2016). Gillick was a landmark decision wherein the House of Lords was called upon to resolve the extent of the parental right to control a minor child, and when, and indeed whether, such a minor could receive contraceptive advice, or consent to medical treatment, against the wishes or knowledge of their parents. The outcome was that a minor will be able to consent to treatment if they demonstrate 'sufficient understanding and intelligence to understand fully what is proposed' (*Gillick v West Norfolk & Wisbeck Area Health Authority* [1986] AC 112 House of Lords).

Fraser guidelines refer to Lord Fraser's involvement with the Gillick case. Lord Fraser stated that a doctor could proceed to give advice and treatment provided they are satisfied with the following criteria:

- That the girl (although under the age of 16) will understand the clinician's advice
- That the clinician cannot persuade her to inform her parents or to allow them to inform the parents that she is seeking contraceptive advice
- That she is very likely to continue having sexual intercourse with or without contraceptive treatment
- That unless she receives contraceptive advice or treatment her physical or mental health are both likely to suffer
- That her best interests require the clinician to give her contraceptive advice, treatment or both without parental consent.

> Eaton, G. (2022) *Law and Ethics for Paramedics: An Essential Guide.*
> Refer to Eaton (2022) for more information about this case.

Emergency Contraception (EC)

Requests for EC are a common presentation in primary care. It is vital to take a full sexual history when consulting with a woman asking for EC. Some patients may find the process of acquiring EC quite distressing or embarrassing. Therefore, it is important to build a good rapport, making the patient feel as comfortable as possible, and to explore their need for EC. See Figure 12.1 for a flowchart demonstrating a consultation with a patient requiring EC.

CHAPTER 12   Contraception and Sexual Health

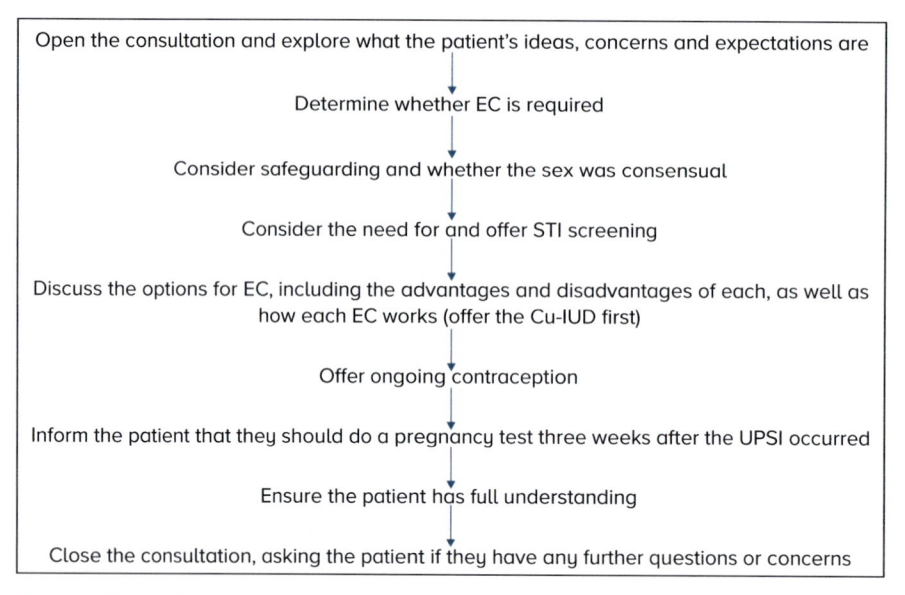

```
Open the consultation and explore what the patient's ideas, concerns and expectations are
                                    ↓
                        Determine whether EC is required
                                    ↓
              Consider safeguarding and whether the sex was consensual
                                    ↓
                   Consider the need for and offer STI screening
                                    ↓
  Discuss the options for EC, including the advantages and disadvantages of each, as well as
                      how each EC works (offer the Cu-IUD first)
                                    ↓
                            Offer ongoing contraception
                                    ↓
    Inform the patient that they should do a pregnancy test three weeks after the UPSI occurred
                                    ↓
                      Ensure the patient has full understanding
                                    ↓
   Close the consultation, asking the patient if they have any further questions or concerns
```

Figure 12.1   Consultation flow chart.

Where is EC available?

- General practice
- Pharmacy (over the age of 16)
- Genitourinary medicine (GUM) clinic
- NHS walk-in centres
- Emergency department (ED) (although this is inappropriate to suggest as an alternative care pathway and not all EDs will offer EC).

Indications for EC

EC should be offered if a woman has had unprotected sexual intercourse (UPSI) on any day of their natural menstrual cycle, or if they think their contraception may have failed and they do not wish to conceive (FSRH, 2020b). This is because pregnancy is theoretically possible after UPSI on most days of the cycle, although risk of pregnancy is highest after UPSI that takes place during the six days leading up to and including the day of ovulation.

It is important to note that EC should be offered to any woman who does not wish to conceive and has had UPSI from day 21 after childbirth (unless the criteria for lactational amenorrhoea has been met). EC should also be offered when UPSI has taken place from day five after abortion, miscarriage, ectopic pregnancy or uterine evacuation for gestational trophoblastic disease.

History

During the history-taking phase of the consultation, consider patients' thoughts and feelings and ask the following questions:

Emergency Contraception (EC)

- When did the UPSI take place?
- Have there been further episodes of UPSI during this cycle?
  - If so, when and how many times?
- Was the sex with a new or regular partner?
- Was the sex consensual?
- Have there been multiple partners?
- Is the patient involved in high-risk sexual activity?
- When was the patient's last menstrual period (LMP)?
  - Was it a normal period for them?
- Where are they in their current cycle?
  - Sometimes women are unsure about this as they have irregular periods, or they have been taking the 'mini pill' and have not had a period for some time. Other patients record their cycle in an app and can clearly tell you the dates of their LMP.
- Was any other contraception used or was there a contraception failure (for example, condom splitting or missed pill).
- If they are not currently taking any contraception, would they like ongoing contraception?
- Ask about their thoughts and feelings about the prospect of being pregnant.
- Have they shared their situation with anyone else?
- Where appropriate, consider the patient's age and the age of their partner.

Safeguarding

As part of your consultation, it is essential that you explore the potential for sexual or domestic abuse. You should always clarify if the sex was with a regular partner and whether it was consensual and without violence. It is important to ask the patient if they feel safe and happy in their relationship(s), and to ensure that the principles of confidentiality are understood (including that in some circumstances they cannot be guaranteed, for example when a crime has taken place). If a disclosure is made to you during the consultation regarding sexual crime or violence, the following approach will enable you to support the patient as you navigate your local safeguarding procedures:

1. Support the disclosure.
   - Provide a quiet and confidential space for the patient to continue the conversation. Acknowledge that it may be difficult to speak about what happened.
   - Provide an interpreter if English is not the person's first language (do not use a family member or friend).
   - Be non-judgemental, supportive and empathetic.
2. Ensure any medical treatment is provided as a priority.
   - This may require assessment at an ED, depending on the injury.
3. Ask the patient what they want to happen next.
   - Inform the patient that they can access an Independent Sexual Violence Advisor (ISVA) who can help them better understand their options. (It is helpful to know how these can be accessed in your local area; it may be via your service, Victim

CHAPTER 12 Contraception and Sexual Health

Support, the police, Rape Crisis Centres or third-sector services.) The role of the ISVA is to provide information and support, particularly around the criminal justice process, to liaise with work or educational settings and to provide therapeutic input.
4. Arrange for police involvement, and find the nearest SARC if they have been sexually assaulted.
5. Ensure that sexual health and medical needs are accounted for:
   - EC (unless it is too late, then ensure you offer pregnancy testing on the first day of the missed period).
   - If indicated, arrange for post-exposure prophylaxis (PEP) to be prescribed.
   - Hepatitis B vaccination may also be indicated. In some situations, the patient will also need a hepatitis B immunoglobin (HBIG) injection along with the hepatitis B vaccine. This should ideally be given within 48 hours but can still be given up until a week after exposure.
   - Assess the wish or need for referral for further assessment and screening, particularly for STIs; this is usually two weeks post possible exposure.
6. Ensure accurate documentation (Luby, 2018).

Examination

Not often required, apart from measuring the patient's BMI.

What Methods of EC Are Available?

In the UK, three methods of EC are currently available: the copper IUD (Cu-IUD), oral ulipristal acetate (UPA) and oral levonorgestrel (LNG).

Copper IUD

The emergency Cu-IUD works by stopping an egg being fertilised or implanting in the uterus. It is toxic to sperm and eggs and therefore prevents implantation. It is ten times more effective than oral EC (FPA, 2020).

Ulipristal Acetate

The emergency contraceptive pill works by stopping or delaying ovulation; therefore it is only likely to work if taken before the egg has been released. It is effective up to 120 hours after UPSI.

Levonorgestrel

The emergency contraceptive pill works by stopping ovulation; therefore it is only likely to work if taken before the egg has been released. Levonorgestrel is licensed for use up to 72 hours after UPSI and has reduced efficacy 96 hours after UPSI.

> Evidence suggests that the oral EC pills (both levonorgestrel and ulipristal) do not disrupt an existing pregnancy and are not associated with fetal abnormality (FSRH, 2020b).

Emergency Contraception (EC)

Choosing the Most Appropriate EC

NICE (2019b) recommends that women who ask for EC should be told that a Cu-IUD is more effective than an oral pill and this should be offered first. However, you should have an open discussion with the patient and identify which EC option would be most appropriate for them, using the FSRH (2020a) guidance to aid the decision making. Remind women that they may still fall pregnant, despite taking the EC pill correctly.

Table 12.2 summarises the mode of action, advantages, disadvantages, risks, cautions and contraindications for each of the three EC methods (FSRH, 2020b; Mason, 2020).

Table 12.2 Comparisons of Emergency Contraception

	Copper IUD	Ulipristal	Levonorgestrel
Mode of action	Plastic and copper coil An inhibitory effect on both fertilisation and implantation	Delays ovulation for five days or more	Inhibits ovulation and causes luteal dysfunction
Advantages	Non-hormonal Can be used as regular contraception for up to ten years Can be inserted up to five days following unprotected sex	No long-term side effects No procedure needed Can be taken up to five days after unprotected sex	No long-term side effects No procedure needed
Disadvantages	An uncomfortable procedure needed to fit the IUD Period-type pain and bleeding are common a few days following fitting Women will need to be given the EC pill in the interim anyway, as it may not be able to be fitted straight away	Less effective than the emergency contraceptive IUD May affect the next period Cannot be taken within five days of taking progesterone (e.g., POP)	Can only be taken up to three days after unprotected sex May affect the next period Less effective than other emergency contraceptive methods
Risks	Small risk of infection, perforation and expulsion	Vomiting and headaches	Vomiting and headaches
Cautions		Use with caution in those with severe asthma, controlled by oral glucocorticoids Use an alternative	Use with caution in those with a BMI of more than 26 or a weight of more than 70 kg

(Continued)

Table 12.2 (Continued)

	Copper IUD	**Ulipristal**	**Levonorgestrel**
Contraindications	Less than 28 days following giving birth Less than five days following a miscarriage or abortion Active STI	Less than 21 days following giving birth Less than five days following a miscarriage or abortion	Less than 21 days following giving birth Less than five days following a miscarriage or abortion
Clinical Pearl	If a woman is referred to have a Cu-IUD inserted, she should be given the EC pill at the time of referral, in case the coil cannot be inserted or the woman changes her mind	The effectiveness of ulipristal is reduced if a women has taken progesterone in the five days after taking it. Additionally, the effectiveness of Ulipristal could theoretically be reduced if a woman has taken progesterone in the seven days prior (e.g., she had missed a pill). A woman can start her ongoing contraception five days after taking the ulipristal. This may not be suitable for women who are young and at high risk of becoming pregnant, and therefore levonorgestrel may be considered instead	A double dose of levonorgestrel should be given to women who are over 70 kg (therefore is it vital to ask or take their weight), as a higher BMI reduces the effects of levonorgestrel

Source: Mason (2020).

> As a paramedic prescriber, it is important to know that enzyme-inducing drugs reduce the effects of both levonorgestrel and ulipristal. Women requiring EC who are using enzyme-inducing drugs should be offered the Cu-IUD if appropriate. A double dose of levonorgestrel can be considered, but the effectiveness of this is unknown. However, a double dose of ulipristal is not recommended.

Emergency Contraception (EC)

This information can be relayed to the patient to enable them to make an informed decision. Additionally, algorithms available from the FSRH (2020a) display the decision-making process that takes place when considering EC.

Regular Use of EC

If a woman has already taken ulipristal once or more in a cycle, she can have ulipristal again after further UPSI in the same cycle. The same can be said for levonorgestrel. However, if a woman has already taken ulipristal, levonorgestrel should not be taken in the following five days. Additionally, if a woman has already taken levonorgestrel in her cycle, ulipristal may be less effective if taken in the following seven days.

EC and Breastfeeding

If the woman is not *exclusively* breastfeeding but is still breastfeeding (perhaps alongside formula milk) or her baby is not under six months old or she has had a period, and she requires EC, further precautions need to be taken. Breastfeeding women have a higher relative risk of uterine perforation during insertion of intrauterine contraception than non-breastfeeding women, although the absolute risk of perforation is low. Breastfeeding women should be advised not to breastfeed and to express and discard milk for a week after they have taken ulipristal. Women who breastfeed should be informed that the limited available evidence indicates that levonorgestrel has no adverse effects on breastfeeding or on infants (BNF, 2021); however, it should be taken immediately after breastfeeding, with nursing avoided for a further eight hours following administration (NICE, 2021b).

Consideration of STIs

When consulting with any female regarding EC, you must consider the risk of an STI and offer screening following taking a comprehensive sexual history (see STI section).

Ongoing Contraception

Women requesting EC should be given information regarding all methods of ongoing contraception and how to access these, as it may be very appropriate to 'quick start' opportunistic ongoing contraception to prevent pregnancy. Patients should be reminded that oral methods of EC do not provide contraceptive cover for subsequent UPSI.

Pregnancy Test

Inform the patient that they should do a pregnancy test three weeks after the UPSI occurred and to contact the GP surgery if it is positive. A 'standard' pregnancy test could 'rule in' or 'rule out' pregnancy with reasonable reliability if undertaken more than 21 days after the last episode of unprotected sex (FSRH, 2020b).

CHAPTER 12   Contraception and Sexual Health

Sexually Transmitted Infections (STIs)

Most methods of contraception do not protect patients from STIs. The impact of STIs remains greatest in young heterosexuals, 15 to 24 years; BME people; and MSM (PHE, 2019). Reliable and correct use of condoms can significantly reduce the risk of STIs and it is important to promote the availability of condoms by local services, including through condom distribution schemes. Individuals who misuse alcohol or drugs, participate in sexual activity at a young age or who persistently have UPSI with multiple partners are also at increased risk (NICE, 2021b). Regular testing for HIV and STIs is essential for good sexual health and patients should be encouraged to have an STI screen annually if they are having condomless sex with new or casual partners (PHE, 2019).

> BASHH (2021) BASHH guidelines [online].
> This is an excellent resource for understanding STIs.

History Taking

It is important to consider the following questions in your consultations:

- Does your patient have any symptoms of an STI? Consider STIs as a differential diagnosis (that is, to a UTI).
  – Are they well in themselves?
- Have they had UPSI with a confirmed case?
- Ask more detail about the sexual contact (sex, age, more than once, high-risk sexual activity, new partner).
- Do they use condoms?
- Have they previously been tested for STIs and HIV?
- Is EC indicated?
- Have they been generally unwell for a long period of time?

Examination

Depending on how the patient is in themselves, it may be appropriate to undertake vital observations. Conditional on the symptoms, it may appropriate to undertake an examination of the external genitalia (always offer a chaperone) (for example, for genital herpes). It may also be appropriate to examine the abdomen (for example, for pelvic inflammatory disease (PID)). Where appropriate, examine for lymphadenopathy and rashes, and consider swabs and urinalysis.

> For all STIs, the patient's current partner must also be treated to reduce the risk of onward transmission, and it is important that the patient is encouraged to have this discussion. If the person is unwilling or unable to have this conversation, advise them that (with their consent) their details can be provided to GUM solely for the purposes of partner notification.

Presentations in Primary Care

Chlamydia

Aetiology
Two-thirds of chlamydia diagnoses are made in young people aged 15–24, with an increase of 2% from 2018 (PHE, 2019). Anyone under 25 who is sexually active should be screened for chlamydia on change of sexual partner or annually. An individual can contract chlamydia even if there is no penetration, orgasm or ejaculation. It can also be contracted from infected semen or vaginal fluid getting into the eye and can be passed by a pregnant woman to her baby.

History and Examination
A detailed history may be sufficient to obtain a diagnosis, but this may be a diagnosis of symptoms, which can include dysuria, abnormal discharge (men and women), lower abdominal pain, post-coital or intermenstrual bleeding in women, deep dyspareunia and pelvic pain in women and pain or swelling of the testicles in men.

> ! Chlamydia presents with no symptoms 70% of the time. If left undetected and untreated, complications such as PID and infertility can occur. It can also increase the risk of ectopic pregnancy. Be alert to the possibility of PID in women who are unwell with a history indicative of and symptoms consistent with chlamydia.

Diagnosis is confirmed with positive swabs in women (nucleic acid amplification tests (NAATs)), either that the patient has taken themselves or that you as the clinician have taken if trained to do so (vulvo-vaginal swab is normally of choice in most women). The swab needs to be inserted about 5 cm into the vagina and gently rotated for 10 seconds. If you are trained to use a speculum, then an endocervical swab can be taken with the swab rotated 360 degrees inside the cervical os. In men, a first-catch urine is the specimen of choice.

> 💡 If the exposure was within the last two weeks, a test should be carried out at presentation, and if negative, repeated two weeks after the exposure.

Management
Chlamydia is treated with antibiotics, and your local antimicrobial prescribing guidelines and NICE guidance should be followed if the prescription is undertaken in primary care, or referral to the GUM clinic. Differences in treatment exist for those with allergies, and for patients who are pregnant or breastfeeding.

For pregnant women, management may be discussed with other healthcare professionals involved in the woman's care (such as the woman's midwife and obstetrician), if the patient consents. If chlamydia is diagnosed in a child under 16 years, then discuss

CHAPTER 12 Contraception and Sexual Health

management with a sexual health specialist or paediatrician. The patient's current partner must also be treated for chlamydia to reduce the risk of onward transmission. Sexual intercourse (including oral sex) should be avoided until the patient and their partner(s) have completed treatment (or waited for seven days if they have been prescribed azithromycin). Reinforce health education and the importance of condom use. Consider full STI screening if the patient consents to this (HIV, hepatitis b and syphilis BT) – NAATs screen for both chlamydia and gonorrhoea.

> Test of cure is not routinely recommended for uncomplicated genital chlamydia infection but *is* indicated in pregnancy, where poor compliance is suspected, and where symptoms persist.
>
> Offer repeat testing to all people under the age of 25 years diagnosed with chlamydia three to six months after completion of treatment to check for re-infection.
>
> Consider offering repeat testing to people over the age of 25 years who are at high risk of re-infection.

If the patient is unwell with PID, refer them to a GUM clinic or ED (NICE, 2022b).

> BASHH (2021) A guide to chlamydia [online].

Genital Herpes

Aetiology

Genital herpes is passed on through vaginal, anal and oral sex and is caused by the herpes simplex virus. It can range from being mild to very painful.

History and Examination

Diagnosis is based on the presence of the following symptoms, in conjunction with a viral swab from the base of one of the lesions formed, which is sent for viral culture:

- Small blisters that burst to leave red, open sores around the genitals, anus, thighs or bottom
- Lesions are usually bilateral and develop four to seven days after exposure to herpes simplex
- Tingling, burning or itching around the genitals
- Dysuria
- Sometimes malaise or fever
- Inguinal lymphadenopathy

- Recurrent infections usually occur in the same area and may be preceded by localised prodromal tingling and burning symptoms up to 48 hours before the appearance of lesions.

Whilst the incubation period is 2–14 days, sometimes symptoms do not appear for years after first exposure (that is, infection is not necessarily from a current or recent partner).

Management

Interpersonal skills are vital to minimise the stigma and address the myths and misconceptions around the herpes virus. Oral antivirals are the primary treatment for genital herpes simplex infection. Treatment should commence within five days of the start of the episode, or while new lesions are forming for people with a first clinical episode of genital herpes. If new lesions are still forming after three to five days, seek specialist advice. Advise individuals about self-care measures, including taking adequate pain relief, cleaning the area with plain or salt water, applying Vaseline or topical lidocaine, increasing fluid intake to dilute the urine and avoiding wearing tight clothing. Advise the patient to abstain from sex until the lesions have cleared. If the infection is severe, the person is systemically unwell or complications are suspected (such as urinary retention), admit for treatment in secondary care (NICE, 2023).

> Herpes simplex virus remains dormant. Some people have no recurrences. In line with BASHH guidance, suppression treatment can be offered to patients who have frequent occurrences (more than six a year). Transmission can occur when there are no symptoms (asymptomatic shedding), but the risk is higher when symptomatic.

Genital Warts

Aetiology

Genital warts are a common STI caused by the human papilloma virus (HPV). This virus is passed on through direct skin-to-skin contact with someone who has HPV on their skin. It can be passed from person to person during vaginal or anal sex.

History and Examination

Genital warts are usually asymptomatic, may be single or multiple and tend to occur in areas of high friction. The patient will present with local irritation and discomfort where warts occur, and warts usually present as soft cauliflower-like growths of varying size.

Management

Refer people with anogenital warts to a sexual health specialist via the GUM clinic. Treatment is often topical (though these cannot be used in pregnancy, are not licensed in children and have a high likelihood of adverse effects). Sometimes, treatment is not always indicated, as in about 30% of people warts disappear spontaneously within

CHAPTER 12   Contraception and Sexual Health

six months. Ablative methods (such as cryotherapy, excision and electrocautery) are accessed via the GUM clinic.

Gonorrhoea

Aetiology

There was a 26% increase in gonorrhoea between 2017 and 2018, especially in young people. It is caused by a bacteria called *Neisseria gonorrhoeae* or *N. gonococcus*. Infection is transmitted vaginally or through oral sex and can occur in the urethra, cervix, rectum, throat and eyes, with an incubation period of 1–14 days. The infection can also be passed from a pregnant woman to her baby. Without treatment, gonorrhoea can cause permanent blindness in a newborn baby (PHE, 2019).

History and Examination

Symptoms present differently in men and women, as outlined in Table 12.3.

An NAAT test should be arranged for the presence of *Neisseria gonorrhoea* in line with local procedures and protocols. In women, a vulvovaginal swab (which may be self taken)

Table 12.3   Symptoms of Gonorrhea in Men and Women

	Symptoms
Men	• Genital gonorrhoea infection is usually symptomatic in men. • Urethral infection causes mucopurulent or purulent urethral discharge in more than 80% of men and dysuria in more than 50% of men within two to five days of exposure; usually there is no effect on frequency or urgency of urination. • Rectal infection is usually asymptomatic but may cause anal discharge (12% of men), acute proctitis, perianal or anal pain or discomfort (7% of men), tenesmus or rectal bleeding. • Pharyngeal infection is asymptomatic in more than 90% of men but may cause cause tonsillitis or pharyngitis. • Other symptoms may be caused by complications of gonorrhoea infection, including prostatitis, epididymitis and orchitis.
Women	• Urogenital gonorrhoea is asymptomatic in up to 50% of women. • Where present, symptoms usually develop within ten days. • Increased or altered vaginal discharge (up to 50% of women). • Lower abdominal pain (up to 25% of women). • Dysuria (up to 12% of women); usually there is no effect on frequency of urination. • Intermenstrual bleeding or menorrhagia (rarely). • Dyspareunia if the infection spreads from the endocervix. • Pharyngeal infection is asymptomatic in 90% of women, but it may cause tonsillitis or pharyngitis.

Source: NHS (2022).

should be used. In men, a first-pass urine specimen should be used. Tests should be taken no earlier than three days after sexual contact with an infected person.

Management

Gonorrheoa is rarely treated in primary care and the patient should be referred to a GUM clinic for treatment. This is because gonorrhoea is treated with an intramuscular (IM) injection that is not readily available in primary care (often ceftriaxone 1 g IM injection as a single dose) (NICE, 2022a).

Hepatitis B

Aetiology

The hepatitis B virus is a major cause of serious, life-threatening liver disease, including liver cancer and cirrhosis. In 2017, the World Health Organization (WHO) estimated that around 250 million people worldwide were chronically infected with hepatitis B virus. Those at risk include people originally from high-risk countries, IV drug users, people who are HIV positive and people who have UPSI with multiple sexual partners. A hepatitis B vaccine is available for people at high risk of exposure to the condition.

History Taking and Examination

Symptoms can be generic, including tiredness, a fever and general aches and pains, which normally begin two to three months after exposure. However, many patients can be asymptomatic. Hepatitis B should be considered in patients with a high risk of exposure and symptoms of:

- Loss of appetite
- Nausea and vomiting
- Diarrhoea
- Abdominal pain
- Jaundice.

Diagnosis is confirmed with hepatitis B serology.

Management

Notify the health protection unit (HPU) promptly to facilitate appropriate surveillance and contact tracing. Admit any person with hepatitis B infection to hospital if they are severely unwell. Manage any pain, itching and nausea and advise the patient to avoid drinking alcohol. Take any necessary steps to minimise transmission. Refer anyone who is found to be hepatitis B positive to a hepatologist or to a gastroenterologist or infectious disease specialist with an interest in hepatology (NICE, 2022c).

> Tracing of previous sexual partner(s) is not recommended for people with anogenital warts in the absence of other STIs (NHS, 2020).

CHAPTER 12 Contraception and Sexual Health

Human Immunodeficiency Virus (HIV)

Aetiology

In the UK, about one in four of all new HIV infections are among youth aged 13 to 24 years and 73% of all infections are male. Heterosexual people over 50 years of age are the fastest increasing group of new diagnoses. People can live well with HIV with early diagnosis and effective treatment, but without adequate treatment AIDs can develop. HIV can be found in vaginal and anal fluids, breast milk, blood and semen; it cannot be transmitted through sweat, saliva or urine. Condomless anal or vaginal sex presents the most common way of transmitting the virus. HIV can also be transmitted through shared needles and between mother and child during pregnancy, birth or breastfeeding. Individuals most at risk include IV drug users, MSM and people with partners from a high-risk country (BHIVA, 2021).

> ❗ Patients at high risk of HIV include those with sexual risk, with physical symptoms, with a partner who has tested HIV positive, having an STI check-up, having an antenatal screening, in a new relationship, stopping condom use, worried well, who have suffered sexual assault and who have had blood donation or operation, medical investigation or occupational exposure.

History and Examination

HIV must be considered in patients from the high-risk groups who have unexplained symptoms that are unusually prolonged, severe or recurrent. Consider HIV in patients with lymphadenopathy, weight loss and persistent pyrexia of unknown origin. Primary HIV infection presents with fever, sore throat, maculopapular rash, malaise, lethargy, arthralgia, myalgia, lymphadenopathy and oral, genital or perianal ulcers; and less commonly with headache, meningitis, cranial nerve palsies, diarrhoea and weight loss.

Conditions associated with longstanding HIV infection can be subtle and people may remain well for some time before developing another condition. Diagnosis is confirmed with HIV serology.

> 💡 The significance of the window period as a repeat test may be necessary. The window period is the time between becoming infected and antibodies appearing; HIV antibodies usually appear four to six weeks after infection but can take up to 12 weeks. Therefore, you may need to repeat the blood test.

Management

Management of the patient depends on whether this is a new diagnosis of HIV or management of a PEP to reduce the chance of developing HIV infection. A patient with a new diagnosis will need to be referred urgently to a specialist HIV clinic, to be seen preferably within 48 hours and at the latest within two weeks of testing positive.

Presentations in Primary Care

> 💡 Arrange admission for urgent specialist assessment if there is concern about the possibility of a serious HIV-related condition such as pneumocystis pneumonia or if the patient is unwell.

Antiretroviral (ARV) therapy stops transmission, and the initiation and management of ARV therapy is largely carried out by specialist HIV services. However, a brief overview is:

- To be taken as soon as diagnosed
- To be taken everyday
- Suppresses viral replication
- Enables immune recovery
- Reduces morbidity and mortality.

Undetectable = untransmittable (U = U). A person living with HIV, who has an undetectable viral load, cannot pass HIV on to their sexual partners.

- Reduces HIV-related stigma
- Improves mental and emotional health for people living with HIV (PLWHIV)
- Reduces barriers to testing
- Reduces time between infection and diagnosis
- Prevents new infections.

Post-exposure Prophylaxis (PEP)

PEP may stop the patient developing an HIV infection if they have been exposed to the virus; however, it does not always work. Direct the patient immediately to GUM clinic or an ED for consideration of PEP following sexual exposure. PEP is a course of anti-HIV medication. The patient must start the treatment as soon as possible after they have been exposed to HIV, ideally within a few hours. The medicines must be taken every day for 28 days (four weeks). PEP is unlikely to work if it is started after three days (72 hours), and it will not usually be prescribed after this time. It is best to start taking PEP within one day (24 hours) of being exposed to HIV.

Pre-exposure Prophylaxis (PrEP)

PrEP is now fully available on the NHS but is currently managed by and only available from specialist sexual health services. It is the single most effective measure for preventing HIV and is up to 100% effective at preventing HIV acquisition. Regimens can be daily or event-based; this is determined by patient preference and risk. All patients are offered three monthly prescriptions, full STI screening including HIV testing and 3–12 monthly renal function checks.

People with HIV attending primary care may require:

- Advice about sources of information and support
- Information on health promotion, screening and immunisation
- Information on sexual and reproductive health

CHAPTER 12   Contraception and Sexual Health

- Management of mental health issues
- Management of HIV-related problems
- Support for end-stage advanced HIV disease.

> To assist with mental health support or if a patient is suffering from a long-term condition, consider engagement with a local health and well-being group or input from a social prescribing link worker.

Syphilis

Aetiology

Syphilis is a bacterial infection caused by the bacterium *Treponema pallidum* and is treated with a short course of antibiotics. It is less common but is increasing in the UK and clinicians should have a lower threshold for testing.

> A patient can catch syphilis more than once. If left untreated, it can spread to the neurological system and cause serious long-term issues.

History and Examination

Syphilis can present with a wide range of non-specific symptoms; in some people infection may be asymptomatic, therefore diagnosis can be delayed or missed. Common symptoms include:

- Small, painless sores or ulcers that typically appear on the penis, vagina or around the anus but can occur in other places such as the mouth
- A blotchy red rash that often affects the palms of the hands or soles of the feet
- Small skin growths (similar to genital warts) that may develop on the vulva in women or around the bottom (anus) in both men and women
- White patches in the mouth
- Tiredness, headaches, joint pains, a fever, lymphadenopathy in the neck, groin or armpits.

Swabs from active lesions and serology confirm diagnosis.

Management

Refer all people with suspected syphilis to a GUM clinic or other specialist local sexual health service, as some tests are not available in primary care and the results are difficult to interpret (NICE 2019a, 2021a).

Presentations in Primary Care

Trichomoniasis
Aetiology
Trichomoniasis is an STI caused by a tiny parasite called *Trichomonas vaginalis*. It is the world's most common non-viral STI, although relatively uncommon in the UK. Although symptoms of the disease vary, most people who have the parasite cannot tell they are infected.

History and Examination
Symptoms of trichomoniasis usually develop within a month of infection; however, 50% of people will not develop any symptoms (though they can still pass the infection onto others). Trichomoniasis is *not* thought to be passed on through oral or anal sex. The symptoms of trichomoniasis are similar to those of many other STIs, and therefore diagnosis can be difficult. There are differences in the symptoms of women and men, which are presented in Table 12.4.

Table 12.4 Symptoms of Trichomoniasis in Men and Women

	Symptoms
Women	• Abnormal vaginal discharge that may be thick, thin or frothy and yellow-green in colour • Producing more discharge than normal, which may also have an unpleasant fishy smell • Soreness, swelling and itching around the vagina • Pain or discomfort when passing urine or having sex
Men	• Pain when urinating or during ejaculation • Needing to urinate more frequently than usual • Thin, white discharge from the penis • Soreness, swelling and redness around the head of the penis or foreskin

Trichomoniasis can usually be diagnosed after an examination of the genitals and a confirmed positive swab taken from the vagina or penis. Although, NAATs are not available and difficult to detect in primary care (40% culture sensitivity) – low threshold for referring to sexual health for more sensitive testing (NHS, 2021e).

Management
Current and other recent partners should be tested and treated following a positive swab. Trichomoniasis is treated with antibiotics (refer to your local prescribing guidelines).

> ! If a patient is infected with trichomoniasis while they are pregnant, the infection may cause the baby to be born prematurely or have a low birth weight (NHS, 2021e).

CHAPTER 12   Contraception and Sexual Health

Chapter Summary

This chapter demonstrates the complexity of sexual health and contraceptive management, and how good sexual health is an extremely important aspect of overall health and well-being. It is vital that paramedics consulting patients with sexual health or contraception issues provide people with the information, confidence and means to develop positive relationships and protect themselves and their partners from infection and unintended pregnancy.

Case Study 1

A 32-year-old female presents to you in out-of-hours asking for the 'morning after pill'.

History

PC: UPSI.
HxPC: She tells you she is not taking any contraception and that her and her husband normally use condoms but this time they did not. Her and her husband had UPSI 12 hours ago; there have been no additional episodes of UPSI this cycle. She is happy in her relationship and the sexual intercourse was consensual. She declines an STI screening and says she is happily married. She declines ongoing contraception and says 'I have tried it all before and none of it works for me'. She has regular periods and is on day six of her cycle.
PMHx/SHx: None, normally fit and well.
DHX: No regular medicines.
SHx: She has three children and does not want any more. She works part time as a hairdresser. Non-smoker. Her BMI is 27.
ROS: NAD.

Examination
- None required.

Preferred Diagnosis
- She requires EC.

Management
- You offer her the Cu-IUD but she declines this.
- She has had UPSI within 12 hours (and therefore under 96 hours), she has not been taking any contraception prior (not recently taken progesterone) and does not wish to have any ongoing contraception. She does not take any enzyme inducers or glucocorticoids. Therefore, ulipristal is most suitable, as it is more effective than levonorgestrel, particularly as her weight is over 70 kg.
- You prescribe this for her (one tablet) and advise her to take it straight away.
- You advise her that she must do a pregnancy test in three weeks' time.

- You also advise her that if she changes her mind regarding ongoing contraception in the future she should call the GP surgery.
- You offer her STI screening.

Case Study 2

A 28-year-old male presents to you with dysuria.

History

PC: Dysuria.
HxPC: He is well in himself with no fever, no abdominal pain, no loin pain and no testicular pain. He tells you there is no discharge, itching, swelling, sores, warts or erythema to his penis. He has never had a UTI before. He has recently had UPSI with two new partners (in the last month). He has had UPSI with multiple partners since he was 18 years old. He tells you that one of the recent partners thought that she might have chlamydia. He tells you that he has never had sexual intercourse with a man.
PMHx/SHx: None, normally fit and well.
DHx: No regular medicines.
SHx: Smokes 20 per day, works as a scaffolder.
ROS: NAD.

Examination

- His urine shows no nitrites, no leukocytes, no blood, no protein and no glucose on dipping. It appears clear.
- His observations are all within healthy ranges.

Preferred Diagnosis

- Chlamydia.

Differential Diagnoses

- UTI
- Trichomoniasis
- Gonorrhoea.

Management

- You strongly suspect an STI (chlamydia) and therefore suggest the GUM clinic, but the patient declines this as he is unable to get into town.
- In men, a first-catch urine is the specimen of choice and a NAAT swab should be sent to the labs to confirm diagnosis, so you arrange this.
- His current partner(s) must also be treated for chlamydia to reduce the risk of re-infection and onward transmission. As he is unwilling or unable to attend a GUM

CHAPTER 12   Contraception and Sexual Health

clinic, advise him that (with his consent) his details can be provided to GUM solely for the purposes of partner notification.
- Sexual intercourse (including oral sex) should be avoided until he and his partner(s) have completed treatment (or waited seven days after treatment with azithromycin).
- You prescribe doxycycline 100 mg twice daily for seven days (first-line treatment) as there are no contraindications (follow local guidance and NICE guidelines).
- You give him written advice (for example, BASHH 'A guide to chlamydia') and discuss safe sex.
- Due to his high-risk sexual activity, he agrees on further screening (gonorrhoea, HIV, Hepatitis B and syphilis).
- He will call for his result to confirm diagnosis. If the exposure was within the last two weeks, a test should be carried out at presentation, and if negative, repeated two weeks after exposure.

References

Association for Young People's Health (AYPH) (2019) Key data on young people, latest information and statistics. Available at: https://www.youngpeopleshealth.org.uk/wp-content/uploads/2019/09/KDYP19-Highlights-booklet.pdf (accessed 28 January 2023).

British Association for Sexual Health and HIV (BASHH) (2021) BASHH guidelines. Available at: https://www.bashh.org/guidelines (accessed 1 May 2021).

British HIV Association (BHIVA) (2021) Current guidelines. Available at: https://www.bhiva.org/guidelines (accessed 1 May 2021).

British National Formulary (BNF) (2021) BNF Levonorgestrel. Available at: https://bnf.nice.org.uk/drug/levonorgestrel.html#breastfeeding (accessed 1 May 2021).

Dennerstein, G.J., Fernando, S., Teo, C.P. et al. (2018) Depot medroxyprogesterone acetate and bone mineral density. *Journal of Clinical Gynaecology and Obstetrics* 7(3): 63–68.

Eaton, G. (2022) *Law and Ethics for Paramedics: An Essential Guide*. 2nd edn. Bridgwater: Class Professional Publishing.

Faculty of Sexual and Reproductive Healthcare (FSRH) (2016) UK medical eligibility criteria. Available at: https://www.fsrh.org/documents/ukmec-2016/ (accessed 1 February 2023).

Faculty of Sexual and Reproductive Healthcare (FSRH) (2019a) Contraceptive choices for young people. Available at: https://www.fsrh.org/standards-and-guidance/documents/cec-ceu-guidance-young-people-mar-2010/ (accessed 1 February 2023).

Faculty of Sexual and Reproductive Healthcare (FSRH) (2019b) Overweight, obesity and contraception. Available at: https://www.fsrh.org/standards-and-guidance/documents/fsrh-clinical-guideline-overweight-obesity-and-contraception/ (28 January 2023).

Faculty of Sexual and Reproductive Healthcare (FSRH) (2020a) Combined hormonal contraception. Available at: https://www.fsrh.org/standards-and-guidance/documents/combined-hormonal-contraception/ (accessed 1 February 2023).

Faculty of Sexual and Reproductive Healthcare (FSRH) (2020b) Emergency contraception. Available at: https://www.fsrh.org/standards-and-guidance/documents/ceu-clinical-guidance-emergency-contraception-march-2017/ (accessed 28 January 2023).

References

Faculty of Sexual and Reproductive Healthcare (FSRH) (2023) Clinical Guideline: Intrauterine Contraception. Available at: https://www.fsrh.org/documents/ceuguidanceintrauterinecontraception/ (accessed 5 May 2023).

Family Planning Association (FPA) (2020) Your guide to contraception. Available at: https://www.fpa.org.uk/download/your-guide-to-contraception/ (accessed 28 January 2023).

Griffith, R. (2016) What is Gillick competency? *Human Vaccines and Immunotherapeutics* 12(1): 244–247.

Luby, R. (2018) Supporting patients who make disclosures of sexual violence on inpatient wards: A practical guide for mental health professionals. Available at: https://www.rcn.org.uk/-/media/royal-college-of-nursing/documents/clinical-topics/mental-health/rachel-luby-disclosures-of-sexual-violence.pdf?la=en&hash=795ED5602DE53E7F21A22B215B696EED (accessed 28 January 2023).

Mason, R. (2020) Emergency contraception counselling – OSCE guide. *Geeky Medics*. Available at: https://geekymedics.com/emergency-contraception-counselling-osce-guide/ (accessed 28 January 2023).

National Health Service (NHS) (2019) What should I do if I miss a pill? Available at: https://www.nhs.uk/conditions/contraception/miss-combined-pill/ (accessed 28 January 2023).

National Health Service (NHS) (2020) Genital warts. Available at: https://www.nhs.uk/conditions/genital-warts/ (accessed 28 January 2023).

National Health Service (NHS) (2021a) Contraceptive patch. Available at: https://www.nhs.uk/conditions/contraception/contraceptive-patch/ (accessed 28 January 2023).

National Health Service (NHS) (2021b) Female condoms. Available at: https://www.nhs.uk/conditions/contraception/female-condoms/ (accessed 17 April 2023).

National Health Service (NHS) (2021c) The progesterone-only pill. https://www.nhs.uk/conditions/contraception/the-pill-progestogen-only/ (accessed 28 January 2023).

National Health Service (NHS) (2021d) The vaginal ring, your contraceptive guide. Available at: https://www.nhs.uk/conditions/contraception/vaginal-ring/ (28 January 2023).

National Health Service (NHS) (2021e) Trichomoniasis. Available at: https://www.nhs.uk/conditions/trichomoniasis/ (accessed 28 February 2023).

National Health Service (NHS) (2022) Gonorrhoea. Available at: https://www.nhs.uk/conditions/gonorrhoea/ (accessed 28 January 2023).

National Institute for Health and Care Excellence (NICE) (2019a) Management of suspected syphilis. Available at: https://cks.nice.org.uk/topics/syphilis/management/management-of-suspected-syphilis/ (accessed 28 January 2023).

National Institute for Health and Care Excellence (NICE) (2019b) Sexual health [QS178]. Available at: https://www.nice.org.uk/guidance/qs178 (accessed 28 January 2023).

National Institute for Health and Care Excellence (NICE) (2021a) Clinical Knowledge Summaries: HIV infection. Available at: https://cks.nice.org.uk/topics/hiv-infection-aids/management/post-exposure-prophylaxis/ (accessed 28 January 2023).

National Institute for Health and Care Excellence (NICE) (2021b) Scenario: Emergency hormonal contraception. Available at: https://cks.nice.org.uk/topics/contraception-emergency/management/management/#postpartum-or-breastfeeding-women (accessed 28 January 2023).

National Institute for Health and Care Excellence (NICE) (2022a) Clinical Knowledge Summaries: Gonorrhoea. Available at: https://cks.nice.org.uk/topics/gonorrhoea/ (accessed 28 January 2023).

CHAPTER 12 Contraception and Sexual Health

National Institute for Health and Care Excellence (NICE) (2022b) Clinical Knowledge Summaries: Management of uncomplicated genital chlamydia. Available at: https://cks.nice.org.uk/topics/chlamydia-uncomplicated-genital/management/management/ (accessed 28 January 2023).

National Institute for Health and Care Excellence (NICE) (2022c) Managing hepatitis B infection. Available at: https://cks.nice.org.uk/topics/hepatitis-b/management/managing-hepatitis-b-infection/ (accessed 28 February 2023).

National Institute for Health and Care Excellence (NICE) (2023) Clinical Knowledge Summaries: Herpes simplex – Genital. Available at: https://cks.nice.org.uk/topics/herpes-simplex-genital/ (accessed 28 January 2023).

NHS Digital (2018) Sexual and reproductive health services England. Available at: https://digital.nhs.uk/data-and-information/publications/statistical/sexual-and-reproductive-health-services/2017-18 (accessed 28 January 2023).

Office for National Statistics (ONS) (2018) Conceptions in England and Wales. Available at: https://www.ons.gov.uk/peoplepopulationandcommunity/birthsdeathsandmarriages/conceptionandfertilityrates/bulletins/conceptionstatistics/2018#:~:text=Conception%20rates%20provide%20a%20better,conceptions%2C%20a%200.9%25%20decrease (accessed 28 January 2023).

Public Health England (PHE) (2018) Teenage pregnancy prevention framework. Available at: https://www.gov.uk/government/publications/teenage-pregnancy-prevention-framework (accessed 28 January 2023).

Public Health England (PHE) (2019) Sexually transmitted infections and screening for chlamydia in England. Available at: https://assets.publishing.service.gov.uk/government/uploads/system/uploads/attachment_data/file/914249/STI_NCSP_report_2019.pdf (accessed 28 January 2023).

Ramdhan, R.C., Simonds, E. and Tubbs, S.R. (2018) Complications of subcutaneous contraceptives: A review. *Cureus* 10(1): e2132.

Sex Wise (2021) Let's talk about sex! [Online] Available at: https://www.sexwise.org.uk/ (28 January 2023).

Obstetric Presentations

13

Aimee Yarrington

Within This Chapter
- Pregnancy diagnosis
- Women who do not wish to continue with their pregnancies
- Types of pregnancy loss
- Early pregnancy issues
  - Abdominal pain
  - Chest infection
  - Headache
  - Nausea and vomiting (N&V)
  - Pruritis
  - Urinary tract infection (UTI)
- Bleeding

Introduction

For the purposes of this chapter, the term pregnant woman/women applies to pregnancies over 20 weeks' gestation, unless explicitly stated. The majority of these cases will be treated exactly the same; however, there is normally a significant difference in the place of treatment when the pregnancy is less than 20 weeks. The term 'woman' is used to describe the person who is giving birth; the author accepts this may not necessarily be the term preferred by the birthing person, and clarity should be sought from the pregnant person as to the pronoun preferred.

Pregnant women are a client group that you may be asked to review and treat in primary care. Maternity care is the one branch of medicine where legislation stipulates that only a registered medical practitioner or a practising midwife can provide care for a pregnant woman (RCN, 2020). However, it is widely accepted that clinicians may be asked to provide treatment for apparently non-pregnancy-related conditions.

Specialist training is required in order to assess a pregnancy. Skills such as auscultation of foetal heart sounds must only be utilised if accredited training and supervision have occurred. Implications of incorrect use of a foetal Doppler can lead to false reassurance of foetal well-being and an increased risk of stillbirth (Chakladar and Adams, 2009).

Maternity cases present with a unique set of issues; pregnant women are vulnerable during illness, and the pregnancy can often mask symptoms that potentially could be fatal

CHAPTER 13   Obstetric Presentations

for both mother and foetus. It is advised that any pregnant woman reviewed and treated by any paramedic, regardless of skill level, should be adequately safety netted and in most cases a direct referral to the most appropriate maternity professional made. If this is not possible, then a minimum of a telephone conversation should take place between the clinician and either an appropriate midwife or obstetrician, as well as a GP for guidance in treatment.

The National Maternity Review (NHS, 2016), also known as 'Better Births', states that it is preferable for every pregnant woman to have a named midwife or team midwife whom they can contact in the case of illness or for advice. However, many women present with problems in the out-of-hours or do not think their illness is related to the pregnancy when actually a large number of illnesses have a direct link or impact upon the pregnancy.

Assessment

During pregnancy, women's bodies go through immense physiological changes which put physical strain on their body. These changes can also mask illness, which the clinician must be aware of to prevent potential mistakes in diagnosis. These changes include (AWMSG, 2018):

- Cardiac output at the end of pregnancy increasing by up to 50%
- Average maternal heart rate increasing by 10–15 beats per minute
- Systolic and diastolic blood pressures dropping by 10–15 mmHg, although by the end of pregnancy these values usually approach the normal range
- Work of breathing increasing, as does respiratory rate, while vital capacity reduces
- Circulating blood volume increasing by 50% (although there is a relative anaemia).

The increase in blood volume results in the pregnant patient tolerating greater blood or plasma loss before showing signs of hypovolaemia. In fact, tachycardia may not develop until blood loss exceeds 1,000 mL, and blood pressure is usually maintained well beyond this level of loss (Bose et al., 2006). However, in order to maintain maternal blood pressure in hypovolaemic states, blood is shunted away from the uterus and placenta, compromising the foetus.

Although these are the physiological changes that the woman's body will go through, the study by Green et al. (2020) found that there are no significant alterations in the mean vital signs of the pregnant woman. Therefore, if there is alteration in the vital signs this should be an indication for further examination. There is currently no National Early Warning Score (NEWS) specifically for the pregnant patient, and 'standard' NEWS tools should not be applied due to the altered physiology associated with pregnancy.

NHS (2016) recommends that any practitioners who are treating women of reproductive age have access to pregnancy testing to assist in diagnostic processes.

When completing an assessment on a pregnant patient, it is important to remember that the pregnancy is often a distraction and can mask underlying physiological conditions. In order to ensure a full assessment is covered, a complete physiology and holistic assessment should be completed. When assessing the pregnant woman, this must also always include blood pressure, urinalysis and abdominal palpation as well as enquiring about foetal well-being. Taking the patient's blood pressure is not only good practice but is particularly important in the pregnant patient as even slight deviations from normal can point to more sinister underlying physiology such as pre-eclampsia (APEC, 2020).

Many of these physiological changes have occurred by the end of the first trimester. Pregnancy duration is divided into three trimesters:

- First trimester: Fertilisation to 12 weeks
- Second trimester: 12–24 weeks
- Third trimester: 24 to birth.

A pregnancy is classified as term at 37 weeks; however, the date given as a due date is at 40 weeks. Weeks of pregnancy are expressed in a woman's notes as /40. So, a woman at 24 weeks and four days into her pregnancy would be expressed as 24 + 4 / 40. Twenty-four weeks is also the point at which viability is reached. Viability is the point at which the foetus is deemed to have the ability to survive outside of the uterus.

Pregnancy Diagnosis

Urine pregnancy test strips are the most convenient way to obtain a rapid pregnancy test result. If the pregnancy is confirmed, then clinicians must be prepared that not all women will respond with positive feelings, as this may not be a wanted pregnancy.

> False positives can be caused by certain medications, including:
> - Anti-anxiety medicines such as diazepam
> - Anticonvulsants
> - Antipsychotic medicines such as clozapine
> - Diuretics
> - Medications used for infertility: Novarel® (Ferring B.V.), Pregnyl® (Merck), Ovidrel® (Merck)
> - Medicines used to treat Parkinson's disease
> - Profasi®
> - Promethazine.

Ovarian cysts, kidney disease, certain cancers, molar pregnancies and peri-menopause may also lead to false positives. If there is a history of any of these, then a serum HCG level should be drawn.

Human chorionic gonadotropin (HCG) used to detect pregnancy is produced by the placenta in small levels around 14 days after fertilisation when implantation of the fertilised ovum occurs. At the point of implantation, a small bleed may also occur; therefore a history of spotting two weeks after the woman's last menstrual period should also be asked. Urine detection levels are not usually high enough until a week after the missed period, but levels can be detected this early. First morning void is recommended, as the levels will be concentrated (Zinaman et al., 2020).

Once the pregnancy is confirmed, the local protocol for referral to booking with maternity services should take place. Local policy will dictate the referral route. This would normally

CHAPTER 13 Obstetric Presentations

involve an email of the referral to the booking coordinator at the desired maternity unit with the woman's details. Details need to include:

- Name
- Address
- DOB
- Last menstrual period (LMP) date
- Number of previous pregnancies
- Pre-existing medical conditions
- Current medications.

These points will assist the booking coordinator to navigate the appropriate pathway for the patient's ongoing care in relation to the appropriate pathways.

Routine care for women includes the assessments at each week of pregnancy shown in Figure 13.1, according to NICE (2020a) guidance.

Women with any of the following conditions will require extra care and contacts during their pregnancies (NICE, 2019a):

- Autoimmune disorders
- Cardiac disease, including hypertension
- Endocrine disorders or diabetes requiring insulin
- Epilepsy requiring anticonvulsant drugs
- Haematological disorders
- Higher risk of developing complications, for example women aged 40 and older, women who smoke
- HIV or BHV infection
- Malignant disease
- Obesity (body mass index (BMI) 30 kg/m² or above at first contact) or underweight (BMI below 18 kg/m² at first contact)
- Psychiatric disorders (being treated with medication)
- Renal disease
- Severe asthma
- Use of recreational drugs such as heroin, cocaine (including crack cocaine) and ecstasy
- Women who are particularly vulnerable (such as teenagers) or who lack social support
- Women who have experienced any of the following in previous pregnancies:
    - Recurrent miscarriage (three or more consecutive pregnancy losses or a mid-trimester loss) or preterm birth
    - Severe pre-eclampsia, (H) haemolytic anaemia, (EL) elevated liver enzymes and (LP) low platelet count (HELLP syndrome) or eclampsia
    - Rhesus isoimmunisation or other significant blood group antibodies
    - Uterine surgery, including caesarean section, myomectomy or cone biopsy
    - Antenatal or postpartum haemorrhage on two occasions
    - Puerperal psychosis

Pregnancy Diagnosis

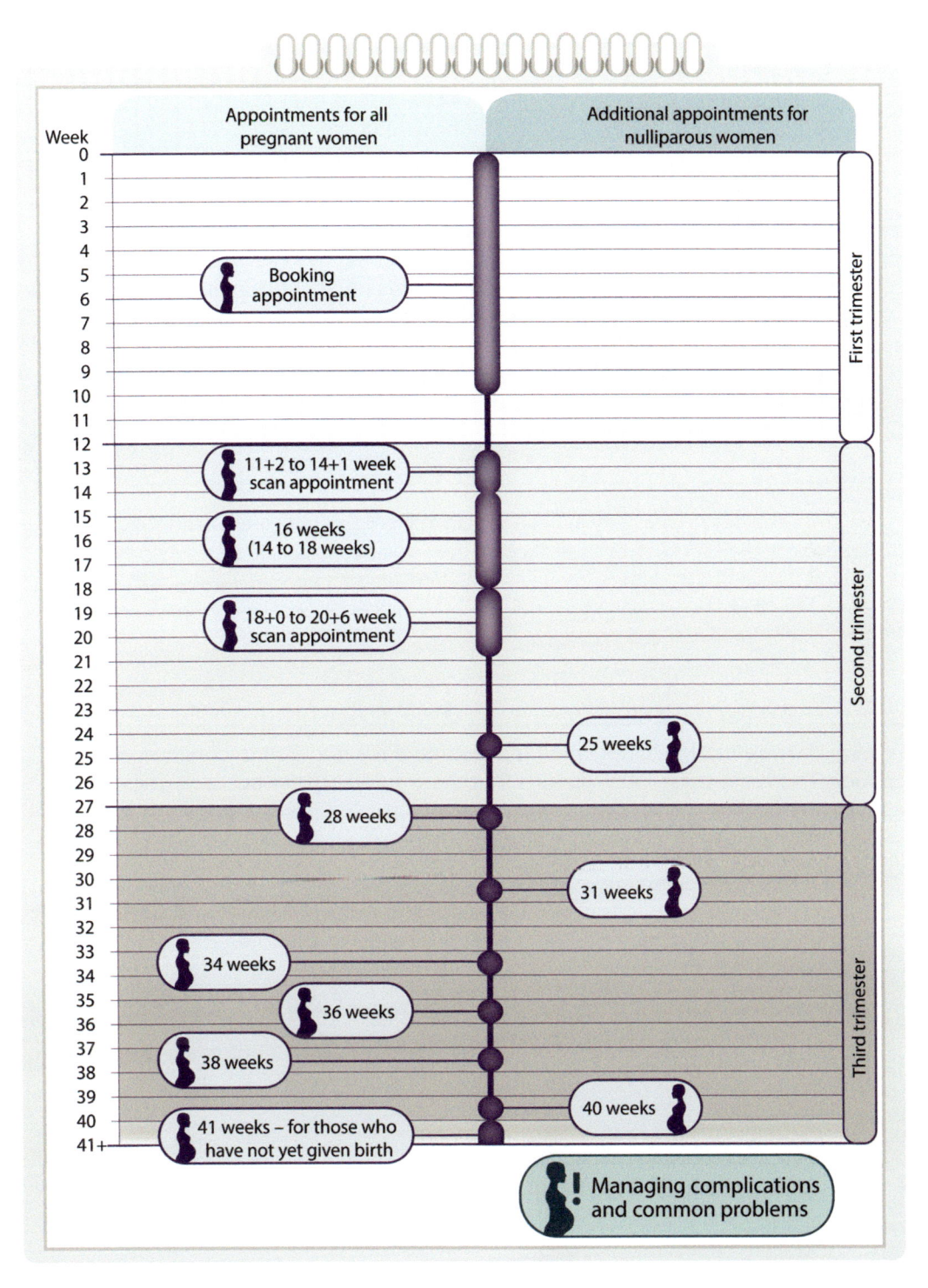

Figure 13.1 Antenatal care for uncomplicated pregnancies.
Source: NICE (2021a).

- Grand multiparity (more than six pregnancies)
- A stillbirth or neonatal death
- A small-for-gestational-age infant (below 5th centile)
- A large-for-gestational-age infant (above 95th centile)
- A baby weighing below 2.5 kg or above 4.5 kg
- A baby with a congenital abnormality (structural or chromosomal).

For each contact that a clinician has with a woman at any point during her pregnancy, the principles of making every contact count (MECC) must be considered. This applies to any contact with any patient at any point, but is especially important in pregnancy when every opportunity for health promotion should be utilised. Women in particularly vulnerable groups such as Black, Asian and minority ethnic, asylum seekers, homeless or women in prison or custody should also be signposted and referrals made where appropriate, as the risks for complication, mortality and morbidity in these groups are greater (Knight et al., 2019; RCM, 2019; Yamamoto et al., 2021).

> To assist patients who need support with their mental health, are lonely or isolated or have complex social needs which affect their well-being, consider engagement with a local health and well-being group or input from a social prescribing link worker.

Women Who Do Not Wish to Continue with Their Pregnancies

There may be the situation faced when the woman does not wish to continue with the pregnancy. There are three main options that the woman has for accessing abortion services on the NHS:

- A referral can be made to local NHS services.
- A local sexual health clinic can also make the referral.
- Self-referral to a national abortion provider: the British Pregnancy Advisory Service (BPAS), MSI Reproductive Choices UK or the National Unplanned Pregnancy Advisory Service (NUPAS).

Abortions in England, Wales and Scotland are normally carried out before 24 weeks. There are limited situations where abortions are carried out above 24 weeks if there is serious risk to the mother or child's life or the baby would be born with a severe disability.

> All women who request an abortion should discuss their options with a trained pregnancy counsellor (NHS, 2020). To assist patients with support with their mental health, consider engagement with a local health and well-being group or input from a social prescriber or link worker.

Types of Pregnancy Loss

Miscarriage is the spontaneous loss of a pregnancy before 24 weeks' gestation.

An ectopic pregnancy is one that develops outside of the womb/uterus. It is identified as a leading cause of foetal death in the first trimester of pregnancy.

A molar pregnancy (also called a hydatidiform mole) is one where an abnormal fertilised egg implants in the uterus. The cells that should become the placenta grow far too quickly and take over the space where the embryo would normally develop. A molar pregnancy may lead to persistent trophoblastic disease and the possible need for chemotherapy (Miscarriage Association, 2023).

Pregnancy of unknown location (PUL) occurs when a woman has a positive pregnancy test, but there is no evidence of an intrauterine or extra-uterine pregnancy or retained products of conception on trans-vaginal ultrasound examination. Management options that will be offered by the obstetric team include:

- Expectant management: Wait and observe for deterioration; 44–69% of PULs settle without intervention.
- Medical management: Methotrexate may be utilised to absorb the pregnancy cells, but this involves several weeks of monitoring.
- Surgical management: A laparotomy may be indicated on the unstable patient with signs of rupture (RCN, 2017).

Early Pregnancy Issues

Abdominal Pain

History and Examination

A pain history as standard for the non-pregnant patient must be carried out, as well as asking about associated factors such as vaginal bleeding and bowel or urinary symptoms.

In the pregnant patient, the following must also be considered:

- In early pregnancy, the risk of miscarriage and ectopic pregnancy must be ruled out – ectopic must be ruled out quickly in a woman with a positive pregnancy test and acute abdominal pain. The rate of ectopic pregnancy is around one in 90 pregnancies – approximately 11,000 pregnancies affected every year (NHS, 2022).
- Musculoskeletal pain – very common in pregnancy due to the effect of relaxin on the smooth muscle tissues. If this is suspected as the cause, it can be managed with simple analgesia and physiotherapy referral.
- Oral iron supplementation can cause abdominal discomfort – this is normally recognised by the distinctive blackened stools.
- Pyelonephritis – can present similarly to appendicitis. In pregnancy, symptoms such as frequency and dysuria may be masked and not present until the infection is severe. UTI must be treated early to prevent the development of preterm labour.
- In the third trimester of pregnancy, pre-eclampsia or HELLP syndrome (a severe variant of pre-eclampsia) may present with abdominal pain and vomiting.

CHAPTER 13 Obstetric Presentations

Hypertension and proteinuria would usually be seen by the time that abdominal symptoms have developed. The first changes diagnostic of HELLP can be seen in the derangement of liver function tests (LFTs) and full blood count (FBC).
- Placental abruption or uterine rupture will present with pain or uterine tenderness. There may or may not be vaginal bleeding; this will often if untreated lead to collapse.
- Chorioamnionitis (an infection within the chorion of the membranes) will cause defuse abdominal pain alongside symptoms of infection. With a history of ruptured membranes or offensive vaginal discharge, this should always be considered; however, it can occur with intact membranes also.
- Braxton Hicks contractions – abdominal pains which are similar to the pain of labour only there is no dilatation of the cervix and they do not culminate in birth. They can start as early as six weeks' gestation and are referred to predominantly as 'false labour' due to the nature of them preparing the uterus for active labour (Raines and Cooper, 2022).
- Labour – pain associated with labour may present as generalised defuse abdominal pain, especially preterm labour, and not the classic waves of contractions normally associated with labour.

A standard abdominal examination will be obscured by the gravid uterus. The degree of displacement will depend upon the gestation. If the gestation is unknown, then the estimation of the fundal height can be made by utilising the symphysio-fundal height measurement, as seen in Figure 13.2; the numbers indicate weeks of pregnancy.

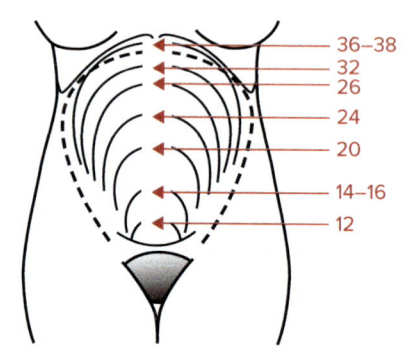

Figure 13.2 Symphysio-fundal height measurement.

Clinical signs may be less distinctive in pregnancy due to the stretching of the retro-peritoneal space.

> Careful assessment of foetal movements should be established, asking pertinent questions regarding pattern, regularity and relation to normality (Knott, 2015).

Early Pregnancy Issues

Differential diagnosis for abdominal pain must take into consideration the conditions that can be both pregnancy and non-pregnancy related.

Non-pregnancy conditions include:

- Appendicitis – in developed countries the risk of appendicitis in pregnancy is 1/800 to 1/1500 and is most common in the second trimester (Rebarber and Jacob, 2021)
- Ovarian cysts or torsion
- Round ligament pain
- Peritonitis
- Gastroenteritis
- Urinary tract infection (UTI)
- Constipation – often worse in pregnancy due to the relaxing effect of progesterone on smooth muscle tissue
- Bowel obstruction
- Pyelonephritis.

Investigations

- Urinalysis
- FBC, LFTs, urea and electrolytes (U&E), amylase and clotting may be considered if patient is suspected bleeding
- Electrocardiogram (ECG) should always be conducted in any epigastric pain.

Management

This will very much depend upon the diagnosis being considered; combined management with the obstetric or midwifery team may be required.

With all of the above, definitive diagnosis can only be made following the full assessment of both maternal and foetal well-being. Foetal well-being, however, can only be assured using a cardiotocography (CTG) after 28 weeks of pregnancy, and interpreted by a competent clinician. If there is no facility for assessment of the presence of a foetal heart by a competent practitioner, then this must be followed up in a maternity unit.

Assessment at an appropriate obstetric facility is recommended to ensure that any signs of preterm labour can be acted on as quickly as possible to prevent preterm birth (NHS England, 2019).

Chest Infection

Aetiology

The maternal immune response is compromised during pregnancy to protect the foetus from maternal rejection. From 13 weeks' gestation there is a reduction in blood monocytes, leaving the mother vulnerable to infection, particularly viral infection. Influenza is still one of the largest causes of maternal death, hence all pregnant women are advised to have a flu vaccine.

CHAPTER 13 Obstetric Presentations

> **BOX 13.1** COVID-19 Considerations
>
> At the start of the coronavirus (COVID-19) pandemic, there was some confusion over the vaccination programme for women who were pregnant, considering pregnancy as well as breastfeeding. Therefore, many women chose not to vaccinate initially. This led to a large number of vulnerable women becoming extremely unwell, with deaths of both mothers and babies. The Royal College of Midwives (RCM) (2022) states that the pregnant woman with COVID-19 symptoms is twice as likely to have a preterm birth, as well as having an increased risk of developing pre-eclampsia, needing an emergency Caesarean section and having a stillbirth.
>
> The Joint Committee on Vaccination and Immunisation (JCVI) advises that it is preferable for pregnant women in the UK to be offered the Pfizer-BioNTech or Moderna vaccines where available.
>
> There is no evidence to suggest that other vaccines are unsafe for pregnant women, but it is acknowledged that more research is needed (PHE, 2021). Both the RCM and the Royal College of Obstetricians and Gynaecologists (RCOG) (2022) strongly recommend vaccination for pregnant women as a priority.
>
> Risk factors which increase the risk of requiring hospital admission include (RCM and RCOG, 2022):
>
> - Being unvaccinated
> - Black, Asian or other ethnic minority background
> - BMI over 25
> - Pre-existing co-morbidity, for example diabetes or chronic hypertension
> - Maternal age over 35
> - Living in socioeconomic deprevation
> - Working in areas where exposure is greater, for example healthcare.

History and Examination

Clinical judgement must always be used to diagnose community-acquired pneumonia because no combination of symptoms or signs is clearly diagnostic.

Cough is the predominant symptom in both acute bronchitis and community-acquired pneumonia. Ask about:

- Onset and duration of symptoms
- The type of cough (dry or productive)
- Additional symptoms such as breathlessness, wheeze, pleuritic pain and fever
- Smoking status

Examine the person, paying particular attention to the chest. Measure the person's temperature, pulse rate and blood pressure and respiratory rate, and assess for signs of confusion.

Chest examination should follow the standard examination of a non-pregnant patient who requires examination. Consider the following factors with specific regard to pregnancy:

- Not allowing the patient to lie flat to reduce risk of aortal caval compression
- In advancing gestations (> 28/40), there may be encroachment of the fundus into the thoracic cage.

Early Pregnancy Issues

Investigations

Pulse oximetry – arrange urgent hospital admission for those who require supplemental O_2. Chest X-ray should not be withheld in cases of suspected pneumonia.

> ⚠ Be aware that pre-existing medical conditions, for example asthma or obesity, may increase the severity of the infection.

Management

Prompt treatment with appropriate antibiotics depending upon allergy status if appropriate and after ruling out viral possibilities. According to NICE (2021b), amoxicillin is the preferred medication, with clarithromycin the choice for penicillin allergies. However, local antibiotic guidance must also be considered and followed where applicable. Do not prescribe doxycycline in women who are pregnant or breastfeeding. Tetracyclines are deposited in growing bone and teeth, which can result in discolouration of teeth and occasionally dental hypoplasia.

> ⚠ Differential diagnosis to consider:
> - Sinusitis
> - Pulmonary embolism (PE).

Headache

Aetiology

Hormonal headaches are often worsened by pregnancy due to the increases in oestrogen and progesterone. If a woman has suffered with menstrual headaches, then she may also encounter these in pregnancy.

> 🚩 Directly related to the pregnancy is blood pressure as the main red flag which should be measured and considered, due to the risk of hypertensive disease in pregnancy.

> ⚠ Hypertension in pregnancy is defined as a systolic of > 140 mm Hg or diastolic of > 90 mm Hg. Care must be taken when assessing the blood pressure and a manual sphygmomanometer should be used. One in ten women will suffer with high blood pressure in pregnancy; medication is not always required, which will be a decision for the obstetric team.

CHAPTER 13   Obstetric Presentations

Hypertensive disorders found in pregnancy are:

- Chronic hypertension: Hypertension that has been previously diagnosed and treated or is present at the booking appointment or before 20 weeks' gestation
- Gestational hypertension: New hypertension (> 140 mm Hg systolic or > 90 mm Hg diastolic) presenting after 20 weeks of pregnancy without significant proteinuria
- Pre-eclampsia: New onset hypertension (> 140 mm Hg systolic or > 90 mm Hg diastolic) after 20 weeks of pregnancy and the coexistence of one or both of the following new-onset conditions:
    - Proteinuria (urine protein:creatinine ratio ≥ 30 mg/mmol, or albumin:creatinine ratio ≥ 8 mg/mmol, or ≥ 1 g/L [2+] on dipstick testing)
    - Other maternal organ dysfunction, including features such as renal or liver involvement, neurological or haematological complications or uteroplacental dysfunction (such as foetal growth restriction, abnormal umbilical artery Doppler waveform analysis or stillbirth) (Webster et al., 2019).

History

A presenting feature of gestational hypertension or pre-eclampsia could be a headache, which is generally frontal in nature. Due to the nature of the hypertension, a presenting complaint may also be the general feeling of malaise and global oedema.

Examination

In cases of severe pre-eclampsia where the blood pressure is 160/110 mmHg or above accompanied by the following red-flag symptoms (NICE, 2019b), ambulance transfer to the nearest obstetric unit must be considered due to the risk of eclampsia:

- Muscle twitches or tremor
- Nausea and vomiting
- Confusion
- Rapidly progressing oedema
- Visual disturbances
- Epigastric or right-sided upper abdominal pain.

Investigations

- Blood pressure
- Blood tests including FBC, U&E, LFT and uric acid levels
- Urinalysis to determine if protein present
- Abdominal assessment ensuring no right upper quadrant tenderness which may indicate liver swelling in later stages of the disease.

Management

If hypertensive and symptomatic, then a direct referral to maternity services should be sought for diagnosis and management.

Early Pregnancy Issues

Chronic Hypertension

Offer pregnant women with chronic hypertension advice on:

- Weight management
- Exercise
- Healthy eating
- Lowering the amount of salt in their diet.

Consider labetalol to treat chronic hypertension in pregnant women. Consider nifedipine for women in whom labetalol is not suitable, or methyldopa if both labetalol and nifedipine are not suitable (NICE, 2019b).

Gestational Hypertension

Pharmacological treatment should be offered if blood pressure remains above 140/90 mmHg (NICE, 2019b).

> NIHR (2019) High blood pressure in pregnancy: Treatment vs no treatment [online]. Research regarding the treatment vs no treatment options for hypertension in pregnancy.

Stroke

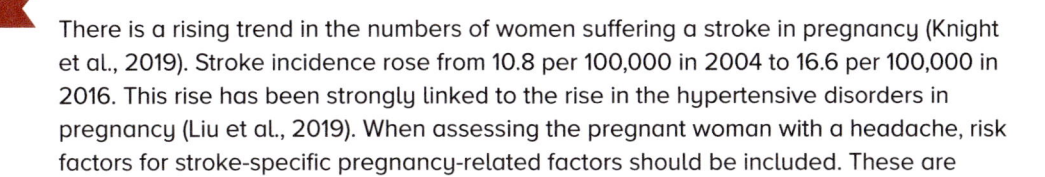

> There is a rising trend in the numbers of women suffering a stroke in pregnancy (Knight et al., 2019). Stroke incidence rose from 10.8 per 100,000 in 2004 to 16.6 per 100,000 in 2016. This rise has been strongly linked to the rise in the hypertensive disorders in pregnancy (Liu et al., 2019). When assessing the pregnant woman with a headache, risk factors for stroke-specific pregnancy-related factors should be included. These are (Scott et al., 2012):
>
> - History of migraine
> - Gestational diabetes
> - Advancing maternal age (age 35 or older)
> - Pre-eclampsia and eclampsia.

Nausea and Vomiting (N&V)
Aetiology

Nausea and vomiting (N&V) affects up to 80% of pregnant women and is one of the most common indications for hospital admission in the first trimester of pregnancy. For many, the symptoms can be controlled in primary care with dietary advice and medication. This should be diagnosed only when onset is in the first trimester and once the other causes of vomiting have been excluded. Reassure women that 90% of women find symptoms resolve by the 20/40. In cases of severe N&V, hyperemesis gravidarum (HG) should be considered. HG affects 1% of women with pregnancy sickness and is a severe and debilitating condition of pregnancy.

CHAPTER 13 Obstetric Presentations

> Further help and support for women can be found on the Pregnancy Sickness Support website: https://www.pregnancysicknesssupport.org.uk.

Transient hyperthyroidism may be present in 60% of women with hyperemesis and is usually self-limiting but may need treatment.

History

Further investigations are required in women who present with N&V and the following onset after 11/40:

- Drug induced – iron, antibiotics, opioids
- Gastrointestinal – gastroenteritis, peptic ulcer, pancreatitis, bowel obstruction, hepatitis, cholelithiasis, cholecystitis, *Helicobacter pylori* infection, appendicitis
- Genitourinary – UTI, uraemia, pyelonephritis
- Metabolic or endocrine – hypercalcaemia, thyrotoxicosis, DKA, Addison's disease
- Neurological – vestibular disease, migraine
- Pregnancy-related conditions – acute fatty liver, pre-eclampsia (if onset in second half of pregnancy)
- Psychological – eating disorders.

Risk factors for HG include:

- HG in a previous pregnancy
- Multiple pregnancy
- Primigravida
- Raised BMI.

Investigations

Blood tests for FBC, U&E, LFTs and thyroid function tests (TFTs) are required to establish any imbalance, and referral to gynaecology services should be considered. Abnormal liver function tests are associated with severe hyperemesis.

Management

Very often, dietary advice and antiemetic treatments can be the most effective. Printable leaflets on dietary advice can be found at the Pregnancy Sickness Support website. This includes advising women that:

- Smaller frequent snacking is preferable to large portions
- Sweet or salty foods are often tolerated better
- If small amounts of food are tolerated, then fortify what is tolerated, for example adding extra calories with butter, creme fraiche, full-fat milk and hard cheese
- Snacking of crisps, crackers and cereal bars should be increased
- Fluids are beneficial – full-sugar soft drinks, milkshakes, tepid water, ice lollies, squash, ice or just holding the fluid in the mouth can help.

Early Pregnancy Issues

Sickness is generally at its worst in the early hormonal change stage between eight and ten weeks, and after this stage it generally settles down. However, drug therapy is often required to assist with management of symptoms.

Antiemetic treatment is not contraindicated in pregnancy and there are several treatment options available. Always consider if suppository medication would be preferable for women who cannot tolerate oral meds. Typically, the most common antiemetic drugs used for pregnancy sickness are:

- Antihistamines – cyclizine and promethazine
- Corticosteroids (prednisolone)
- Domperidone
- Metoclopramide
- Ondansetron
- Prochlorperazine
- Doxylamine/pyridoxine.

NICE (2020a) recommends that inpatient management should be considered if there is at least one of the following:

- Continued N&V and unable to keep down liquids or oral antiemetics
- Continued N&V with ketonuria or weight loss (greater than 5% of body weight), despite treatment with oral antiemetics
- A confirmed or suspected comorbidity (for example, unable to tolerate oral antibiotics for a UTI).

The threshold for admitting to hospital or seeking specialist advice should be lower for women with co-existing conditions (for example, diabetes).

Admission or specialist advice may also be required if there is suspicion of an alternative diagnosis or complications requiring specialist management.

Pruritis

Aetiology

Itching in pregnancy can be a normal complaint often suffered by women as the skin around the abdomen stretches to accommodate the pregnancy.

History and Examination

Careful assessment of the itching needs to take place and questioning regarding the location of itching needs to rule out intrahepatic cholestasis of pregnancy (ICP) or obstetric cholestasis (OC). Although rare, OC affects 1:140 pregnant women. The presentation of the condition is normally late second or third trimester, often after 30 weeks' gestation. The woman may also have noticed dark urine or a pale stool. This disease is specific to pregnancy and can be summarised by these three key points:

- Generalised pruritis without rash
- Elevated serum bile acids
- Abnormal LFTs.

CHAPTER 13 Obstetric Presentations

The main presenting symptom of OC is itching or pruritis, usually without a rash. This is often more noticeable on the palms of the hands or the soles of the feet, although it can be anywhere on the body. Typically, the itching is worse at night. Dark urine is also usually present in many cases. There would also be the presence of elevated serum bile acids and possibly abnormal LFTs. In very rare presentations, jaundice can also occur.

Causes are unknown, but factors affecting OC include (Tommy's, 2017):

- Hormones: Pregnancy hormones oestrogen and progesterone are thought to affect how the liver works. Oestrogen has a particularly cholestatic effect, which may be the route of the risk factors (in other words, oestrogen peaks later in pregnancy). Oestrogen peaks in ovarian hyper stimulation as seen in IVF and in multiple pregnancies, putting them at greater risk. Women who have oral oestrogen contraceptive post OC pregnancy may also be at risk.
- Genetics: OC has familial links as well as with certain ethnic groups, such as South American, Indian or Pakistani.
- Environment: OC is more common in the winter months, which is why dietary factors may be involved including lack of vitamin D and selenium levels, but the evidence for this is unclear.

> Risk factors for developing the condition include:
> - Age above 35
> - Multiple pregnancy
> - Conception after IVF
> - Pre-existing liver disease
> - Personal or family history of cholestasis
> - History of OC in previous pregnancies.

Investigations

Differentiation is to consider if this is OC or an actual rash. Blood work that is important and of note in OC are:

- Elevations in AST/ALT, alk phos and bilirubin
- LFTs are, however, normally deranged in pregnancy, so use pregnancy values
- There are no structural changes on imaging.

Management

If OC is suspected, then immediate referral to maternity services should be sought.

Foetal well-being must be assessed by CTG, not just hand-held doppler, as there is a 1:4 risk of still birth with OC (RCOG, 2011) as the bile acids can cross the placental barrier causing accumulation in the foetus and amniotic fluid. There is also the increased risk with pregnancy of comorbid gestational diabetes, pre-eclampsia/HELLP syndrome and acute fatty liver.

Early Pregnancy Issues

> HELLP syndrome is a serious complication of severe pre-eclampsia
> It is associated with:
>
> - Haemolysis – micro-angiopathic haemolytic anaemia
> - Elevated liver enzymes – secondary top parenchymal necrosis
> - Low platelets – increased platelet consumption.
>
> It affects 20% of pregnancies complicated by severe pre-eclampsia. Maternal mortality is 1–10%. Management of HELLP syndrome involves control of blood pressure, monitoring and correcting coagulation disorders and safe delivery of the foetus.

Urinary Tract Infection (UTI)

Aetiology

UTI is the most common bacterial infection during pregnancy (Cunningham et al., 2018). UTIs can cause significant morbidity, such as preterm labour, sepsis, adult respiratory distress syndrome and ultimately mortality if left untreated (Johnston et al., 2017). Asymptomatic bacteriuria occurs in 2–10% of pregnancies and, if not treated, up to 30% of mothers may develop acute pyelonephritis (Smaill and Vazquez, 2015). Clinical guidelines (EAU, 2022; NICE, 2019a; PHE, 2018) agree that asymptomatic bacteriuria in pregnancy should be treated in an attempt to prevent the associated co-morbidity. All pregnant women undergo screening at the initial booking appointment with their midwife to assess if there is any underlying bacteriuria present.

History and Examination

A pregnant patient presenting with symptoms of UTI: Frequency, pain on micturition, offensive smelling urine, cloudy urine or the feeling of inadequately emptying the bladder should always be seen and examined further. Pain history should also be taken to rule out any possibility of preterm labour.

Investigations

From urinalysis, observe for presence of leucocytes. However, should not be considered in isolation; nitrates are more specific for diagnosis. If there is 1+ or more proteins, then send for polymerase chain reaction (PCR) also.

Management

For uncomplicated first lower UTI in a pregnant woman (NICE, 2022):

- Give advice on self-care measures: Simple analgesia such as paracetamol can be used for pain relief.
- Encourage intake of enough fluids to avoid dehydration.
- A patient information leaflet 'Treating your infection – Urinary tract infection (UTI)' is available from the Royal College of General Practice (RCGP) eLearning website.

CHAPTER 13   Obstetric Presentations

- Send a midstream urine sample for culture and sensitivities before antibiotics are taken.
- Offer an immediate antibiotic prescription, taking account of previous urine culture and susceptibility results, previous antibiotic use (which may have led to resistant bacteria) and local resistance patterns – if unsure, discuss with a specialist. Treatment with antibiotics should follow local guidelines.

As first choice antibiotic, consider prescribing:

- Nitrofurantoin **(avoid at term)** 100 mg modified-release twice a day for seven days if eGFR ≥ 45 mL/minute.

As second choice (no improvement in lower UTI symptoms on first choice taken for at least 48 hours or when first choice not suitable), consider prescribing:

- Amoxicillin (only if culture results available and susceptible) 500 mg three times a day for seven days
- Cefalexin 500 mg twice a day for seven days.

For alternative second choices, discuss with local microbiologist.

> ❗ Trimethoprim should be avoided – there is a teratogenic risk in the first trimester of pregnancy (folate antagonist).

> ❗ Nitrofurantoin is not known to be harmful in pregnancy, but clinical guidelines (NICE, 2018) and the British National Formulary (BNF) recommend that it should be avoided at term, because of the risk of neonatal haemolysis. This includes women with threatened preterm labour (All Wales Medicines Strategy Group, All Wales Antimicrobial Guidance Group, 2018). Amoxicillin and cefalexin are not known to be harmful in pregnancy (NICE, 2022).

Following the diagnosis, the woman should be advised to contact her named midwife to inform them of the diagnosis and to seek an obstetric review if their symptoms get worse or they do not improve in 48 hours. Further specialist help should be sought if the following are present:

- Recurrent lower UTI
- Catheter associated UTI
- The culture reveals an atypical bacteria
- An underlying structural or functional abnormality or comorbidity which increases the risk of complications or treatment failure
- Suspected underlying malignancy or renal disease.

Bleeding

Bleeding in pregnancy is abnormal. Any blood loss in pregnancy, regardless of the gestation, should be investigated and treated if appropriate. The classification used to describe the bleed depends on the gestation of the foetus:

- < 24 weeks' gestation bleeding is termed either miscarriage or threatened miscarriage.
- > 24 weeks' gestation bleeding is now described as an antepartum haemorrhage.

The point of viability differentiates the terms.

Early Pregnancy Bleeding

Aetiology

Early pregnancy loss, before 12 weeks, unfortunately is common. Miscarriage will affect 25% of women under 39 who have been pregnant (Farren et al., 2016). Not all cases of bleeding will lead to miscarriage. Differential diagnosis must include:

- Ectopic pregnancy
- Vaginal infections (thrush, bacterial vaginosis)
- Cervical ectropion or polyps
- Sexual intercourse
- History of a recent speculum examination
- Subchorionic bleeding
- Implantation bleeding.

BOX 13.2　Key Facts

The below highlights some key facts of early pregnancy bleeding from the RCN (2017):

- 50% of pregnant women will have some vaginal bleeding in the first 12 weeks of pregnancy.
- 75% of these women will carry on with their pregnancy.
- One in four pregnancies in the first trimester will miscarry.
- One in 80 pregnancies will result in an ectopic pregnancy.
- One in 600 are molar pregnancies.
- One in 100 pregnancies in the second trimester miscarry.
- One in 100 women have recurrent miscarriage.

History and Examination

Pregnant patients who present with bleeding or pain before 15/40 of pregnancy must be treated cautiously, due to the potential for pregnancy loss (NICE, 2021b). Where a woman presents without a history of an ultrasound scan (USS), the potential for complications is greater due to the unconfirmed pregnancy location.

CHAPTER 13 Obstetric Presentations

Key presentations and information to be explored within the patient history taking include:
- Pain – especially duration and location
- Bleeding – amount and if clots or mucus present
- Previous history of pregnancy loss, especially if previous ectopic pregnancy
- Natural or artificial conception due to raised miscarriage risk with assisted conception.

Internal or speculum examination is not indicated and should not be performed by a non-qualified clinician (Bora et al., 2014). A referral should be sought to an appropriate early pregnancy or gynaecology assessment unit for a USS. This should ideally be arranged directly with the assessment unit to prevent unnecessary A&E admission. Unfortunately, many assessment units are not operational out of hours, so the woman must be made aware that she may have to wait up to two days for the USS.

Management

Expectant management is used for women with a pregnancy that is confirmed to be of less than six weeks' gestation who are bleeding but not in pain, and who have no risk factors, such as a previous ectopic pregnancy. Advise these women:

- To return or recontact if bleeding continues or pain develops
- To repeat a urine pregnancy test after seven to ten days and to return if it is positive
- A negative pregnancy test means that the pregnancy has miscarried.

Women should be advised that bleeding will be as a heavy period and they may also pass clots. Period cramping pain is normal, as well as contraction-type pain, as the uterus contracts to remove the content.

Referral immediately to an early pregnancy assessment unit or out-of-hours gynaecology service should be made for any woman who has:

- Had a previous ectopic pregnancy
- Pregnancy of six weeks' gestation or more
- Pregnancy of uncertain gestation
- Pain and abdominal tenderness
- Pelvic tenderness.

The urgency of the referral will be based on the clinical findings in your examination. Remember – a third of all women with an ectopic pregnancy will have no known risk factors.

Women Who Have Miscarried at Home

Women who have miscarried without a medical practitioner present often find themselves in a situation of extreme distress. Foetal remains have no legal status, so it is the parents who decide how they wish to dispose of them. This may be at home or, dependent upon the gestation, they may be asked to take them to the nearest hospital for disposal. The Miscarriage Association has produced a letter template that can be provided to women so that they are able to use the services of burial or cremation should they wish, as this is not offered for miscarriages under 24 weeks. The Institute of Cemetery & Crematorium Management (ICCM) guidance on the sensitive disposal of foetal remains and its charter for the bereaved can be found at www.iccm-uk.com, and the letter template that parents may ask for you to provide can be found at https://www.sands.org.uk/forms-and-certificates.

Bleeding After 24 Weeks: Antepartum Haemorrhage

After 24 weeks, the foetus is viable and has legal status if born with signs of life, so bleeding is treated slightly differently. Bleeding is still abnormal and will require further investigation as to its cause. There are several reasons that the woman may bleed. These include:

- Cervix problems: Inflammation or growths on the cervix can cause light bleeding. This is usually not serious.
- Infection, such as severe thrush: Can cause bleeding, which is normally light and scant.
- Placental abruption: The placenta detaches or partially detaches from the uterine wall before or during labour. This may occur with or without bleeding, and pain is normally severe.
- Placenta previa: The placenta is sited low in the uterine cavity and partly or completely covers the cervix. Bleeding is normally frank, and usually happens without pain.
- Vasa previa: Some of the placenta's blood vessels go across the cervix.
- Premature labour: Bleeding can occur in premature labour.
- Show: The show, mucus plug or operculum can be heavily blood stained.

In cases of bleeding over 24 weeks, foetal well-being must be clearly established, so referral to the appropriate obstetric facilities would need to be sought in these situations.

> Immediate red-flag conditions that must be referred directly to maternity:
> - Reduced or altered pattern of foetal movements
> - No foetal movements
> - Spontaneous rupture of membranes (SROM) or suspected rupture of membranes, regardless of gestation
> - Fresh frank bleeding over 20 weeks
> - Any abdominal pain which is constant
> - Active labour
> - Any case where the clinician feels they need extra support.

Chapter Summary

This chapter has discussed the most common pregnancy-related presentations in primary care. This is by no means an exhaustive guide, and if there are any doubts or concerns then these should be escalated to a maternity or obstetric professional. It is important to remember that sometimes just the discussion of a case with a maternity or obstetric clinician can result in an alternative diagnosis that was previously not considered. Safety netting is an important step and must be remembered with every presentation. Women should also be reminded of the importance of keeping regular midwife appointments in line with their pregnancy recommendations.

CHAPTER 13   Obstetric Presentations

Case Study 1

You are working in a GP surgery and are asked to see a 34-year-old female who states that she is pregnant and has started bleeding PV.

History

PC: Patient reports that as she went to the toilet this morning when she wiped there was a streak of blood on the paper and in the toilet. Now there is around 10–20 mL on the pad she is wearing.
HxPC: 9/52 pregnant G3P1.
PMHx/SHx: Previous miscarriage at 8/52 last year and full-term pregnancy two years ago. No other medical complaints or surgery.
DHx: Folic acid.
SHx: Lives with husband and two-year-old daughter.
FHx: Cardiac disease.
ROS: All systems reviewed, no deviations observed.

Examination

- Vital signs: BP 110/60 mmHg; HR 90 bpm; RR 18/min; SpO_2 98%; pain score 2–3/10; temperature 37°C.
- No constant pain reported, other than occasional mild cramping.
- Abdominal assessment: No palpable uterus, non-tender lower abdomen.

Preferred Diagnosis

- Threatened miscarriage.

Differential Diagnoses

- Complete miscarriage
- Vaginal infections (thrush, bacterial vaginosis)
- Cervical ectropion or polyps
- Sexual intercourse
- Speculum examination
- Subchorionic bleeding
- Implantation bleeding.

Management

- Referral to an early pregnancy assessment unit or out-of-hours gynaecology service should be made for the next available appointment.
- The patient should also be advised that bleeding may increase and be as a heavy period and they may pass clots also. Period cramping pain is normal as well as contraction-type pain as the uterus contracts to remove the content.
- Simple analgesics should be advised also.

- They should be advised that if pain increases before they attend for the scan to recontact, as possible emergency admission may be required if ectopic is suspected.

Case Study 2

You are working in the out-of-hours walk-in centre when a 21-year-old female presents with pain on urination.

History
HxPC: Patient is 36/40 pregnant G1P0 and for the last 24 hours has noticed disurea, frequency and abdominal pain.
PMHx/SHx: Asthmatic well controlled, minimal use of treatment. Tonsillectomy age 12.
DHx: Ferrous sulphate, pregnancy vitamins.
SHx: Lives with partner.
FHx: None.
ROS: All systems reviewed, no deviations observed.

Examination
- Vital signs: BP 120/70 mmHg; HR 98 bpm; RR 20/min; SpO_2 98%; pain score 4/10; temperature 37.8°C.
- Gravid uterus observed, foetal movements seen. Tender over supra pubic region.
- Urinalysis: Blood + leucocytes +++ nitrates strongly positive.

Preferred Diagnosis
- UTI, +/− early labour.

Differential Diagnosis
- Labour.

Management
- Due to the patient being almost term and with lower abdominal pain there should be a conversation with the on-call obstetric team regarding treatment, as nitrofurantoin should be avoided at term. The degree of pain should be addressed and if there is a suspicion of labour then direct referral to maternity triage should be made.
- Ensure MSSU is sent for culture and sensitivity.
- Inform the woman that if the pain increases or becomes intermittent (contraction type), she must immediately contact maternity services. Remember this patient is a primigravida so will not know what experiencing contractions feels like.

CHAPTER 13   Obstetric Presentations

Case Study 3

You are working in a primary care centre where a 38-year-old female has been sent in from a triage call who is complaining of itchy hands.

History

HxPC: Patient has a three-day history of itchy hands, worse at night. She is 34/40 pregnant and a G2P1.
PMHx/SHx: None of note, normally FAW.
DHx: Pregnancy vitamins, iron tablets.
SHx: Lives with husband, four-year-old son and her in-laws.
FHx: Cardiovascular disease and diabetes in maternal history.
ROS: All systems reviewed, no deviations observed.

Examination

- Vital signs: BP 100/60 mmHg; HR 62 bpm; RR 19/min; SpO_2 99%; pain score 0/10; temperature 36.8°C.
- Gravid uterus noted, with rash over lower portion also noted.
- Itching over skin of the abdomen as well as the palms of the hands. No change in soaps/detergents.
- No obvious signs of contact dermatitis.
- Foetal movements reported but she cannot be certain they have not slowed over the past two days.

Preferred Diagnosis

- Obstetric cholestasis (OC).

Differential Diagnoses

- Contact dermatitis
- Allergic reaction.

Management

- Immediate referral to maternity services must be arranged with a same-day appointment. This is not just because of the risk that OC may be present but also because the patient is reporting reduced foetal movement and, combined with the possible diagnosis of OC, this puts her at increased risk of stillbirth.

References

Action on Pre-eclampsia (APEC) (2020) Why blood pressure and urine are tested during pregnancy: A woman's guide to screening for pre-eclampsia. Available at: https://action-on-pre-eclampsia.org.uk/wp-content/uploads/2018/10/Why-Blood-Pressure-and-Urine-are-Tested-During-Pregnancy.pdf (accessed 28 January 2023).

References

All Wales Medicines Strategy Group, All Wales Antimicrobial Guidance Group (AWMSG) (2018) Primary care empirical urinary tract infection treatment guidelines. Available at: https://phw.nhs.wales/services-and-teams/harp/urinary-tract-infection-uti-resources-and-tools/uti-downloads/primary-care-empirical-urinary-tract-infection-treatment-guidelines-all-wales-medicines-strategy-group-awmsg/ (accessed 28 January 2023).

Bora, S., Kirk, E. and Bourne, T. (2014) Do women with pain and bleeding in early pregnancy require a speculum examination as part of their assessment? *Gynaecology and Obstetric Investigation* 77(1): 29–34.

Bose, P., Regan, F. and Paterson-Brown, S. (2006) Improving the accuracy of estimated blood loss at obstetric haemorrhage using clinical reconstructions. *International Journal of Obstetrics and Gynaecology* 113(8): 919–924.

Chakladar, A. and Adams, H. (2009) The dangers of listening to the fetal heart at home. *British Medical Journal* 339: 1112–1113.

Cunningham, F., Leveno, K., Bloom, S. et al. (eds) (2018) *Williams Obstetrics*. 25th edn. London: Mc Graw Hill.

European Association of Urology (EAU) (2022) Urological infections. Available at: https://uroweb.org/guidelines/urological-infections (accessed 2 February 2023).

Farren, J., Jalmbrant, M., Ameye, L. et al. (2016) Post-traumatic stress, anxiety and depression following miscarriage or ectopic pregnancy: A prospective cohort study. *BMJ Open* 6(11): e011864.

Green, L., Mackillop, L. Salvi, D. et al. (2020) Gestation-specific vital sign reference ranges in pregnancy. *Obstetrics and Gynaecology* 135(3): 653–664.

Johnston, C.L., Johnston, M.J., Corke, A. et al. (2017) A likely urinary tract infection in a pregnant woman. *British Medical Journal* 357: j1777.

Knight, M., Bunch, K., Tuffnell, D. et al. (2019) *Saving Lives, Improving Mothers' Care – Lessons Learned to Inform Maternity Care from the UK and Ireland Confidential Enquiries into Maternal Deaths and Morbidity 2015–17*. Oxford: National Perinatal Epidemiology Unit, University of Oxford.

Knott, L. (2015) Abdominal pain in pregnancy. Available at: https://patient.info/doctor/abdominal-pain-in-pregnancy (accessed 10 April 2023).

Liu, S., Chan, W., Ray, J. et al. (2019) Stroke and cerebrovascular disease in pregnancy incidence, temporal trends, and risk factors. *Stroke* 50: 13–20.

Miscarriage Association (2023) Types of pregnancy loss. Available at: www.miscarriageassociation.org.uk/information/types-of-pregnancy-loss (accessed 28 January 2023).

National Health Service (NHS) (2016) National maternity review. Better Births: Improving outcomes of maternity services in England; A five year forward view for maternity care. Available at: https://www.england.nhs.uk/wp-content/uploads/2016/02/national-maternity-review-report.pdf (accessed 28 January 2023).

National Health Service (NHS) (2022) Overview: Ectopic pregnancy. Available at: https://www.nhs.uk/conditions/ectopic-pregnancy/ (accessed 28 January 2023).

National Health Service (NHS) (2020) Abortion overview. Available at: https://www.nhs.uk/conditions/abortion/ (accessed 12 July 2021).

National Institute for Health and Care Research (NIHR) (2019) High blood pressure in pregnancy: Treatment vs no treatment. Available at: https://action-on-pre-eclampsia.org.uk/wp-content/uploads/2019/11/high-blood-pressure-in-pregnancy-infographic-web.pdf (accessed 28 January 2023).

CHAPTER 13 Obstetric Presentations

National Institute for Health and Care Excellence (NICE) (2018) Urinary tract infection (lower): Antimicrobial prescribing [NG109]. Available at: https://www.nice.org.uk/guidance/ng109 (accessed 28 January 2023).

National Institute for Health and Care Excellence (NICE) (2019a) Antenatal care for uncomplicated pregnancies [CG62]. Available at: https://www.nice.org.uk/guidance/cg62 (accessed 28 January 2023).

National Institute for Health and Care Excellence (NICE) (2019b) Hypertension in pregnancy: Diagnosis and management [NG133]. Available at: https://www.nice.org.uk/guidance/ng133/chapter/Recommendations#management-of-gestational-hypertension (accessed 28 January 2023).

National Institute for Health and Care Excellence (NICE) (2021a) Antenatal care. Guideline NG201. Available at: https://www.nice.org.uk/guidance/ng201/resources (accessed 28 January 2023).

National Institute for Health and Care Excellence (NICE) (2021b) Chest infections – Adult. Available at: https://cks.nice.org.uk/topics/chest-infections-adult/ (accessed 28 January 2023).

National Institute for Health and Care Excellence (NICE) (2022) Urinary tract infection (lower) – Women. Available at: https://cks.nice.org.uk/urinary-tract-infection-lower-women#!scenario:3 (accessed 1 February 2023).

NHS England (2019) *Saving Babies' Lives Care Bundle Version 2: A Care Bundle for Reducing Perinatal Mortality.* London: NHS England.

Public Health England (PHE) (2018) UK standards for microbiology investigations: Investigation of urine. Available at: https://www.gov.uk/government/publications/smi-b-41-investigation-of-urine (accessed 28 January 2023).

Public Health England (PHE) (2021) Press release: JCVI issues new advice on COVID-19 vaccination for pregnant women. Available at: https://www.gov.uk/government/news/jcvi-issues-new-advice-on-covid-19-vaccination-for-pregnant-women (accessed 28 January 2023).

Raines, D. and Cooper, D. (2022) Braxton Hicks contractions. Available at: https://www.ncbi.nlm.nih.gov/books/NBK470546/ (accessed 28 January 2023).

Rebarber, A. and Jacob, B. (2021) Acute appendicitis in pregnancy. *UpToDate*. Available at: https://www.uptodate.com/contents/acute-appendicitis-in-pregnancy (accessed 28 January 2023).

Royal College of General Practitioners (RCGP) (2021) Treating your infection – Urinary tract infection (UTI). Available at: https://elearning.rcgp.org.uk/mod/book/view.php?id=12652&chapterid=468 (accessed 28 January 2023).

Royal College of Midwives (RCM) (2019) Position statement: Perinatal women in the criminal justice system. Available at: https://www.rcm.org.uk/media/3640/perinatal-women-in-the-criminal-justice-system_7.pdf (accessed 28 January 2023).

Royal College of Midwives (RCM) (2022) Guidance for pregnant women. Available at: https://www.rcm.org.uk/coronavirus-hub/covid-vaccines-for-pregnant-women/vaccine-facts/ (accessed 28 January 2023).

Royal College of Midwives (RCM) and Royal College of Obstetricians and Gynaecologists (RCOG) (2022) Coronavirus (COVID-19) infection in pregnancy: Information for healthcare professionals. Available at: https://www.rcog.org.uk/media/kbknl3z3/2022-03-07-coronavirus-covid-19-infection-in-pregnancy-v15.pdf (accessed 28 January 2023).

Royal College of Nursing (RCN) (2017) Clinical nurse specialist in early pregnancy care. Available at: https://www.rcn.org.uk/professional-development/publications/pub-006394 [archived].

References

Royal College of Nursing (RCN) (2020) Advanced practice standards. Available at: https://www.rcn.org.uk/professional-development/advanced-practice-standards (accessed 28 January 2023).

Royal College of Obstetricians and Gynaecologists (RCOG) (2011) *Obstetric Cholestasis Green-top Guideline No. 43*. London: RCOG.

Royal College of Obstetricians and Gynaecologists (RCOG) (2022) Coronavirus (COVID-19), infection in pregnancy: The impact of new evidence and changes in policy – specifically related to the Omicron variant – is being reviewed on a weekly basis. Available at: https://www.rcog.org.uk/media/ftzilsfj/2022-12-15-coronavirus-covid-19-infection-in-pregnancy-v16.pdf (accessed 28 January 2023).

Scott, C., Bewley, S., Rudd, A. et al. (2012) Incidence, risk factors, management, and outcomes of stroke in pregnancy. *Obstetrics and Gynaecology* 120(2): 318–324.

Smaill, F. and Vazquez, J. (2015) Antibiotics for asymptomatic bacteriuria in pregnancy. *Cochrane Database of Systematic Reviews* 8: CD000490.

Tommy's (2017) Intraheptic cholestasis of pregnancy (ICP). Available at: https://www.tommys.org/pregnancy/complications/obstetric-cholestasis (accessed 10 April 2023).

Webster, K., Fishburn, S., Maresh, M. et al. (2019) Diagnosis and management of hypertension in pregnancy: Summary of updated NICE guidance. *British Medical Journal* 366: l5119.

Yamamoto, A., Gelberg, L., Needleman, J. et al. (2021) Comparison of childbirth delivery outcomes and costs of care between women experiencing vs not experiencing homelessness. *JAMA Network Open* 4(4): e217491.

Zinaman, M., Warren, G. and Johnson, S. (2020) HCG and FSH levels during early pregnancy and reproductive aging. *Obstetrics and Gynaecology* 135(14S).

Musculoskeletal Presentations

14

Sarah Jardine and Georgette Eaton

> **Within This Chapter**
> - Minor injury
> - Pain
> - Redness
> - Spasticity
> - Stiffness
> - Swelling

Introduction

Musculoskeletal (MSK) conditions have been estimated to account for approximately 20% of primary care consultations (Keavy, 2020), with re-presentations accounting for just under 70% of all MSK consultations. For many of these patients, pain or a functional abnormality will exist, which may be the reason for their attendance. Whilst primary care is rapidly seeking the inclusion of specialist allied health professionals, such as MSK physiotherapists, a good understanding of the broad presentation areas and examination skills is crucial for paramedics in order to explore presenting complaints and the safe onward referral of patients who present to paramedics in primary care.

Assessment

The MSK system is the mechanism by which the body performs all mechanical functions. Each joint is designed to perform a specific set of motions, and there is a complicated system of bones, muscles, joints and connective tissues that join these structures (Totora and Derrickson, 2017) to produce and facilitate delivery of the mechanical forces required to either move or stabilise an area. An abnormality in any of these structures will produce a malfunction, and so examination should seek to understand the problem in order to provide a solution.

History

Arguably the most important part of the assessment is the history, where both the presenting complaint and the context (in this case the patient's current health, past medical history and social circumstances) in which it presents itself should be explored.

CHAPTER 14 Musculoskeletal Presentations

It is only by understanding how the condition developed that consideration can be given to the underlying structures involved. And it is only by understanding what the patient needs to be able to do that you can begin to work on an appropriate management plan with them.

> Management plans should be devised *with* the patients, not *for* them. This is to ensure their individual circumstances and requirements form part of the shared decision-making process.

During the history, investigation of the exact presenting complaint and the circumstances that led to it, along with any associated features such as paraesthesia or referred pain, are important. This may require some quite detailed questioning about the timings and sequence of onset, or around mechanism of injury. This will help you to work out if it is related to an injury, and you can then explore the forces that the joint has been subjected to and therefore work out which structures may have been affected, or if it is the result of a medical condition.

> The greater your knowledge of the underlying anatomy and the common injury presentations for a particular area, the more competent you will be in interpreting your findings and preparing for your physical assessment.

Inspection

As you begin the consultation, visually note any gross abnormalities – either in deformity or gait.

Once the reason for the consultation has been clarified, gain as much information from inspection as you can. Inspect the problem area, and then the joint above and below for observable abnormalities such as discolouration (for example ecchymoses, redness), soft tissue swelling, bony enlargement, muscle wasting and deformity (abnormal angulation, subluxation). While noting these changes, attempt to determine whether they are limited to the joint or whether they involve the surrounding structures (for example tendons, muscles, bursae). This will help with the approach to movement screening.

Regardless of abnormality observed, the remaining examination process will not only delineate the extent of gross abnormalities present, but also ascertain subtle anomalies that may not have been apparent on the initial inspection. Use the opposite side for comparisons: it is easier to spot subtle differences as well as identify symmetrical problems.

Palpation

To perform an examination of the muscles, bones and joints, use the classic technique of palpation. A good way to start this is by dividing the MSK system into functional parts and working distally-proximally. With practice, you will establish an order of approach that works for you, but for the beginner, starting distally and working proximally (or, in a

Assessment

localised area, away from the pain towards the pain) is a helpful approach to add structure to the MSK examination.

For a full-body examination, begin distally with the upper extremity from the fingers, working proximally through hands, wrist, elbow and up to the shoulder. Moving to the temporomandibular joint, pass on to the cervical spine, the thoracic spine, the lumbar and sacral spine and the sacroiliac joints. Finally, in the lower extremity, again begin distally with the toes and the foot, proceeding proximally through the knee to the pelvis and hip.

In primary care, the patient will often present with pain in a specific area or localised to one joint. In this case, it is usually sufficient to palpate the joints immediately distal and proximal to the pain, before palpating the painful area directly. The same methodical approach should be taken to the palpation of a single joint or area so that you can visualise the structures under your fingers as you work.

> 💡 Observe the patient's eyes while palpating the joints and the surrounding structures. One of the most objective indicators of the magnitude of tenderness produced by palpation is involuntary muscle movements about the eyes.

Note areas of tenderness to pressure and, if possible, identify the anatomic structures over which the tenderness is localised – this will help inform an impression regarding the functionality of the associated joint and thus your approach to assessing movement.

Movement

Equipped with information from the history, inspection and palpation, you will likely start the movement assessment with an indicative diagnosis, for which you are looking to determine the impact on joint functionality.

You may already have an idea of the patient's functional ability from when you first met them and watched them approach you and settle themselves in the consultation room. Your aim now is to get an objective view of the range of movement and functional compromise of the areas directly affected.

Active movement is approached initially, asking the patient to perform a complete active range of motion with each joint or set of joints. Comparing these movements to those on the unaffected side will give you a good idea of any deficit. Take note of the range of movement that the patient can perform for each individual movement, and also of what is stopping them from moving further. Is it pain, stiffness, weakness or a combination of factors?

> 💡 Pain on active movement does not help you identify which structure is causing the pain. This is because both the muscles and joints (and the structures stabilising the joints, such as ligaments) are involved in the movement. In order to identify the structure, you will need to put together information about the mechanism of injury and the results of your palpation.

CHAPTER 14   Musculoskeletal Presentations

Passive range of motion can be helpful in pinpointing the injured structures. A true passive movement occurs when the patient completely relaxes and allows you to take over the work of their muscles. If the patient is in pain, then remember that this will be difficult for them, and that they will most likely have some muscle activation in order to protect the painful area. Good patient-handling skills will help to produce a more effective passive movement, so be aware of how you are interacting with and holding the patient. If you can perform a true passive movement, then you are taking the contractile tissues, the muscles, 'out of the equation', and are testing the joints and the surrounding structures. If the pain of a passive movement is less or the range movement is more than in an active movement, this indicates that the muscles have been injured. Whilst this does not rule out joint or ligament involvement, it does give you a good place to start. If the pain and range of movement remain the same, then it indicates that the joint has been injured. Passively moving a joint also gives you the opportunity to feel for crepitus and for the stability of the joint.

Lastly, assessing resisted movement performs two functions. It can determine the muscle power around the joint which can add to the neurological assessment of the condition, along with reflexes and dermatome testing. It can also add to the information about whether the pain is originating from the muscles or the joint. A resisted movement should be performed in such a way that it prevents the joint moving. In this way, the muscles are activated and can be tested, but the joint is taken 'out of the equation'. If a resisted movement, that is, the muscle contraction, causes less pain than the active movement, then it indicates that the pain is originating in the joint and surrounding structures rather than in the muscle.

> 💡 To encourage a patient to keep their joint still during a resisted movement, try encouraging them to 'stop' you performing a movement, rather than asking them to actually perform that movement. For example, 'Stop me straightening your elbow', rather than 'Bend your elbow'. Both instructions encourage activation of the elbow flexors, but one discourages movement and one encourages it.

Presentations in Primary Care

Minor injury

Aetiology

Minor injury presentations can be many and varied. Some of the most common soft tissue injuries are to the following structures, although this list is by no means exhaustive.

Tendons and Muscles

Strain: A partial or complete rupture of a tendon or muscle. Patients with underlying conditions such as rheumatoid arthritis may be prone to strains without the expected injury history.

Overuse injuries: Sometimes known as repetitive strain injuries (RSIs). For example, tendonitis, which is inflammation of the tendon itself; or tenosynovitis, which is roughening of the tendon and the inner layer of the synovial sheath, causing pain and crepitus on movement (Purcell, 2016).

Ligaments
Sprains: A partial or complete rupture of a ligament. Injury to collateral ligaments, those which prevent side-to-side movement at a joint, is particularly common, and injuries to ankles and knees are frequently seen in primary care. Injury is caused by a joint being forced beyond its normal range of movement, either by direct or indirect force. Ligaments are slow to heal and can cause ongoing problems if not managed well in the early stages of an injury.

Cartilage
Tears: The most common presentation of cartilage injury is to the menisci of the knee. This is caused by forceful rotation of the knee, such as in sports, or direct stress on the knee when squatting or kneeling.

Bursa
Inflammation: Bursitis – discussed in the 'swelling' section.

Fascia
Inflammation: Fasciitis – the most-seen presentation is plantar fasciitis, a common cause of heel pain. This can develop spontaneously or as an overuse injury.

History and Examination
The history of a soft tissue injury is very important, as the mechanism of injury or development of the condition will give clear clues as to the origin of the pain and the structure(s) involved. The past medical history of the patient will also help you to understand whether injury may have occurred without the usual, or expected, forces being present. Some soft tissue injuries, particularly those caused by overuse, may not have a clear history of injury and may require a careful and systematic exploration of the history of the presenting complaint and the patient's occupation and activities.

Sprains and Strains
These types of injury usually present with a history of injury and pain on palpation of the affected structures. Pain, and perhaps weakness, is also present on resisted movement (strains) and passive stretching (sprains). Complete rupture of either tendons or ligaments is often associated with the patient hearing a noise, a snap or crack, which they may attribute to bony injury rather than soft tissue injury. The pain of a complete rupture may be less than expected, and palpation may reveal a space, where tissue is no longer present, due to the movement of the structure that is now no longer anchored at both ends. This is particularly

CHAPTER 14   Musculoskeletal Presentations

the case for the contractile tissue of muscles and tendons. Note that swelling around the area in reaction to the injury may prevent this sign being as obvious on palpation as one might expect it to be.

Overuse Injuries

These can be hard to diagnose, as the patient may not be aware of the factors involved, particularly if the onset has been gradual. Careful exploration of the history and examination of the affected area is needed.

Injury to the Menisci in the Knee

This is the shock-absorbing cartilage located on the tibial plateau. When injured, it is often associated with a history of 'locking' or 'giving way' of the knee. This may be after an injury, or may be a chronic issue that the patient is unable to pinpoint to a specific event. The menisci have poor blood supply and do not heal themselves, so can cause pain associated with swelling, and can move or fold, causing the 'locking' and 'giving-way' sensations.

Plantar Fasciitis

This can be an extremely painful and difficult to treat presentation. It is characterised by pain in the heel felt in the morning and on weight bearing. It is not usually associated with an injury event. Pain will be felt on palpation of the calcaneal insertion of the plantar fascia, on the sole of the foot.

Management

Minor injuries can generally be managed with analgesia, protection (for example crutches, splints, shoe modifications), rest (relative to the phase of healing), ice, compression (dependent on the guidelines in your department) and elevation. It is important, however, not to become complacent about this management and to remember, and stress to the patient, that poorly managed minor injuries can lead to significant pain and functional compromise for many months. It may be necessary for the patient to be referred to physiotherapy if the injury does not resolve.

> The acronym PRICE (protection, rest, ice, compression, elevation) is a commonly used and understood guide for treatment of soft tissue injuries. This does not mean it is a 'one size fits all' approach though, and advice still needs to be tailored to your patient, their expectations and needs and the presentation of the injury in front of you (Bleakley, 2013). A discussion around the 'rest' element is particularly important to ensure that the injury is rested sufficiently in the initial stages of healing, but that gentle exercise is introduced carefully as early as possible to reduce stiffness and encourage optimal healing (Purcell, 2016).

If you suspect a completely ruptured tendon or ligament, or a meniscus which has folded over resulting in an acutely 'locked' knee, then onward referral for surgery is appropriate.

Presentations in Primary Care

> When considering the management of minor injuries, it is essential to understand how this injury affects the patient, and what level of function they need to return to. Patients respond differently to advice, so understanding the factors influencing the patient, such as whether they are entitled to paid sick leave or are keen athletes, is vital if you want to engage them and empower them to 'own' their management plan.

Pain

Aetiology

Pain from the back, neck, shoulder or knee are four of the most common presentations to primary care, with the additional problem of multi-site pain across these joints (Hill et al., 2020). Pain is typically categorised by the damage that causes it, and within MSK presentations here we are focused on nociceptive pain (caused by tissue damage).

> Dubin, A.E. and Patapoutian, A. (2010) Nociceptors: The sensors of the pain pathway.

History and Examination

> History taking should include screening for suspicion of infection, malignancy, fracture, inflammatory causes of pain, severe and progressive neurological deficit and serious conditions that masquerade as MSK pain (such as myocardial infarction or aortic aneurysm).

The examination should include an assessment of mobility, movement, strength, position and proprioception – combining the examination principles outlined within this chapter with those outlined in Chapter 5 – Neurological Presentations (pp. 95–119).

If a fracture is clinically suspected, the examination should also feature a referral for imaging.

> Radiological imaging is discouraged unless serious pathology is suspected or imaging is likely to change management (Lin et al., 2020).

Blood tests may also be a useful indicator of MSK health:

- Vitamin D status: Low vitamin D levels may lead to clinical manifestations, including bone pain, muscle weakness, falls, low bone mass and fractures.

CHAPTER 14 Musculoskeletal Presentations

- Calcium: A high level of calcium in the blood (hypercalcaemia) can develop in people with multiple myeloma because too much calcium is released from affected bones into the bloodstream. Unexplained, persistent, dull achy bone pain is one of the defining features of multiple myeloma.

However, they do have a varying degree of reliability in diagnosis, and should be used in conjunction with the whole clinical picture.

Management

Management should be patient centred, and tailored to their individual contexts (for example employment, social considerations and expectations). The management strategy below outlines a general plan that can be adapted to specific sites:

- Physical activity or exercise therapy can be effective for relieving pain and improving function for MSK pain.
- Manual therapy (such as massage) can be used as an adjunct but should not be used in isolation (Lin et al., 2020).
- Non-steroidal anti-inflammatory drugs (NSAIDs) and opioids reduce pain in the short term but the benefits and burdens of efficacy and the side effects should be considered in each case (Babatunde et al., 2017).
- Injury to deep tissues can cause both referred and neuropathic pain, and muscle spasm. In some patients, it may be appropriate to consider the use of adjunctive therapies such as anticonvulsants, antidepressants or muscle relaxants. However, the effect size is modest and the potential for adverse effects needs careful consideration and discussion with the patient.
- Corticosteroid injections may be beneficial for short-term pain relief among patients with knee and shoulder pain (Babatunde et al., 2017). However, optimal dose, intensity and frequency are dependent on other patient comorbidities, and the injection should only be undertaken by clinicians trained in its use. Referral to MSK physiotherapists in primary care may be useful here.

Redness

Aetiology

Redness associated with an MSK problem is caused by hyperaemia (increased blood flow) in superficial capillaries – which also causes the area to be warm. This may occur on its own (as a response to changes in temperature or direct trauma). More typically, redness is also associated with an inflammatory response. Cells become damaged due to bacteria, heat, trauma or toxins, then heat up and so release chemicals including histamine, bradykinin and prostaglandins. These chemicals cause blood vessels to leak fluid into the tissues, causing local swelling to the soft tissues.

History and Examination

During palpation, as you proceed from distal to proximal, the skin temperature gradually warms. Therefore, during palpation, note areas of increased warmth. Using the most

Presentations in Primary Care

heat-sensitive portion of the hand (usually the dorsum of the fingers) start distally and lightly passing over the area of concern. If you find an area becoming slightly warmer, this represents increased heat (and will likely be red), so an infective source must be considered. A reactive effusion, a swelling that comes up several hours or the next day after an injury, is often accompanied by redness and heat.

If you discover an area of swelling around a joint that appeared immediately after an injury and is *not* red, consider a haemarthrosis. This is when there is significant bleeding into a joint. This is more common in patients with haemophillia but can also happen in patients without this underlying condition if the mechanism of injury is sufficiently forceful. A haemarthrosis will usually need onward referral for orthopaedic review.

Management

> ! Redness rarely occurs on its own, so the history and examination should work to determine the underlying cause and therefore consider the appropriate management plan.

Once an infection is ruled out, inflammation and reactive effusions can usually be managed with appropriate rest, ice and elevation.

Spasticity

Aetiology

Spasticity is a condition which is caused by interruption of the nerve impulses which control muscle movement. This results in stiff, tight muscles which remain contracted and resist being stretched. Spasticity itself is not an MSK condition but a clinical feature of a neurological condition such as a spinal cord injury, a brain injury or a condition such as multiple sclerosis or cerebral palsy (NINDS, 2019).

Spasticity can, however, be associated with many MSK presentations such as joint pain, stiffness, reduced range of movement and functional compromise.

History and Examination

It is vital to ascertain if this is the first presentation of spasticity for this patient, as if so, onward referral for a neurological assessment is essential. If the patient has a known neurological condition and the spasticity is causing other MSK symptoms, then these will need to be assessed within the context of the severity and stage of the patient's condition. This may present a challenge to the primary care practitioner without prior knowledge of the patient. A comprehensive history and open discussion with the patient will assist with devising an appropriate physical assessment.

Management

Ongoing management of neurological conditions is often best carried out by a multidisciplinary team (Ward, 2003). If the patient has a pre-existing condition, then they will, in all likelihood, already be under the care of some such team and referral back to this team would be appropriate once any immediate concerns have been addressed.

Spasticity is managed in a variety of ways, including medications such as baclofen, diazepam or clonazepam, physiotherapy such as muscle stretching and range-of-movement exercises and injections of botulinum toxin. Surgery, splinting and plastering can also be used (NINDS, 2019).

Stiffness

Aetiology

Stiffness can occur in a number of situations, and is often accompanied by pain or a reduction in range of movement. Stiffness has two main points of origin – muscle stiffness or joint stiffness.

Muscle Stiffness

Muscle or tendon strains and delayed onset muscle soreness (DOMS) after unaccustomed exercise are common causes of muscle stiffness. DOMS usually presents 12–24 hours after exercise (Braun and Sforzo, 2011). Medical conditions such as underlying myopathies, for example polymyalgia rheumatica, or neuromuscular disorders, or such as Parkinson's disease and myasthenia gravis, should also be considered.

Joint Stiffness

Joint stiffness can be caused by injury to the joint affecting the surrounding ligaments or cartilage. Underlying conditions can include rheumatoid arthritis, osteoarthritis, lupus, bursitis, gout and bone cancer.

History and Examination

Much of the information that will enable you to diagnose the cause of the presenting stiffness will come from a full history, including a detailed exploration of the timings of the stiffness, for example, worse in the morning for 30 minutes, and aggravating and easing factors. You will be able to differentiate between an injury or presentation of DOMS and an underlying medical condition.

If you suspect an undiagnosed underlying pathology, then blood tests, as discussed above, and referral on for nerve conduction testing may be appropriate.

Blood tests – full blood count (FBC), calcium, erythrocyte sedimentation rate (ESR), anti-cyclic citrullinated protein (anti-CCP), urate, autoimmune, antibodies, C-reactive protein (CRP), vitamin D, rheumatoid factor.

Physical examination will need to consider specifically range of movement, quality of movement (that is, fluidity of movement) and pain.

Management

If an underlying pathology is suspected, management will initially consist of symptom control and onward referral, as discussed in the section on 'swelling'.

If the stiffness originates from an injury, be that muscle, tendon, ligament or cartilage, then analgesia, relative rest and ice will be appropriate.

Presentations in Primary Care

> 💡 'Relative rest' is an important concept, as complete immobility is not advised since this in itself can be a cause of stiffness.

In a patient who presents with a history of subacute injury and stiffness, an exploration of their management of the condition so far would be appropriate. It may be that too much rest has caused the presenting stiffness, and that you will need to advise on how they should integrate appropriate levels of movement into their management plan.

Suspected DOMS as the cause of stiffness can be managed by alleviating the symptoms while the muscles repair themselves. Massage after exercise, specifically 48 hours post workout, can be helpful (Guo et al., 2017), as can a warm bath (Petrofsky et al., 2017). The effect of over-the-counter analgesics seems to be minimal (Barlas et al., 2000), but gentle movement and stretching may help.

Swelling

Aetiology

The aetiology will depend on the site of the swelling, and whether it is bony or soft tissue in origin. Table 14.1 outlines a range of conditions and relevant aetiology.

History and Examination

Whilst palpating joints and surrounding structures, carefully note the presence of any enlargement and its boundaries. You can then decide whether this is due to bony widening; effusion into the joint capsule; soft tissue swelling; thickening of the synovial lining of a joint; or nodule formation, which might be in a tendon sheath, subcutaneous tissue or other structures around a joint.

Blood tests are useful to assist in the diagnosis to confirm the cause of swelling:

- Anti-CCP: Antibodies commonly produced by the immune system in people with rheumatoid arthritis.
- CRP: Assesses levels of inflammation in the body.
- ESR: Assesses levels of inflammation in the body.
- FBC: Anaemia is common in people with rheumatoid arthritis.
- Rheumatoid factor: Measures rheumatoid factor proteins and is an indicator of rheumatoid arthritis.
- Urate: To determine the level of uric acid, an indicator of gout.

In uncertain situations, radiographic imaging is frequently performed to evaluate the extent of the swelling and confirm the diagnosis. However, considerations should be given to the visibility of some bony swelling on plain forms — bone marrow oedema, one of the earliest pathological features of bone sarcomas and osteomyelitis, is not visible on plain films. In soft tissue swelling, cross-sectional imaging, such as computed tomography and magnetic resonance imaging, provides detailed anatomic information in the evaluation of soft tissues due to their inherent high spatial and contrast resolution. However, this will depend on accessibility and ability to refer locally. Plain radiography continues to be an appropriate first line, useful for excluding other differentials such as fractures, and for assessing the progression of disease by comparing changes seen on follow-up films with the initial radiograph (RCR, 2017).

CHAPTER 14 Musculoskeletal Presentations

Table 14.1 Conditions Related to Swelling and Their Aetiology

Condition	Aetiology
Osteoarthritis	Characterised by a degenerative cascade of progressive cartilage loss. Subsequent calcification of the surrounding articular cartilage reduces the thickness of and eventually destroys the cartilaginous matrix (Senthelal et al., 2022)
Rheumatoid arthritis	This is an autoimmune systemic inflammatory disorder. The degradation of cartilage and, eventually, bone is preceded by endothelial cell activation and synovial cell hyperplasia (Senthelal et al., 2022)
Septic arthritis	Typically, an inflammatory response to a mono-bacterial infection. Bacterial entry into the synovial fluid triggers a release of cytokines, chemokines and proteases that degrade cartilage and trigger hyperplasia of the synovial membrane (Senthelal et al., 2022)
Bone marrow oedema	Occurs when fluid builds up in the bone marrow, which is typically a response to an injury such as a fracture or conditions such as osteoarthritis
Bursitis	Prolonged pressure, whereby the bursa is stressed between a hard surface and a bony prominence, is the most common cause of bursitis. Repetitive motions can also irritate the bursa and result in bursitis. The second most common cause of bursitis is trauma when direct pressure is applied to the bursa (Williams et al., 2022)
Gout	Prolonged hyperuricaemia leads to uric acid deposition in joints, which then leads to joint inflammation (Senthelal et al., 2022)
Osteomyelitis	An acute or chronic inflammatory process involving the bone and its structures secondary to infection (Momodu and Savaliya, 2022)
Bone sarcoma	Several different types of tumour can grow in bones: primary bone tumours, which form from bone tissue and can be malignant or benign, and metastatic tumours. Malignant primary bone tumours (primary bone cancers, such as osteosarcoma, Ewing sarcoma and chondrosarcoma) are less common than benign primary bone tumours. Both types of primary bone tumours may grow and compress healthy bone tissue, but benign tumours usually do not spread or destroy bone tissue (NICE, 2020b)
Soft tissue sarcoma	A broad term for cancers that start in soft tissues (muscle, tendons, fat, lymphatic vessels, blood vessels and nerves). These cancers can develop anywhere in the body, but are found mostly in the arms, legs, chest and abdomen (NICE, 2020b)

Presentations in Primary Care

Management

Management will depend on the underlying cause of swelling, and the involvement of associated structures.

Osteoarthritis

Patients with osteoarthritis should be offered an individualised management plan, based on their circumstances, expectations and goals.

> Further information for considerations in the management of osteoarthritis is available from NICE (2022).

Rheumatoid Arthritis

Suspected rheumatoid arthritis will typically be managed initially by referral to rheumatology, with NSAIDS at the lowest effective dose, alongside a proton pump inhibitor (NICE, 2020b).

Bone Marrow Oedema

Bone marrow oedema is managed conservatively, but efforts should be made to categorically rule out osteomyelitis. Identification of the underlying cause is advocated during the progression of the management plan (Baumbach et al., 2020).

Bursitis

Bursitis is typically managed conservatively until symptoms improve. This may include rest, ice and reduced activity, as well as NSAIDs for analgesia (NICE, 2021). Aspiration may be considered to improve function and comfort if the effusion is large and you are clinically confident that the bursitis is non-septic. Septic bursitis requires aspiration and oral antibiotics initially, followed by ongoing conservative management and review.

Gout

Where the patient has a clear history of previous gout, treatment is with NSAIDs. In a typical case of gout or pseudogout where the patient is well, has no systemic symptoms of infection and no risk of chronic kidney disease, a short course of NSAIDs and review within a week is appropriate management.

Osteomyelitis and Septic Arthritis

> ⚠️ Osteomyelitis and septic arthritis are diagnoses not to miss. For both of these, there is no history of trauma (or no history of insignificant trauma for the degree of pain) and the patient cannot move the joint at all, strongly resisting any passive movements (FitzSimmons and Wardrope, 2004). For these patients, refer for further opinion via the emergency department – who may involve orthopaedics or rheumatology.

CHAPTER 14 Musculoskeletal Presentations

Sarcomas

Suspected bone sarcomas should have an urgent (48 hours) direct access X-ray. Similarly, suspected soft tissue sarcomas should have an urgent (two-week) direct-access ultrasound scan (NICE, 2020a). If either are deemed a possibility, both require a pathway referral for suspected cancer within two weeks.

Chapter Summary

MSK presentations make up a fifth of consultations in primary care, with repeat attendances for the same problem making up about three-quarters of these (Keavy, 2020). The MSK assessment requires a systematic approach to assess the impact of the concerning symptom on joint functionality and the extent to which this affects the patient's life. Devising a management plan with the patient which addresses their concerns and is tailored to meet their individual needs and expectations should help prevent unnecessary re-presentation. Using the range of professionals within primary care (such as MSK physiotherapists) also ensures patients get access to further examination and rehabilitation in a timely manner.

Case Study 1

You are working in a minor injury unit when a patient presents with a three-week history of a swelling to the left elbow, which has started to develop heat and redness.

History

PC: Left elbow swelling.
HxPC: Swelling to left elbow, developing in size over three weeks. Over the past few days, redness has developed, with a gradual feeling of warmth over the last few days. The patient reports no reduction in movement or functionality, with swelling being the primary concern.
PMHx/SHx: None.
DHx: None.
SHx: Works remotely at home in business consultancy. Plays rugby league with friends at weekends with some weekday training sessions.
FHx: None.
ROS: Denies recent illness.

Examination
- Inspection: Obvious egg-shaped swelling at the olecranon process. No bruising. Redness is present at the elbow tip.
- Palpation: No pain to the fingers, hand, wrist or forearm. During palpation of the proximal forearm and moving into the elbow, the patient denies pain but you notice that they scrunch their eyes. The swelling is firm and immobile, with some warmth noted in comparison to the forearm or upper arm. There is no pain beyond the elbow, moving to the shoulder.

- Movement: During active movement, you notice that full extension is reduced at 10°, with a limit in flexion to 120°. The patient reports this as an inability to move the limb further, rather than pain. No further reductions in movement are found on passive or resisted movement.

Preferred Diagnosis
- Olecranon bursitis.

Differential Diagnoses
- Septic bursitis
- Septic arthritis
- Bone tumour.

Management
- Rest, ice and reduced activity.
- Paracetamol or a NSAID for analgesia.
- Consider aspiration (if the expertise and equipment are available) to improve function and comfort, particularly if the effusion is large.
- Encourage a low threshold for return if there is increasing pain, increasing heat and spreading inflammation or redness (NICE, 2021).

Case Study 2

You are working in a minor injury unit when a patient presents with a 24-hour history of knee pain. The joint has swollen overnight.

History

PC: Right knee pain.
HxPC: Knee injured yesterday whilst playing football. The patient was tackled and was struck by his opponent's body on the lateral aspect of his knee. The patient was wearing football boots and his foot was on the ground when the impact occurred. Pain was felt immediately on the medial aspect of the knee but the patient was able to play on until the end of the match. Overnight, the joint has swelled and feels stiff and painful. No pain in the hip or ankle. No referred pain. No paraesthesia or anathaesia.
PMHx/SHx: None.
DHx: None.
SHx: Lives in a maisonette with two flights of stairs to the bedroom. Bedroom and bathroom on the same floor. Works as a frontline paramedic. Plays football and attends the gym regularly.
FHx: None.
ROS: Nil of note.

Examination
- Inspection: Antalgic gait on entrance to the consultation room. General swelling around the knee joint, more obvious on the medial aspect of the knee. No bruising.
- Palpation: No pain on palpation of the quadriceps, hamstrings, calf muscles or patella. No pain on palpation of the fibula head or in the popliteal fossa. Pain evident on palpation of the medial aspect of the knee joint line.
- Movement: Active movement shows full range of motion in extension and flexion, although the patient carries this out carefully. Pain is consistent throughout the movement. Passive movement elicits much the same results, but resisted movement, without movement of the joint, is less painful.

Preferred Diagnosis
- Medial collateral ligament sprain.

Differential Diagnoses
- Mensicus injury
- Tendon strain
- Tibial plateau fracture.

Management
- Protection (including discussion about how to manage stairs at home), rest (incorporating discussion about absence from work and gradual introduction of movement), ice and elevation when seated.
- Paracetamol or a NSAID for analgesia.
- Discussion surrounding the expected progression of healing is important, and the patient should be encouraged to access further support, either via the GP or directly to a physiotherapist, if the healing appears delayed or they are concerned.

References

Babatunde, O., Jordan, J., Van der Windt, D. et al. (2017) Effective treatment options for musculoskeletal pain in primary care: A systematic overview of current evidence. *PloS One* 12(6): e0178621.

Barlas, P., Craig, J.A., Robinson, J. et al. (2000) Managing delayed-onset muscle soreness: Lack of effect of selected oral systemic analgesics. *Archives of Physical Medicine and Rehabilitation* 81 (7): 966–972.

Baumbach, S.F., Pfahler, V., Bechtold-Dalla Pozza, S. et al. (2020) How we manage bone marrow edema: An interdisciplinary approach. *Journal of Clinical Medicine* 9(2): 551.

Bleakley, C.M. (2013) Acute soft tissue injury management: Past, present and future. *Physical Therapy in Sport* 14(2): 73–74.

Braun, W. and Sforzo, G. (2011) Delayed onset muscle soreness (DOMS). Available at: acsm.org/docs/default-source/files-for-resource-library/delayed-onset-muscle-soreness-(doms).pdf?sfvrsn= 8f430e18_2 (accessed 28 January 2023).

References

Dubin, A.E. and Patapoutian, A. (2010) Nociceptors: The sensors of the pain pathway. *The Journal of Clinical Investigation* 120(11): 3760–3772.

FitzSimmons, C. and Wardrope, J. (2004) Assessment and care of musculoskeletal problems. *Emergency Medicine Journal* 22(1): 68–76.

Guo, J., Li, L., Gong, Y. et al. (2017). Massage alleviates delayed onset muscle soreness after strenuous exercise: A systematic review and meta-analysis. *Frontiers in Physiology* 8: 747.

Hill, J.C., Garvin, S., Chen, Y. et al. (2020) Stratified primary care versus non-stratified care for musculoskeletal pain: Findings from the STarT MSK feasibility and pilot cluster randomized controlled trial. *BMC Family Practice* 21(1): 30.

Keavy, R. (2020) The prevalence of musculoskeletal presentations in general practice: An epidemiological study. *British Journal of General Practice* 70(Suppl 1): bjgp20X711497.

Lin, I., Wiles, L., Waller, R. et al. (2020) What does best practice care for musculoskeletal pain look like? Eleven consistent recommendations from high-quality clinical practice guidelines: Systematic review. *British Journal of Sports Medicine* 54: 79–86.

Momodu, I.I. and Savaliya, V. (2022) Osteomyelitis. Available at: https://www.ncbi.nlm.nih.gov/books/NBK532250/ (accessed 28 January 2023).

National Institute for Health and Care Excellence (NICE) (2020a) Clinical Knowledge Summary: Rheumatoid arthritis. Available at: https://cks.nice.org.uk/topics/rheumatoid-arthritis/management/suspected-ra/ (accessed 28 January 2023).

National Institute for Health and Care Excellence (NICE) (2020b) Bone and soft tissue sarcoma – Recognition and referral. Available at: https://cks.nice.org.uk/topics/bone-soft-tissue-sarcoma-recognition-referral/ (accessed 10 April 2023).

National Institute for Health and Care Excellence (NICE) (2021) Olecranon bursitis. Available at: https://cks.nice.org.uk/topics/olecranon-bursitis/ (accessed 28 January 2023).

National Institute for Health and Care Excellence (NICE) (2022) Clinical Knowledge Summary: Osteoarthritis. Available at: https://cks.nice.org.uk/topics/osteoarthritis/management/management/ (accessed 2 February 2023).

National Institute of Neurological Disorders and Stroke (NINDS) (2019) Spasticity information page. Available at: ninds.nih.gov/disorders/all-disorders/spasticity-information-page (accessed 10 April 2023).

Petrofsky, J., Berk, L., Bains, G. et al. (2017) The efficacy of sustained heat treatment on delayed-onset muscle soreness. *Clinical Journal of Sport Medicine* 27(4): 329–337.

Purcell, D. (2016) *Minor Injuries: A Clinical Guide*. 3rd edn. Amsterdam: Elsevier.

Royal College of Radiologists (RCR) (2017) *iRefer: Making the Best Use of Clinical Radiology*. 8th edn. London: RCR.

Senthelal, S., Li, J., Goyal, A. et al. (2022) Arthritis. Available at: https://www.ncbi.nlm.nih.gov/books/NBK518992/ (accessed 2 February 2023).

Totora, G. and Derrickson, B. (2017) *Tortora's Principles of Anatomy and Physiology*. 15th edn. Orlando, FL: Wiley.

Ward, A.B. (2003) Long-term modification of spasticity. *Journal of Rehabilitation Medicine* 41: 60–65.

Williams, C.H., Jamal, Z. and Sternard, B.T. (2022) Bursitis. Available at: https://www.ncbi.nlm.nih.gov/books/NBK513340/ (accessed 28 January 2023).

Dermatological Presentations

Vanessa Smeardon

15

Within This Chapter

Acute Skin Conditions
- Contact dermatitis
- Intertrigo
- Pityriasis rosea
- Urticaria

Bacterial Skin Conditions
- Cellulitis and erysipelas
- Folliculitis
- Hidradentis suppurativia
- Impetigo
- Lyme disease

Chronic Skin Conditions
- Acne vulgaris
- Eczema
- Stasis or varicose eczema
- Psoriasis
- Rosacea

Exanthems of Childhood
- Chickenpox
- Hand, foot and mouth
- Measles
- Molluscum contagiousum
- Roseola
- Rubella
- Scarlet fever
- Slapped cheek syndrome

Fungal Skin Infections
- Angular cheilitis
- Candidiasis
- Oral candidiasis
- Pityriasis versicolor
- Tinea
  - Tinea capitis
  - Tinea corporis and tinea cruris
  - Tinea pedis

Infestations
- Scabies

Lesions
- Actinic keratosis
- Sebaceous keratosis

Skin Cancer
- Skin cancer (non-melanoma)
  - Basal cell carcinoma
  - Squamous cell carcinoma
- Malignant melanoma
  - Acral lentiginous melanomas and subungal melanomas
  - Lentigo maligna melanoma
  - Nodular melanoma
  - Superficial spreading melanoma

Skin Emergencies
- Erythroderma
- Necrotising fasciitis
- Stevens-Johnson syndrome
- Vasculitis

Viral Skin Infections
- Herpes simplex
- Shingles (herpes zoster)

383

CHAPTER 15   Dermatological Presentations

Introduction

Skin conditions are a common presenting complaint within the primary care setting. They account for approximately 13 million GP consultations a year (King's Fund, 2014). This is not surprising, as the skin is the largest organ in the body. It is a protective layer, providing a barrier against infection and ultra-violet (UV) damage. It also helps maintain bodily fluids and regulate temperature, and is involved in the production of vitamin D (McCance and Huether, 2018). It is comprised of three main layers: the outer layer, the epidermis; the dermis; and the inner layer, the subcutaneous layer.

> The anatomy of the skin is often missed from undergraduate paramedic courses. Consider your level of knowledge and whether you need to undertake further reading in this area.

Many skin complaints seen in primary care are minor ailments that either will self-resolve or can be treated with over-the-counter medications. It is, however, important to be able to identify more serious conditions such as skin cancers where referral can be time critical.

Assessment

The following questions are pertinent to cover when undertaking a history related to a skin condition:

- Onset:
  - When did the rash first appear?
- Provoking or alleviating factors:
  - Any alleviating or exacerbating features – for example, is it associated with hot weather, sweating or exercise?
  - Triggered by chemicals, sun exposure or stress?
- Distribution of the rash:
  - Where on the body did it first start?
  - Has it spread slowly or rapidly, does it come and go?
  - Does the lesion appear as it is now or has it changed in appearance, such as the size, shape, colour, sensation?
  - If there are multiple lesions, where did the first one appear?
- Timings of the rash:
  - Were there any prodromal symptoms or recent illness prior to the rash?
  - Were there any obvious triggers?
  - How long has it been present?
  - Does it come and go?
  - Has the patient had it before?
- Past medical history:
  - Comorbidities
  - Immunosuppression
  - History of atopy

- Any history of recent trauma, such as cuts, bites, any breach of integrity in the skin
- Does the past already have a diagnosis? Have they had it before?
- Medication:
  - Any new medications
  - Has the patient tried any treatment? If so, what have they tried and has it been effective?
- Occupation:
  - Occupational exposure to any allergens, such as chemicals
- Social history:
  - History of smoking or alcohol use
  - Hobbies, swimming, gym, hot tub use
  - Walking, such as recent walks in wooded areas
  - Have any contacts had a similar rash?
  - Any pets? Presence of fleas or mites?
  - Diet: alcohol, caffeine, spicy foods?
- Family history:
  - Any skin conditions in family?
  - Genetic link, such as psoriasis.

Description of the Rash

It is important to accurately describe the rash. This includes the distribution of the rash, and the colour, size and shape of any lesions.

The description of the rash should include:

- Site: The areas of the body involved
- Distribution: Is it localised or generalised, and is the distribution symmetrical or is the rash more on one side of the body than the other? Is it bilateral or unilateral?
- Onset
- Colour
- Blanching or non-blanching
- Surface: Texture of the skin surface – for example, is it dry or scaly?
- Description of lesion, number of lesions and their distribution (for example, are they grouped in clusters or widespread), type of lesions, texture of lesion, border, colour and shape of lesion and size (where possible).

> Photographic documentation can be invaluable, as it can clearly show how a rash has progressed and indeed clearly shows treatment failure or success. It can be particularly useful with skin lesions, as it can document changes that may show a lesion has become malignant. Likewise, no change can be reassuring to a patient.

Terminology

The terminology used to describe dermatological presentations can be quite specific and so it will be useful to familiarise yourself with the terms in Table 15.1 to increase accuracy when describing presentations.

CHAPTER 15   Dermatological Presentations

Table 15.1   Terminology Related to Dermatological Presentations

Term		Description
Flat lesions	Macule	Not raised above the surface of the skin, feels smooth, no change in the skin felt on palpation, with a diameter of less than 1 cm
	Patch	Flat lesion that has a diameter of greater than 1 cm
Raised lesions	Plaque	Slightly raised thickened area of skin, rough to palpation (usually to fine scale or crust), e.g. as seen in psoriasis
	Papule	Raised firm lesion that is less than 1 cm in diameter
	Nodule	Raised firm lesion that is greater than 1 cm in diameter
Fluid-filled lesion	Pustule	Raised lesion that is filled with pus and is less than 1 cm in diameter
	Vesicle	Raised fluid-filled lesion that is less than 1 cm in diameter, e.g. blister
	Bulla	Blister greater than 1 cm in diameter
Other descriptors	Atrophy	Thinning of the surface of the skin
	Excoriation	Linear loss of the epidermis, e.g. scratch
	Fissure	Linear crack, deeper than excoriation as passes into the dermis
	Erosion	Non-linear loss of the epidermis, e.g. following a ruptured vesicle
	Ulcer	Loss of the epidermis and dermis
	Eschar	Dead tissue that sheds or falls from the skin

Source: Nast et al. (2016).

> Online resources including Dermnet NZ and the Primary Care Dermatology Society have an extensive library of images where the terminology outlined here can be visualised.

Primary Care Presentations
Acute Skin Conditions
Contact Dermatitis
Aetiology

Contact with an allergen which causes inflammation and well-defined patches of eczema.

Primary Care Presentations

History and Examination
The skin will be affected at the site that has come into contact with the allergen. The rash may mimic the shape of the allergen – for example, contact with metal on a belt buckle or hands commonly affected due to contact with chemicals.

Treatment
- Avoid contact with allergen where possible, using protective equipment as necessary
- Emollients
- Topical corticosteroids
- Refer to dermatology if patient suffers frequent flares (Oakley, 2017).

Intertrigo
Aetiology
Intertrigo results from the friction of two moist areas of skin rubbing together and typically affects skin folds. The rash is commonly found sub-mammary, in lower abdominal skin folds or the groin.

> Due to inflammation from the rubbed skin, areas of intertrigo can commonly become infected with bacteria or *Candida* (yeast) known as 'candida intertrigo'.

History and Examination
Causes painful bright red skin that is localised to the areas of rubbing. Predisposing factors include obesity and warm weather.

Management
- Lifestyle advice: Encourage weight loss
- Mild to moderate topical steroids
- Combination treatments can be used if an associated *Candida* infection is suspected.

> To assist with weight loss, consider engagement with local health and well-being groups or input from a social prescribing link worker.

Pityriasis Rosea
Aetiology
The cause of pityriasis rosea is unknown but it is commonly associated with viruses or as an adverse drug reaction.

History and Examination
Usually appears in children or young adults and starts from a single large salmon-coloured plaque 2–3 cm in diameter, called 'the herald patch'. The rash then develops elsewhere on

CHAPTER 15   Dermatological Presentations

the body within two weeks after the initial plaque. The rest of the rash tends to appear as smaller macules or plaques with smaller pink papules. It is usually distributed on the trunk but can appear on the thighs (Eisman and Sinclair, 2015).

Management
- A self-limiting rash that should resolve completely within five months
- It can be itchy, so manage with antihistamines, emollient and topical steroid (mild to moderate potency if required).

> If it develops in pregnancy, discuss urgently with a dermatologist as it can cause adverse effects including miscarriage in the first trimester (NICE, 2020).

Urticaria
Aetiology
Urticaria develops in response to an allergen, although the trigger is often unknown. It is caused by the release of histamine and other inflammatory meditators.

History and Examination
Urticaria presents as an itchy rash with hives – areas of erythema with skin swelling that form papules or plaques.

> It is important to consider the presence of other symptoms of allergy, as outlined in Chapter 9 – Respiratory Presentations, and to be aware of the signs and symptoms of anaphylaxis.

Management
- Rash often self-resolves rapidly when contact with the allergen has been removed.
- Treatment with over-the-counter antihistamines (such as cetirizine, loratadine or fexofenadine) can be helpful to relieve itching

> For frequent flares, encourage patients to keep a diary in order to consider and outline any potential triggers.

Bacterial Skin Conditions
Cellulitis and Erysipelas
Aetiology
Cellulitis is an infection of the skin, affecting the dermis and subcutaneous tissue. It is most commonly caused by *Streptococcus pyogenes* or *Staphylococcus aureus* entering the skin through a break in the barrier.

Erysipelas is a superficial form of cellulitis that affects the dermis and does not spread into the deeper tissues.

History and Examination

Most commonly effects lower limbs in adults and the face in children. Upper limbs can also be involved, particularly with intravenous drug users. Cellulitis is usually unilateral, and it is rare for both limbs to be affected (this is more likely to be varicose eczema). It presents as a spreading area of erythema that can be hot to touch, swollen, tender and can cause red shiny skin with blistering.

Erysipelas tends to have more defined borders than cellulitis and facial infections are more commonly erysipelas rather than cellulitis.

> Mark the area of the rash with a pen so it is clear to see if it has spread.

Predisposing factors to consider during history taking:

- Diabetes
- Immunocompromised
- IV drug use
- Obesity
- Pregnancy
- Previous cellulitis
- Skin trauma.

Management

- Treatment is typically with oral antibiotics
- Analgesia to ease pain
- If cellulitis occurs in the legs, elevation of the legs can reduce oedema.

> Emergency referral required if systemically unwell, rash spreading and not responding to oral antibiotics or with facial (unless mild) or all cases of periorbital cellulitis.

Folliculitis

Aetiology

Inflammation of the hair follicles; this can occur with or without infection. The most common bacterial infection associated with it is *Staphylococcus aureus*. However, pseudomonas is the likely cause in hot tub-associated folliculitis (Dermnet NZ, 2021).

History and Examination

Causes erythema and pustules that can become widespread. The rash can be itchy and painful. Can appear on any part of the body that has hair follicles.

CHAPTER 15   Dermatological Presentations

Predisposing factors to consider during history taking:

- Hot tubs
- Oily ointments
- Restrictive clothing
- Shaving
- Waxing.

Management

- Mild infections usually self-resolve and can be managed with topical antiseptics.
- If infections are widespread or associated with local infection, oral antibiotics are required.

Hidradenitis Suppurativa

Aetiology

Caused by blocked follicles obstructing gland ducts. This stops secretions escaping, resulting in inflamed hair follicles that then rupture and become infected.

History and Examination

Appears as papules, pustules and inflammatory nodules and in severe cases abscesses. It is commonly distributed to the axilla, groin and inner thighs. The cause for the blocked follicles is unknown and it is not linked to poor hygiene, but the following are thought to be predisposing factors:

- Crohn's disease
- Sex (three times more likely in women)
- Genetics
- Hormones (does not occur prior to puberty or post menopause)
- Obesity
- Smoking.

Management

Management is typically in a stepwise approach and features:

- Antimicrobial emollient or topical antiseptic
- Topical antibiotic
- Prolonged courses of tetracyclines.

> Abscesses at risk of infection should be referred to surgical on call for incision and drainage.

Primary Care Presentations

Impetigo

Aetiology
Impetigo is a common bacterial skin infection. It is usually caused by *Staphylococcus aureus*. It can occur at any age but is most common in childhood. It presents in two forms – bullous and non-bullous (most common).

History and Examination
Starts as small vesicles and pustules that evolve into yellow-crusted plaques. The initial area of infection can spread rapidly. Predisposing factors include eczema and breaks in the skin, such as from bites, trauma or burns. Non-bullous impetigo is usually distributed on the face, around the mouth and nose. Bullous impetigo infects intact skin, causing vesicles filled with clear fluid that then burst. More common in under two-year-olds and can occur on all sites of the body.

Management
- If localised and non-bullous, treat with a topical treatment – either hydrogen peroxide 1% or a topical antibiotic such as fusidic acid 2% – applied three times a day for five days (NICE, 2022e).
- For more widespread impetigo or if it has not responded to topical treatment, try oral antibiotics.
- All bullous impetigo should be treated with oral antibiotics.
- Public Health England advises staying off work or school until the lesions are dry and have crusted or for 48 hours after antibiotics have been started (PHE, 2023).

> Food handlers are required, by law, to inform employers immediately if they have impetigo (PHE, 2023).

> In recurrent infections, consider nasal swabs as the nose is one of the main sites to be colonised with *Staphylococcus aureus*.

Lyme Disease

Aetiology
A bacterial infection caused by the *Borrelia burgdorferi* bacteria. Transmission to humans occurs through tick bites. These ticks usually live on deer or sheep. It is the most common vector-borne disease in England and Wales (PHE, 2022).

History and Examination
Normally appears as a single circular lesion, an area of expanding area erythema with a central puncture (from initial bite). The rash can take a month to develop but usually

CHAPTER 15 Dermatological Presentations

appears within one week of the initial bite. It often has the appearance of a bullseye on a dartboard, with an area of darker erythema surrounded by a lighter pigment. The classic bullseye rash (Erythema migrans) is diagnostic of Lyme disease and people presenting with this rash should be treated even if they are otherwise asymptomatic. This rash, however, only appears in 70–80% of people infected with Lyme disease (Dermnet NZ, 2015). Initially can present with flu-like symptoms, including headache, malaise and aching joints. If untreated, it can cause neurological disorders, cardiac conditions including peri and myocarditis, chronic fatigue and arthritis.

Predisposing factors to consider during history taking:

- Areas of long grass
- Pets that can bring ticks into the home
- Walking in areas with the usual host deer or sheep
- Walking in wooded areas
- Walking with shorts and short sleeves.

Management

Lyme disease is a bacterial infection that can be successfully treated with antibiotics (NICE, 2022f). The use of antibiotics reduces the risk of further symptoms. Most patients will have no long-lasting symptoms.

> Those without the rash but who are symptomatic should have an enzyme-linked immunosorbent assay (ELISA) blood test.

Chronic Skin Conditions

Acne Vulgaris

Aetiology

Acne is a chronic skin condition of a pilosebaceous unit, characterised by blockage of a sebaceous follicle and subsequent inflammation. A single blocked sebaceous follicle is known as a comedo. As follicles burst, they cause inflammation, resulting in papules and pustules. An excess inflammatory response can lead to the development of nodules and cysts which as they heal leads to scarring (Ashton and Leppard, 2021). Acne is characterised by mild, moderate and severe forms, outlined in Table 15.2.

History and Examination

Acne is most prevalent in teens but can continue into older age groups (Oakley, 2017). It is commonly found on the face, chest and back. The skin appears greasy and depending on the severity of the acne there will be non-inflamed lesions (comedones), inflamed lesions (papules and pustules) and, in severe forms, nodules, cysts and scarring. A change in pigmentation of the skin may also be seen.

Table 15.2 Types of Acne

Mild	Moderate	Severe
Comedones (non-inflamed lesions)	Papules and pustules	Large numbers of papules and pustules, presence of nodules, cysts and scarring
Whitehead: Comedones can either be open or closed. A closed comedo is known as a whitehead		
Blackhead: An open comedo is known as a blackhead. The pigment of blackheads comes from oxidised sebum and not dirt		

Predisposing factors to consider during history taking:

- Diet (high in dairy and sugar)
- Drugs (such as steroids and anticonvulsants)
- Genetic
- High humidity
- Hormones
- Occlusive cosmetics
- Polycystic ovary syndrome (PCOS).

> 💡 If PCOS is suspected in females, testing for free testosterone could be beneficial.

Management

The primary aim of treatment is to reduce the number of lesions, minimise scarring and reduce the psychological impact of the disease. Treatment is dependent on the form of acne, and all patients should be advised that treatment can take several months to be effective (NICE, 2021a).

Mild to moderate acne: First-line treatment options are usually topical and include topical retinoids to reduce comedones, topical antibiotics or azelaic acid.

> ❗ Avoid use of topical retinoids in pregnancy or in those planning to conceive.

Moderate acne: Oral antibiotics (tetracyclines for a period of three months) in combination with a topical retinoid. For women, consider adding dianette in addition to the treatments mentioned above.

Severe acne: Should be referred to dermatology. Patients should be followed up at 8–12 weeks to assess for efficacy.

CHAPTER 15   Dermatological Presentations

> ❗ Seek further advice on management with multiple treatment failure in primary care, and consider skin swabs, for microscopy, culture and sensitivity.

Patients should be advised to:

- Avoid picking or squeezing spots to reduce the risk of scarring
- Avoid greasy cleansers and wash twice daily with warm water and fragrance-free soap
- Follow a healthy diet
- Use non-occlusive cosmetics.

Eczema

Aetiology

A history of atopy can predispose patients to eczema, as these patients often have an impaired skin barrier that leads to drying of the skin and increased inflammation due to penetration of irritants (PCDS, 2021b).

History and Examination

An itchy erythematous rash, often poorly defined without discrete borders. It can present at any age but atopic eczema tends to develop in early childhood. It can be widely distributed, although usually affects the flexures and tends to spare the groin.

Predisposing factors for eczema include:

- Allergens, such as dust mites, food, pollen, detergents
- Infection
- Stress
- Weather.

Management

The mainstay of management is the use of regular emollients, both directly to the skin and as a soap substitution for bathing. The frequency of flare-ups and the need for topical steroids can be reduced with regular application of emollients. The patient should be advised to avoid irritants and use fragrance-free products.

> 💡 Ointments tend to be more effective than creams, as the layer of grease prevents evaporation of water (NICE, 2022c). However, patients may not like greasy preparations, so it is a personal choice.

> 📄 Check to see if your local area has an emollient and steroid ladder for the treatment of eczema.

394

Primary Care Presentations

Antihistamines can be useful to reduce the itching, particularly at night.

Flare-ups should be treated promptly with a topical steroid. The potency of the steroid used is dependent upon the severity of the flare, the site and the age of the patient (NICE, 2022k).

> The amount of steroid to use can be determined by the fingertip unit. A fingertip unit (FTU) is the amount cream or ointment squeezed out along the length of an adult's fingertip. One FTU = approximately 500 mg; two FTUs = 1 g (Long and Finlay, 1991).

> If eczema is not responsive to treatment, skin swabs and scrapings may be undertaken for identification of fungal infection.

Stasis or Varicose Eczema

Aetiology

Most often seen in elderly patients, affecting one in five people over 70 (Oakley, 2017). Caused by venous insufficiency, leaky valves in the veins of the lower legs cause blood to pool in the legs; this can leak into surrounding tissue, causing cell death and irritation of the skin.

History and Examination

Affects both lower legs, causing areas of erythema and sometimes brown pigmentation that is itchy. It can be become blistered and weep. It may be mistaken for cellulitis but venous eczema can affect both lower limbs at the same time, whereas cellulitis is normally unilateral.

Predisposing factors:

- History of cellulitis
- History of deep vein thrombosis (DVT) in the affected limb
- Oedema
- Varicose veins.

Management

As per other forms of eczema, emollients are the mainstay of management, with topical steroids only used for flare-ups (National Eczema Society, 2019; PCDS, 2021b).

Management of the venous insufficiency also needs to take place, which includes regular exercise and elevation of affected limbs at rest.

> Compression hosiery is indicated in patients with venous eczema that do not have arterial disease in the legs (NICE, 2022b). The patient should be referred to a practice nurse for appropriate sizing and to check the ankle-brachial pressure index prior to using.

CHAPTER 15   Dermatological Presentations

Psoriasis

Aetiology

The development of this skin condition is thought to be linked to both genetic and environmental factors, and a proliferation of epidermal cells leads to immature keratin that is scaly (Ashton and Leppard, 2021; BAD, 2018).

History and Examination

Characterised by well-defined, red scaly plaques. The scale becomes silvery when scratched. Often the lesions are symmetrical.

History taking should determine the presence of predisposing factors:

- Alcohol
- Comorbidities including cardiovascular disease, arthritis and inflammatory bowel disease
- Drugs (beta blockers, non-steroidal anti-inflammatory drugs (NSAIDs))
- Genetic
- Post infection: Streptococcal tonsillitis can lead to guttate psoriasis that normally resolves within a few months
- Smoking
- Stress
- Sunlight (usually beneficial but can aggravate psoriasis in some people)
- Trauma.

The severity of psoriasis can be determined by assessing the extent of body coverage, degree of erythema and thickness of lesions. It is also important to assess the impact on a patient's quality of life, including physical, social and psychological impact.

> The Psoriasis Area and Severity Index (PASI) can aid in this assessment. A PASI score of less than 10 indicates mild psoriasis, a score of greater than 10 moderate psoriasis (BAD, 2021).

Management

Management differs according to the type of psoriasis, and is outlined in Table 15.3 (BNSSGCCG, 2021; NICE 2022h; Psoriasis Association, n.d.).

Generally, patients need to be advised that it is a chronic condition, prone to flares, but is not contagious.

> Provide lifestyle advice, including exercise, weight loss and reducing alcohol and cigarette intake.

Primary Care Presentations

Table 15.3 Types of Psoriasis and Corresponding Management

Types of psoriasis	Description	Management
Plaque psoriasis	The most common psoriasis can appear anywhere on the body. Lesions with well-defined borders. Red background with a silvery scale	Use emollients as maintenance treatment to reduce scale For thick scale, a salicylic acid treatment may be required Initially use a combination treatment of vitamin D analogue and a potent topical corticosteroid If treatment fails after four weeks try separate steroids and vitamin D analogues or use a vitamin D analogue on its own
Scalp psoriasis	Thick scale often initially mistaken for dandruff. Red plaques in hairline, neck and behind ears. Often the first site for psoriasis to appear	Coal tar shampoos are used as maintenance treatment If required, use a treatment such as salicylic acid, olive oil or coconut oil to remove thick scale Potent topical corticosteroids to treat inflammation, in formulations suitable for scalp application, e.g. gel or foam Combination treatments of potent topical steroid and vitamin D analogue if topical steroid not effective after four weeks
Nail psoriasis	Features pitting of the nail, discolouration of nail bed, possible separation of nail from nail bed and sublingual hyperkeratosis (a build-up of keratin under the nail)	Difficult to treat Often no treatment required in mild cases Send off nails for mycology to exclude fungal infection Keep nails as short as possible Advise patient to avoid manicures and the use of prosthetic nails In severe cases, refer to dermatology
Flexural psoriasis	Affects flexures. Skin appears bright red and can look moist. Has well-defined borders. Affects flexural surfaces, e.g. sub-mammary, groin, axilla and buttocks. Can be colonised with *Candida*.	Emollients to ease itching and reduce scale. Use of mild or moderate topical corticosteroids

(Continued)

397

CHAPTER 15 Dermatological Presentations

Table 15.3 (Continued)

Types of psoriasis	Description	Management
Guttate psoriasis	Associated with streptococcal throat infection. Small, red (up to 1 cm diameter), well-defined plaques with scale. Appears approximately two weeks after infection and usually resolves within four months	Emollients are often sufficient to reduce the itch. Coal tar preparations can be used in addition. If widespread, consider referral to dermatology and the use of vitamin D analogues Advise patient that it should resolve within four months

Rosacea

Aetiology

A chronic inflammatory skin condition. The cause is unknown, but it has been linked to chronic vasodilation and migraines (PCDS, 2022c).

History and Examination

Normally presents with a flushed appearance. It can appear similar to acne but affects an older age group. It is more common in people with fair skin and is usually distributed on the forehead, cheeks, nose and chin.

The rash can be exacerbated by the following factors, which could be considered in history taking:

- Alcohol
- Cold weather
- Spicy food
- Stress
- Sun exposure
- Topical steroids
- Vasodilators.

Management

For erythema, topical brimonidine and if papules or pustules are present consider a topical antibiotic such as metronidazole 0.75% (NICE, 2021b).

Exanthems of Childhood

A viral exanthem is a rash associated with viruses. The rashes are often associated with a fever, malaise and headaches. They are sometimes referred to as a non-specific viral rash.

Table 15.4 outlines the seven viral exanthems associated with childhood (although rarer, these can also occur in adulthood).

Primary Care Presentations

Table 15.4 Viral Exanthems

	Measles	Rubella	Slapped cheeked syndrome	Hand, foot and mouth	Roseola	Chickenpox	Scarlet fever	Molluscum contagiousum
Virus	Paramyxovirus	Rubella virus	Parovirus B19	Coxsackie A viruses	Herpes virus (types 6 and 7)	Herpes varicella-zoster virus	Streptococcal A	Pox virus
Usual age of onset	< 5 years Rare due to vaccination programme	< 2 years Rare due to vaccination programme	4–10 years	< 10 years	< 3 years	< 3 years	< 8 years	< 15 years
Incubation period	10 days	21 days	10 days	3–5 days	10 days	21 days	Up to 7 days	N/A
Transmission	Respiratory droplets	Respiratory droplets	Respiratory droplets	Respiratory droplets; faecal transmission; contact with fluid in blisters	Respiratory droplets	Respiratory droplets; contact with fluid from blisters	Respiratory droplets	Direct skin-to-skin contact
Contagious period	4 days after onset of rash	1 week before symptoms start to 4 days after rash appears	No longer infectious once rash appears	Until blisters have healed	Whilst febrile	Until vesicles have crusted over	Infectious for 7 days prior to onset of symptoms and for 24 hours after starting antibiotics. Without antibiotics patients can remain contagious for up to 3 weeks	Continuous
Time of onset of rash	2–4 days after initial symptoms Usually resolves within a week	Within 5 days of initial symptoms	7 days after initial symptoms	1–2 days after initial symptoms	3–5 days after fever	Rash often first symptom	1 day after initial symptoms	2–6 weeks after viral exposure
Distribution of rash	Face first then spreads to the trunk and limbs	Face, neck and behind ears, then trunk and limbs Rash clears in same order as it appeared (face downwards)	Face followed by trunk and limbs	Oral lesions normally start first, followed by lesions to the hands and feet	Appears on trunk (after fever has subsided) before spreading to face and limbs	Can start anywhere – scalp, face, oral cavity and trunk usually affected, with limbs less commonly affected	Rash usually develops on trunk before spreading elsewhere	Occurs in clusters, which can disappear and reappear

(Continued)

399

CHAPTER 15 Dermatological Presentations

Table 15.4 (Continued)

	Measles	Rubella	Slapped cheeked syndrome	Hand, foot and mouth	Roseola	Chickenpox	Scarlet fever	Molluscum contagiousum
Characteristic of rash	Erygetamatous maculopapular rash Itchy Koplik spots – blue-white spots in oral cavity (not everyone gets these but for those that do it is diagnostic)	Pink macular rash	Marked facial erythema to the cheeks (spares nasolabial folds and eyelids), followed by lace-like reticular rash elsewhere	Round lesions in mouth look like ulcers with red borders. Grey blisters with red halo on fingers and toes	Red maculapapular rash	Red papules that evolve into vesicles and then crust over Itchy New spots appear whilst others are becoming vesicles or crusting over	Erythema to the face with pallor around the mouth (circumoral pallor) Furring and strawberry-like appearance of tongue. Rash on trunk and limbs is red fine papules with a sandpaper texture	Small (up to 5 mm) skin-coloured lesions that are raised and circular in shape with an umbilicated centre
Associated symptoms	Rash is normally preceded by pyrexia, cough, conjunctivitis, child often looks unwell	Mild fever, conjunctivitis, lymphadenopathy (post-auricular, cervical and occipital). Aching fingers and wrists	Symptoms usually mild and may be absent, low-grade fever, sore throat and malaise	Prodromal symptoms include low-grade fever, malaise, sore mouth 1–2 days prior to onset of rash	Fever, and occasional malaise and coryza, but normally otherwise well	Often mild fever, malaise, loss of appetite, feeling generally unwell	Fever and sore throat precede rash. Swollen tonsils, often with exudate and painful lymphadenopathy in the neck	Itching (occasional)
Complications	Diarrhoea, convulsions, otitis media and pneumonia and in rare cases encephalitis. Infection during pregnancy can lead to miscarriage or foetal abnormalities	Significant risk during pregnancy, as a high chance of foetal abnormalities (particularly in the first trimester)	Infection during pregnancy can lead to foetal abnormalities	Complications are rare but can include meningitis and encephalitis, although this is rare	Febrile convulsions	Secondary streptococcal skin infection, viral pneumonia – immunosuppressed and pregnant patients most at risk of severe complications	Rheumatic fever (leading to valve stenosis), pneumonia, ear infections, sinusitis, tonsillar abscess	Rarely bacterial infection (requiring antibiotics)

Primary Care Presentations

Management	Self-care; maintain hydration	Self-care; maintain hydration	Self-care; maintain hydration.	Self-care; maintain hydration (avoid acidic drinks like fruit juice)	Self-care; maintain hydration	Self-care; avoid ibuprofen as this may cause secondary skin infection; consider calamine lotion and antihistamines to ease the itching	Treatment with antibiotics Consider calamine lotion and antihistamines to ease the itching	Self-limiting, with no treatment normally required
Resolution period	Within a week	Within a week	Facial rash will resolve with 2 weeks, rash on body can last for a month	Within 10 days	Within 2 days	5 days after spots appear	Within a week	18 months
Notifiable disease	Yes	Yes	No	No	No	No	Yes (except in Scotland)	No
Isolation period	Stay home for 4 days after onset of rash	Stay home for 5 days after onset of rash	None	None (but most infectious 5 days after symptoms start)	Only whilst febrile	Until vesicles have crusted over	24 hours after starting antibiotics	None but patients do need to be advised that it is contagious

Source: Middlemiss (2002).

CHAPTER 15   Dermatological Presentations

Fungal Skin Infections

Angular Cheilitis

Aetiology

Inflammation of the corners of the lips caused by a *Candida* infection or bacterial infection (usually *Staphylococcus aureus*) (PCDS, 2021a).

History and Examination

Cheilitis is inflammation of the lips. In angular cheilitis, only the corners of the lips are involved. This can cause soreness, cracking and fissures at the edge of the mouth.
   Predisposing factors include:

- Anaemia
- Dental braces
- Dry lips
- Ill-fitting dentures
- Vitamin B12 deficiency.

Management

- Topical antifungals. Miconazole treats *Candida* as well as having some bacteriostatic action (NICE, 2022a).
- If not improving with antifungals, treat with fusidic acid.
- Denture wearers should remove them at night and store in an appropriate solution. If they are ill-fitting, they should be replaced.

> Skin swabs should be taken if not responding to topical antifungals (to check for a staphylococcal infection).

Candidiasis

Aetiology

Candida is a yeast that forms part of the normal flora of the human gastrointestinal tract. Infection can occur when the host's defences are lowered or there is a disruption in the skin or mucosal barrier.

History and Examination

A bright red rash that is often painful; differs from intertrigo as has papules and pustules that extend beyond the main rash. Can occur at any age but most common in young children and the elderly. Affects all flexures, axilla, sub-mammary, groin and toe webs.
   Predisposing factors to consider during history taking include:

- Antibiotic use
- Diabetes

- High-oestrogen oral contraceptive
- Immunosuppression
- Iron deficiency
- Obesity
- Pregnancy.

Management
- Topical antifungal or a combination treatment such as Daktacort® if more inflamed (NICE, 2022a)
- If more widespread or not responding to topical treatment, consider an oral antifungal in persistent infection.

> ⚠️ If not responding to treatment or infection is recurrent:
> - Skin scrapings for mycology
> - Bloods to check for diabetes or iron deficiency.

Oral Candidiasis

Infection of the oral mucosa can cause white furring to the tongue, white spots and plaques to the oral mucosa. Can be painful and cause a burning sensation in the mouth.

History and Examination

Predisposing factors (in addition to those for candidiasis):

- Common in babies
- Denture use
- Smoking
- Use of inhaled corticosteroids.

Management
- An oral solution or gel such as nystatin
- Rinsing mouth after use of inhaled corticosteroids
- Cleansing of dentures and ensuring they are correctly fitted (NICE, 2022a).

Pityriasis Versicolor

Aetiology

> ⚠️ A common superficial skin complaint caused by the proliferation of the Malassezia fungus. It is most common in healthy young adults or teenagers. The yeast is lipophilic, so proliferates in areas dense with sebaceous glands.

CHAPTER 15   Dermatological Presentations

History and Examination
It is non-contagious and appears as dry, flaky patches with a fine scale that are often hypo-pigmented. It is usually asymptomatic. It is most distributed on the upper trunk but can appear elsewhere.

Predisposing factors to consider during history taking:

- Immunosuppression
- Increased physical activity
- Increased sweating
- Malnutrition
- Occlusive clothing
- Warm weather.

Management
- For localised areas, an antifungal cream can be used.
- If topical treatment is ineffective, an oral antifungal can be considered.
- Patients should be advised that areas of hypo-pigmentation can take several months to resolve after treatment (Hay, 2016).
- If widespread, then an antifungal shampoo (ketonconazole 2% or selenium sulphide 2.5%) should be applied to the affected skin (NICE, 2022g).

> Refer to dermatology:
> - If symptoms do not respond to treatment in primary care
> - For further management or advice with patients in treatment failure who are pregnant or breastfeeding, as options limited in primary care
> - If pityriasis versicolor is extensive.

> Skin scrapings should be taken if not responding to topical treatment and to confirm diagnosis prior to oral treatment.

Tinea Infection
Aetiology
Tinea, also known as ringworm, is a common fungal infection. Tinea infections are contagious and can be spread by skin-to-skin contact, contaminated surfaces or from infected animals. Some of the common sites of infection and their presentation are described in Table 15.5.

Management
- Topical or oral antifungals (dependent on the severity).

Primary Care Presentations

Refer:

- If rash is extensive
- Treatment failure
- Immunosuppressed patients (apply clinical judgement).

> 💡 Topical steroids can mask the symptoms of a fungal infection. This is known as 'Tinea Incognito'. If a localised rash is not resolving with topical steroids, it is worthwhile trying a topical antifungal instead.

Table 15.5 Types of Tinea Infection

Type of tinea	Site	History and examination	Management and treatment	Red flags
Tinea capitis	Scalp	Causes hair loss, scaling and broken hair. Broken hairs can appear like black dots. Itchy but not usually painful. Kerions (inflamed lesions that can appear like boils and cause boggy areas of inflamed tissue)	To confirm diagnosis, send plucked hairs off for mycology	Children should be referred to dermatology for oral antifungals (NICE, 2022d)
			Oral antifungals	Kerions: areas where the fungal infection has progressed deep into the scalp – refer urgently to dermatology (BNSSGCCG, 2020c)
			Antifungal shampoos help to reduce transmission of the fungus	
Tinea corporis and tinea cruris	Trunk and limbs (corporis) and groin (cruris)	Lesions are often circular, erythematous and dry with scale. The scale and erythema is more pronounced at the borders	Topical antifungal cream. For extensive rashes, systemic treatment may be required with oral antifungals	
Tinea pedis	Feet	Erythema and scaling to soles and between digits and can cause blisters	Topical antifungals	Even mild fungal nail infections should be treated in immunosuppressed patients and those with comorbidities such as diabetes (BNSSGCCG, 2020c)

Source: Moriarty et al. (2012).

405

CHAPTER 15   Dermatological Presentations

Infestations

Scabies

Aetiology

Scabies is caused by the Sarcoptes scabiei mite. The mite burrows into the skin to lay its eggs which results in an intensely itchy rash that is often worse at night.

> 💡 The mite is transmitted through prolonged skin contact and is often passed between partners, so always suspect it if multiple close contacts are itching or have a similar rash.

History and Examination

The rash develops approximately four to six weeks after initial infestation. It can appear across the trunk and limbs and can affect the genitals but usually spares the back and face (except in infants). It is commonly associated with a rash on the hands or wrists, and it is also important to check finger webs for a rash. It is made up of red papules and excoriations. Burrows appear as a linear or s-shaped papule approximately 5 mm in length and are usually found on the sides of fingers or the wrists.

Predisposing factors to consider during history taking:

- Care facilities
- Military barracks
- Multiple sexual partners
- Overcrowding.

Management

- Treat patients over the age of two months with a topical insecticide.
- Decontaminate clothing, bedding and towels by washing them at over 60 degrees, dry cleaning them or sealing them in a plastic bag for over 72 hours.
- Itch can be treated with an antihistamine; a sedating one may be beneficial at night.
- Advise patients that the itch may last for at least a month after treatment of the mite. Eurax HC can be used for the treatment of the itch (BNSSGCCG, 2020a).

> 💡
> - If left untreated, secondary skin infections can occur.
> - It is essential to treat all members of the family to clear an infestation. Sexual partners and other close contacts within the past month should also be treated, even if they are asymptomatic (NICE, 2022i). For notification of sexual partners, refer patients to a GUM clinic.

> 🚩
> - In patients aged under two months, advice from a paediatric dermatologist needs to be sought (BNSSGCCG, 2020a).
> - Beware of crusted scabies – hyper-infestation of mites resulting in an abnormal immune response.

Primary Care Presentations

Lesions
Actinic Keratosis
Aetiology
Abnormal skin growth following DNA damage caused by chronic sun exposure (Oakley, 2017).

History and Examination
Rough scaly papules. The areas tend to be felt more easily than seen. They can appear without scaling and present as a pink macule. Common sites are areas of high sun exposure such as the scalp, face, ears and the dorsum of the hands.
Predisposing factors:

- Aged over 50
- Chronic UV exposure
- Fair skin.

Management
- Actinic keratoses are considered premalignant, although the potential for this to occur is low. Patients, however, should be advised to monitor for any changes and alert accordingly.
- Treatment in primary care is usually topical with either diclofenac or fluorouracil cream; further options include treatment with liquid nitrogen and curettage of the lesion.

> If there is change in colour, size, tenderness, bleeding or treatment failure, then undertake a referral to dermatology under two-week wait (2WW) criteria.

Sebaceous Keratosis
Aetiology
A benign lesion that becomes more common with advancing age. Especially common in over 60s.

History and Examination
Have a warty appearance, with a waxy surface, and appear stuck onto the surface of the skin. Range in appearance from skin-coloured to brown pigment. Can grow large to be several centimetres in size.

Management
- As a benign lesion, there is no treatment required; if patients wish to have it excised this would normally be done at a private clinic.

> Any diagnostic uncertainty, seek further review or 2WW referral.

CHAPTER 15   Dermatological Presentations

Skin Cancer

A suspicious lesion is one that has changed in size, shape, colour or sensation, is non-healing, bleeds, oozes or is inflamed and tends to have one or more of the following (ABCDEFG) (NICE, 2021c; Oakley, 2017; PCDS, 2021c).

- Asymmetry: The appearance of one half is different to the other. Look for asymmetry in shape and colour.
- Borders: The borders are not even; they may be irregular or jagged.
- Colour: The colour is not uniform. Any lesion with three or more pigments, or that has a colour that is different to other moles, is suspicious.
- Dimensions: It is increasing in size either horizontally or vertically.
- Elevated: The lesion is growing upwards.
- Firm: It is firm to palpation; benign moles tend to be softer or more wobbly to palpation.
- Growth: Any lesion that is persistently growing.

> Patients can be referred for mole mapping if they have large numbers of moles (> 50) or have a significant family history of melanoma in one or more second-degree relatives. Referral criteria for mole mapping may differ across the UK, so refer to local guidance.

> MySkinSelfie [online].
> This skin monitoring app was created by dermatologists and can be downloaded by patients to help them monitor their moles.

Skin Cancer (Non-melanoma)
Basal Cell Carcinoma
Aetiology

The commonest form of skin cancer. It is caused by exposure to UV but can also develop in old scars (PCDS, 2022a). About 75% of non-melanoma skin cancers are basal cell carcinomas (Cancer Research UK, 2022).

History and Examination

They are slow-growing, and a patient may have had the lesion for many years before they present with it. They often present as nodules that are shiny or pearlescent in appearance. The edges of the lesion appear rolled and the centre may be depressed. There are visible blood vessels on the surface. They can also be subtle in appearance, presenting as scaly plaques or a waxy plaque with lighter pigment.

Primary Care Presentations

Management

As basal cell carcinomas rarely metastasise, appropriate management is routine referral to dermatology rather than via a 2WW (NICE, 2021c).

> Exceptions to this are if there is significant clinical concern, in which case they should be referred as a 2WW, such as if the lesion is on the head or neck **and** there is rapid growth, the lesion is on or near the eye, nose, lip or ear, has a diameter > 2 cm or is incompletely excised or recurrent (BNSSGCCG, 2020b).

Squamous Cell Carcinoma

Aetiology

A malignant lesion that usually arises from areas of sun-damaged skin. They can also occur at areas of low sun exposure, sites of radiotherapy, scars or ulcers. About 20% of skin cancers are squamous cell carcinomas (Cancer Research UK, 2023).

History and Examination

Usually present on areas of high sun exposure – scalp, face, ears or dorsum of the hands.
Tend to grow quickly over several months. Often present as firm crusted lumps that are increasing in size. Can be tender and may bleed and ulcerate.
Predisposing factors to be considered during history taking:

- Actinic keratosis
- Age
- Chronic inflammation
- Fair skin
- Sex (men more affected than women)
- Genetic
- Immunosuppression therapy
- Sun exposure.

Management

> All patients who have this as a differential need to be referred as a 2WW.

Malignant Melanoma

Aetiology

Caused by abnormal and uncontrolled growth of melanocytes (pigment cells), it is a malignant tumour. Can occur from previously normal-appearing skin or develop from existing moles or freckles.

409

CHAPTER 15 Dermatological Presentations

There are four common subtypes of melanoma:
- Acral lentiginous melanoma: Melanomas that appear on the soles of the feet or palms of the hand, present as small, slow-growing patches of pigmentation that become irregular in border and pigmentation and can later ulcerate and bleed. Subungal melanomas are acral lentiginous melanoma that appear under the nail bed. They can appear as a linear area of pigmentation or may have no pigmentation and are noticed when the nail bed breaks down.
- Lentigo maligna melanoma: A malignant melanoma that grows in the epidermis (lentigo maligna) before spreading into the dermis (lentigo maligna melanoma). Usually found on the head, neck and back of hands. More common in elderly patients. Grows slowly over many years and tends to appear as a brown pigmented patch that slowly expands.
- Nodular melanoma: Usually appears as a firm, dark-pigmented nodule that is growing rapidly. The melanocytes spread downwards rather than superficially, so prognosis is usually poorer than with other melanomas, and it can progress deep into the skin within a few months. It can also present as pink or red nodules (known as an amelanotic melanoma). As it grows, the lesion can bleed, ooze and become ulcerated.
- Superficial spreading melanoma: Has a good prognosis. Malignant melanocytes migrate horizontally, staying in the epidermis and dermis. Appears as a flat brown plaque that is increasing in diameter. As it grows, the borders become irregular and it develops uneven pigmentation; it can become inflamed with altered sensation.

History and Examination

Melanomas often appear markedly different to surrounding lesions. They can present anywhere, including on lips, genitals and nails.

> 💡 Healthy moles tend to be symmetrical, uniform in colour and to have smooth borders. So, look out for the 'ugly duckling', the one that sticks out from the crowd.

Predisposing factors to consider during history taking:
- Advancing age
- Fair skin and blue or green eyes
- Family history of melanoma
- History of sunburn
- Large number of moles
- Light or red hair
- Previous skin cancer
- Sun exposure
- Use of sunbeds.

Primary Care Presentations

> There is a weighted seven-point checklist for assessment of pigmented skin lesions, and to determine referral (NICE, 2021c; 2022j):
>
> Major features of the lesion (two points each):
> - Change in size
> - Irregular shape or border
> - Irregular colour.
>
> Minor features of the lesion (one point each):
> - Largest diameter 7 mm or more
> - Inflammation
> - Oozing or crusting of the lesion
> - Change in sensation (including itch).

Suspicion is greater for lesions scoring three points or more. However, if there are strong concerns about cancer, any one feature is adequate to prompt urgent referral under the 2WW rule.

> Any growing nodule where you are uncertain of the diagnosis should be referred as a 2WW.

Management

> Any suspicious lesion needs to be referred via 2WW criteria.

Advise monitoring and using photos to clearly document any change. Consider advising on sun care, using resources aimed at patients. In particular, advise to monitor for any one feature of ABCDEFG and ask the patient to return if they notice a suspicious change in their lesion.

> 💡 If you are confident a lesion is benign, it is prudent to book in a review with another member of the clinical team (such as someone with a specialist interest in dermatology). This will reassure the patient.

Skin Emergencies

Erythroderma

Aetiology

> Erythroderma is an inflammatory skin disease. Thirty per cent of cases are idiopathic (Dermnet NZ, 2016).

CHAPTER 15   Dermatological Presentations

History and Examination
Widespread erythema affecting 90% of the body surface. The erythema spreads quickly and can become thick and scaly. The rash is often intensely itchy. The skin can be warm to touch.

Management
Erythroderma should be referred urgently to the on-call dermatologist.
 If the patient is systemically compromised, or is high risk (elderly and living alone or is in poor general health), they will need to be admitted to hospital urgently.

Necrotising Fascitis
Aetiology

> An acute infection of the subcutaneous fat and deep fascia. The bacteria releases toxins, causing thrombosis of blood vessels in the skin and then subsequent necrosis.

History and Examination
It can initially appear like cellulitis, but over several days the skin becomes purple before becoming necrotic.

> 💡 Suspect in patients whose cellulitis is not improving with oral antibiotics or who are developing areas of purple pigment within the rash.

Management
Requires urgent admission for debridement.

Stevens-Johnson Syndrome
Aetiology

> An extremely rare reaction to medication that causes an acute and life-threatening skin reaction. It can occur several months after taking a medication, but onset is normally quicker. It is seen more frequently with drugs with a longer half-life, and is associated with allopurinol, anticonvulsants, NSAIDs and antibiotics.

History and Examination
Prodromal symptoms prior to the rash include a fever and flu-like illness; the patient may also have a cough, diarrhoea and photosensitivity. Causes a widespread painful red rash

with widespread erythema, macules and target-like lesions that come on acutely. Starts on the trunk and spreads to the face and limbs. The scalp, soles and palms are usually spared. Causes sheet-like loss of the skin, as well as blisters, and skin erosion occurs with gentle rubbing (the Nikolsky sign). Also affects the mucosal surfaces, causing ulcers to affected areas including mouth, lips and genitals.

Management

This is a medical emergency and needs to be discussed urgently with the on-call dermatologist.

Vasculitis

Aetiology

> Refers to inflammation of blood vessels and can lead to necrosis of vessels. This can be localised, affecting the skin, or systemic. Systemic vasculitis is life-threatening. It can be caused by drug reactions, infections both viral and bacterial and malignancy, autoimmune disorders, and be associated with sepsis, Henoch-Schonlein purpura and Kawasaki disease (Dermnet NZ, 2016; PCDS, 2021d).

History and Examination

The clinical presentation varies greatly but can cause a non-blanching purpuric rash, itching and pain.

Management
- Undertake bloods and urinalysis to look for an underlying cause.
- Bloods should include full blood count (FBC), liver function tests (LFTs), urea and electrolytes (U&E) and estimated glomerular filtration rate (eGFR).
- Discuss management with dermatology if the patient is systemically stable.

> If a patient is acutely unwell and a systemic cause is suspected, then refer urgently for admission.

Viral Skin Infections

Herpes Simplex

Aetiology

Rash caused by the herpes simplex virus, transmitted through direct contact with vesicles or contact with droplets. There are two main types of herpes simplex – HSV1 and HSV2. Both types can affect any site; however, HSV1 tends to affect the face and mouth (cold sores) and HSV2 is more likely to affect the genitals (PCDS, 2022b).

CHAPTER 15   Dermatological Presentations

History and Examination
Prodromal symptoms include itching, burning and tingling prior to the onset of a group of vesicles on an erythematous background. These vesicles burst and then crust.

> 💡 Herpes simplex can appear similar to impetigo but is the more likely diagnosis in an adult patient.

Management
- Most instances resolve within seven to ten days without treatment.
- Topical cyclovir can help shorten flare-ups but should be applied as soon as possible after the prodromal tingling starts.
- Oral cyclovir can be used for extensive infections or those that reoccur frequently (screen for immunosuppression in frequent or extensive infections) (NICE, 2023).

Shingles (Herpes Zoster)
Aetiology
Shingles (or, herpes zoster) occurs in patients who have previously had chickenpox. It is a reactivation of the varicella zoster virus that has laid dormant. The virus travels down cutaneous nerves, causing pain or a tingling burning sensation in the skin. It then infects the epidermal cells, resulting in the formation of the characteristic vesicles.

> 💡 People can catch chickenpox from those with shingles but cannot catch shingles as it is a reactivation of a previous chickenpox virus (Ashton and Leppard, 2021).

History and Examination
An erythematous rash with clusters of vesicles that weep and crust over. The rash has a dermatomal distribution, is unilateral and does not cross the midline of the body. It is usually distributed on the trunk, with dermatomes T1–L2 most commonly affected.
Predisposing factors to consider during history taking:

- Comorbidities: Including asthma, diabetes, arthritis, depression, lupus
- Female
- Immunocompromised
- Older age
- Stress.

Be aware of complications, such as post-herpetic neuralgia (pain at site of rash that persists for 90 days or more) and secondary skin infections.

Management
- Manage mild pain with simple oral analgesia.

Chapter Summary

> ⚠ NICE (2022j) recommends considering antiviral treatment (ideally within 72 hours of the onset of the rash) in:
> - All patients over 50
> - Immunocompromised patients.

- – Patients with moderate to severe pain
- – Patients with a moderate to severe rash
- – Rash that is not on the trunk.
- Elderly patients are at higher risk of developing post-herpetic neuralgia, hence vaccination is available in the UK for patients aged between 70 and 80.
- In children, antivirals are not recommended (unless the child is immunocompromised).

Advise patients:

- Lesions are contagious until they are dry and crusted over.
- They should cover up exposed lesions.
- There is no need to stay off work or school (unless the rash cannot be covered).
- They should avoid contact with immunosuppressed people, pregnant women, children younger than a month and those that have not had chickenpox (Phuc and Rothberg, 2022).

> 💡 For recurrent herpes zoster or simplex infections, consider screening for immunosuppression, including HIV screening. Swab recurrent infections to confirm simplex or zoster infection and offer prophylaxis antivirals in herpes simplex.

> ⚠ Ramsay Hunt syndrome is herpes zoster that has infected the facial nerve (cranial nerve VII). This can cause facial paralysis and lesions in the ear. The patient often has hearing and vestibular symptoms (Younghoon and Lee, 2018). Patients with this should be discussed with ear, nose and throat (ENT) specialist on call.

> 🚩 Herpes zoster opthalmicus occurs when the virus infects the ophthalmic branch of the trigeminal nerve. Any patient with this, especially those with visual symptoms, red eye or Hutchinson's sign, should be admitted. Hutchinson's sign is a rash on the tip, side or root of the nose and is indicative of later eye inflammation and permanent corneal denervation (Phuc and Rothberg, 2022).

Chapter Summary

Skin conditions are a common presenting complaint in primary care. Many conditions can be treated with over-the-counter medications, and patient information leaflets allow patients to take ownership of their condition and management plan. Paramedics can safely manage

CHAPTER 15   Dermatological Presentations

these conditions, but to do so safely an awareness of red flags is essential for identifying patients that require rapid referral. The key to management is working within your own knowledge base whilst utilising the expertise of those around you – including colleagues with a specialist interest in dermatology or referral to local dermatology services.

Case Study 1

You are working in a walk-in centre when a patient presents with a three-week history of soreness to the left of their mouth, which has started to develop heat and redness.

History

PC: Soreness to left side of mouth.
HxPC: Over the past few days, redness has developed, with a gradual feeling of warmth over the last 12 hours. The patient reports no pain, with their appearance being their primary concern.
PMHx/SHx: None.
DHx: None.
SHx: Works as a hairdresser and make-up artist.
FHx: None.
ROS: Denies recent illness.

Examination

- Inspection: Obvious crusting to the left corner of the mouth, with cracks in the centre.
- Palpation: Slight tenderness, crusting in raised and there is no heat. Movement of the mouth creates pressure and increases the soreness.

Preferred Diagnosis

- Angular cheilitis.

Differential Diagnoses

- Cold sore
- Herpes simplex.

Management

- Advise good oral hygiene.
- Prescribe topical miconazole (NICE, 2022k).
- Advise review if does not respond to antifungal cream.
- Avoid make-up for duration of treatment.

Case Study 2

You are working in out-of-hours when a 50-year-old patient presents with a 12-hour history of rash developing to their legs.

History

PC:	Rash to lower legs.
HxPC:	Noted rash to the lower legs started to develop following the first day of discharge following admission, which ended with hospital-acquired pneumonia. Twelve hours since discharge, started to experience abdominal and lower-back pain. Also notes dark urine, described as 'sludgy'.
PMHx/SHx:	Hypertension; diabetes; rheumatoid arthritis; recent chest infection.
DHx:	Ramipril, metformin, diclofenac, recent infusion of cefuroxime.
SHx:	Semi-retired car salesperson.
FHx:	None.
ROS:	Notes to be sweating slightly, walking as normal.

Examination

- Vital signs: BP 140/90 mmHg; HR 107 bpm; RR 12/min; temperature 39.9 °C.
- Inspection: Exposure of the patient reveals a maculopapular rash on their trunk, and palpable purpura remarkable in the lower extremities.
- Urinalysis showed proteinuria (++) without pyuria or bacteriuria.

Preferred Diagnosis

- Henoch-Schönlein purpura.

Differential Diagnoses

- Vascultiis
- Allergic reaction to cefuroxime.

Management

- Stop diclofenac.
- Refer to emergency department for urgent blood tests to determine kidney function and renal impairment.
- Paracetamol for analgesia until seen by other healthcare professional.

References

Ashton, R. and Leppard, B. (2021) *Differential Diagnosis in Dermatology*. 5th edn. Abingdon: CRC Press.
British Association of Dermatologists (BAD) (2018) Psoriasis: An overview. Available at: https://www.skinhealthinfo.org.uk/condition/psoriasis/ (accessed 28 January 2023).
British Association of Dermatologists (BAD) (2021) Psoriasis Area and Severity index (PASI) worksheet. Available at: https://www.bad.org.uk/shared/get-file.ashx?itemtype=document&id=1654bad.org-psorasis worksheet (accessed 16 November 2022).
Cancer Research UK (2023) Skin cancer types. Available at: https://www.cancerresearchuk.org/about-cancer/skin-cancer/types (accessed 28 January 2023).
Dermnet NZ (2015) Lyme disease. Available at: https://dermnetnz.org/topics/lyme-disease/ (accessed 28 January 2023).

CHAPTER 15 Dermatological Presentations

Dermnet NZ (2016) Erythroderma. Available at: https://dermnetnz.org/topics/erythroderma/ (accessed 28 January 2023).

Dermnet NZ (2021) Spa pool folliculitis. Available at: https://dermnetnz.org/topics/spa-pool-folliculitis/ (accessed 28 January 2023).

Eisman, S. and Sinclair, R. (2015) Pityriasis rosea. *British Medical Journal* 351: h5233.

Hay, R.J. (2016) Fungal infections. In Chalmers, R., Barker, J., Griffiths, C. et al. (eds) *Rook's Textbook of Dermatology*. 9th edn. Hoboken, NJ: John Wiley & Sons.

King's Fund (2014) How can dermatology services meet current and future patient needs while ensuring that quality of care is not compromised and that access is equitable across the UK? Available at: https://www.bad.org.uk/shared/get-file.ashx?id=2347&itemtype=document (accessed 16 November 2022).

Long, C.C. and Finlay, A.Y. (1991) The finger-tip unit – a new practical measure. *Clinical and Experimental Dermatology* 16(6): 444–447.

McCance, K.L and Huether, S.E. (2018) *Pathophysiology: The Biologic Basis for Disease in Adults and Children*. 8th edn. Maryland Heights, MO: Mosby.

Middlemiss, P. (2002) *What's That Rash?* London: Hamlyn.

Moriarty, B., Hay, R. and Morris-Jones, R. (2012) The diagnosis and management of tinea. *British Medical Journal* 345: e4380.

MySkinSelfie (2023) Available at: https://myskinselfie.org.uk (accessed 14 April 2023).

Nast, A., Griffiths, C.E.M., Hay, R. et al. (2016) The 2016 International League of Dermatological Societies' revised glossary for the description of cutaneous lesions. *British Journal of Dermatology* 174(6): 1351–1358.

National Eczema Society (2019) Topical Steroids factsheet. Available at: https://eczema.org/wp-content/uploads/Topical-steroids-Sep-19-1.pdf (accessed 28 January 2023).

National Institute for Health and Care Excellence (NICE) (2020) Clinical Knowledge Summaries: Pityriasis rosea. Available at: https://cks.nice.org.uk/topics/pityriasis-rosea/ (accessed 28 January 2023).

National Institute for Health and Care Excellence (NICE) (2021a) Clinical Knowledge Summaries: Acne vulgaris. Available at: https://cks.nice.org.uk/topics/acne-vulgaris/ (accessed 28 January 2023).

National Institute for Health and Care Excellence (NICE) (2021b) Clinical Knowledge Summaries: Rosacea. Available at: https://cks.nice.org.uk/topics/rosacea/ (accessed 10 April 2023).

National Institute for Health and Care Excellence (NICE) (2021c) Clinical Knowledge Summaries: Skin cancers recognition and referral. Available at: https://cks.nice.org.uk/topics/skin-cancers-recognition-referral/ (accessed 10 April 2023).

National Institute for Health and Care Excellence (NICE) (2022a) Clinical Knowledge Summaries: Candida Oral. Available at: https://cks.nice.org.uk/topics/candida-oral/ (accessed 28 January 2023).

National Institute for Health and Care Excellence (NICE (2022b) Clinical Knowledge Summaries: Compression stockings. Available at: https://cks.nice.org.uk/topics/compression-stockings/ (accessed 28 January 2023).

National Institute for Health and Care Excellence (2022c) Clinical Knowledge Summaries: Eczema – atopic. Available at: https://cks.nice.org.uk/topics/eczema-atopic (accessed 28 January 2023).

National Institute for Health and Care Excellence (NICE) (2022d) Clinical Knowledge Summaries: Fungal skin infection scalp. Available at: https://cks.nice.org.uk/topics/fungal-skin-infection-scalp/ (accessed 28 January 2023).

References

National Institute for Health and Care Excellence (NICE) (2022e) Clinical Knowledge Summaries: Impetigo. Available at: https://cks.nice.org.uk/topics/impetigo/ (accessed 28 January 2023).

National Institute for Health and Care Excellence (NICE) (2022f) Clinical Knowledge Summaries: Lyme disease. Available at: https://cks.nice.org.uk/topics/lyme-disease/ (accessed 28 January 2023).

National Institute for Health and Care Excellence (NICE) (2022g) Clinical Knowledge Summaries: Pityriasis versicolor. Available at: https://cks.nice.org.uk/topics/pityriasis-versicolor/ (accessed 28 January 2023).

National Institute for Health and Care Excellence (NICE) (2022h) Clinical Knowledge Summaries: Psoriasis. Available at: https://cks.nice.org.uk/topics/psoriasis/ (accessed 28 January 2023).

National Institute for Health and Care Excellence (NICE) (2022i) Clinical Knowledge Summaries: Scabies. Available at: https://cks.nice.org.uk/topics/scabies/ (accessed 28 January 2023).

National Institute for Health and Care Excellence (NICE) (2022j) Clinical Knowledge Summaries: Shingles. Available at: https://cks.nice.org.uk/topics/shingles/management/management/ (accessed 28 January 2023).

National Institute for Health and Care Excellence (NICE) (2022k) Clinical Knowledge Summaries: Topical corticosteroids. Available at: https://cks.nice.org.uk/topics/eczema-atopic/prescribing-information/topical-corticosteroids (accessed 28 January 2023).

National Institute for Health and Care Excellence (NICE) (2023) Clinical Knowledge Summaries: Herpes simplex. Available at: https://cks.nice.org.uk/topics/herpes-simplex-oral/ (accessed 28 January 2023).

NHS Bristol, North Somerset and South Gloucestershire CCG (BNSSGCCG) (2020a) Remedy: Scabies. Available at: https://remedy.bnssgccg.nhs.uk/adults/dermatology/scabies/ (accessed 28 January 2023).

NHS Bristol, North Somerset and South Gloucestershire CCG (BNSSGCCG) (2020b) Remedy: Skin suspected cancer 2WW. Available at: https://remedy.bnssgccg.nhs.uk/suspected-cancer-2ww/skin-2ww/ (accessed 29 March 2021).

NHS Bristol, North Somerset and South Gloucestershire CCG (BNSSGCCG) (2020c) Remedy: Tinea. Available at: https://remedy.bnssgccg.nhs.uk/adults/dermatology/tinea/ (accessed 28 January 2023).

NHS Bristol and North Somerset and South Gloucestershire CCG (BNSSGCCG) (2021) Remedy: Psoriasis. Available at: https://remedy.bnssgccg.nhs.uk/adults/dermatology/psoriasis/ (accessed 28 January 2023).

Oakley, A. (2017) *Dermatology Made Easy*. Banbury: Scion.

Phuc, L. and Rothberg, M. (2022) Best Practice Guidance: Herpes zoster infection. Available at: https://bestpractice.bmj.com/topics/en-gb/23 (accessed 28 January 2023).

Primary Care Dermatology Society (PCDS) (2021a) Angular cheilitis (syn. Angular stomatitis). Available at: https://www.pcds.org.uk/clinical-guidance/angular-chelitis/ (accessed 28 January 2023).

Primary Care Dermatology Society (PCDS) (2021b) Concise guidance: National primary care treatment and referral guidelines for common skin conditions: Eczema – atopic and discoid. Available at: https://www.pcds.org.uk/desktop-treatment-guide (accessed 28 January 2023).

Primary Care Dermatology Society (PCDS) (2021c) Concise guidance: National primary care treatment and referral guidelines for common skin conditions: Skin cancer (BCC, SCC, melanoma), and common benign lesions. Available at: https://www.pcds.org.uk/desktop-treatment-guide (accessed 28 January 2023).

CHAPTER 15   Dermatological Presentations

Primary Care Dermatology Society (PCDS) (2021d) Vasculitis. Available at: https://www.pcds.org.uk/clinical-guidance/vasculitis-and-capillaritis (accessed 28 January 2023).

Primary Care Dermatology Society (PCDS) (2022a) Basal cell carcinoma. Available at: https://www.pcds.org.uk/clinical-guidance/basal-cell-carcinoma-an-overview (accessed 28 January 2023).

Primary Care Dermatology Society (PCDS) (2022b) Herpes simplex. Available at: https://www.pcds.org.uk/clinical-guidance/herpes-simplex (Accessed 28 January 2023).

Primary Care Dermatology Society (PCDS) (2022c) Rosacea. Available at: https://www.pcds.org.uk/clinical-guidance/rosacea (accessed 28 January 2023).

Psoriasis Association (n.d.) Available at: https://www.psoriasis-association.org.uk (accessed 28 January 2023).

Public Health England (PHE) (2022) Lyme disease epidemiology and surveillance. Available at: https://www.gov.uk/government/publications/lyme-borreliosis-epidemiology/lyme-borreliosis-epidemiology-and-surveillance (accessed 28 January 2023).

Public Health England (PHE) (2023) Health protection in schools and other childcare facilities. Chapter 9: Managing specific infectious diseases. Available at: https://www.gov.uk/government/publications/health-protection-in-schools-and-other-childcare-facilities/chapter-9-managing-specific-infectious-diseases (accessed 28 January 2023).

Younghoon, J. and Lee, H. (2018) Ramsay Hunt Syndrome. *Dental Anaesthesia and Pain Medicine* 18(6): 333–337.

Endocrine Presentations

16

Ant Kitchener

> **Within This Chapter**
> - Adrenal disease
>   - Addison's disease
>   - Cushing's syndrome
> - Diabetes insipidus (DI)
> - Diabetes mellitus
> - Overactive thyroid disease
> - Parathyroid disease
> - Underactive thyroid disease

Introduction

The endocrine system is composed of glands that secrete hormones which the bloodstream carries to organs and tissues to regulate functions such as metabolism, digestion, blood pressure and growth. Some of the endocrine system's most important glands are the pineal gland, hypothalamus, pituitary gland, thyroid, ovaries and testes.

Although the endocrine system is not directly linked to the nervous system, the two interact in several ways. They're linked by the hypothalamus – the part of the brain that controls human behaviour, including emotional and stress responses. It is also involved in basic drives such as hunger, libido, sleep and thirst. Importantly, the hypothalamus controls the pituitary gland, which in turn regulates the release of hormones from other glands in the endocrine system. This activates based on information that makes it back to the brain in a feedback system.

The endocrine system is not a part of the nervous system, but it is just as essential to communication throughout the body. We can think of endocrine communication like a love letter you send to everyone in your neighbourhood (see Box 16.1) – but the message inside only has 'meaning' for the one person. With this analogy we can think about hormones in a much more complex way, in that they are secreted into the blood with this message, will then travel to the whole neighbourhood around the body, but will only activate certain receiving receptors where they have an effect – or to stay with the analogy, where meaning is intended. The communication of hormones is catalytic for one of three things. They firstly

CHAPTER 16 Endocrine Presentations

> **Box 16.1   Hormonal Love Letters from the Pituitary Gland**
>
> **F**ollicle-stimulating hormone (FSH)
> **L**eutinising hormone (LH)
> **A**drenocorticotrophic hormone (ACTH)
> **T**hyroid-stimulating hormone (TSH)
> **P**rolactin
> **E**ndorphins and encephalins
> **G**rowth hormone (GH)

encourage growth or repair; secondly, they deal with stress on the body; and thirdly, they enable reproduction.

Every hormone in the body has a normal range needed to achieve its goal, known as a homeostatic range. Where there is too much or too little, there is a disease outcome. An example is that TSH travels like a love letter in the blood, and it is detected by the thyroid because it has meaning there. Where the homeostatic range is met, the outcome is that it makes thyroxine. Thyroxine is used to set the metabolic rate and too little thyroxine would be a representative proxy of hypothyroidism. Too much thyroxine would be a representative proxy of hyperthyroidism, and each causes a pattern of disease due to too much or too little of the hormone.

Many conditions of hormone imbalance, either too high or too low, may be due to an autoimmune process, so it is important to check autoantibodies to help determine longevity of imbalance and treatment need.

Presentations in Primary Care

Adrenal Disease

Aetiology

The adrenal gland is suprarenal and produces a variety of hormones, including adrenaline and steroid hormones (aldosterone and cortisol), each of which deal with the stress response. The instructional hormone that needs to be released is produced in the pituitary gland and is called adrenocorticotrophic hormone (ACTH). Producing too few of these hormones from the adrenal gland, or excreting too many of the hormones from the pituitary gland, would be considered an adrenal insufficiency. Conversely, if too many stress hormones are produced, this would cause an over-stimulation of respondents. Primary adrenal insufficiency, where the problem is with the adrenal gland, is called Addison's disease and is often of autoimmune aetiology. Too much steroid response is termed Cushing's disease and can occur from tumours or as a result of steroid therapy. These conditions are usually managed under a shared care arrangement with hospital endocrinology services.

> There are some great resources available for healthcare professionals through Addison's UK (www.addisonsdisease.org.uk) and the Pituitary Foundation (www.pituitary.org.uk).

Presentations in Primary Care

Addison's Disease

History and Investigation

Addison's disease can be tough to diagnose. Symptoms may include darker areas of skin pigmentation (hyperpigmentation); severe fatigue; unintentional weight loss; gastrointestinal symptoms such as nausea, vomiting and abdominal pains; joint and muscle pains; and salt cravings (Wass et al., 2013).

> ❗ Hyponatraemia and hyperkalaemia are common imbalances associated with Addison's disease. This water imbalance can also present as a hypotension or dizziness.

Cortisol and ACTH (which cause the stress response) are stimulated through a synACTHen test. Normally an early morning (8–10am) blood test to check cortisol levels is offered and, if this is high enough, then the synACTHen test is not required. Oestrogen-containing contraceptives or replacement therapies should be stopped for six weeks prior to the synACTHen test and the test is contraindicated in pregnancy. Any other steroid- or aldosterone-related medications need stopping 48 hours prior to the test. Whether this can be done in primary care will depend whether the synACTHen is on the prescribing 'red list', in which case if the early morning cortisol is low, referral to endocrinology services is required for further diagnostics (Arlt and Allolio, 2003).

Management

Direction for management should be from the hospital endocrinology services; however this generally falls into two parts – glucocorticoid replacement and mineralocorticoid replacement. The common replacement therapy for the glucocorticoid is oral hydrocortisone (usually in an adult dose of 10 mg twice daily), and the common replacement for the mineralocorticoid is fludrocortisone (most often 100 µg daily). Treatment will be lifelong. Dehydroepiandrosterone is also produced in the adrenal glands, which turns into testosterone and may need monitoring.

> 👥 Utilisation of social prescribing initiatives, such as referral to self-help and support groups, is often valuable.

> 💡 Sick-day rules should be given to the patient to follow. If the person is sick and not vomiting, they can adjust their oral dose of corticosteroid. If they have a vomit or recurring vomiting, they must administer their intramuscular hydrocortisone and present as a medical emergency. This should be treated as an Addisonian crisis.

> ❗ Infection that is trivial for the average patient with no comorbidities is easily fatal to those with this condition.

CHAPTER 16 Endocrine Presentations

Cushing's Syndrome

Conversely to Addison's, Cushing's syndrome refers to a group of clinical symptoms that occur as the result of persistently and inappropriately raised glucocorticoid levels. The origin can be pituitary gland in nature, but it can also be induced by the over-prescription of steroids.

History and Investigation

Symptoms can include palpably thin skin with easy bruising and oedema; a moon-shaped face; proximal muscle weakness that causes struggle with squatting and rising; osteoporosis leading to back pain and spinal fracture; kyphosis; and avascular necrosis of the head of femur.

Management

If gland related, treatment is surgical. If pharmacologically induced, it will require cessation of the responsible drugs. In either case, direction for management should be from the hospital endocrinology services.

Diabetes Insipidus (DI)

Aetiology

The lack of production of anti-diuretic hormone (ADH, also known as vasopressin) means the kidney cannot make enough concentrated urine, and too much urine is passed.

> 💡 Cranial diabetes insipidus (DI) is when the issue is at the pituitary gland, whereas nephrogenic DI is where ADH is produced but the kidneys fail to respond to it.

History and Examination

The common history is around going to the toilet too much and needing to drink lots due to excessive thirst. This condition is a water-balance condition associated with voiding urine too much and becoming dehydrated. In severe disease, a person can void 20 litres of urine a day and thus has electrolyte imbalance risk. Therefore, dehydration and electrolyte imbalance are the most significant clinical findings in presentation.

> ❗ The presentation could be secondary to head injury, hypothalamic damage, post infection, post operation or post brain tumour.

As the condition shares symptoms with diabetes, a diabetic screen is needed. The condition can affect electrolytes, predominantly due to excessive urination and oral rehydration, so a kidney function and electrolyte check are also required. A 24-hour urine osmolality test can determine urine volume, and dilution can be diagnostic.

Management

Referral to endocrinology services for confirmation and an ongoing treatment plan is needed. The patient will need to maintain hydration by ensuring adequate fluid intake. Nephrogenic causes are often treated with thiazide diuretics, which reduce the amount of urine the kidney produces, whilst cranial DI may be managed with desmopressin through endocrinology.

Diabetes Mellitus

Diabetes is a major public health concern with increasing prevalence (Khan et al., 2020).

Diabetes mellitus is a dysfunction of the endocrine pancreas, in which we observe insufficient production of insulin, reduced cellular response to insulin (known as 'insulin resistance') or a mixture of both pathologies. There are two generic descriptors for diabetes:

- Type I early onset diabetes mellitus (T1DM), a form of insulin-dependent diabetes mellitus (IDDM) (Achenbach et al., 2005). T1DM is thought to be autoimmune in nature.
- Type II (2) diabetes mellitus (T2DM) where a later onset is generally associated with visceral adiposity. T2DM may become IDDM through progression.

Aetiology

There are strong genetic indicators for diabetes; however, it has a complex and multi-factorial aetiology including genetics, epigenetics and environmental factors. Those with a T1DM are often diagnosed in childhood and this type of diabetes is thought to be autoimmune in nature. Insulin reduces blood sugar levels, so in a dysfunctional pancreas this lack or insufficiency of insulin leads to chronically raised sugar levels. In the older patient, T2DM is predominant, with genetics and obesity acting as the most common culprits. Here, obesity has a significant impact on tissue sensitivity to insulin and the higher the body mass, the more insulin resistance occurs. Thus, we can observe a direct correlation between weight and diabetes risk (Lee and Olefsky, 2021).

> Prior to this, however, there is an at-risk phase of raised blood sugar levels termed 'pre-diabetes', and this is a particular area where healthcare advice and social prescribing initiatives may be able to influence the progression of the disease process.

> NICE (2020) Diabetes in Pregnancy: Management from Preconception to the Postnatal Period [NG3].
> In addition to type 1 and type 2 disease, diabetes can also occur during pregnancy, which is known as gestational diabetes.

There are a number of other types of diabetes, such as those that occur secondary to pancreatic removal or surgery or that which is secondary to cystic fibrosis (cystic fibrosis-related diabetes mellitus, CFDM).

CHAPTER 16 Endocrine Presentations

History and Examination

Diabetes should be considered when the four Ts of diabetes feature in a presentation:

- Thirst (polydipsia)
- Toileting (polyuria)
- Tiredness
- Thinness.

A diabetes screen is a common primary care screening test and should be considered pathognomonic with cardiovascular risk. Therefore, anyone with cardiac risk factors has diabetes risk (McAlister et al., 2002). Those with diabetes also have a raised vascular risk as well (Department of Health, 2001). Further to this, findings in new onset diabetes are often picked up through a random capillary blood glucose test, urinalysis or a blood test. However, first presentations of disease may be a diabetic crisis in the form of diabetic ketoacidosis (DKA). This may include symptoms of vomiting, abdominal pain, deep-sighing breathing and reduced levels of consciousness. Ketones in the urine, when associated with hyperglycaemia, should prompt the paramedic to consider the possibility of a metabolic acidaemia which will require urgent same-day admission for treatment. Knowing this, a capillary blood glucose test should be performed on non-specific unwell people to exclude glycaemic emergencies, especially those in early teen years with the four Ts above and when a T1DM diagnosis is more common.

There is also the possibility of a hyperosmolar hyperglycaemic state (HHS), which tends to be associated with T2DM where blood sugars are very high, but without significant ketoacidosis (Kitabchi et al., 2009). Symptoms include weakness, leg cramps, visual problems and reduced levels of consciousness. Capillary blood glucose monitoring (CBGM) may be useful, but often sugar readings are too high for these machines and may default to just show as a 'hi' level.

> In undiagnosed individuals, recurring infections such as balanitis, urinary tract infection or thrush should prompt the clinician to consider checking for diabetes.

Investigations

There are four diagnostic tests for diabetes:

- HbA1c blood test (diabetes = > 48 mmol/mol)
- Fasting plasma glucose blood test (diabetes = > 7 mmol/L)
- Oral glucose tolerance test (blood test > 75 g glucose > blood test)
- Random plasma glucose blood test (diabetes = > 11 mmol/L).

In the asymptomatic patient, a single abnormality should be confirmed through a repeat test or an alternative to confirm the presence of abnormality. If the second is in range, then regular monitoring should follow. Generally, HbA1c is an easy test to perform, but there are a range of people where this test is not recommended for diagnosis.

In those where HbA1c can be considered a reliable test, once diagnosis of diabetes is established, the test should be repeated up to quarterly. The HbA1c test is useful as it reflects longevity of blood sugar levels, estimated at 8–12 weeks – the approximate life span of a red cell – compared to a plasma glucose test which shows only a moment in time. An aim should be to reduce the HbA1c below the 48 mmol/mol target.

> Once on insulin therapy, the HbA1c blood test becomes less useful as the disease has progressed to the stage where there is no further treatment.

Investigation of end-organ damage and cardiovascular disease is important, and you may want to take damage control actions, such as starting reno-protective medicines like angiotensin-converting enzyme (ACE) inhibitors and calculating QRISK. Arrange for the following screens at diagnosis (NICE, 2011):

- An electrocardiogram (ECG)
- Diabetic foot check
- Retinopathy screening
- Urine albumin creatinine ratio (UrACR) and serum creatinine.

> QRISK is a UK-specific, multi-ethnic scoring system used to estimate the risk of an individual having a cardiovascular event within ten years. It is advocated by NICE and can be found at: https://qrisk.org/three/index.php.

Management

For a new diagnosis of T1DM, refer the same day as an acute admission for confirmation of diagnosis. People without initial insulin therapy will potentially die in hours to days, and thus are not for community treatment. Insulin will not correct the acidaemia (BSPED, 2013). Shared care will be established after diagnosis, with the primary care team taking responsibility for prescribing insulin, blood glucometers and associated items such as sharps bins, lancets and testing strips.

T2DM is more commonly managed in a 'stepwise fashion' by the primary care team and can be reviewed within a patient-centred care model, which allows the patient to own their healthcare experience. This generally will always include lifestyle advice and there are good sources of information on culinary adaptations which may help in diabetes (Holt and Kumar, 2010).

> Of note, there is higher prevalence of T2DM in the Asian community, and dietary elements here are often calorific with high levels of complex carbohydrate sugars (Yang et al., 2019). Directing to social prescribing initiatives and culturally appropriate self-help groups can offer viable and sustainable alternatives for the patient. Community exercise programmes may also be available as part of commissioned services and this will help to reduce visceral weight (NICE, 2013b).

CHAPTER 16 Endocrine Presentations

Table 16.1 Anti-diabetic Drugs

Drug group	Example drug
Biguanides	Metformin (Glucophage®)
Sulfonylureas	Glipizide (Glucotrol®), glyburide (Glynase®, Micronase®), chlorpropamide (Diabinese®) and tolbutamide (Orinase®)
Alpha-glucosidase inhibitors	Acarbose (Precose®) and miglitol (Glyset®)
Thiazolidinediones	Pioglitazone (Actos®)
DPP-4 inhibitors	Sitagliptin (Januvia®), saxagliptin (Onglyza®) and vildagliptin (Galvus®)
GLP-1 receptor agonists	Exenatide (Byetta®) and liraglutide (Victoza®)

Capillary blood glucose measurement is not routinely offered in T2DM management unless there is progression to an IDDM or if there is a DVLA driving requirement to do so (for example, for heavy goods vehicle drivers).

If diet and exercise fail to address diabetes, then drug therapy may be an addition, and a maximum of three groups should be tried before considering progression to injectable formats (see Table 16.1 for anti-diabetic drug groups). Referral to a diabetes education course has also been shown to be beneficial in the reduction of HbA1c, so is recommended (Kim and Han, 2020).

Where patients are on insulin, the care tends to be shared with the community or hospital diabetology teams.

> HHS will require emergency admission and is often associated with intensive care stays.
>
> Alongside acute issues associated with hyperglycaemia, the long-term negative sequelae of raised blood sugars include micro- and macrovascular changes, which can cause:
>
> - Depression
> - Diabetic feet issues
> - Diabetic neuropathy
> - Diabetic retinopathy
> - Erectile dysfunction
> - Increased cardiovascular disease and myocardial infarction (MI) risk (including silent MI)
> - Increased stroke risk
> - Prone to infections
> - Skin changes.
>
> Any patients with diabetes should be considered for screening for these conditions, or for health information and promotion strategies to prevent their occurrence.

Presentations in Primary Care

Overactive Thyroid Disease

Aetiology

Hyperthyroidism is predominant in the female population and has a peak age of occurrence between the 20s and 30s. High thyroxine levels are often autoimmune in nature, known as Grave's disease, or may be caused by a cancer, known as adenoma (BTA, 2006). An inflamed thyroid, referred to as thyroiditis, may also cause over-stimulation. Some diets, such as those with high seafood content, can cause too much iodine and this can contribute to too much thyroxine production.

> As an iatrogenic aetiology, consumption of too much levothyroxine may cause toxic levels and this may be a good first check when considering the cause of hyperthyroidism.

Summary of most common aetiologies:

- Adenoma (thyroid, pituitary)
- Drugs (levothyroxine excess, amiodarone)
- Grave's disease
- Post-partum thyroiditis
- Toxic multinodular goitre
- Viral thyroiditis.

History and Examination

You should look for general signs of agitation, such as being fidgety, and be alert to fine tremors and acropachy of the hands (a form of finger clubbing). Also check for palmar erythema and excessive sweating, which could be a sign of raised thyroid levels. A pulse check may indicate tachycardia or atrial fibrillation (AF) and prompt you to perform an ECG. Check the eyes to see if they protrude, known as exophthalmos, and finally check for a goitre (Selmer et al., 2012).

Thyrotoxicosis is a toxic form of hyperthyroidism causing symptoms such as tachyarrhythmia, palpitations, AF and anxiety. The clinical presentation may only show one of the symptoms, such as anxiety, so what appears to be a mental health consultation may in fact uncover a biological cause, such as thyroid disturbance, if the patient is properly checked for biochemical imbalances. This is important before assuming that it is mental ill health and highlights the importance of the biopsychosocial model of care. Palpitations are another common reason for primary care consultation and could be the outcome of an overactive thyroid. Sometimes swallowing issues also present and this is due to an enlarged goitre (neck swelling related to the enlarged thyroid gland).

> Excessive symptoms would be called a 'thyroid storm' and warrant immediate intervention. A thyroid storm is often precipitated by an underlying infection and can cause fast AF, hyperpyrexia, heart failure and collapse. Treatment would involve symptom control of the storm, as well as addressing the underlying thyroid issues (Bahn et al., 2011).

CHAPTER 16 Endocrine Presentations

Investigations

In overactive thyroid disease, blood tests will show low TSH as there is too much thyroxine in the blood. Biologically, this means the pituitary is asking for less thyroxine production and it will also show a high T4, which is the actual thyroxine.

Requesting a TSH is a surrogate for T4, as it is cheaper and faster to gain a result. When replacing thyroxine after successful suppression of the thyroid output, titrate replacement, increase it gently and repeat the TSH test every 10–14 days until back in homeostatic range. If TSH is deranged, check thyroid peroxidase (TPO) antibodies as this will tell you whether this has an autoimmune origin. If positive, this is likely to be a lifelong issue for this patient.

Management

There are three traditional methods for treating hyperthyroidism:

- Pharmacological (carbimazole or propylthiouracil)
- Radioiodine treatment
- Surgical treatment.

Beta blockers are commonly used for symptom control of acute thyroid storm (Franklyn and Boelaert, 2012), including a referral to an endocrinologist to treat the cause. Long-term treatment options are consultant led and include radiotherapy, drug control or a surgical cut out (De Groot, et al., 2012). In the meantime, you may consider suppression with oral carbimazole, as this will 'kill the thyroid output', and then titration to replace thyroxine with oral levothyroxine.

> Advice and guidance from the endocrinology team may be prudent if you do not have experience of starting thyroid suppression therapy.
> The caution with carbimazole is it places the patient at risk of pancytopenia, which wipes out their white cells, and thus they become at risk of trivial infections having sinister infection processes, such as sepsis.

> Be cautious when seeing patients taking anti-thyroid medications and presenting with the following:
>
> - High fever
> - Flu-like symptoms
> - Mouth ulcers
> - Sore throat.
>
> This may be an indication of neutropenia. Patients must immediately stop the medication and have an urgent full blood count (FBC) check. If neutropenic, admission for more invasive treatment and endocrinological advice may be needed.

Presentations in Primary Care

> ❗ Overactive thyroid could be a cancer presentation and may be referred under the head-and-neck two-week wait (2WW) pathway (NICE, 2020).

Parathyroid Disease

Aetiology

The parathyroid sits behind the thyroid and pokes out like butterfly wings to show four small glands. It produces parathyroid hormone (PTH). As with all balancing of hormones, disease can present as too high (hyperparathyroidism) or, much more rarely, too low (hypoparathyroidism). Most commonly, 'primary hyperparathyroidism' is caused by adenoma of the parathyroid gland; however, cancer may also occur. Hyperparathyroid levels are linked with vitamin D levels and calcium levels, so it can present as altered levels of any one of these three aspects – PTH, calcium or vitamin D.

History and Examination

When considering hyperparathyroidism, symptoms predominantly originate from the resultant hypercalcaemia and may be vague or absent in many cases, with many individuals being picked up through routine screening. Some historical features may however present, such as abdominal pain, lethargy, nausea, muscle weakness and mild confusion. As calcium is needed for muscle contraction, including that of cardiac myocytes, derangement can lead to convulsions, arrhythmias, tetany and peripheral paraesthesia (Bilezikian et al., 2018).

> 💡 Hyperparathyroidism may also present with psychiatric presentations, secondary to the resultant hypercalcaemia. Hence, consideration for calcium-level testing to check for biochemical imbalances before making presumptions of mental ill health is prudent.

As too much calcium can cause stone formation, patients may present with renal stone, gall stone or salivary stone presentations on physical examination. In addition, assessment of hydration status and cognitive impairment is warranted. With regards to the hypercalcaemia, patients can present as asymptomatic, or with mild, moderate or severe symptoms depending on their levels. These symptoms are:

- Myopathy
- Irritability or confusion
- Paralytic ileus leading to abdominal pain, constipation, anorexia, nausea and vomiting
- Pancreatitis secondary to ectopic calcification
- Dehydration
- Renal stones
- Polyuria and polydipsia
- Renal failure.

CHAPTER 16   Endocrine Presentations

Investigations

There is a triad of linked items, all of which can be tested:

- PTH
- Vitamin D (25 hydroxyvitamin D)
- Calcium levels.

Checking the thyroid level is also useful, as thyrotoxicosis causes excessive osteoclast activity, known more commonly as bone breakdown. Renal function checks are useful in addition, as renal failure leads to parathyroid hypertrophy.

> 💡 If calcium is high, with a normal PTH, this is suspicious of cancer elsewhere, so checking for bony destruction, renal, ovarian and lung pathology, as well as a DEXA bone scan, skin cancer check and breast examination may be useful (Marcocci et al., 2013).

Management

Hypercalcaemia with symptoms requires emergency medical admission. If minimal symptoms or asymptomatic, and parathyroid malignancy is suspected, you should refer under the 2WW pathway for head and neck. There is an 80% parathyroid origin vs. 20% bone destruction malignancy (Clines, 2011). Other malignancies that can cause hypercalcaemia include lung, oesophagus, skin, breast, kidney and bladder cancer. Where an obvious cause is not apparent, but the cancer referral pathways criterion is not met, referral to endocrinology services for further investigations is required.

You should also stop drugs, such as thiazide diuretics, lithium, vitamin D, vitamin A and calcium (including those within antacids), as these may be a cause for the hypercalcaemia (Griebeler et al., 2016). If a primary hyperparathyroidism is found, then a referral for endocrinological surgery may be warranted.

Underactive Thyroid Disease

Aetiology

Underactive thyroid disease is more common than overactive thyroid disease. This condition is commonly autoimmune in nature, again affecting women more than men. In existing thyroid disease, it may be due to under-dosing with levothyroxine replacement therapy.

Summary of the most common aetiologies:

- Autoimmune thyroiditis (most commonly 'Hashimoto's disease')
- Hypopituitarism
- Post radioiodine treatment
- Post thyroidectomy
- Viral thyroiditis.

History and Examination

With effective screening strategies and widely available thyroid function testing, many cases of hypothyroid are picked up when symptoms are mild, non-specific or even when the patient is asymptomatic. Those who are symptomatic commonly present to primary care with 'tired all the time' symptoms. This complaint has a variety of causes and commonly turns out to be low thyroid levels. Other primary care presentations of low thyroid may include dry skin presentations, weight gain, hair loss, constipation, cold intolerance, depressive symptoms, memory loss, irregular periods or loss of libido.

> In postpartum thyroiditis, there is a hypothyroidism phase, which is three to eight months post birth, so gestation history is important (Lazarus, 2011).

In older people, symptoms are often subtle or even absent (Boelaert et al., 2010).

The diagnosis is based on the degree of clinical symptoms. When thyroid levels are low, low-density lipoproteins are not broken down, so cholesterol goes up. Therefore, signs of raised cholesterol and vascular disease should also be considered. Otherwise, examination findings often relate to advanced disease (for example, hair loss, heart failure, prolonged tendon jerk relaxation).

Investigations

TSH is inverse to the actual amount of T4, so it may be high if T4 levels are low. Considerations of alternative causes of 'tired all the time' aetiology must be made, so a FBC for anaemia and a liver and renal screen are often completed simultaneously. Given the effects of low thyroid on cholesterol risk, a lipid profile and subsequent QRISK may be required.

A repeat TSH and a clinical review should be made at six to eight weeks after initiation or dose change, giving adequate time to respond to the new levels. An additional check after six months of reaching a euthyroid state is required, as metabolism of thyroxine differs in euthyroid state compared to underactive thyroxine level (Garber and Cobin, 2012). Checking TPO antibodies will tell you whether this has an autoimmune origin and, if positive, this is likely to be a lifelong issue for this patient. It is worth checking their medicines list, as some medicines reduce thyroxine levels, such as amiodarone.

Management

The goal of management is to:

- Resolve the symptomology of presentation
- Normalise the blood values within their ranges
- Avoid over-treatment, especially with the older patient.

Unlike overactive thyroid disease, which will need an intervention to manage and subdue the overactive element, the majority of low thyroid cases can be managed in primary care.

CHAPTER 16 Endocrine Presentations

> ❗ You may wish to consider a more specialist endocrinology opinion if the patient presents with a goitre or nodules of the thyroid gland, which may suggest malignancy – check the 2WW head and neck pathway (NICE, 2021b).

If they have other endocrine conditions, this will make them more complex, and specialist advice would be needed (for example, in cases of co-existing Addison's disease). Those who are planning pregnancy or are pregnant may need specialist advice. If the TSH does not respond to levothyroxine, and where reversible causes such as adherence, drug interaction and malabsorption have been excluded, these patients again may need a specialist endocrine opinion (Roberts and Ladenson, 2004).

Sub-clinical Hypothyroidism

In those patients with an autoimmune presentation, you may have a sub-acute phase of hypothyroidism in that their TSH is raised but the T4 has not yet dropped (Collet et al., 2012). If the patient is symptomatic, you may choose to initiate treatment in this group for symptom resolution (Cooper and Biondi, 2012). With raised TPO antibodies, it will likely be a matter of time before the T4 levels drop, so a three-monthly check is warranted, or sooner if symptoms evolve (NICE, 2021a).

Chapter Summary

Endocrinology is about the production and balance of hormones. Levels that are too high or too low can cause imbalance pathologies. The most common conditions for the paramedic in primary care to manage will be thyroid disease and diabetes mellitus, with the aim of gaining a rebalance of homeostatic range being the cornerstone of treatment. This may be through advice, social prescribing signposting, medical prescribing or surgical interventions. The advice and guidance facility available from most endocrinology services is a useful support mechanism for this complex area of medicine. Shared care and referral to endocrinology services are helpful for definitive diagnosis, condition exploration and expert care planning.

Case Study 1

You see a 45-year-old female who presents with feeling tired all the time.

History

PC: Feeling tired all the time.
HxPC: She has a busy working life as a school teacher and she is not sure whether she is just exhausted as it progresses towards the end of the school term. She reports no menorrhagia or other bleeding sources, and describes slightly low mood and lethargy, even at weekends when she is off from school.
PMHx: She has an autoimmune skin condition called vitiligo (which may make other autoimmune presentations more likely). She reports often struggling to get warm,

despite having the central heating on at home. Sometimes struggles to go to the toilet. Her periods are slightly erratic.
DHx: She takes over-the-counter vitamins.
SHx: Ex-smoker (now vapes), social alcohol use only, no recreational drug use.
FHx: Mother had medication for a thyroid condition.
ROS: Nil of note.

Examination
- Unremarkable, no goitre.
- You arrange for her to have an initial panel of bloods, which show no anaemias but a raised TSH level with a low T4 level.
- You also run TPO antibodies which come back raised.

Preferred Diagnosis
- Autoimmune hypothyroidism.

Differential Diagnoses
- Low-mood presentations are often confused for hypothyroidism. Other causes of 'tired all the time' presentations include lupus, multiple sclerosis, rheumatoid arthritis, polymyalgia rheumatica, diabetes and chronic fatigue syndrome (amongst many others).

Management
- Thyroid replacement therapy, titrated against response (with regular blood monitoring as needed).

Case Study 2

You are on call and see a 13-year-old male who has been brought in by his mum as he is vomiting with abdominal pain. He seems quite lethargic and presents as tachycardic but with normal blood pressure.

History
PC: Vomiting with abdominal pain.
HxPC: Some abdominal pain, feeling very thirsty and passing urine a lot over the past two weeks, before becoming acutely unwell today.
PMHx: Also a history of balanitis over the past two months, as well as a recurring boil in the right groin. Otherwise, no major disease of note.
DHx: Is on a clindamycin gel for acne vulgaris.
SHx: Normally attends school, non-smoker.
FHx: Father died of cardiovascular disease (aged 62), mother alive with a history of hypertension.
ROS: He is a thin-looking character and reports urinating at least once an hour which has been ongoing for a number of months.

CHAPTER 16 Endocrine Presentations

Examination
- Vital signs: BP 90/40 mmHg; HR 122 bpm; no (high) temperature.
- You undertake a capillary blood glucose test which shows a capillary glucose level of 18.2 mmol/L.
- You have him undertake a urine dip test which shows Ketones+++ of the dip.
- He has non-specific abdominal pain, not localised or guarded.
- No renal angle pain.
- Normal bowel sounds.
- Visibly diaphoretic.

Preferred Diagnosis
- DKA

Differential Diagnoses
- Similar symptoms may present in cerebral oedema, stroke, epilepsy, electrolyte imbalance, hypoglycaemia (although CBGM would be low in this case), metabolic disorders or lactic acidosis (amongst many other presentations).

Management
- Acute admission for management.
- This patient will require insulin therapy as well as management of their electrolytes and acidotic state.
- An emergency ambulance transfer should be booked for this patient.

References

Achenbach, P., Bonifacio, E., Koczwara, K. et al. (2005) Natural history of type 1 diabetes. *Diabetes* 54(2): 25–31.

Arlt, W. and Allolio, B. (2003) Adrenal insufficiency. *Lancet* 361(9372): 1881–1893.

Bahn, R.S., Burch, H.B. and Cooper, D.S. (2011) Hyperthyroidism and other causes of thyrotoxicosis: Management guidelines of the American Thyroid Association and American Association of Clinical Endocrinologists. *Endocrine Practice* 17(3): 456–520.

Bilezikian, J.P., Mrandi, M. and Eastell, R. (2018) Guidelines for the management of asymptomatic primary hyperparathyroidism: Summary statement from the fourth international workshop. *Lancet* 391(10116): 168–178.

Boelaert, K., Torlinska, B., Holder, R.L. et al. (2010) Older subjects with hyperthyroidism present with a paucity of symptoms and signs: A large cross-sectional study. *Journal of Clincial Endocrinology* 95(6): 2715–2726.

British Society for Paediatric Endocrinology and Diabetes (BSPED) (2013) *BSPED Recommended DKA Guidelines 2009 (Minor Review 2013)*. London: British Society for Paediatric Endocrinology and Diabetes.

British Thyroid Association (BTA) (2006) *UK Guidelines for the Use of Thyroid Function Tests*. London: British Thyroid Association.

References

Clines, G. (2011) Mechanisms and treatment of hypercalcemia of malignancy. *Current Opinions in Endocrinology, Diabetes, and Obesity* 18(6): 339–336.

Collet, T.H., Gussekloo, J. and Bauer, D.C. (2012) Subclinical hyperthyroidism and the risk of coronary heart disease and mortality. *Archives of Internal Medicine* 172(10): 799–809.

Cooper, D.S. and Biondi, B. (2012) Subclinical thyroid disease. *Lancet* 379(9821): 1142–1154.

De Groot, L., Abalovich, M., Alexander, E.K. et al. (2012) Management of thyroid dysfunction during pregnancy and postpartum: An Endocrine Society clinical practice guideline. *Journal of Clinical Endocrinology and Metabolism* 97(8): 2543–2565.

Department of Health (2001) *National Service Framework for Diabetes: Standards.* London: Department of Health.

Franklyn, J.A. and Boelaert, K. (2012) Thyrotoxicosis. *Lancet* 379(9821): 1155–1166.

Garber, J. and Cobin, R. (2012) Clinical practice guidelines for hypothyroidism in adults: Cosponsored by the American Association of Clinical Endocrinologists and the American Thyroid Association. *Endocrine Practice* 18(6): 998–1028.

Griebeler, M.L., Kearns, A.E. and Ryu, E. (2016) Thiazide-associated hypercalcaemia: Incidence and association with primary hyperparathyroidism over two decades. *Journal of Clinical Endocrinology and Metabolism* 101(3): 1166–1173.

Holt, T. and Kumar, S. (2010) *ABC of Diabetes – Types of Diabetes.* New York: Wiley Blackwell.

Khan, M.A.B., Hasim, M.J., King, J.K., et al. (2020) Epidemiology of Type 2 Diabetes - Global Burden of Disease and Forecasted Trends. *Epidemiological Global Health* 10(1): 107–111.

Kim, E.J. and Han, K. (2020) Factors related to self care behaviours amongst patients with diabetic foot ulcers. *Journal of Clinical Nursing* 29(9): 1712–1722.

Kitabchi, A.E., Umpierrez, G.E., Miles, J. et al. (2009) Hyperglycemic crises in adult patients with diabetes. *Diabetes* 32(7): 1335–1343.

Lazarus, J.H. (2011) The continuing saga of postpartum thyroiditis. *Journal of Clinical Endocrinology and Metabolism* 96(3): 614–616.

Lee, Y.S. and Olefsky, J. (2021) Chronic tissue inflammation and metabolic disease. *Genes and Development* 1(35): 307–328.

Marcocci, C., Bollerslev, J., Khan, A. et al. (2013) Medical management of primary hyperparathyroidism: Proceedings of the fourth international workshop on the management of asymptomatic primary hyperparathyroidism. *Journal of Clinical Endocrinology and Metabolism* 6(2465): 1116–1119.

McAlister, F.A., Zarnke, K.B. and Campbell, N.R. (2002) The 2001 Canadian recommendations for the management of hypertension: Part two – Therapy. *Canadian Journal of Cardiology* 18(6): 625–641.

National Institute for Health and Care Excellence (NICE) (2020) Diabetes in Pregnancy: Management from Preconception to the Postnatal Period [NG3]. Available at: https://www.nice.org.uk/guidance/ng3 (accessed 28 January 2023).

National Institute for Health and Care Excellence (NICE) (2021a) Clinical Knowledge Summary: Hypothyroidism. Available at: https://cks.nice.org.uk/topics/hypothyroidism/management/subclinical-hypothyroidism-non-pregnant/ (accessed 28 January 2023).

National Institute for Health and Care Excellence (NICE) (2021b) Suspected Cancer: Recognition and Referral [NG12]. Available at: https://www.nice.org.uk/guidance/ng12 (accessed 28 January 2023).

Roberts, C.G. and Ladenson, P.W. (2004) Hypothyroidism. *Endocrine Practice* 363(9411): 793–803.

CHAPTER 16 Endocrine Presentations

Selmer, C., Olesen, J.B. and Hansen, M.L. (2012) The spectrum of thyroid disease and risk of new onset atrial fibrillation: A large population cohort study. *British Medical Journal* 345: e7895.

Wass, J., Howlett, T. and Arlt, W. (2013) *Diagnosing Addison's: A Guide for GPs.* London: Addison's Self Help Group.

Yang, J.J., Danxia, Y., Wanquing, W. et al. (2019) Association of Diabetes With All-Cause and Cause-Specific Mortality in Asia. *Journal of the American Medical Association Open* 2(4): e192696.

Palliative and End-of-Life Care Presentations

Karina Catley and Joseph St Leger-Francis

17

Within This Chapter

- Introduction to palliative and end-of-life care
- Assessment
  - History taking
  - Psychosocial assessment
  - Religion and spirituality
- Assessment and management of symptoms
  - Agitation
  - Constipation
  - Dyspnoea
  - Nausea and vomiting
  - Pain
- Acute oncological emergencies in palliative patients
  - Neutropenic sepsis
  - Malignant spinal cord compression (MSCC)
  - Hypercalcaemia
  - Superior vena cava obstruction (SVCO)
- Regonition and management of the dying phase
  - Terminal restlessness or agitation
  - Anticipatory medications
  - Breaking bad news
- Care after death
  - Verification of death

Introduction

'The way we die lives on in the memory of those who survive.'
(*Dame Cicely Saunders, founder of the modern hospice movement*)

Palliative care is an approach that improves the quality of life both of patients facing a life-limiting condition and of their families, through prevention and relief of symptoms causing suffering. This is achieved through early identification, assessment and management of physical and psychosocial signs and symptoms utilising a holistic, biopsychosocial approach (WHO, 2020). Importantly, whilst the terms 'palliative' and 'end-of-life' care are used interchangeably within the UK health system, it is clinically relevant to appreciate the difference between the two. Palliative care refers to individuals requiring identification, assessment and management of physical, psychological, spiritual and social needs as a result of suffering with one or multiple long-term, life-limiting conditions, and thus individuals receiving palliative care are not solely those who are at the end of their life and dying (WHO, 2020). Conversely, end-of-life care is generally referred to as the care provided to patients within the last weeks and days of life (LACDP, 2014). Having outlined this, the terms 'palliative' and 'end-of-life' care will be used synonymously moving forward in this chapter, as in clinical practice.

CHAPTER 17   Palliative and End-of-Life Care Presentations

Broadly speaking, generalist palliative care is provided by the usual clinical professionals involved in the patient's care where the complexity of needs is low. As such, paramedics working in primary care would be expected to provide generalist palliative care and refer to, or seek advice from, specialist palliative care professionals for more complex presentations. Generalist palliative care has no clear definition; however, generalist providers can be expected to:

- Provide symptom control and other interventions to improve or maintain quality of life.
- Communicate with the patient and their family to ensure needs are met.
- Respect patient autonomy and choice in place of care and death, as well as treatment options.

Alternatively, specialist palliative care is provided by those trained in the speciality for patients with more complex needs. This includes complex symptomology, as well as challenging social situations that would benefit from specialist input to coordinate care. Specialist palliative care in the UK can be sourced from hospices or hospital teams, and, importantly, community services and in-patient units provided by specialist palliative care vary dependent on location, so it is crucial to be aware of the palliative care services within your local area.

When managing those transitioning towards the end of life, adopting a patient-centred approach to decision making is vital to ensuring needs are met in line with patient preferences. In particular, assessment of pain should incorporate physical, psychological, social and spiritual elements which can all contribute to suffering. This concept is described as 'total pain' (Figure 17.1) and demonstrates a holistic approach to healthcare for those at the end of life.

Social pain
- Loss of role/status
- Loss of job
- Dependency

Psychological pain
- Depression
- Fear
- Anxiety

Total pain

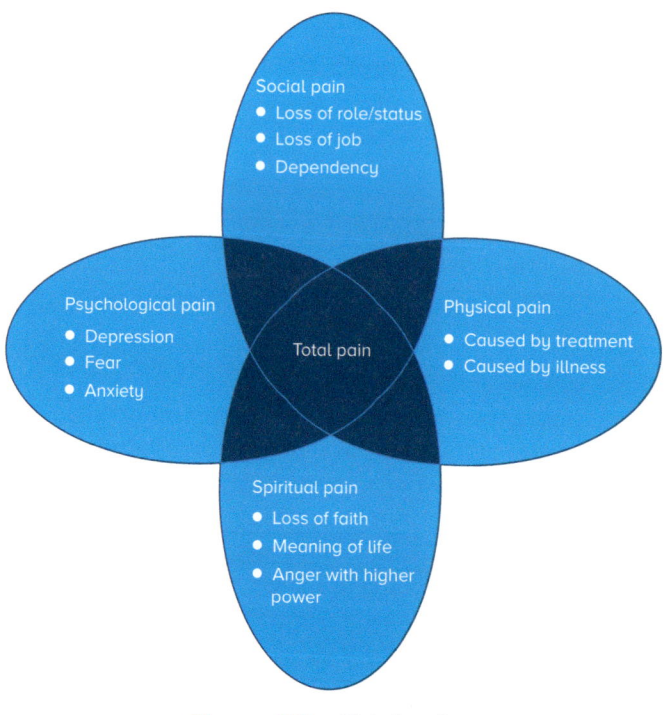

Physical pain
- Caused by treatment
- Caused by illness

Spiritual pain
- Loss of faith
- Meaning of life
- Anger with higher power

Figure 17.1   Total pain.

Assessment

This chapter is therefore written with the aim of furthering the reader's knowledge and understanding with regards to the assessment and management of common palliative care presentations in primary care settings.

Assessment

In addition to managing individuals who are under palliative care services and thus have already been identified as having palliative care needs, the paramedic in primary care should be cognisant of presentations where referral to the patient's primary healthcare professional for consideration of palliative care is warranted. This is most often when the patient is identified as being within the last 12 months of life.

> This is not a simple task and is outside the scope of this chapter; however, helpful tools such as the following exist to improve decision making in this area:
> - SPICT4-ALL (2018) Supportive and palliative care indicators tool.
> - Gold Standards Framework (2018) GSF proactive identification guidance.

History Taking

When taking a history from an end-of-life care patient or their family, two pieces of key information to obtain early in the consultation are:

- The history of the disease progression
- Any recent trend in deterioration.

This may not only assist in establishing the patient's current baseline health status but also offer insight into the patient and their family's awareness of the patient's illness. In addition, it is important to find out patients' awareness of their disease progression to ensure you can sensitively obtain a thorough patient history.

Other factors requiring particular attention in the end-of-life care patient group include:

- Social and family support – to ensure early referrals for additional care can be implemented if required
- Preferences for care – both at the present time and when the patient is approaching the end of life.

Patient preferences for care can include decisions such as preferred place of care, preferred place of death and levels of treatment or intervention they would find acceptable. These discussions may not have taken place or may be in the early stages, as it often takes time to have these difficult conversations for those experiencing a life-limiting illness. When discussions have taken place, usually with the patient's general practitioner (GP) or palliative care clinician, they should be documented formally in what is known as an Advance Care Plan (ACP).

CHAPTER 17 Palliative and End-of-Life Care Presentations

Advance care planning is the patient-led process of making formal decisions regarding their future care, and these decisions can be used at a time when a patient loses capacity or can no longer communicate (NICE, 2018). Advance care planning is a term used for any documentation of patient preference or clinical decisions for future care and can include specific documentation such as:

- Advance decisions to refuse treatment (ADRT)
- Advance statements
- Do not attempt cardiopulmonary resuscitation (DNACPR)
- Lasting power of attorney for health and welfare
- Treatment escalation plan.

See Table 17.1 for a summary of ACP documentation with reference to the legal structures underpinning such documentation.

Table 17.1 Advance Care Planning

Type of advance care plan	What is it?	Is it legally binding?
Advance decisions to refuse treatment (ADRT)	Enables a person to refuse pre-specified medical treatment. This is done in advance so if the time comes when a patient loses capacity or is unable to consent to or refuse medication treatment, the ADRT will convey their wishes and treatment plan	Yes
Lasting power of attorney for health and welfare	A document which allows a person to nominate another person/persons to make decisions about their healthcare on their behalf should they lose capacity. If a patient still holds capacity, treatment is in line with their current wishes	Yes
Advance statement	A person's wishes for their care, which can be used to inform best decision making by healthcare professionals involved in their care if that person lacks capacity at a later date	No
Do not attempt cardiopulmonary resuscitation (DNACPR)	A clinicial decision made by a senior clinician that CPR would be futile as the person is dying as a result of advanced, irreversible disease **or** adults with capacity can choose to have a DNACPR. Clinicians must always consult with a patient and/or their family before recording a DNACPR decision	No. However, you must have robust evidence for overriding a DNACPR

Source: Mallinson (2022).

Assessment

In the ACP process, patients have had courageous conversations with healthcare professionals. It is therefore vital that these care plans are read and taken into account when considering any management plan during consultations. In particular, consulting clinicians should be aware of agreed ceilings of treatment for patients. To capture this information, treatment escalation plans may have been created by primary care or specialist clinicians and these documents can vary greatly from general statements surrounding ceilings of treatment to specific instructions in the event of expected symptoms such as breathlessness or pain. In primary care, paramedics may be able to create, access and update ACPs through central or electronic palliative care coordination systems (EPaCCS).

Psychosocial Assessment

> A holistic approach to end-of-life care includes consideration to the psychological and social impact of the illness on the patient and family members or loved ones. Anxiety and depression are common amongst those with advanced disease. Consolations assessing psychological distress can be challenging, so consider using assessment tools such as the Hospital Anxiety and Depression Scale (HADS) for patients, to assess for presence of psychological distress.

> For patients experiencing pain, it can be helpful to ask: 'I know you are experiencing physical pain; other than this, is there anything else that is causing you distress?'.
> This can help to open up the conversation to identify any areas of psychological or social distress that the patient may be experiencing. Evidence is limited for the treatment of anxiety and depression in the palliative care population; therefore assessment and management as per NICE guidelines is recommended (NICE, 2011).

> Assessment of the social network important to the patient is good practice. This can be particularly helpful to identify who the main caregivers are, so appropriate support can be offered to reduce the risk of caregiver burden becoming overwhelming. Family can also be at risk of complicated grief, a prolonged grief response after the death of a loved one impacting on the normal functioning of the person and even leading to suicidal thoughts (WHO, 2023). It is worth being aware of the early signs of complicated grief and offering referral to bereavement counselling services, even prior to the death.

Religion and Spirituality

When taking care of patients at the end of their life, it is important to consider a person's spirituality, which may be in the form of a specific religion, to ensure these needs are met. Spirituality is defined as:

CHAPTER 17 Palliative and End-of-Life Care Presentations

Those beliefs, values and practices that relate to the human search for meaning in life. For some people, spirituality is expressed through adherence to an organised religion, while for others it may relate to their personal identities, relationships with others, secular ethical values or humanist philosophies.

(NICE, 2021b)

There is no one definitive approach to the assessment of spiritual needs; however, is it important to ask questions around faith and what type of support patients would like for their religious or spiritual needs. This could be practical assistance such as transport to get to their place of worship or requests for a religious leader to be present when approaching the end of life. Assessment tools can be useful to help guide discussions, such as the FICA Spiritual History Tool detailed in Table 17.2. Discussions should be led by the patient in this assessment and take an individualised approach to spirituality and religion. This means being wary of making assumptions and always asking the patient how they interpret and practice their faith. Equally be aware that during advanced illness religion or spirituality may become more prominent in patients and their families' lives, even for those who earlier on in their illness did not disclose a strong sense of spirituality.

Table 17.2 FICA Spiritual History Tool©

F – Faith, Belief, Meaning	• 'Do you consider yourself to be spiritual?' or 'Is spirituality something important to you?' • 'Do you have spiritual beliefs, practices or values that help you to cope with stress, difficult times or what you are going through right now?' (contextualise to visit) • 'What gives your life meaning?'
I – Importance and Influence	• 'What importance does spirituality have in your life?' • 'Has your spirituality influenced how you take care of yourself, particularly regarding your health?' 'Does your spirituality affect your healthcare decision making?'
C – Community	• 'Are you part of a spiritual community?' • 'Is your community of support to you and how?' For people who don't identify with a community, consider asking 'Is there a group of people you really love or who are important to you?' • (Communities such as churches, temples, mosques, family, groups of like-minded friends or yoga or similar groups can serve as strong support systems for some patients.)
A – Address/ Action in Care	• 'How would you like me, as your healthcare provider, to address spiritual issues in your healthcare?' (With newer models, including the diagnosis of spiritual distress, 'A' also refers to the 'Assessment and Plan' for patient spiritual distress, needs and/or resources within a treatment or care plan

Source: © Christina Puchalski, MD, and The George Washington University 1996 (updated 2022). All rights reserved. Adapted from: Puchalski and Romer (2000). Reused with permission.

Assessment and Management of Symptoms

The presence of symptoms can be ascertained through undertaking a thorough patient history. Once identified, symptoms must be assessed for severity to guide conversations with patients around management options. Consideration of what impact these symptoms have on the patient's quality of life is vital when weighing up potential treatment options. Four common symptom presentations are discussed below, with tips on how to assess these in the end-of-life patient.

The following section gives an overview of common symptoms experienced by palliative care patients and management options. This is not a definitive list, but these are the key symptoms where the management is novel within this patient group that you are likely to encounter working in the primary care setting.

Agitation

Agitation can occur towards the end of life and is characterised as:

- An inability to settle
- Fidgeting
- Moaning or calling out in distress.

It is important to establish any underlying causes for the agitation, including pain, constipation or urinary retention (Watson et al., 2016). It would in most cases be appropriate to conduct an abdominal examination on the agitated patient to rule out any retention as well as consider any symptoms that might be causing pain. If agitation is still present once any underlying causes have been ruled out or managed appropriately, then pharmacological management would be appropriate. Patients at higher risk of agitation are those with brain metastasis, older age and pre-existing cognitive impairment (Todd and Teale, 2017).

Agitation is a distressing symptom for the patients experiencing it, as well as for family members and caregivers that witness it. Below gives a summary of the common causes and both pharmacological and non-pharmacological management options.

Common Causes

Common causes include medication toxicity or withdrawal, dehydration, constipation, urinary retention, pain, electrolyte disturbance, infection, hypoxia and cerebral tumour (Watson et al., 2016).

Identification and treatment of the underlying cause is vital in the management of the agitated patient. If all other causes have been corrected or ruled out and agitation continues, consider management below. For agitation in the dying patient, please refer to 'terminal restlessness' in the Recognition and Management of the Dying Phase section.

Pharmacological Intervention

Anxiolytic medications are the first-line treatment for agitation where underlying causes have been rectified and agitation persists. Midazolam or haloperidol are recommended (Hosker and Bennett, 2016). Second-line medication is levomepromazine if agitation

CHAPTER 17 Palliative and End-of-Life Care Presentations

is considered severe. Seek specialist advice on doses and drug interactions prior to prescription or administration of anxiolytic medications.

> It is important to explain to patients and family the chance of sedative effect on the patient to prepare them, especially if within the last few days of life, to ensure family are able to converse with patient if they wish prior to administration.

Non-pharmacological Intervention

Ensure environment is kept quiet and low-level lighting is implemented, as noise and bright lights can exacerbate symptoms. Communication with patient and family about likely cause is key to promoting understanding and reducing anxiety about the symptoms. Reassurance for the patient and family will help ease anxiety.

Constipation

Constipation is a common symptom in the palliative and end-of-life care patient and is characterised by the cessation or infrequent passing of stools or the passing of painful, hard stools. It is important to conduct a full abdominal assessment on patients presenting with abdominal discomfort or a change in bowel habit. During this assessment, if any red flags (for example, silent bowel) are noted then imaging is usually required to check for bowel obstruction. The history of any laxatives taken and their effectiveness should also be noted. A rectal examination may be indicated in a patient presenting with constipation to guide clinical decision making (Larkin et al., 2008).

> Assessment tools such as the Bristol Stool Chart can be helpful to monitor a change in normal bowel habits.

Common Causes

- Opioid, diuretic and antimuscarinic medications
- Poor nutrition or hydration
- Immobility and weakness
- Emergency presentations should be considered in an end-of-life care patient presenting with constipation, including hypercalcaemia and bowel obstruction.

Pharmacological Intervention

First line it is recommended to choose a stimulant agent combined with a stool softener. If patient is not responsive to this, specialist palliative care advice should be sought if considering either rectal treatments or increased dosages of oral medications that are off licence (Table 17.3).

Assessment and Management of Symptoms

Table 17.3 Pharmacological Treatment of Constipation

Function	Drug
Predominantly softening	Macrogols, e.g. Movicol®, Laxido® Lactulose Docusate sodium
Predominantly stimulating	Senna Bisacodyl

Source: NICE (2023).

Non-pharmacological Intervention

Encouragement of fluid intake and increasing mobilisation (where possible) may assist in return of normal bowl movements in mild cases. Applying gentle abdominal massage or hot water bottle or pack on abdomen can be utilised as a comfort measure.

Dyspnoea

Dyspnoea is the subjective experience of breathlessness or breathing discomfort experienced commonly in palliative care patients, especially towards the end of life.

> There are many tools that can be used to assess dyspnoea, such as the Borg Dyspnoea Scale. Assessment should include questioning the functional impact of the breathlessness, associated symptoms, exacerbating factors and any emotional or physiological involvement (NICE, 2018).

A full respiratory assessment is indicated, except for those experiencing dyspnoea within the dying phase.

Dyspnoea can often be managed effectively in the end-of-life care patient with a range of techniques and medication. Always consider reversible emergencies that can cause dyspnoea, and ensure invasive treatment is balanced against the patient's preferences, ACP and prognosis.

Common Causes (NHS Scotland, 2020)

- Exacerbation of chronic condition (chronic obstructive pulmonary disease (COPD) or heart failure)
- Infection
- Pulmonary embolism, effusion or oedema
- Primary or secondary tumour in lung
- Superior vena cava obstruction (SVCO)
- Fatigue or muscle weakness
- Anxiety.

CHAPTER 17 Palliative and End-of-Life Care Presentations

Pharmacological Intervention

If anxiety is believed to be the underlying cause, consider benzodiazepines. If hypoxic, give oxygen therapy in line with the British Thoracic Society guidelines (O'Driscoll et al., 2016). Morphine is commonly prescribed by palliative care specialists to manage dyspnoea and may be available to administer within the anticipatory medications. Bronchodilators can be utilised for suspected bronchoconstriction, even in the absence of a wheeze (NICE, 2022). Corticosteroids are appropriate if the history and presentation suggests cancer is the likely cause.

Non-Pharmacological Intervention

Fan therapy is a helpful technique, utilising a handheld or standing fan or open window to blow cool air over a patient's face which is thought to stimulate the trigeminal nerve, reducing the sensation of breathlessness (Kako et al., 2018). Consider coaching the patient using breathing techniques and assisting with changing their positioning to sitting upright if possible. Patients with long-term chronic lung conditions may have a particular breathing technique they are familiar with. Anxiety-reduction techniques can be considered where the primary cause is thought to be anxiety related. Longer-term patients may benefit from referrals for physiotherapy or pulmonary rehabilitation. For anxiety-related causes, consider offering referral for cognitive behavioural therapy.

Nausea and Vomiting

Nausea and vomiting increases in prevalence towards the end of life, with up to 60% of patients experiencing symptoms during their illness and it being a common presentation in the final week of life (Watson et al., 2016).

Common Causes

Causes are often multifactorial in advanced disease, encompassing (but not limited to):

- Chemically induced nausea – drugs, toxins, metabolic
- Gastric stasis – ascites, ulcer, gastritis
- Raised intracranial pressure (ICP)
- Movement associated
- Anxiety
- Constipation
- Bowel obstruction.

> ! It is vital that likely cause and the pathway by which the cause(s) trigger the vomiting reflex are identified in order to appropriately prescribe a suitable antiemetic. Consultation with a palliative care team should be considered if the cause is not clear.

Assessment and Management of Symptoms

Table 17.4 Pharmacological Treatment of Nausea and Vomiting

Syndrome	Causes	Drug treatment
Anxiety	Anticipatory anxiety	Lorazepam
Gastric stasis	Gastric outlet obstruction Cancer Opioids Ascites	Metoclopramide Domperidone Levomepromazine
Gastric irritation	Bowel obstruction	Cyclizine Haloperidol Levomepromazine Steroids
Biochemical	Hypercalcaemia Liver disease Opioids Chemotherapy Antibiotics	Haloperidol Levomepromazine
Raised inter-cranial pressure	Cancer – primary/secondary Meningeal disease Bleeding	Steroids Cyclizine
Vestibular	Cancer – primary/secondary	Cyclizine Prochlorperazine

Source: NICE (2021a).

Pharmacological Intervention

Table 17.4 summaries the main medications available dependent on the cause of the nausea or vomiting. If unable to identify the cause of the symptom and non-pharmacological techniques are ineffective, consider haloperidol. Please refer to the NICE guidelines for further details.

Non-pharmacological Intervention

Ensure environment will not induce nausea – avoid cooking smells and unpleasant odours. Encourage cold carbonated drinks, as often these are easier to consume than still or warm drinks.

Pain

The concept of 'total pain' can be adopted to assess patients' level of distress holistically, taking into account physical, social, psychological and spiritual domains of pain. Physical pain can result from the underlying aetiology of the disease or side effects from treatment.

CHAPTER 17 Palliative and End-of-Life Care Presentations

> When assessing physical pain, ensure you use a pain assessment tool appropriate for the patients' needs, such as the Abbey Pain Scale for patients with cognitive impairment. It is also helpful to ask family or carers how a patient with cognitive impairment normally expresses pain, to ensure you pick up on indications that the patient is distressed. Changes in the type of pain and the number of breakthrough (acute) pain episodes should be noted and may indicate that a change in dose or type of pain medication is required.
>
> When managing pain in those towards the end of life, it is useful to refer to the WHO analgesic ladder (Figure 17.2). This provides a stepwise approach to prescribing analgesia for the management of pain. It is worth noting that caution should be taken when prescribing any analgesic medication in those with likely or confirmed hepatic or renal impairment, and it is recommended you seek advice from specialist palliative care teams in such circumstances.

Common Causes

There are many causes of pain in the end-of-life care patient group, but these can be broadly categorised by onset (chronic or acute) and type of pain:

- Nociceptive
- Neuropathic.

Pharmacological Intervention

Patients towards the end of life may be on very high doses of opioid medications. As such, there is a risk of opioid toxicity, which in severe cases should be managed with naloxone.

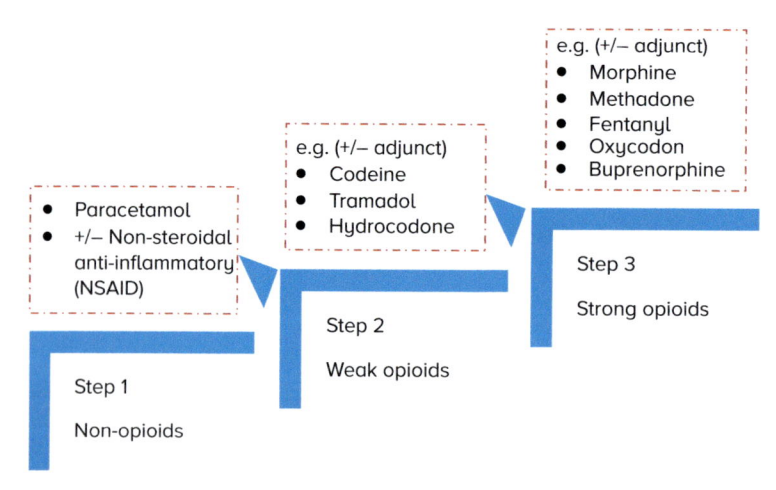

Step 1 Non-opioids
- Paracetamol
- +/− Non-steroidal anti-inflammatory (NSAID)

Step 2 Weak opioids
- e.g. (+/− adjunct)
  - Codeine
  - Tramadol
  - Hydrocodone

Step 3 Strong opioids
- e.g. (+/− adjunct)
  - Morphine
  - Methadone
  - Fentanyl
  - Oxycodon
  - Buprenorphine

Figure 17.2 WHO analgesic ladder.
Source: WHO (1986).

Toxicity typically occurs after conversion to an alternative opioid, a rapid increase in titration or if the patient becomes unwell and develops renal failure impacting on drug excretion (Watson et al., 2016). Consider discussing your management plan with a specialist palliative care clinician prior to switching or increase opioids.

Non-pharmacological Intervention

Consider referral to specialist palliative care teams for assessment of suitability if you believe the patient would benefit from interventions such as complementary therapies, acupuncture or transcutaneous electrical nerve stimulation (TENS). Comfort measures include cold or warm packs at the site of pain and distraction techniques.

Acute Oncological Emergencies in Palliative Patients

Neutropenic Sepsis

Aetiology

A potentially life-threatening complication of anti-cancer or other immunosuppressant drug treatment. It is typically associated with chemotherapy treatment, which can be given in a palliative care context for symptom management. The period of most risk for patients is 10–14 days post chemotherapy treatment, as this is when the immune response is at its lowest; however, suspect all patients that have a recent history of treatment (6–8 weeks) and the following symptoms to be septic (JRCALC, 2022).

Examination

Common presentations include typical signs of sepsis:

- Indication of possible infection (dysuria, diarrhoea, productive cough)
- Chills and shivering
- Decreased consciousness level
- Hypotension
- Tachycardia.

> ⚠️ These signs and symptoms are similar to those within the dying phase. The key to distinguishing between the dying phase and neutropenic sepsis lies in the history of an acute deterioration. Some hospices can manage neutropenic sepsis on in-patient units, so this should be considered in line with patients' advance care plan.

In these patients, their immune response is usually diminished due to anticancer treatment so they may not present with a temperature above 38°C and could be hypothermic (NHS Scotland, 2020).

CHAPTER 17   Palliative and End-of-Life Care Presentations

Management

Management involves contacting the local oncology department and urgent hospital transfer for intravenous antibiotics and oxygen therapy to people with reduced oxygen saturation or with an increase in oxygen requirement over baseline, to maintain oxygen saturation above 94% unless contraindicated (NICE, 2020).

Malignant Spinal Cord Compression (MSCC)

Aetiology

Malignant spinal cord compression (MSCC) occurs when cancer metastasises to the spine or epidural space cause secondary compression of the spinal cord through direct compression or interruption to the blood supply. Approximately 5–10% of patients with cancer go on to develop MSCC (NHS Scotland, 2020). If left untreated, it can lead to paraplegia and symptoms that seriously affect quality of life. Vertebral metastases are most common in prostate, breast and lung cancers.

Examination

Common presentations include:

- Back pain
- Limb weakness
- Sensory deficit
- Bladder or bowel dysfunction
- Reduced mobility (history of recent falls).

> Sensory deficit is a late sign of MSCC and often patients are only referred at this late stage. Do not delay in referring patients with initial signs of compression or suspicion of spinal metastasises, to give the best chance of neurology reversal.

Management

Management is an urgent admission of oncological management and urgent MRI scan of the whole spine, analgesia, high-dose steroids and radiotherapy, chemotherapy or surgical intervention (NHS Scotland, 2020). The impact of MSCC on a patient's quality of life should be discussed with the patient and their family alongside the impact of the management plan. Consider the patient's prognosis, wishes and involvement of specialist palliative care teams when managing these patients.

Hypercalcaemia

Aetiology

Hypercalcaemia refers to an increased plasma calcium concentration above 2.6 mmol/L. Hypercalcaemia occurs through several processes, and in malignancy is mainly associated with increased parathyroid hormone-related protein (PHTrp) secretion and increased bone reabsorption (Watson et al., 2016) (Figure 17.3).

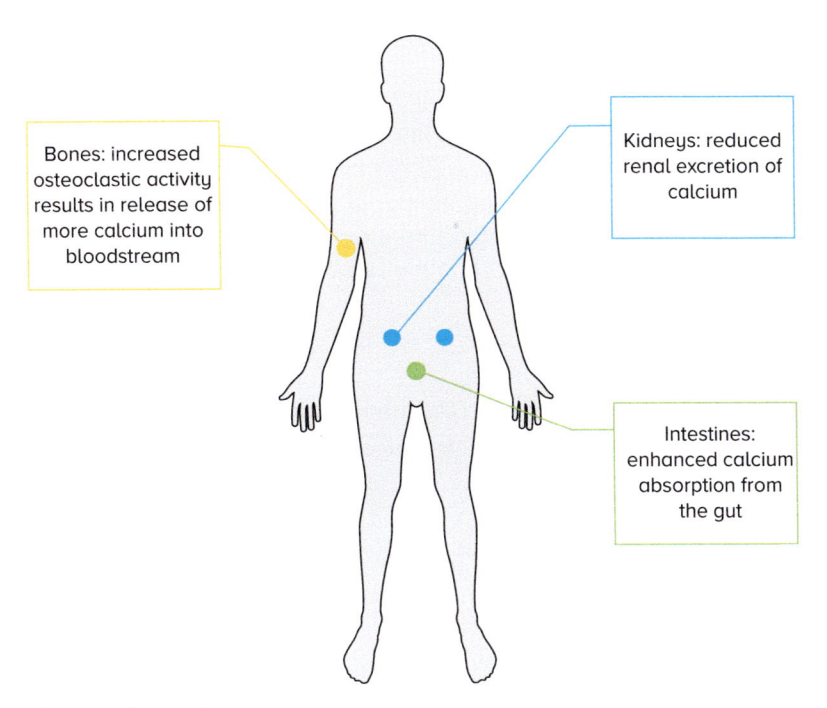

Figure 17.3 Hypercalcaemia.

Examination

Hypercalcaemia is notoriously difficult to diagnose in the community setting due to the common symptoms associated with it, and if under any suspicion management should be actioned in line with the patient's preferences and plan of care.

Patient presentations include:

- Gastrointestinal (GI): Dry mouth, nausea and vomiting, constipation
- Neurological: Confusion, weakness, seizures
- Renal: Polyuria, thirst, dehydration
- Cardiac: Arrhythmias.

Management

Management should focus on good symptom control (for example, antiemetic for nausea or vomiting) and offer emergency hospital admission for those with symptomatic hypercalcaemia for intravenous fluid replacement and bisphosphonate therapy. Asymptomatic hypercalcaemia can be managed in the community and may not warrant invasive treatment if a patient is nearing the end of life. Liaise with the patient's palliative care team if there is any uncertainty regarding ongoing management.

CHAPTER 17 Palliative and End-of-Life Care Presentations

Superior Vena Cava Obstruction (SVCO)

Aetiology

SVCO commonly occurs in patients with a primary lung cancer, but those with lymphoma, breast, colon, oesophagus and testicular cancers are also at risk. SVCO occurs when blood flow is impaired either due to compression of the superior vena cava by external metastases or through direct invasion by a tumour or thrombus (NHS Scotland, 2020). The obstruction leads to a reduction in venous return from the head, thorax and upper limbs to the right atrium of the heart.

Examination

Obstruction of the superior vena cava causes the following presentations:

- Dyspnoea
- Headache or dizziness
- Visual disturbance
- Swelling of the face and upper limbs – reddening of the skin
- Periorbital oedema
- Dilated veins on the chest and arms
- Dilated neck veins (non-pulsatile).

Management

Place patient in sitting upright position, provide high-flow oxygen and contact local specialist oncology centre for immediate transfer. Consider administering morphine for breathlessness if prescribed by specialist team. Onward treatment may include stent insertion, chemotherapy or radiotherapy.

There are three medication-related emergencies to be aware of:

- Opioid toxicity
- Serotonin syndrome
- Neuroleptic malignant syndrome.

> Buckley, N.A. (2014) Serotonin syndrome.
> Knott, L. and Bonsall, A. (2021) Neuroleptic malignant syndrome [online].
> See for further reading on these medical-related emergencies.

Recognition and Management of the Dying Phase

Signs that a person may be entering the dying phase, the last few days or hours of life, are illustrated in Table 17.5. Dying is a natural process and is indicated by organ failure, which will present abnormal observations upon assessment. Where the deterioration is sudden and unexpected, then a prompt clinical review, in line with the patient's preferences, should be performed to rule out any reversible emergencies. Where the deterioration is expected,

Recognition and Management of the Dying Phase

Table 17.5 Signs and Symptoms of Dying

Signs/symptoms of dying	Presentation
Change in respiratory pattern	• Shortness of breath • Cheyne-Stokes breathing (irregular, shallow breathing with periods of apnoea) • Respiratory secretions – noisy, rattling sound from upper airway ('death rattle')
Reduced hydration and nutrition	• Reduced food and fluid intake • Difficulty swallowing • Anorexia • Dehydration
Reduced cardiac output	• Cardiac arrhythmias • Hypotension • Central and peripheral cyanosis • Loss of peripheral pulses • Mottled/waxy skin
Functional decline	• Profound weakness • Bedbound • Requiring assistance with day-to-day care • Unconscious or reducing consciousness level
Renal functioning	• Oliguria or anuria • Incontinence or retention • Dark-coloured urine

communicating effectively with the dying person is key – involve them and their family in decision making and assess and support their needs in line with their preferences.

All non-essential observations should be withheld when assessing a dying patient (NICE, 2015), and any spiritual or religious wishes should be actioned in line with a patient care plan, such as contacting a religious leader.

Prognosticating a specific timeframe for patients can be distressing, as often this is predicted incorrectly which can have a negative impact on the well-being of patients and their loved ones. If asked prognostication questions, explain the difficulty in making this predication. Broadly speaking, the deterioration over weeks or days is an indicator of how long a person has left. For example, if a person is deteriorating from week to week, then often they are expected to die within weeks; if a deterioration is from day to day then they likely only have days left (Neuberger, 2013).

Terminal Restlessness or Agitation

Terminal restlessness is a symptom that may be experienced by patients in the last days and hours of life whereby they can be unsettled, agitated or present as acutely distressed. This is thought to be due to a multitude of factors, including 'total pain' distress, side effects of medications or existential suffering experienced by a patient as they are nearing the end of life (Marie Curie, 2022). Steps should be taken to rule out causes for this restlessness in the same fashion as described with agitation. In severe cases of refractory restlessness, specialist teams will offer palliative sedation.

Anticipatory Medications

In the final weeks or months of life, anticipatory medication may be prescribed by the patient's GP or palliative care team to manage symptoms in this final stage. Anticipatory medications cover the four As:

- Analgesia
- Anxiolytics
- Antiemetics
- Antisecretories.

> Many medications prescribed for end-of-life care patients are done so 'off licence', and therefore doses or indications for drugs may be different from regular practice. It is usually only specialists within palliative care or GPs with a background in this field that can prescribe in this way, and you must adhere to your organisation's prescribing protocols.

Paramedics can administer anticipatory medication to the patient if the Medication Authorisation and Administration Record (MAAR) is available and signed. Any administrations must be recorded on this chart, and it is good practice to consult with the palliative care team, where possible, prior to administration of any unfamiliar drug.

Breaking Bad News

Bad news can refer to significant information that negatively alters a person's expectations or perceptions of their future (Fallowfield and Jenkins, 2004). Within palliative care, this could be delivering information about a terminal diagnosis or a deterioration in condition or informing family that a patient has died. Some key tips to effective communication of bad news are:

- Start with a warning shot: Prepare the patient and family that bad news is coming – 'I'm sorry to have to tell you this'; 'I have some difficult news to tell you about your condition'.
- Simple language: Do not use medical jargon or phrases that could be misinterpreted, e.g. 'gone' instead of 'died'.
- Pause: After delivering bad news, allow silence whilst the patient or family member processes the information, and wait for a response.
- Assess their understanding: Ask the receiver to summarise the information to ensure the message has been delivered clearly and any misinterpretations are resolved.
- Give an opportunity for questions: Be honest if you do not have an answer at that time and advise you will get back to them.

- Action plan: Next steps, including signposting to relevant services and identification of coping strategies. It can be helpful to document this information for the patient or family so they can refer back to it when they have had some time to process the information given (Watson et al., 2016).

Care After Death

Training on and familiarisation with your organisation's verification of death process is recommended. Consider offering bereavement support services to family and loved ones and be prepared to answer practical questions relating to death certifications and removal of the deceased.

Verification of Expected Death

Verification of expected death is the process undertaken by a registered healthcare professional, performing an assessment to confirm and record that a person has died. Once verification has taken place, the patient's GP can issue the Medical Certificate of Cause of Death (MCCD). The purpose of the assessment is to ascertain that there is no circulatory, respiratory or cerebral activity. This involves the following steps (BMA, 2020):

1. Confirm the death was expected – is there an advance care plan or DNACPR in place? If unexpected or suspicious circumstances, referral to the coroner is required.
2. Check the patient's pupillary reflexes with a pen torch. The pupils should be unreactive to light, fixed and dilated.
3. Check for no chest wall movements for three minutes by observing the chest. Confirm absent breath sounds using a stethoscope.
4. Palpate the carotid pulse and check that pulse is absent for at least one minute.

Wait ten minutes and repeat steps 2–4.

5. Complete accurate patient records, noting:
    - Time of verification of death
    - Patient details: name, date of birth, address, NHS number, next of kin
    - Name of person in attendance
    - Other people present
    - Circumstances of death
    - Name of guiding clinician (the clinician performing the verification process).

Care of the deceased and family is particularly important. Ensure you take adequate time to perform the verification of death process alongside providing support for family members, including signposting to bereavement services as appropriate.

Chapter Summary

This chapter outlines the principles of palliative and end-of-life care that can be applied in paramedic practice within a primary care setting. A patient-centred, holistic approach to assessment and management is best practice for all patient care;

CHAPTER 17 Palliative and End-of-Life Care Presentations

however, with those towards the end of life this care can impact significantly on quality of life. Symptom control should incorporate comfort measures and non-pharmacological treatments where appropriate, and advice sought from specialist palliative care teams for complexity or shared decision making. Paramedics working in primary care are likely to encounter many palliative patients within the last 12 months of life and can make a difference through provision of care to maintain quality of life and support a good death.

Case Study

You are conducting a home visit after a family member has called the surgery concerned about the behaviour of an 80-year-old female patient.

History

PC: Appears distressed and agitated.
HxPC: 3/7 change in behaviour, crying out appears distressed and more confused, unable to settle. Patient is advanced dementia, doubly incontinent and monosyllabic speech.
PMHx/SHx: Advanced dementia, osteoarthritis, hyperlipidaemia, chronic kidney disease Stage 3.
DHx: Memantine, naproxen, atorvastatin.
SHx: Lives with elderly husband, hospital bed downstairs. Carers x 4 daily. Awaiting referral for nursing home as husband now unable to cope with ongoing carer duties.
FHx: Nil relevant.
ROS:
  CV: Nil chest pain or peripheral oedema.
  Resp: Nil DIB or SOB, clear bilateral air entry, nil cough.
  GI: Frequent constipation, small hard bowel movement 2/7, oliguria 3/7.
  MSK: Nil recent injury or fall, nil pain.
  Neurological: Non-compliant with neurological examination.

Examination

- Vital signs: BP 112/74 mmHg; HR 90 bpm; RR 20/min; SpO_2 98%; temperature 37.6°C.
- GCS: 10 (eyes: 3; verbal: 2; motor: 5).
- Abdominal examination:
  - I: Appears slightly distended
  - A: Hypoactive bowel sounds
  - P: Dull on percussion, nil fluid
  - P: Global pain on palpation.

Preferred Diagnosis

- Agitation due to urinary retention or constipation. Need to rule out urinary tract infection due to change in behaviour and low-grade fever.

Differential Diagnoses
- Dehydration
- Electrolyte disturbance
- Cerebral tumour
- Other neurological cause.

Management
- Constipation: Stimulant and stool softener combination.
- Urinary retention: Referral to district nurses for catheter, or apply catheter.
- Review required and if agitation does not resolve after successful treatment of constipation or urinary retention, consider pharmacological management with first-line anxiolytics.

References

British Medical Association (BMA) (2020) Guidance for Remote Verification of Expected Death (VoED) out of hospital. Available at: https://www.bma.org.uk/media/2323/bma-guidelines-for-remote-voed-april-2020.pdf (accessed 27 January 2023).

Buckley, N.A. (2014) Serotonin syndrome. *British Medical Journal* 348: g1626.

O'Driscoll, B.R., Howard, L.S., Earis, J. et al. (2016) BTS guideline for oxygen use in adults in healthcare and emergency settings. *BMJ Thorax* 72(1): i1–i90.

Fallowfield, L. and Jenkins, V. (2004) Communicating sad, bad and difficult news in medicine. *The Lancet* 363(9405): 312–319.

Gold Standards Framework (2018) GSF proactive identification guidance. 6th edn. Available at: https://www.goldstandardsframework.org.uk/cd-content/uploads/files/PIG/NEW%20PIG%20-%20%20%2020.1.17%20KT%20vs17.pdf (accessed 27 January 2023).

Hosker, C.M.G. and Bennett, M.I. (2016) Delirium and agitation at the end of life. *British Medical Journal* 353: i3085.

Joint Royal College Ambulance Liaison Committee (JRCALC) (2022) *JRCALC Clinical Guidelines 2022*. Bridgwater: Class Professional Publishing.

Kako, J., Morita, T., Yamaguchi, T. et al. (2018) Fan therapy is effective in relieving dyspnea in patients with terminally ill cancer: A parallel-arm, randomized controlled trial. *Journal of Pain and Symptom Management* 56(4): 493–500.

Knott, L. and Bonsall, A. (2021) Neuroleptic malignant syndrome. Available at: https://patient.info/doctor/neuroleptic-malignant-syndrome#nav-0 (accessed 27 January 2023).

Larkin, P.J., Sykes, N.P., Centeno, C. et al. (2008) European Consensus Group on Constipation in Palliative Care. The management of constipation in palliative care: Clinical practice recommendations. *Palliative Medicine* 22(7): 796–807.

Leadership Alliance for the Care of Dying People (LACDP) (2014) One chance to get it right. Available at: https://www.gov.uk/government/uploads/system/uploads/attachment_data/file/323188/One_chance_to_get_it_right.pdf (accessed 27 Janaury 2023).

Mallinson, T. (2022) Law and ethics in palliative medicine and end of life care. In Eaton, G. (ed.) *Law and Ethics for Paramedics*. 2nd edn. Bridgwater: Class Professional, pp. 179–192.

CHAPTER 17 Palliative and End-of-Life Care Presentations

Mannix, K. (2004) Palliation of nausea and vomiting. In Doyle, D., Hanks, G., Cherny, N. et al. (eds) *Oxford Textbook of Palliative Medicine*. 3rd edn. Oxford: Oxford University Press, pp. 459–467.

Marie Curie (2022) Agitation. Available at: https://www.mariecurie.org.uk/professionals/palliative-care-knowledge-zone/symptom-control/agitation (accessed 27 January 2023).

National Institute for Health and Care Excellence (NICE) (2011) Common mental health problems: Identification and pathways to care [CG123]. Available at: https://www.nice.org.uk/guidance/cg123 (accessed 27 January 2023).

National Institute for Health and Care Excellence (NICE) (2015) Care of dying adults in the last days of life [NG31]. Available at: www.nice.org.uk/guidance/ng31 (accessed 27 January 2023).

National Institute for Health and Care Excellence (NICE) (2018) Advance care planning [NG94]. Available at: https://www.nice.org.uk/guidance/ng94/evidence/15.advance-care-planning-pdf-172397464602 (accessed 27 January 2023).

National Institute for Health and Care Excellence (NICE) (2020) Clinical Knowledge Summary: Neutropenic sepsis. Available at: https://cks.nice.org.uk/topics/neutropenic-sepsis/management/management/ (accessed 27 January 2023).

National Institute for Health and Care Excellence (NICE) (2021a) Clinical Knowledge Summaries: Palliative care: Nausea and vomiting. Available at: https://cks.nice.org.uk/topics/palliative-care-nausea-vomiting/ (accessed 27 January 2023).

National Institute for Health and Care Excellence (NICE) (2021b) End of life care for adults: Quality statement 6: Holistic support – spiritual and religious [QS13]. Available at: https://www.nice.org.uk/guidance/qs13/ (accessed 27 January 2023).

National Institute for Health and Care Excellence (NICE) (2022) Clinical Knowledge Summaries: Palliative care – dyspnoea. Available at: https://cks.nice.org.uk/topics/palliative-care-dyspnoea/ (accessed 31 January 2023).

National Institute for Health and Care Excellence (NICE) (2023) Treatment summaries: Constipation. Available at: https://bnf.nice.org.uk/treatment-summaries/constipation/ (accessed 27 January 2023).

NHS Scotland (2020) Scottish palliative care guidelines: Palliative emergencies. Available at: https://www.palliativecareguidelines.scot.nhs.uk/guidelines/palliative-emergencies.aspx (accessed 27 January 2023).

Neuberger, J. (2013) *More Care, Less Pathway: A Review of the Liverpool Care Pathway*. London: Department of Health and Social Care.

Puchalski, C. and Romer, A.L. (2000) Taking a spiritual history allows clinicians to understand patients more fully. *Journal of Palliative Medicine* 3(1): 129–137.

SPICT4-ALL (2018) Supportive and palliative care indicators tool. Available at: https://www.spict.org.uk/the-spict/spict-4all/ (accessed 27 January 2023).

Todd, O. and Teale, E. (2017) Delirium: A guide for the general physician. *Clinician Medicine* 17(1): 48–53.

Watson, M., Armstrong, P., Back, I. et al. (2016) *Palliative Adult Network Guidelines*. 4th edn.

World Health Organization (WHO) (1986) WHO's Pain Relief Ladder.

World Health Organization (2020) WHO definition of palliative care. Available at: https://www.who.int/news-room/fact-sheets/detail/palliative-care (accessed 27 January 2023).

World Health Organization (WHO) (2023) ICD-11 for mortality and morbidity statistics: Prolonged grief disorder. Available at: https://icd.who.int/browse11/l-m/en#/http%3a%2f%2fid.who.int%2ficd%2fentity%2f1183832314 (accessed 27 January 2023).

A Note on Assessing and Managing Chronic Pain

Jim Huddy and Keith Mitchell

Introduction

Treating chronic pain in primary care is difficult, time-consuming and frustrating for clinicians and patients. All too often, important positive outcomes are not achieved. Once pain pathways become 'hard wired', there are knock-on behavioural, emotional and psychological changes leading to complex biopsychosocial problems which are not easily untangled. Usually, there is no quick fix that will take it all away; instead, as clinicians, we must persistently nudge patients in the direction of wellness using different approaches.

There is a temptation for clinicians to reach for the prescription pad when faced with patients with chronic pain, which is completely understandable because they do not know what to offer patients as an alternative and are often undertrained in this speciality. This, however, can lead to ever-escalating doses of harmful drugs. Understanding and managing of chronic pain has undergone dramatic changes in recent years. For example, after three to six months, tissue damage is usually healed and persistent pain is more due to maladaptive changes in the pain pathways and the nervous system, especially the spinal cord (McGreevy et al., 2011).

Treating chronic pain is now much more directed at self-management where, with the help of reframing, patients learn the skills necessary to perceive their pain differently – more compassionately and less judgementally. Then, with lifestyle adaptations, the patient can carve out a life which is acceptable to them. This contrasts with the traditional model of the clinician assuming the burden of rendering the patient pain-free using increasing doses of drugs. This approach does not work. It can add to patients' problems and has resulted in hundreds of thousands of deaths worldwide from the opioid epidemic (Gregory and Collins, 2019).

> 💡 We use the term 'skills, not pills' to describe this approach.

Epidemiology

Chronic pain is very common. A systematic review in the UK shows that the prevalence of chronic pain is 35–51%, and the prevalence of moderate–severe disabling long-term pain is 10–14% (Fayaz et al., 2016). Long-term pain is more frequent in the elderly population

CHAPTER 18 A Note on Assessing and Managing Chronic Pain

but can happen in any age group. Globally, lower back pain is the leading cause of years lived with disability (Vos et al.., 2015), and in the UK chronic pain accounts for 4.6 million GP appointments per year at a cost of £69 m (Hart et al., 2015). Pain most often affects the musculoskeletal system. Other pain syndromes are neuropathic pain, chronic headaches and irritable bowel, though these are less-frequent conditions.

What Chronic Pain Is, and What It Is Not

Acute pain is easy to understand. If you get kicked in the shin, it hurts. In medical terms, tissue injury excites nociceptive nerve fibres, which transmit signals up the spinal cord to the brain, which then enter your awareness and conscious perception.

Chronic pain is completely different. It is about as different to acute pain as type II diabetes is to type I. They both result in a raised blood glucose, but the mechanisms bear little resemblance.

Chronic pain is somewhat arbitrarily defined as pain which lasts more than three months (NICE, 2021). It is not usually caused by ongoing tissue damage. Pain arises when the body feels the need to protect a particular area. In some people, for reasons which are not clear, this protection system becomes oversensitive and overactive; the patient has the sensation of pain when there is no good physiological reason behind it.

Some make the analogy that chronic pain is like a faulty smoke detector. Sometimes when a smoke detector goes off, it is not because of a serious fire. In relation to pain, there is some sort of short circuit in the neural networks which when added to our thoughts, beliefs, fears and cognitions can lead to the experience of persistent pain.

> You might notice that we talk about 'the formation of pain in the mind' or 'the experience of pain'. Some patients can read that as 'it's all in your mind' or 'you're inventing it', which is not surprising when often they have been through years of unsatisfying and sometimes dismissive or damaging therapeutic relationships.

Purposeful fabrication of pain is rare, and it is always safest and wisest to believe what you are being told and work on that. Just because medical tests do not show pathology, it does not mean that the subject is not experiencing pain. Migraine is a good example: blood tests, X-rays and imaging are all normal, but we believe the patient that the pain is severe.

Imagine having daily severe pain which the medical profession cannot help with and that, on occasion, professionals do not even believe. It may wear the patient down, make them depressed; they may have trouble sleeping, lose relationships and even jobs. Once you understand this, you can begin to appreciate how difficult this must be for the patient. So, take time to listen, to believe, to care and to understand. Those are the first steps to a successful therapeutic journey.

A Template for Consultations

Chronic pain does not fit the basic consultation template of history, examination, investigations, diagnosis and treatment. Chronic pain is a long-term condition which requires long-term work, a bit like type II diabetes. Let us explore that.

The pharmaceutical industry would love to have a pill or an injectable which would reverse and negate all the causes and consequences of insulin insensitivity and the metabolic syndrome. However, type II diabetes is a phenotype which is the end result of a perfect storm of genetics, environment, behaviour, beliefs, culture, the sugar industry and the microbiome. Therefore, 'treatment' is actually 'management' of all these different things in different ways. There is no fix. More challenging than that, whereas most diabetics and healthcare professionals understand the multifactorial aetiology of diabetes, in the field of chronic pain there is a great deal of ignorance. In addition, the treatment of chronic pain is not a political priority, and so there simply are not enough practitioners within this speciality to be part of the multidisciplinary management for the sheer number of patients it affects.

But that does not mean we cannot try. In fact, most of the pieces are in place and you, as the paramedic in primary care, can set patients on the right path by understanding the patient, their condition and what is available in your area to help them.

To start with, split your consultation into three phases:

Phase 1

Listen. Listen a bit more; do not speak, just listen.

OK, you can talk a bit but focus on taking the history. Find out how it started, how it has been, what has been tried, what has worked, what has not. What is their understanding and explanation of the symptoms? And most importantly, *how much does it affect them*? We like the question 'how bothersome is it?'. Sometimes, you will find that it is no bother at all, they are just interested in why it is there or what it represents. Knowing this from the outset can save hours when addressing their ideas concerns and expectations.

Then stop, and congratulate them for being patient with the process. It may seem like a small thing, but this may be the first time they will have experienced this acknowledgement.

Phase 2

Depending on time and context, phase 2 may be in a second consultation, or it may flow in the same consultation as phase 1. If it is the former, pick up where you left off and introduce the self-management of chronic pain (outlined below). Explain that there is a different way to living a fruitful existence, though it might not be the existence the patient would have picked initially. Then introduce the Health Needs Assessment (HNA) questionnaire which is depicted in Box 18.1.

> The HNA is a useful tool to open up conversations about what matters most to the patient, and gives a basis for onward referrals to relevant services. This may be a direct referral to services, or it may be a review with the link worker social prescriber.

CHAPTER 18 A Note on Assessing and Managing Chronic Pain

> **BOX 18.1** The Health Needs Assessment Questionnaire
>
> Pain can affect people's lives in many ways. This checklist shows some of the problems due to longstanding pain.
>
> Please help us understand the main problems at present that you feel are important to improve your quality of life and self-manage with more confidence.
>
> Please follow the two steps below. Tick ✓ the boxes below related to your needs.

Name		Date of birth
Step 1	Do you have any problems or difficulties with	
	1 ☐	Walking or moving about, lack of fitness and stamina
	2 ☐	Balance or recurrent falls
	3 ☐	Side effects or problems with current pain medication, e.g. tablets etc.
	4 ☐	Pain symptoms or pain relief
	5 ☐	Understanding why persistent pain occurs
	6 ☐	An unhelpful cycle of activity of less pain, so do too much, so more pain, so rest more often or for longer
	7 ☐	Eating the right sort of foods, weight changes
	8 ☐	Disturbed sleep, tiredness or lack of energy
	9 ☐	Managing mood changes of depression, anger, anxiety or worry
	10 ☐	Relationship difficulties; with partner, family, work etc., or sex-life concerns
	11 ☐	Remaining in work or returning to work and/or training
	12 ☐	Financial or money difficulties
	13 ☐	Other difficulties important to change, e.g. concerns about housing, hobbies, leisure or social events with friends, family issues or visiting the church, temple or mosque. Please describe here: ....
Step 2		If you ticked more than three areas of your life and health, please circle the three most important to change at present. Thank you for helping us understand your needs and issues around pain.

Self-management of Chronic Pain

Patients living with chronic pain will experience some or all of 12 sequelae outlined within it. Ask them to pick their top three to work on as their initial priorities.

In our experience, the most frequently chosen are:

- Help with emotions
- Be more active
- Sleep better
- Understand pain and medications better.

It may be that you need to let them go away to consider and fill out the HNA questionnaire. If this is the case, arrange a review appointment in a timely manner.

Phase 3

Now, tackle the three priorities the patient has outlined on the HNA questionnaire. You could do this using the 'ten footsteps' model (on p. 467) and develop a bespoke patient-centred chronic pain management plan, which can then be revisited and reviewed as the patient needs.

> If social prescribers were not engaged in phase 2, this is definitely the point to engage them, as well as your other local resources (local physiotherapists, counsellors) as the patient needs.

Remember that for complex cases who might be on high doses of deleterious drugs with significant mental health and social issues, your local pain team is able to offer advice.

Self-management of Chronic Pain

When self-management of chronic pain is discussed, sometimes patients hear 'modern medicine is not very good at treating this condition, I cannot help you, it is your pain, goodbye'. One way of approaching these conversations is using the pain cycle (Figure 18.1). The pain cycle is a visual aid that can be used to help navigate conversations with patients to recognise how pain can affect different aspects of their life in negative and self-reinforcing ways.

Using the pain cycle relies on listening to the patient's story, and really understanding them – their values, their preferences and what they want as they live with chronic pain. This is a fundamental component of evidence-based practice, and also supports in the development of trusting relationships between paramedic and patient. This also lays the foundation to look at local community groups or resources that the patient may benefit from.

> Social prescribers and link workers are often well situated to support patients with chronic pain. A good approach to opening discussions regarding social prescribing is something like: 'Modern medicine often struggles to improve or cure pain like this and sometimes treatments make people worse. An alternative is for me to put you in contact with resources and professionals who can help you learn new skills to live better with the pain you carry'.

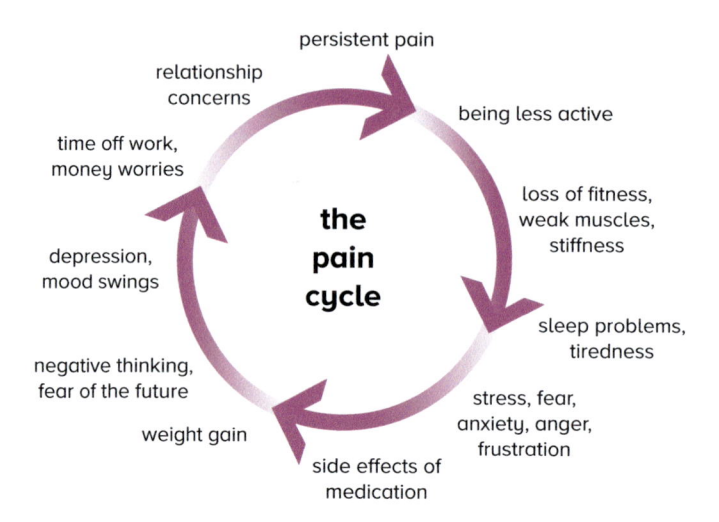

CHAPTER 18 A Note on Assessing and Managing Chronic Pain

Figure 18.1 The pain cycle.

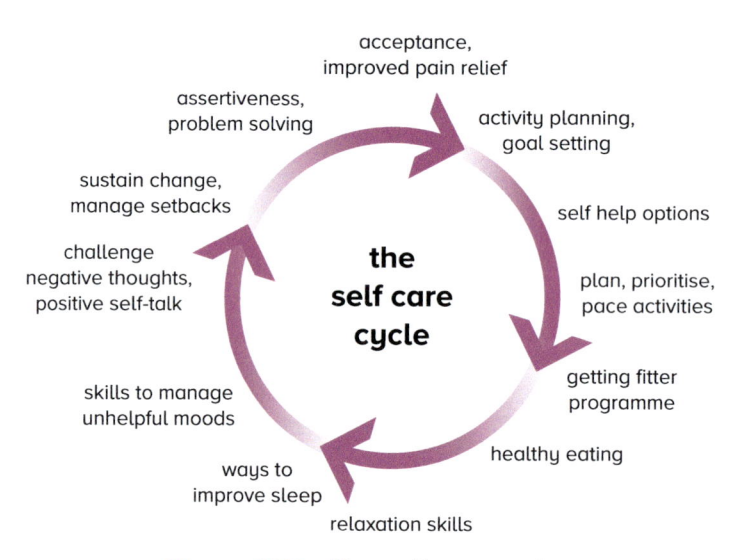

The pain cycle: persistent pain → being less active → loss of fitness, weak muscles, stiffness → sleep problems, tiredness → stress, fear, anxiety, anger, frustration → side effects of medication → weight gain → negative thinking, fear of the future → depression, mood swings → time off work, money worries → relationship concerns → persistent pain.

Figure 18.2 The self-care cycle.

The self care cycle: acceptance, improved pain relief → activity planning, goal setting → self help options → plan, prioritise, pace activities → getting fitter programme → healthy eating → relaxation skills → ways to improve sleep → skills to manage unhelpful moods → challenge negative thoughts, positive self-talk → sustain change, manage setbacks → assertiveness, problem solving → acceptance, improved pain relief.

A companion to the pain cycle is the self-care cycle (Figure 18.2). This cycle shows the positive outcomes of adopting a range of self-management approaches to undo or limit the impact of pain.

Self-management is teaching and learning these skills to become fitter and stronger, to sleep better, to start to understand pain and medications, to pace oneself and deal with setbacks, to get help for relationships and moods and for finances when needed. Together, these can help to re-build a life.

The journey to acceptance of the very significant diagnosis of chronic pain is difficult and life-changing. Sometimes it can take years. Sometimes it is never achieved. Often, people see it as 'giving up' to start with. But in time they realise that without adapting to who you are at present then you will always struggle and battle against your symptoms.

However, embedding sustained changes to beliefs, behaviours, emotions and cognitions can take a huge amount of work by the patient and by the various practitioners required to perform holistic changes – and remember that those practitioners are often not even in existence in many areas for the sheer size of the patient group. There is a woeful imbalance of patients versus professionals who are trained to help those in chronic pain. Because persistent pain does not kill people, it is under-represented in political health policy, unlike conditions like cardiac disease and cancer. But we are now in the technical era of online resources and web-based group therapy so we hope that we can reach and help more and more people.

Ten Footsteps

To guide the self-management of chronic pain, there are 'ten footsteps', developed by Dr Frances Cole (co-founder of Live Well with Pain), to support patients on their journey to live well with pain (Cole, 2017).

The footsteps are centred around:

1. Building knowledge about pain
2. Acceptance that the pain exists, and is part of everyday life
3. Finding the balance of activity and rest breaks (pacing)
4. Goal setting to support change in response to the pain cycle
5. Getting fit and staying active
6. Managing moods
7. Achieving a healthier sleep pattern
8. Healthy eating, managing relationships and coping with work
9. Relaxation and mindfulness
10. Managing setbacks.

Together, these footsteps can help patients start the journey of the self-care cycle and continue on that cycle to manage their pain.

> A range of further resources is available on the Live Well with Pain website, aimed at both patients and clinicians: https://livewellwithpain.co.uk.

The Role of Medications

Chemicals have been used to treat pain for thousands of years, and that is not going to stop. And it should not stop, because some chemicals are life-changing for some people with pain. For example, break your ankle and feel the difference when 10 mg of intravenous morphine hits your mu-receptors. Similarly, see the patient with bony metastases from prostate cancer who can get up and walk again with a sensible dose of a transdermal opioid. No side effects, lots of benefits and it is good medicine. However, the benefits in the context of chronic pain are rarely so clear. Improvement in pain and function is less likely and side effects and risks accrue over time.

There are three broad categories of analgesic medications:

- Non-opioid analgesics, which includes non-steroidal anti-inflammatory drugs (NSAIDs) and paracetamol
- 'Adjuvant analgesics', which are a diverse group of drugs (which includes neuropathic agents) that have primary indications other than pain relief but may be analgesic in selected circumstances
- Opioid analgesics.

Non-opioid Analgesics

Paracetamol

Often considered a stable first step on the analgesic ladder, paracetamol has limited side effects (BNF, 2023a). However, the evidence is that it probably does not work at all for chronic pain, where large, independent clinical trials and reviews from the Cochrane Library show it to be no better than placebo for chronic back pain or arthritis (Saragiotto et al., 2016). Whilst it may be limited in effect, it is dangerous in overdose, and careful attention needs to be given to the frequency of administration (both prescribed and as taken by the patient in an effort to reduce their pain).

NSAIDs and COXII Inhibitors

This group of drugs provide their analgesic properties via their anti-inflammatory properties, blocking the cyclo-oxygenase pathway, and are therefore particularly useful for the treatment of patients with chronic disease accompanied by pain and inflammation. They are also suitable for the relief of pain caused by secondary bone tumours, many of which produce lysis of bone and release prostaglandins. Due to the risks of upper gastrointestinal bleeding, provocation of cardiovascular events and acute kidney injury, they should be used with caution in those at risk, and depending on their degree of risk (Coxib and traditional NSAID Trialists' (CNT) Collaboration, 2013). For example, if a patient has had mild dyspepsia with NSAID in the past, then this is not a contraindication. However, if they have previously been hospitalised with a bleeding peptic ulcer then NSAIDs should not be used. In a patient with hypertension as a single cardiovascular risk factor, who tells you that NSAID makes their joints so much better that they can get out and about and enjoy their life, then on balance of the risk and benefit, a prescription is justified. However, such patients must be aware of the risks and a shared decision made. For patients who have had a heart attack or have heart failure, then the risk is too great (Davis and Robson, 2016).

Prescriptions should be risk assessed and closely monitored using the lowest dose for the shortest time and gastro-protection when required. It is important that the patient is aware of the risks and accepts them. And the drugs should not be prescribed if the risks are too high.

Nefopam Hydrochloride

This is often prescribed when there has been no relief from paracetamol or basic NSAIDs, and the British National Formulary (BNF) recommends it may have a place in the relief of persistent pain unresponsive to other non-opioid analgesics (BNF, 2023b). It causes little or no respiratory depression, but sympathomimetic and antimuscarinic side effects may be troublesome.

Adjuvant Analgesics

These types of drugs are usually tried when the pain is neuropathic in nature, due to direct damage or irritation to the peripheral or central pain neurones rather than from the stimulation of nociceptors. Neuropathic pain has typical features, being described as burning, tingling, electric, stabbing, unrelenting and independent of activity and position. Neuropathic pain medications provide little instant pain relief and are best used regularly 'by the clock' to enable pain relief to accrue gradually over time. In addition to their potential benefits, all of these drug classes are associated with various adverse effects, though experiences of these do tend to reduce over time (Portenoy, 2020).

> 💡 When determining whether pain may be neuropathic in nature, the associated features can be a clue. Look for allodynia (pain resulting from a non-painful stimulus, for example light stroking of the skin or a cold wind) and hyperaesthesia (oversensitivity).

NICE (2020) guidance outlines that a choice of tricyclic antidepressants (for example, amitriptyline), gabapentinoids (for example, gabapentin or pregabalin) or duloxetine should be offered as initial treatment for neuropathic pain (except trigeminal neuralgia). If the first one offered does not work, swap to a different drug. Again, if that does not work, swap to another, and so on.

> 💡 The choice of the first drug offered might depend on if there are co-existing problems, for example if sleep is poor then amitriptyline would be good; alternatively if the patient experiences co-existent depression, then try duloxetine.

A standard approach to trialling these medications is:
1) Prescribe the drug, but do not activate repeat prescription.
2) Titrate dose as appropriate.
3) The patient may experience side effects, but these will hopefully diminish over time.
4) After 2–4 weeks on final dose, review the patient and ask them whether their quality of life has increased since starting these drugs.
5) If the answer is clearly 'yes', continue the medication, reviewing the continuing need for the medication every few months.

If the answer is not yes, wean and discontinue the medication, and look to start an alternative.

CHAPTER 18 A Note on Assessing and Managing Chronic Pain

Tricyclic Antidepressants (TCAs)

Amitriptyline has the best evidence regarding neuropathic pain, though there have been concerns regarding overestimation of treatment effect in its use for chronic pain (Moore et al., 2015). Therefore, it is important for paramedics to be cognisant of the fact that only a small number of people will achieve satisfactory pain relief using this medicine.

> Gabapentin and pregabalin are Schedule 3 controlled drugs under the Misuse of Drugs Regulations 2001, and Class C of the Misuse of Drugs Act 1971.
>
> As well as a reduction in pain, possible additional benefits include improved sleep and, at higher doses, improved mood (it is, after all, an antidepressant). However, if it causes excessive sedation, consider nortripyline which is less sedating.

Gabapentinoids

Over half of those treated with gabapentinoids will not have worthwhile pain relief and may experience adverse events. Dizziness, sleepiness, water retention and problems with walking all occurred in about one in ten people who took gabapentin, according to the most recent Cochrane review (Wiffen et al., 2017). Similar findings occur with pregabalin, where dizziness and sleepiness occurred in about one to three in ten people who took it (Derry et al., 2019). It is therefore important that a discussion on the side effects of the medicine is had prior to starting either prescription as a drug of choice. As it is not possible to know beforehand who will benefit and who will not, a short trial (of perhaps four weeks) is recommended.

> Slightly more people taking gabapentinoids stop taking it because of its side effects; however, serious side effects are normally uncommon.

There is no significant difference between the two drugs for decreasing pain and adverse events (Davari et al., 2020).

Duloxetine

Duloxetine is a drug that is licensed for use in treating clinical depression as well as urinary incontinence that is caused by stress. In the context of treating neuropathic pain, it also has a possible additional benefit of mood improvement. Although duloxetine is beneficial in the treatment of neuropathic pain and fibromyalgia, there is little evidence from trials comparing duloxetine to other antidepressant drugs as to which is better. Most people taking duloxetine will have at least one side effect (Lunn et al., 2014). These are mostly minor, and the most common are feeling sick, being too awake or too sleepy, headache, dry mouth, constipation or dizziness. About one in six people stop duloxetine because of side effects, but again serious problems caused by duloxetine are very rare.

Opioids

Opioid analgesics have a good reputation in acute and cancer-related pain, but there is little evidence that they are helpful for long-term pain. Indeed, the use of opioids for chronic pain can be a disaster. This problem is they do work well, to start with. There are a large number of randomised control trials and systematic reviews that conclude that opioids reduce pain for some patients in the short and medium term (usually less than 12 weeks) for a number of chronic painful conditions (Hauser et al., 2015). However, after that golden 12 weeks, the original pain symptoms start creeping back in as the neural networks readjust their sensitivity to the effect of the chemical on the receptors. So, after a couple of months the symptoms are back to square one *and* the patient is now on an opioid. If you stop the opioid now, you will have an unpleasant eight weeks of worsened pain before stabilising back to baseline – the opposite of starting it. So, what often happens after two to three months is that the dose is increased and again there is an eight-week 'honeymoon' period of improved pain and function. Despite there being no good evidence of long-term benefit of opioids in chronic pain, patients end up being prescribed higher and higher doses (FPM, 2023).

Should We Not Use Opioids for Chronic Pain?

The human body loves opioids. They give a feeling of calm, euphoria, relaxation and a lifting of (physical and emotional) pain, often called the 'warm hug'. When the human body has been exposed to opioids for a few weeks, it starts getting used to the warm hug and sometimes it wants more. Or, if the opioid is withdrawn, then there is the opposite feeling – the 'cold sting' where one feels anxious, jittery, sweaty, experiences diarrhoea and widespread pain. To avoid the cold sting and to seek the warm hug, the human body will desire more opioids. This is called dependence. This is not a character flaw or the sign of a weak or defective personality; this is basic pharmacology, physiology and psychology. Sometimes, the body's desire for opioids becomes so strong that the person's behaviours change. They start prioritising opioids over other parts of their life, work and family life can disintegrate and they might beg, borrow or steal to get opioids. This change in behaviour is called addiction – different from dependence (although the words are often used interchangeably).

With the evidence we have, a therapeutic trial of traditional opioids can be used in modest doses over about two to four weeks (FPM, 2023). The drug should be tried cautiously and watched closely for improved function and side effects, and misuse should be caught early. If there is a sustained overall benefit in function (not just pain levels) without side effects or misuse, then a repeat prescription with regular review is reasonable. Side effects or misuse should terminate opioid prescribing, with warnings for the future in the patient notes.

> There are some patients (such as those with a previous history of drug misuse) where initial prescribing of any opioid is just too hazardous. Do not put them in that position, and encourage the trial of alternatives.

CHAPTER 18   A Note on Assessing and Managing Chronic Pain

The Opioid Therapeutic Trial

Despite the problems, regular use of a potent opioid may be appropriate for certain cases of chronic non-malignant pain. Regardless of whether you are going to try a weak, medium or strong opioid, the strategy is the same. Start at a dose where you would hope for or expect to see a benefit. Review every week or two for a few weeks. Increase up to the highest dose you and the patient feel comfortable with. If after a few weeks there is not significant functional improvement, wean and stop the drug. And do not try it again – the trial has failed.

If there is improvement, then, if you are both happy, continue with another review in about two months. If the significant functional improvement persists, continue; if not, wean and stop – the trial has failed.

Then review two to four times a year. Always look for opportunities to climb down the ladder, for example if the patient is making headway with self-management tools.

> BNF (2023a) Analgesics [online].
> This analgesic treatment summary outlines the range of opioids that can be suitable for use in pain management.

Remember that these drugs have killed an enormous number of people worldwide – the 'opioid epidemic', most notably in the USA. From 1999 to 2020, opioids were responsible for more than 500,000 deaths, and prescription opioids account for more than a quarter of these (CDC, 2022).

Chapter Summary

You cannot use principles like the analgesic ladder when treating someone who experiences chronic pain. Pharmacological treatment can help (sometimes), but the essence of management is for the patient and paramedic to understand what it is and what it is not, and to identify what facets of chronic pain are most important to that patient.

With the ten footsteps self-management resource and wise prescribing, you can start your patient on a journey towards a life that they find acceptable and rewarding whilst protecting them from the risks of unnecessary drugs and healthcare interventions so prevalent with the current management of chronic pain in primary care.

Acknowledgements

We are forever indebted to Dr Frances Cole, a retired GP, who has made her life's work the understanding and promotion of self-management strategies for chronic pain. She has received a lifetime achievement award from the British Pain Society. She has written various books, and hosts the Live Well with Pain website for patients and clinicians alike. Thank you, Frances.

References

British National Formulary (BNF) (2023a) Analgesics. Available at: https://bnf.nice.org.uk/treatment-summary/analgesics.html (accessed 28 January 2023).

British National Formulary (BNF) (2023b) Nefopam hydrochloride. Available at: https://bnf.nice.org.uk/drug/nefopam-hydrochloride.html (accessed 28 January 2023).

Centers for Disease Control and Prevention (CDC) (2022) Understanding the epidemic. Available at: https://www.cdc.gov/drugoverdose/epidemic/index.html (accessed 28 January 2023).

Cole, F. (2017) *An Introduction to Living Well with Pain*. London: Little, Brown.

Coxib and traditional NSAID Trialists' (CNT) Collaboration (2013) Vascular and upper gastrointestinal effects of non-steroidal anti-inflammatory drugs: Meta-analyses of individual participant data from randomised trials. *Lancet* 382(9894): 769–779.

Davari, M., Amani, B., Amani, B. et al. (2020) Pregabalin and gabapentin in neuropathic pain management after spinal cord injury: A systematic review and meta-analysis. *The Korean Journal of Pain* 33(1): 3–12.

Davis, A. and Robson, J. (2016) The dangers of NSAIDs: Look both ways. *British Journal of General Practice* 66(645): 172–173.

Derry, S., Bell, R., Straube, S. et al. (2019) Pregabalin for neuropathic pain in adults. *Cochrane Database of Systematic Reviews* 2019(1): CD007076.

Faculty of Pain Medicine (FPM) (2023) Clinical use of opioids. Available at: https://fpm.ac.uk/opioids-aware/clinical-use-opioids (accessed 28 January 2023).

Fayaz, A., Croft, P., Langford, R.M. et al. (2016) Prevalence of chronic pain in the UK: A systematic review and meta-analysis of population studies. *BMJ Open* 6: e010364.

Gregory, A. and Collins, D. (2019) Britain's opioid epidemic kills five every day. *The Times*. Available at: https://www.thetimes.co.uk/article/britains-opioid-epidemic-kills-five-every-day-83md7wc3k (accessed 28 January 2023).

Hart, O., Uden, R.M., McMullen, J.E. et al. (2015). A study of National Health Service management of chronic osteoarthritis and low back pain. *Primary Health Care Research & Development* 16(2): 157–166.

Hauser, W., Bernardy, K. and Maier, C. (2015) Long-term opioid therapy in chronic noncancer pain: A systematic review and meta-analysis of efficacy, tolerability and safety in open-label extension trials with study duration of at least 26 weeks. *Schmerz* 29(1): 96–108.

Lunn, M.P.T., Hughes, R.A.C. and Wiffen, P.J. (2014) Duloxetine for treating painful neuropathy, chronic pain or fibromyalgia. *Cochrane Database of Systematic Reviews* 2014(1): CD007115.

McGreevy, K., Bottros, M.M. and Raja, S.N. (2011) Preventing chronic pain following acute pain: Risk factors, preventive strategies, and their efficacy. *European Journal of Pain Supplements* 5(2): 365–372.

Misuse of Drugs Act (England and Wales) 1971. Available at: https://www.legislation.gov.uk/ukpga/1971/38/contents (accessed 28 January 2023).

Moore, R.A., Derry, S., Aldington, D. et al. (2015) Amitriptyline for neuropathic pain in adults. *Cochrane Database of Systematic Reviews* 2015(7): CD008242.

National Institute for Health and Care Excellence (NICE) (2020) Neuropathic pain in adults: Pharmacological management in non-specialist settings [CG173]. Available at: https://www.nice.org.uk/guidance/cg173/chapter/Recommendations#key-principles-of-care (accessed 28 January 2023).

CHAPTER 18   A Note on Assessing and Managing Chronic Pain

National Institute for Health and Care Excellence (NICE) (2021) Chronic pain (primary and secondary) in over 16s: Assessment of all chronic pain and management of chronic primary pain [NG193]. Available at: https://www.nice.org.uk/guidance/ng193/chapter/Context#:~:text=Chronic%20pain%20(sometimes%20known%20as,pain%20can%20also%20be%20primary (accessed 28 January 2023).

Portenoy, R.K. (2020) A practical approach to using adjuvant analgesics in older adults. *Journal of the American Geriatrics Society* 68: 691.

Saragiotto, B.T., Machado, G.C., Ferreira, M.L. et al. (2016) Paracetamol for low back pain. *Cochrane Database of Systematic Reviews* 2016(6): CD012230.

The Misuse of Drugs Regulations (England and Wales) 2001. Available at: https://www.legislation.gov.uk/uksi/2001/3998/contents/made (accessed 28 January 2023).

Vos, T., Allen, C. and Arora, M. (2016) Global, regional, and national incidence, prevalence, and years lived with disability for 310 diseases and injuries, 1990–2015: A systematic analysis for the Global Burden of Disease Study 2015. *Lancet* 388(10053): 1545–1602.

Wiffen, P.J., Derry, S., Bell, R.F. et al. (2017) Gabapentin for chronic neuropathic pain in adults. *Cochrane Database of Systematic Reviews* 2017(6): CD007938.

Safeguarding Considerations   19

Karen Kitchener

Introduction

Safeguarding is not just the responsibility of one practitioner. It takes a team to identify concerns and issues that may arise within any healthcare setting to ensure the safety of their patients. Of crucial importance here is the acknowledgement that the safeguarding 'team' does not simply consist of a centralised group of specialist safeguarding leads, but includes the frontline clinician seeing the patient and members from other health sectors, such as midwives, school nurses, health visitors, social workers, key workers and mental health practitioners. Thus the mantra 'safeguarding is everyone's responsibility'.

As the role of the paramedic in primary care evolves, it is necessary to understand where we fit into this form of multi-agency working and how we can safely treat our patients. Reports from national statistics indicate that there has been a steady rise in reported incidences of safeguarding referral for children and adults, which is thought to possibly indicate better use of reporting systems and an increased awareness of needs amongst practitioners. This is shown in Figure 19.1 for children and Table 19.1 for adults.

This chapter is designed as a guide to help understand the process of safeguarding and how to raise concerns in primary care. It does not cover the elements of safeguarding for children or adults that are covered in mandatory safeguarding training and benchmarked in the inter-collegial framework document, and paramedics in primary care are encouraged to ensure completion of regular training on this subject.

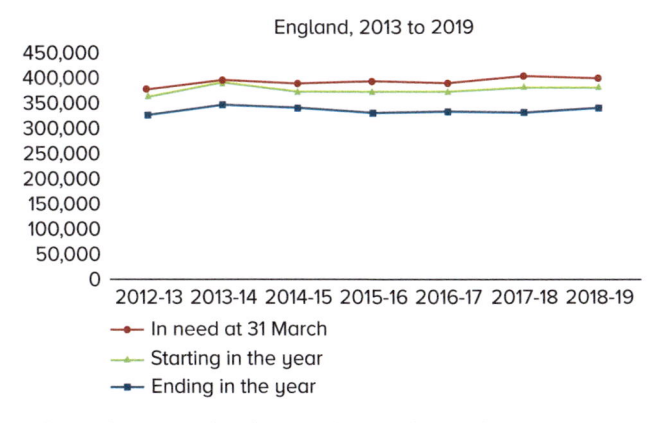

Figure 19.1 Reported incidences of safeguarding referral for children.

CHAPTER 19 Safeguarding Considerations

Table 19.1 Reported Incidences of Safeguarding Referral for Adults

Measure	2015–2016	2016–2017	2017–2018
Count of safeguarding concerns	231,220	364,605	394,655
Count of section 42 enquiries	99,805	133,265	131,860
Count of other safeguarding enquiries	11,655	17,895	18,210

Source: Safeguarding Adults Collection Table SG1f, NHS Digital (2021).

Safeguarding Adults

The pre-requisite for any healthcare practitioner working with adults is Level One and Level Two safeguarding training. Any healthcare practitioner who is involved in care planning assessing, intervening and evaluating adult safeguarding concerns requires Level 3. Level 3-trained practitioners could be named safeguarding leads. Designated professionals would require Levels 4 and 5 and these should all be reviewed on a regular basis to ensure all training needs are met. Figure 19.2 clearly shows the training needs of practitioners in primary care.

Level 5: Specialist roles, designated professionals within commissioning organisations, providing advice and guidance across the health and social care community

Level 4: Specialist roles, such as named GP/Practitioner Lead of Children/Adult Safeguarding

Level 3: Registered healthcare professionals, HCPC, NMC, GMC, GPC

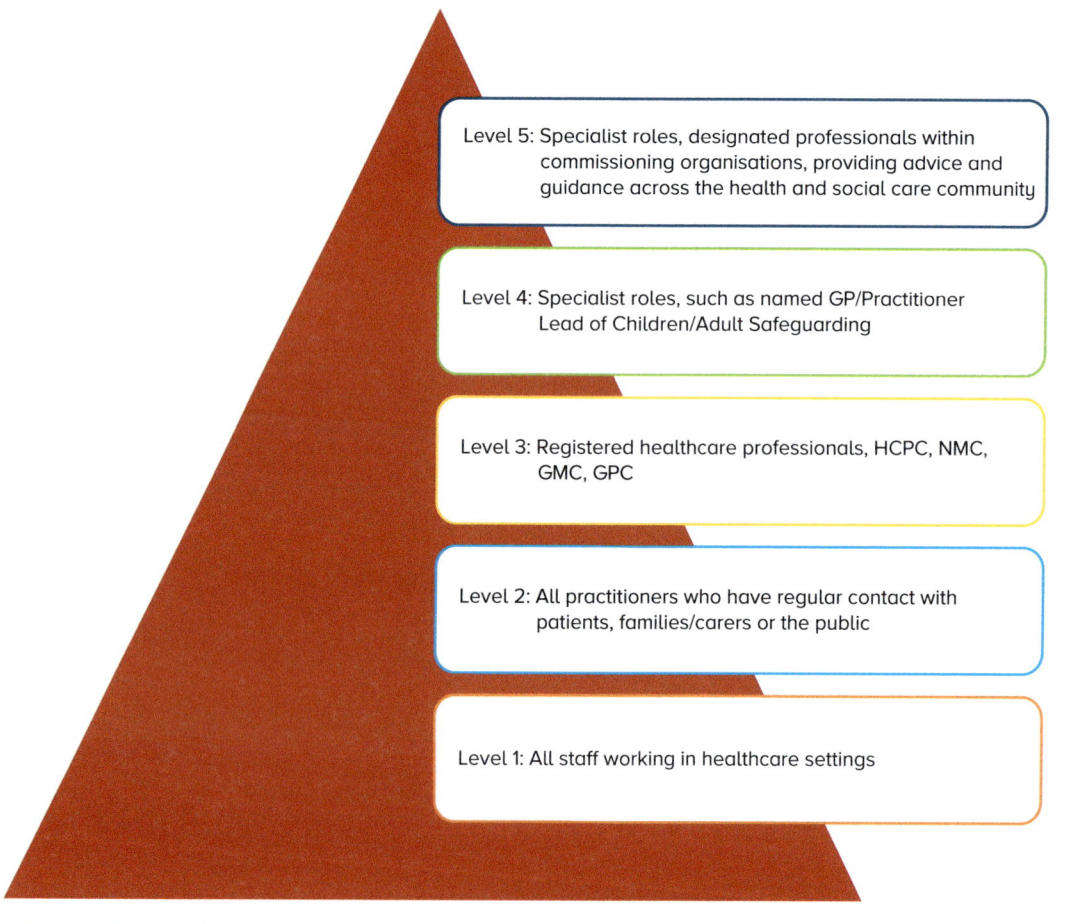

Level 2: All practitioners who have regular contact with patients, families/carers or the public

Level 1: All staff working in healthcare settings

Figure 19.2 Safeguarding training requirements for healthcare professionals.

Safeguarding Adults

In 2018, groundbreaking adult safeguarding guidance was launched by the Royal College of Nursing (RCN), with the support of the Royal College of General Practitioners (RCGP), providing professional guidance and standards that should be met by all healthcare professionals looking after adults over 18 years of age. This document outlines six principles that underpin adult safeguarding (RCN, 2018):

1. Empowerment: Personalisation and the presumption of person-led decisions and informed consent.
2. Prevention: It is better to take action before harm occurs.
3. Proportionality: Proportionate and least-intrusive response appropriate to the risk presented.
4. Protection: Support and representation for those in greatest need.
5. Partnership: Local solutions through services working with their communities. Communities have a part to play in preventing, identifying and reporting neglect and abuse.
6. Accountability: Accountability and transparency in delivering safeguarding.

Table 19.2 is a brief outline of concerns, and identifies suitable courses of action with each type of abuse that may be encountered whilst working in primary care and attending home visits. In particular, home visits provide a unique opportunity to establish concerns and risks to patients' overall well-being.

Identifying Safeguarding Issues and Concerns

In most cases of concern, patients will present multiple times with minor injuries or illness to multiple and different healthcare providers. Sometimes this is to avoid detection. Where concerns are raised in consultation, due to the presentation of the patient and information shared, it is worth considering several factors:

- The environment you are in
- Whether it is safe for the patient to talk
- Never discuss with family members or friends, or with children over two years of age present
- The ability to create an opportunity to ask questions in a safe setting, and whether the patient feels able to discuss
- If language is a barrier, use a professional interpreter (never a family member or friend).

> ! Safeguarding concerns should be considered for every presentation – even the first one.

These may give further insight or indication of multiple types of abuse and may cause you to raise a safeguarding concern. It is important to remember that the patient may not be willing to disclose information for fear of reprisal. It is always worth reviewing the medical history of the patient and the safeguarding node of their clinical notes to see if concerns have previously been raised, particularly as these may match the information that is now

CHAPTER 19 Safeguarding Considerations

Table 19.2 Responding to Safeguarding Concerns

Types of abuse	Safeguarding referral may be required – speak to lead	Safeguarding referral – police may be required	Safeguarding referral – referral to police
Physical (falls)	Fall occurring when in receipt of care (long bone fracture)	Fall causing significant harm to person where previous concerns identified – insufficient prevention methods identified, numerous falls affecting more than one person in the same setting	One fall causing catastrophic harm to one person, possible hospitalisation, irreversible damage or death where previous concerns identified
Physical	Inexplicable marking or lesions, burns, cuts or grip marks on a number of occasions	Inappropriate restraint, inexplicable fractures or injuries to any part of the body at various stages of healing	Assault or grievous bodily harm leading to significant harm, irreversible damage or death
Physical (pressure ulcers)	High frailty index not risk assessed for pressure concerns, failure to follow advice from professionals, preventable pressure ulcers **If affecting more than one person in setting, consider organisational abuse**	As per previous box **If affecting more than one person in setting, consider organisational abuse**	Catastrophic harm, injury or death with regards to pressure ulcer risk and management, failure to provide suitable pressure-relieving equipment **If affecting more than one person in setting, consider organisational abuse**
Medication	One-off medication error to more than one person – no harm caused Medication error resulting in healthcare intervention Appearance of over-medication or ineffectiveness of medication	Deliberate misadministration of medication Covert administration without proper medical supervision	Reoccurring errors, or incidence of deliberate misadministration, resulting in ill health or death Catastrophic harm to more than one person

Sexual	Isolated incident where inappropriate sexual remark is made to an **adult** Verbalised sexual teasing that causes offence (Victim should be offered referral to police)	One-off or reoccurring sexualised touch or isolated or reoccurring masturbation without consent Attempted penetration by any means without consent Sexual harassment Sexualised relationship between staff and patients	Sex in a relationship characterised by authority, inequality or exploitation Rape Being made to look at pornographic material without consent Being subject to indecent exposure
Psychological	Treatment that undermines dignity and damages self-esteem Denying or failing to recognise adult's choice or opinion Frequent verbal outbursts Withholding information to disempower	Humiliation Emotional blackmail (threats of abandonment or harm) Taunts or verbal outbursts that cause distress	Denial of human rights or civil liberties Prolonged intimidation Vicious personalised verbal attacks
Deprivation of liberty	Lack of policy or practices that recognise deprivation of liberty	Restriction of liberty repeatedly unreported	Deprivation of liberty so significant that there is evidence of neglect or physical harm
Self-neglect	Consider both decisional and executive capacity; a self-neglecting person who recognises an action is required but lacks the ability to undertake it, or a person lacking ability to refrain from self-harming behaviour If the person does not have capacity and there is perceived harm, or refuses interventions to prevent harm	Organisational approach to self-neglect is of concern (consider organisational abuse)	Organisational approach to self-neglect is of concern (consider organisational abuse)
Domestic abuse	Refer to local domestic abuse, stalking and honour-based violence (DASH) risk assessment	Sexual, emotional, financial or physical abuse from family members or intimate partners	Forced marriage 'Honour' violence

(Continued)

CHAPTER 19 Safeguarding Considerations

Table 19.2 (Continued)

Types of abuse	Safeguarding referral may be required – speak to lead	Safeguarding referral – police may be required	Safeguarding referral – referral to police
Modern slavery	Discuss with local lead DASH assessment	Not applicable	Any concerns about slavery, human trafficking, forced labour or domestic servitude must be reported to police
Financial	Adult's money in joint account without access or arrangement for equal access Adults denied access to own funds Staff and carers personally benefiting from support offered to service users	Misuse or misappropriation of property, possessions or benefits by person of trust or control Personal finances removed from adult's control	Fraud exploitation relating to income benefits, property or will Theft
Neglect (clinical care plans)	Poor-quality clinical care plans, affecting one person, causing harm or distress Previous concerns about clinical care plans not addressed locally	Poor-quality clinical care plans, affecting more than one person, causing harm or distress (Consideration of organisational abuse)	Poor clinical care plans, leading to catastrophic harm of one person – hospitalisation, irreparable harm or death Causing significant harm to more than one person Insufficient prevention measures in place
Neglect (discharge from a clinical setting)	Poor discharge from clinical setting, leading to support services not being set up, causing harm or distress	Poor discharge from clinical setting, leading to no referral to support services and to significant harm	Poor discharge from clinical setting, leading to no referral to support services, and to catastrophic harm
Organisational	Rigid inflexible routines, dignity undermined, care planning not person centred, poor or no continuity of care or handovers, no policies in place that recognise safeguarding	Bad practice unreported and unchecked Unsafe, unhygienic living environments	Staff misusing position of power, over-medication or restraint used to manage behaviour and widespread ill treatment or poor access to treatment within institutional setting

Safeguarding Adults

shared in the consultation. This may highlight a pattern of multiple healthcare attendances or frequent non-attendance to appointments for clinics or at the surgery.

Other indicators of abuse may be identified through the appearance and presentation of the patient, such as:

- Bruising injuries in various stages of healing
- Mental capacity to make a decision
- Delays in presentation or evidence of obstacles in seeking or receiving treatment or care
- Hydration and nutrition (over or underweight)
- Personal presentation (well-groomed or dishevelled)
- Reaction to other people present at the consultation.

Vulnerable patients and those at risk of abuse can fall into several categories. These include but are not limited to:

- Drug or alcohol abuse
- Immigration status – legal or asylum
- Language barriers
- Learning disabilities
- Limited family or friend networks
- Low-income families
- Mental health concerns.

> These patients may not be aware of the support available to them, such as advocacy services, specific support services and alcohol and drug services. As a result, they may present in primary care with low mood or anxiety issues, which require support through outreach teams or support workers. Social prescribing initiatives are also very useful in these circumstances, and it is worth identifying the resources available in your own area of practice.

One of the main under-reported concerns is domestic violence and physical abuse of the adult.

Recently updated legislation – the Domestic Abuse Act 2021 – outlines that domestic abuse can occur between two people who are 'each aged 16 or over and are personally connected to each other'. This supersedes the requirement of being, or having been, in a relationship or being family members, and has some important ramifications in scenarios where friends or family members are co-habiting. The presentation of these patients may be for minor ailments, chronic and non-specific complaints or other concerns, and patients may present on multiple occasions.

> It is exceptionally easy to miss the underlying cause for presentations as a safeguarding concern if we are not already considering safeguarding for each patient within our biopsychosocial model of assessment.

CHAPTER 19 Safeguarding Considerations

Equally, system-based issues such as time constraints of the consultation, distracting performance indicators or attitudes of the practitioner can equally funnel us into considering the medical aspect of assessment and management, without consideration of safeguarding concerns. Of equal note is having a suspicion of a safeguarding issue but assuming that this will be raised elsewhere.

> 💡 If safeguarding reports are received from a number of different agencies, this will assist with building a more holistic picture and elevate the concern more quickly.

As clinicians with a duty of care to our patients, it behoves us to take on the responsibility of raising concerns when we have them and never assuming that this will be done by someone else.

> 📄 There are many toolkits available online to help the practitioner and patient needing advice. The main suggested application is the NHS safeguarding one, which can take you through a multitude of questions and resources. As always, it is worth finding out which kinds of support are available in your area of work.

When you are unsure whether an issue should be escalated to a referral, the following issues should be considered:

- The seriousness, nature and degree of concern of the alleged incident
- Whether there has been an appropriate response to meet the needs of the adult at risk
- The impact on the individual
- The likelihood and severity of re-occurrence
- The complexity of the situation requiring a multi-agency response
- Where poor-quality care or practice by a care provider or individual is considered to be extensive (for example, missed calls over a weekend leaving a service user in bed without food or medication).

> 💡 Even 'accidental' or non-malicious harm or neglect should be referred, as these experiences, whilst considered minor, can be a learning experience for the perpetrator.

Reporting

When a concern has been identified or there is a need for further support, you will need to gain the consent from the patient before acting. You should provide awareness that you have concerns and, to protect the patient, you now need to share these concerns. Understanding of an individual's capacity to consent and of deprivation of liberty

Safeguarding Adults

safeguarding is required of all practitioners working with patients and services users. If the patient does not consent to information being shared, you are still required to document all concerns in the patient notes and notify the safeguarding lead for your area. This person may be advised that a referral is made for the safety of the patient, and of any children living at the address or associated with the patient and perpetrator (or perpetrators), or for that of services users if an organisation is involved.

In all cases of safeguarding concerns, you should be aware of the safeguarding lead for your area, and all concerns should be discussed with them. This usually requires a referral process to social services or the Multi-Agency Safeguarding Hub (MASH) through the multi-agency framework as detailed in Figure 19.3. If concerns are related to domestic violence or abuse, then a separate form, known as the referral to the Independent Domestic Violence

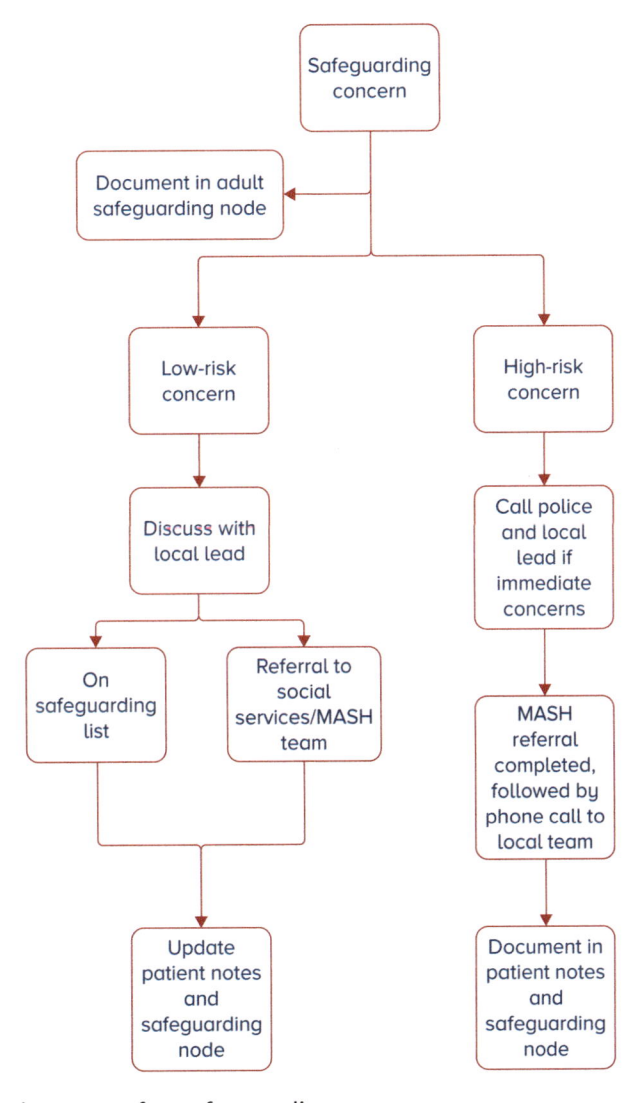

Figure 19.3 Referral process for safeguarding concern.

483

CHAPTER 19 Safeguarding Considerations

Advisor (IDVA) form, should be used which is then sent to the Multi-Agency Risk Assessment Conference (MARAC).

The police will need to be notified if there is immediate concern of harm and danger to the patient or family. Contact numbers and processes are specific to each county and will need identifying in the workplace. Once a referral has been made, Figure 19.4 shows how that information is used to help investigate concerns.

Once all areas have been assessed and a plan has been put in place, there will often be regular reviews as to whether this has supported the patient sufficiently.

> NHS England (2019) Safeguarding adults [online].

Safeguarding Children

The RCN (2018) safeguarding guidance identifies six levels of competence, and it is suggested that clinical staff with some degree of contact with children should have a minimum of Level 2 safeguarding training. Clinical staff working with children, young people and their parents or carers, or any adult who could pose a risk to children, who could potentially contribute to assessing, planning, intervening or evaluating the needs of a child or young person or parenting capacity, where there are safeguarding or child protection concerns, should have at least Level 3 training. Levels 3 and upwards is for named professionals, designated professionals and experts. These training levels are a pre-requisite for working in primary care, and it is a requirement that all staff update these qualifications regularly.

As with adult safeguarding, you should be aware of the safeguarding leads in your area and your mandatory safeguarding training should make you aware of how to identify concerns. Identification of safeguarding concerns can be more difficult with children, as there can be many additional factors, such as language and age; and there can be increased likelihood of accidents, due to their developing motor skills and curiosity in development, that are not a safeguarding concern.

Identifying Safeguarding Concerns

Defining vulnerable families can be very difficult, and it is important to remember that this is often subjective. A generic understanding is that a vulnerable family could be thought of as a familial living situation that is considered problematic and may require professional support. In most cases, it requires the identification of families at risk of significant harm or neglect and so requiring support to prevent incidences from occurring.

Generally, a vulnerable family can be identified through different categories such as:

- Alcohol dependence
- Drug dependence
- Families experiencing problems with housing
- Families with a parent or child with a disability

Safeguarding Children

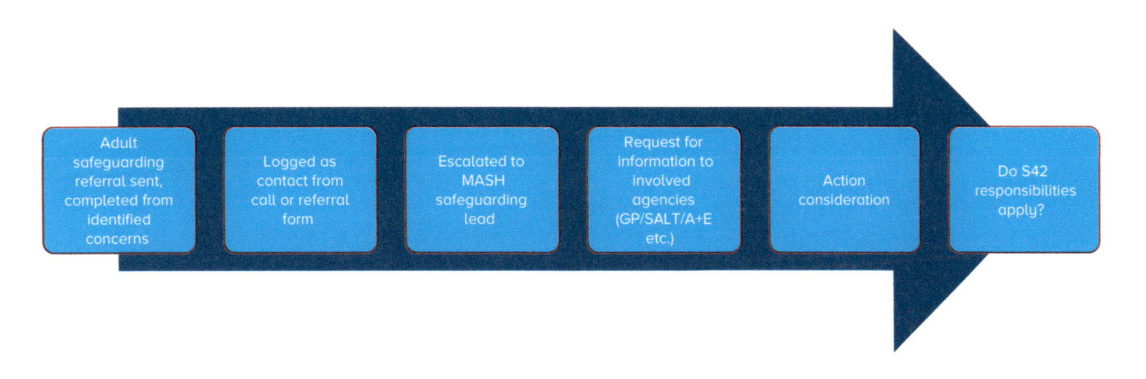

Adult safeguarding referral sent, completed from identified concerns → Logged as contact from call or referral form → Escalated to MASH safeguarding lead → Request for information to involved agencies (GP/SALT/A+E etc.) → Action consideration → Do S42 responsibilities apply?

The Care Act 2014 (Section 42) requires that each local authority must make enquiries, or cause others to do so, if it believes an adult is experiencing, or is at risk of, abuse or neglect. An enquiry should establish whether any action needs to be taken to prevent or stop abuse or neglect, and if so, by whom.

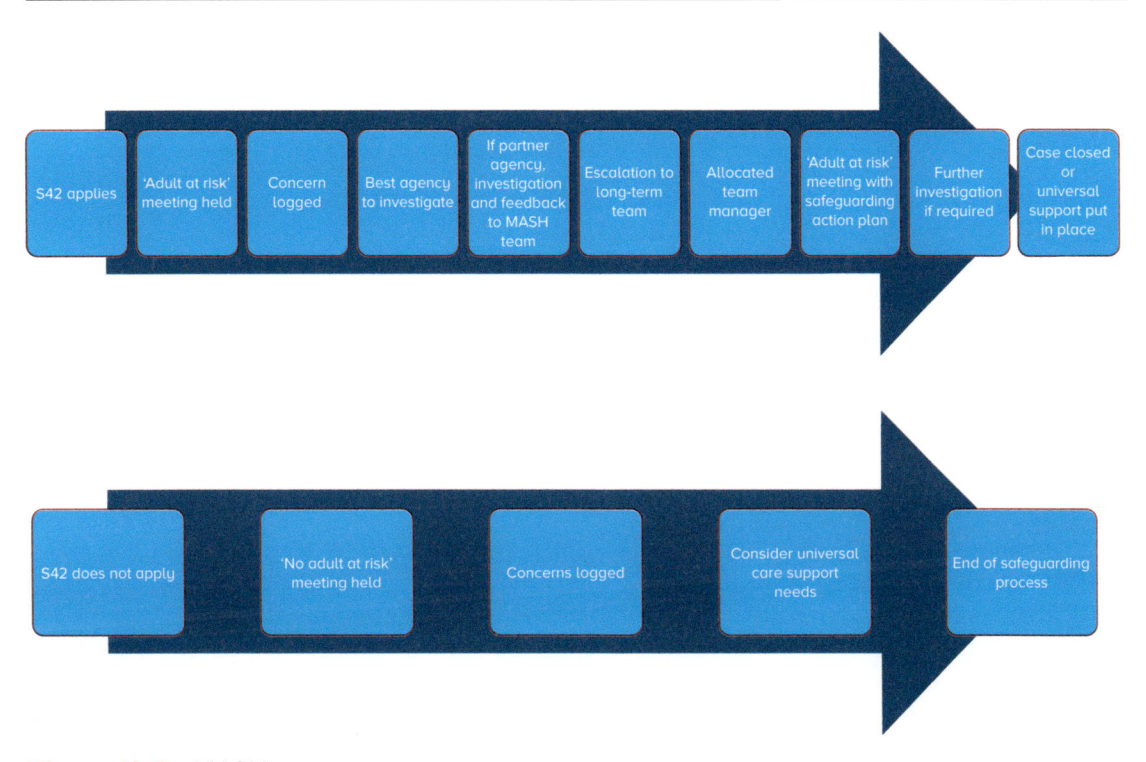

S42 applies → 'Adult at risk' meeting held → Concern logged → Best agency to investigate → If partner agency, investigation and feedback to MASH team → Escalation to long-term team → Allocated team manager → 'Adult at risk' meeting with safeguarding action plan → Further investigation if required → Case closed or universal support put in place

S42 does not apply → 'No adult at risk' meeting held → Concerns logged → Consider universal care support needs → End of safeguarding process

Figure 19.4 MASH process.

- Low-income families
- Mental health concerns (parent or care provider)
- Single-parent families
- Young carers
- Young-parent families.

485

CHAPTER 19   Safeguarding Considerations

Other concerns to note are whether the family has previously had involvement with social services or health visitors. This information can be found on the clinical tree in SystmOne and EMIS, and may indicate a higher level of concern. Early reporting is in the child's best interests, to allow support to be gained early to protect the family and children's well-being.

This is not an exhaustive list, and a family that fits into one or more of these categories is not necessarily a cause for concern or requiring of professional support. However, these categories serve as a useful indicator if there is suspicion of neglect or harm.

In most cases of concern, patients will present multiple times with minor injuries or illnesses to multiple different healthcare providers to avoid detection. Where concerns are raised in consultation due to presentation of the patient and information shared, it is worth considering several factors:

- The environment you are in
- Whether it is safe for the patient to talk
- Never discuss with family members or friends, or with children over two years of age present
- The ability to create an opportunity to ask questions in a safe setting, and whether the patient feels able to discuss
- If language is a barrier, use a professional interpreter (never a family member or friend).

These may give further insight or indication of multiple types of abuse occurring that may give rise to a safeguarding concern as they may not be willing to disclose information for fear of reprisal. It is worth looking at the medical history of the patient and at the safeguarding node of their clinical notes to see if concerns have been raised previously that match the information being shared in the consultation; this may highlight the pattern of multiple healthcare attendances or frequent non-attendance to appointments for clinics or at the surgery.

Other indicators of abuse may be identified through the appearance and presentation of the patient, such as:

- Bruising injuries in various stages of healing
- Mental capacity
- Cultural differences
- Delays or evidence of obstacles in seeking or receiving treatment or care
- Developmental delays, including in social, educational, hygiene, relationships
- Hydration and nutrition (over or underweight)
- Personal presentation (well-groomed or dishevelled)
- Reaction to other people present in the consultation.

If a parent attends for a consultation related to low mood or mental health concerns, and is requiring treatment, it is worth seeking support for the family early on. You must always ensure that you gain consent to discuss with the health visitor or specialist nurse, dependent on the age of the child (or children), to allow discussions to happen with relevant third parties. This ensures that any changes in the child's behaviour are identified early and

Safeguarding Children

addressed to prevent neglect or harm to them, and that early intervention and support is provided.

> There are many processes that can occur once a need has been identified. In the first instance, it is important to record and report the concern to the child safeguarding lead in the practice, making sure that it is well documented in the safeguarding node on the system.

Involvement of Other Healthcare Professionals

Information about safeguarding concerns may be received from multiple sources. One of these could be the ambulance service, and reports of this kind are sent to the local social services and also sometimes to the patient's primary care provider, such as the registered doctor or safeguarding lead. Child Protection-Information Sharing (CP-IS) alerts, accessible via the patient's summary care records, will alert clinicians to the child's status as a 'looked-after child' or if the child is subject to a Child Protection Plan (CPP). It is important to check these notes because it builds a wider picture for healthcare working and allows notification of environmental factors that may be of concern.

Health visitors, midwives and school nurses are also able to share concerns about children through their medical reports and safeguarding node on the patient's clinical notes. In most cases, meetings are held between the surgery safeguarding leads and the home visitor or specialist nurse to discuss ongoing concerns or to identify risks that the others may not be aware of. This allows for better information sharing and so better multi-agency support for the families.

Reporting

In the event that a referral is made to social services, there will be many information-gathering processes undertaken to ensure a whole picture is gained of a child's circumstances. This usually includes requests for information from all agencies involved in the child's well-being, such as primary care, school nurses, health visitors and hospital clinics (which might include specialist teams such as speech and language therapy or diabetes clinics). These requests are usually made through the MASH or police services who, depending on the circumstances, may use the domestic abuse, stalking and honour-based violence (DASH) assessment model. This can take the form of two types of requests – Section 17 or Section 47.

Section 17 (Child in Need)

This places a general duty on all local authorities to 'safeguard and promote the welfare of children within their area who are in need'. Basically, a 'Child in Need' (CIN) is a child who needs additional support from the local authority to meet their potential. Information can be

CHAPTER 19   Safeguarding Considerations

shared in a multi-agency arena, with consent from the parents, if they are under Section 17 of the Children Act (1989). This should be completed within 48 hours of request.

Section 47 (Child Protection)

This requires the local authority to investigate the child's circumstances where they have 'reasonable cause to suspect that a child [...] is suffering, or is likely to suffer, significant harm' and to 'take any action to safeguard or promote the child's welfare'. Local authorities have a duty to provide a range of services to safeguard children and promote their welfare. Consequently, a local authority must investigate any concerns or allegations that suggest a child is likely to suffer physical, emotional or sexual abuse, or neglect, and to take action to prevent this. This should be completed in 24 hours of request.

> 💡 If the family is on a child protection (Section 47) arena, professionals have a statutory duty to share information in order to safeguard the welfare of the child. Whilst it is preferable to obtain parental consent in this setting, it is not mandatory if the clinician feels that disclosing this information would place the child or themselves at risk. If you are unsure about sharing information but are clear that you are acting in the best interests of the child, then you are protecting the child and you should clearly document your rationale for sharing. Consider police intervention if the child needs to be removed immediately.

When a child or family is put under either a CIN plan or a CPP, there may be multiple review points where up-to-date information can be requested. Examples of this are shown in Boxes 19.1, 19.2, 19.3 and 19.4.

BOX 19.1   Name of the Adult

1. Does the adult have any ongoing health concerns?
2. Do you have comments to make regarding parent–child relationships?
3. Are any other health professionals involved with this family? If so, what are the details?
4. Any other information you would like to share?

Signature:

Print Name:

Date:

Safeguarding Children

BOX 19.2 Request for Information

Name:

1. When did they register at the practice?
2. Are immunisations up to date?
3. Have they been diagnosed with any condition?
4. Any support offered previously if there is any?
5. Any CAHMS referral? If yes, what is the outcome?
6. Are they on any regular medication?
7. Have they attended all of their appointments?
8. When were they last seen?
9. Any safeguarding concerns?
10. Are any other health professionals involved with this family? If so, is there any other information you would like to share?

Signature:

Please print your name:

Date:

BOX 19.3

Family name:		Date of meeting:
GP's name		Contact details

Forename	Surname	Date of birth	Sex	Address	Ethnicity/ language	Additional needs	School / other setting

Other household members and those of importance to the child or young person:

Full name	Relationship	Parental responsibility	Address (if not the same as above)

CHAPTER 19   Safeguarding Considerations

> **BOX 19.4**   The Report
>
> Are you worried about?
>
> > For example: What has happened to these child(ren) or young person(s), adult issues impacting on the development of the child(ren) or young person(s). What harm might happen to the child(ren) or young person(s); if there is no change, then what concerns do you have?
>
> What is working well?
>
> > For example: Attendance at school or other setting, communication with the adults, changes in family functioning
>
> What needs to change?
>
> > For example: What do you think needs to change in order to make things better for the child(ren) or young person(s)?
>
> Any other comments
>
> Have you shared this report with the child(ren) or young person(s) and their family?

If you are still not clear on these processes, you should contact the lead safeguarding professional in your practice, or the designated team, for advice. It is important to keep a balance between the need to maintain confidentiality and the need to share information to protect others, but safeguarding is always paramount. Any decisions to share information must always be based on professional judgement about the safety and well-being of the individual and in accordance with legal, ethical and professional obligations.

There may be many codes within SystmOne or EMIS relating to safeguarding concerns. These codes are attributed to the different levels of concern, and they require auditing or review to capture all information when writing reports. This is mainly entered by safeguarding administration teams but may require you to review before reports are sent. Once these reports have been sent, a meeting usually follows to look at all information gathered, to identify the level of risk or concern and to put in place a plan for care or support. This information is then shared with all agencies involved to allow collaborative multi-agency working.

Documentation

For both adults and children, it is imperative that all information is documented concisely and consistently at the time of the concern. This should include:

- Who attended with the patient to the consultation (names and relationship)?
- What were the interactions like – warm, affectionate, rude, interruptive?
- Body language: Did they appear withdrawn, nervous, hesitant to discuss concerns, open, happy? It is worth noting that if they are hesitant to discuss certain issues, whether adult or children, it may be advisable to separate them and use a chaperone to investigate further concerns or allow the patient to explain any concerns they may have.
- Any injuries that might be visible, and explanation of patient or carer of these – are they consistent with what has been explained?

Serious Case Review or Multi-agency Review

These reviews happen after a serious case or in the event of serious injury to a child or adult. This process brings together all parties involved with the family to identify where concerns were not highlighted or where processes may be changed to prevent further incidences from occurring. This can be a useful reflective tool to improve information sharing and support.

> Shacklock, J. (2019) Good practice safeguarding in general practice [online]. The RCGP has published a series of workbooks to enable GPs and their practices to safeguard children and young people. This includes systems and operational arrangements, downloadable tools and information on particular areas of concern. They can be found on the RCGP website.

Chapter Summary

This chapter has highlighted that safeguarding is everyone's responsibility and there is a need to identify concerns early, whilst considering the six principles of safeguarding. It is imperative that there is a documentation of concerns and discussions with your safeguarding leads, to facilitate ongoing investigation and management of these concerns, ensuring that your documentation is contemporaneous, clear and concise. It is also a necessity to ensure that all training in this area is kept up to date, to enable any changes in the process to be followed and to ensure that individuals and families are identified and supported at the earliest opportunity.

CHAPTER 19   Safeguarding Considerations

References

Cooper, A. and White, E. (2017) *Safeguarding Adults Under the Care Act 2014 – Understanding Good Practice.* London: Jessica Kingsley Publishers.

Department of Education (2020) Characteristics of children in need 2018–2019. Available at: https://www.gov.uk/government/statistics/characteristics-of-children-in-need-2018-to-2019 (accessed 28 January 2023).

HM Government (2018) Statutory guidance. Available at: https://assets.publishing.service.gov.uk/government/uploads/system/uploads/attachment_data/file/779401/Working_Together_to_Safeguard-Children.pdf (accessed 28 January 2023).

Koubel, G. (2016) *Safeguarding Adults and Children – Dilemmas and Complex Practice.* London: Palgrave.

NHS Digital (2021) Safeguarding adults, England, 2020–21. Available at: https://digital.nhs.uk/data-and-information/publications/statistical/safeguarding-adults/2020-21 (accessed 28 January 2023).

NHS England (2019) Safeguarding adults. Available at: https://www.england.nhs.uk/wp-content/uploads/2017/02/adult-pocket-guide.pdf (accessed 28 January 2023).

Robson, S. and Sherwen, E. (2017) *Adult Safeguarding Best Practice Guidance for Providers of Healthcare in East Anglia and Essex.* Cambridge: National Health Service.

Royal College of Nursing (RCN) (2018) Adult safeguarding: Roles and competencies for health care staff. Available at: https://www.rcn.org.uk/Professional-Development/publications/adult-safeguarding-roles-and-competencies-for-health-care-staff-uk-pub-007-069 (accessed 28 January 2023).

Royal College of Paediatrics and Child Health (UK) (n.d.) Child protection and safeguarding. Available at: https://www.rcpch.ac.uk/key-topics/child-protection (accessed 28 January 2023).

Shacklock, J. (2019) Good practice safeguarding in general practice. Available at: https://www.rcgp.org.uk/clinical-and-research/safeguarding.aspx (accessed 28 January 2023).

Social Care Institute for Excellence (2018) Adult safeguarding practice questions. Available at: https://www.scie.org.uk/safeguarding/adults/practice/questions (accessed 28 January 2023).

Legislation

Care Act (England and Wales) 2014.
Children Act (England and Wales) 1989.
Domestic Abuse Act (England and Wales) 2021.

Making Every Contact Count: Health Promotion in Primary Care

20

Andrew Hichisson

Introduction

Promoting good health in society is not a new concept and has been considered for hundreds of years. The foundations of modern healthcare were laid by the Ancient Greeks and Romans, who established links between ill health and human behaviour, as well as wider societal and environmental influences. However, health promotion as a recognised area of healthcare is a relatively modern development. In simple and traditional terms, health promotion should be considered as a method to help reduce preventable illness, disability and death. However, as healthcare has advanced, health promotion has also evolved. Contemporary views now recognise that helping individuals live well with chronic illness, preventing disease progression and avoidable complications is also an integral part of the field.

At the first International Conference on Health Promotion in Ottawa, Canada, the World Health Organization (WHO) declared the first, and most widely used, definition: 'Health promotion is the process of enabling people to increase control over, and to improve, their health' (WHO, 1986: 1). The rest of their statement highlights that good physical, mental and social well-being cannot be achieved by health services alone and is the responsibility of society. This should not be interpreted as suggesting that health services cannot improve the health of individuals, but is instead a recognition that taking a joined-up approach to tackle the wider determinants of health will deliver the most improvement to the widest possible population.

The benefits of effective health promotion are wide. At an individual level, the personal burden of ill health can be reduced, which helps individuals to live well for longer. This interlinks and benefits wider society by reducing the reliance of healthcare and welfare services, along with associated financial costs.

Health promotion is closely linked, although not interchangeable, with health prevention. It is useful to consider the three levels of health prevention and how this informs the approaches that health promotion programmes may take:

- 'Primary' prevention seeks to prevent illness, disease or injury before it occurs. This is often undertaken at a society or government level by providing education, delivering an intervention, or encouraging or discouraging an activity. Examples may include health warnings on tobacco products, childhood immunisation programmes or sexual health education.

CHAPTER 20 Making Every Contact Count: Health Promotion in Primary Care

- 'Secondary' prevention aims to identify illness, disease or injury at the earliest opportunity to limit the impact or progression. This may be undertaken as part of a national programme or by individual clinical teams. Examples may include mammography for early identification of breast cancer, NHS health checks to identify heart disease, diabetes and hypertension or screening for abdominal aortic aneurysm.
- 'Tertiary' prevention attempts to limit the progression or the impact of an illness, disease or injury after it has been identified. Examples may include weight loss programmes to tackle obesity, smoking cessation advice and interventions for chronic respiratory diseases or cardiac rehabilitation exercise programmes following a myocardial infarction.

Health Promotion Theories and Models

Many elements of the psychological, social and behavioural sciences have been used to inform and help develop theories and models for contemporary health promotion. Three of the most common are the health belief model (Becker, 1974); the stages of change (transtheoretical) model (Prochaska and DiClemente, 1984); and the social cognitive theory (Bandura, 1986).

Although all distinctly different, they share similarities in that behaviour change is often centred around personal motivations and capacity to makes changes. This will differ between individuals depending on many factors, such as social and cultural background, health literacy, stage of life and support network of family and friends. Lifestyle changes are more likely to become embedded if an individual is motivated to change and if support is available from their network of family and friends. Taking time to understand the current lifestyle of an individual, their individual circumstances, barriers or enablers and any personal goals for the future is an important part of health promotion.

> 💡 When a patient is seeking help for a medical condition, their motivation to get better and prevent a recurrence is likely to be higher. This may be a good opportunity to ask about any current lifestyle choices that may be affecting the presentation, and can lead to opportunities to offer information about support that is available to help. Even if the support is not taken immediately, it may provide the foundation for the individual to seek help at a later time.

UK Policy

It has been recognised by healthcare leaders and policy makers across the United Kingdom (UK) that the NHS needs to change its approach and develop strategies to prevent ill health, rather than just focusing on treatments. Key policy across the four nations, such as the *NHS Long Term Plan* (NHS England, 2019) the *NHS Recovery Plan 2021–2026* (NHS Scotland, 2021), *A Healthier Wales: Our Plan for Health and Social Care*

Health Promotion in Primary Care

(Welsh Government, 2022) and *Health and Wellbeing 2026: Delivering Together* (DHNI, 2016), highlights the importance of moving towards population and preventative health approaches, of which health promotion is a component.

Increasing health promotion education and training for allied health professionals, including paramedics, is also contained within the 'UK Allied Health Professions Public Health Strategic Framework 2019–2024' (AHPF, 2019) and 'Rethinking the Public Health Workforce' (RSPH, 2015) reports. Whilst it is likely that tangible results will take time to be seen, the aim is for a modern health service which helps to prevent ill health, with reduced reliance on treating the effects of preventable illness and disease. It is important to caveat that healthcare is often subject to changes in priority, but these plans indicate an important change in direction.

Health Promotion in Primary Care

Health promotion is already well established in primary care. Whilst some principles of health promotion may now be covered in the undergraduate curriculum for paramedics (College of Paramedics, 2020), paramedic training has historically had more of a reactive, rather than proactive, approach befitting of its preparation for emergency ambulance services.

> Take a few minutes to consider times when you may have offered advice to individuals about their health condition or tried to give practical help. Would you consider these to be health promotion?

If you take an objective look at your past interactions with individuals, there are likely to be many examples of health promotion that you have already been undertaking without necessarily realising. Examples may include:

- Assisting an individual to understand their medication regimen and the importance of taking them correctly
- Encouraging an individual with higher-risk co-morbidities to have the influenza vaccination
- Making a referral to a falls service for an individual who is frail or disabled
- Suggesting to an individual with hypertension that they book a review with their GP practice team
- Teaching cardiopulmonary resuscitation in the community
- Trying to help a homeless individual access a shelter.

As you gain experience and develop within primary care, it is likely that much of your focus will initially be on increasing your clinical knowledge and assessment skills as well as trying to refine this into the time constraints of an appointment list. However, looking at factors that may be causing or aggravating a condition should also be incorporated into your practice. This may seem unnatural at first, but over time it will likely become a

CHAPTER 20 Making Every Contact Count: Health Promotion in Primary Care

routine part of your consultation skills and you will start to recognise some of the links between ill health and lifestyle choices. The significance of both physical and mental health, and how these are interlinked, should also be understood, with the aim of helping an individual to achieve an overall level of health and well-being that is as high as possible.

Making Every Contact Count (MECC)

Health promotion does not need to be formal, and every interaction with individuals provides an opportunity to provide practical support and signpost to relevant services. For example, when you ask about smoking status for an individual that presents with symptoms of a lower respiratory tract infection, or whether the individual with depression undertakes any regular social activities, what do you do with the information? If the answer is nothing, then this is a missed opportunity to help an individual improve their health and well-being. There isn't an expectation that you will be an expert in health promotion, but even just signposting to relevant services can make a difference, especially when individuals are receptive to seeking help.

Making Every Contact Count (MECC) is a useful tool that can be used to make the most of the small interactions that take place every day to support positive changes to improve physical and mental health and well-being (PHE, 2016). MECC has been developed to be used by all staff across the NHS, regardless of their clinical grade or practice setting. As someone who may be new to the concept of health promotion, this is an ideal introduction and is simple to introduce into your wider clinical practice.

MECC has been developed around the COM-B model of behaviour. COM-B consists of three main components, **C**apability, **O**pportunity and **M**otivation, which interact and influence a **B**ehaviour. This model provides a more simple and practical approach that can be easy to apply practically to clinical encounters. The success of any behaviour change requires an action for one or more of these three components:

- Capability: Does the individual know how to change? Are there any barriers to change? Are any new skills required for change to be successful?
- Opportunity: What support is currently available? Can additional support from family, friends or through other services be utilised?
- Motivation: What are the reasons why an individual wants to change? Is there a longer-term goal that can be the focus for change?

The MECC framework itself encompasses three elements that can be used to guide conversations around improving health and well-being – Ask, Assist and Act.

> Chisholm, A. et al. (2020) Online behaviour change technique training to support healthcare staff 'Make Every Contact Count'. *BMC Health Services Research*.
> eLearning packages are available via the e-Learning for Health platform, and these have been shown to be an effective way of teaching this health-promotion technique.

Ask

As part of your history taking, ask about a health condition when an opportunity arises. This may be proactive, such as when you notice something relevant to the presentation that may be impacting on the individual, or reactive if they discuss that they are concerned about something (e.g. stress, weight). Try to highlight the link between lifestyle factors and the individual's health concerns.

Assist

During your conversation, assist the individual to understand that there are potential solutions to their health concerns and how these may lead to improvements. Use open questions, utilise active listening skills and be guided by what the individual is receptive to discussing rather than trying to force a fixed message. Try to be consistent with the messages you convey.

Act

Offer information about services that are available in the area to support change. Ask the individual what their next steps are or if they are considering an action plan, and always try to be positive in conversations. Even if the actions they are suggesting seem small, it is important to recognise that the first steps are being taken which may lead to more change in the longer term. If the individual decides not to take action, then that decision needs be respected, and pressure should not be applied. However, it would be reasonable to consider offering some website addresses or leaflets to read at another time in case their thoughts change in the future. Achieving full physical or mental health may not be realistic, so your focus should be on what is important to the individual.

There is no expectation that you will become an expert in health promotion, and MECC is centred around having informal conversations based around an individual's motivations, needs and beliefs. MECC is not about giving advice, but it can be an opportunity to offer information about what services are available locally. It can be useful to spend some time getting to know what is available in your area or nationally. Make sure that information is up to date and services are available before passing this on.

> Some primary care settings may have a directory of services available that accept direct referrals such as smoking cessation, drug and alcohol services and social prescribing.

MECC can encompass all the elements of health prevention discussed previously but is ultimately about preventing individuals from deteriorating or getting ill in the first place, and helping those with illness, disease or injury live well for longer. The impact can seem small, or even unnoticeable at the time, but it can lead to healthier lifestyles which reduces the impact of ill health later in life. As you are likely to have ongoing or repeated interactions with individuals in primary care, there is more opportunity to see long-term benefits, which can be rewarding and increase your own motivation to help others. This is very different

CHAPTER 20 Making Every Contact Count: Health Promotion in Primary Care

from the ambulance service setting, and is one of the many reasons why primary care can be an interesting and rewarding environment to work in.

Immunisation Programmes

Providing access to protection against illness and disease is an important and well-established function of healthcare. Primary care plays a vital role by helping to deliver the majority of vaccinations as part of national immunisation programmes. It is also often the first place that individuals will go to for advice and information when they have questions or concerns.

The value of immunisation has been known since the 18th century, and vaccines for many common illnesses have been developed since Edward Jenner first used the cowpox virus to protect against smallpox. There have been global successes since, most notably the eradication of smallpox and significant progress towards achieving the same status for polio. More recently, the global effort to rapidly develop and mass-produce vaccines that are effective against the SARS-CoV-2 (COVID-19) virus shows how society can be offered protection through organised immunisation programmes.

The effectiveness of immunisation programmes is dependent on the proportion of the population who are vaccinated against an illness or disease. This is known as 'herd immunity', and the amount of coverage required varies depending on a number of factors. However, misinformation and hesitancy about vaccines has become an increasing issue. The 1999 study published by Andrew Wakefield and his colleagues which suggested a link between autism and the measles, mumps and rubella (MMR) combined vaccination is a pertinent example. Although now discredited, the findings were widely reported throughout the media and it is one factor which has led to the reduction in uptake of the vaccine which still exists today. After the UK was declared measles free by WHO in 2016, this status was subsequently lost in 2018 and vaccination rates are still below the required threshold to eliminate community transmission in the UK. Disinformation and conspiracy theories have also influenced the uptake of the COVID-19 vaccination.

> Take a few minutes to consider what your views on vaccines are. Where do you get your information from – official sources or the internet? Do you feel comfortable explaining the benefits whilst also recognising that there may be concerns? Do any of your own beliefs influence these discussions?

As part of a multidisciplinary team, it is vital that you are able to hold conversations about vaccinations, and health promotion plays an important role here. To be able to hold effective and informed discussions, it is essential that you have an understanding of how vaccines work, how they benefit the individual and how they benefit wider society. You should be prepared to answer questions and dispel common myths, regardless of your own views. This is not to say that concerns should be dismissed, as this is unlikely to increase confidence. However, vaccines are generally safe for the majority of the population, and you should have confidence in promoting these during your clinical practice.

> The vaccines offered as part of immunisation programmes differ between age groups and in some cases between areas of the UK, such as the Bacillus Calmette-Guérin (BCG) vaccine for tuberculosis. These are regularly reviewed, so it is important to ensure that your knowledge of this is up to date. Official guidelines, both national and local, are available online and should be consulted for more information.

Chapter Summary

Health promotion is an essential part of primary care and should be incorporated into your practice, particularly if you are transitioning away from the traditional ambulance service setting. Having conversations that aren't necessarily focused on the immediate clinical presentation can feel unusual and possibly uncomfortable at first. However, as you develop your consultation skills, this will become more routine and the MECC framework can be used as a tool to guide your conversations. There is no expectation for you to become an expert in health promotion, and signposting to relevant services is a better approach than offering formal advice. Having a good knowledge of what is available in your area will help you to provide the most appropriate support. Health promotion also includes supporting immunisation programmes by promoting the uptake of vaccinations. Understanding how vaccines work and the principle that they are safe for the overwhelming majority of individuals is essential to help dispel myths and counter misinformation and conspiracy theories.

Some key things to remember are:

- Health promotion is an integral part of primary care, and paramedics should adopt this into their own practice.
- Health promotion does not need to be formal, and MECC is a tool that can be used to focus on signposting to relevant services.
- Immunisation programmes are an important tool for healthcare services to protect individuals against illness and disease.
- Paramedics can play a vital role in promoting the uptake of vaccinations and dispelling myths and misinformation.

References

Allied Health Professions Federation (AHPF) (2019) UK allied health professions public health strategic framework 2019–2024. Available at: http://www.ahpf.org.uk/files/UK%20AHP%20Public%20Health%20Strategic%20Framework%202019-2024.pdf (accessed 28 January 2023).

Bandura, A. (1986) *Social Foundations of Thought and Action: A Social Cognitive Theory.* Englewood Cliffs, NJ: Prentice-Hall.

Becker, M.H. (1974) The health belief model and personal health behavior. *Health Education Monographs* 2: 324–473.

Chisholm, A., Byrne-Davis, L., Peters, S. et al. (2020) Online behaviour change technique training to support healthcare staff 'Make Every Contact Count'. *BMC Health Services Research* 20(1): 1–11.

CHAPTER 20 Making Every Contact Count: Health Promotion in Primary Care

College of Paramedics (2020) *Paramedic Curriculum Guidance*. 5th edn. Bridgwater: College of Paramedics.

Department of Health Northern Ireland (DHNI) (2016) Health and wellbeing 2026: Delivering together. Available at: https://www.health-ni.gov.uk/sites/default/files/publications/health/health-and-wellbeing-2026-delivering-together.pdf (accessed 28 January 2023).

NHS England (2019) NHS long term plan. Available at: www.longtermplan.nhs.uk (accessed 12 April 2023).

NHS Scotland (2021) NHS recovery plan 2021–2026. Available at: https://www.gov.scot/binaries/content/documents/govscot/publications/strategy-plan/2021/08/nhs-recovery-plan/documents/nhs-recovery-plan-2021-2026/nhs-recovery-plan-2021-2026/govscot%3Adocument/nhs-recovery-plan-2021-2026.pdf (accessed 28 January 2023).

Prochaska, J. and DiClemente, C. (1984) *The Transtheoretical Approach: Crossing Traditional Boundaries of Therapy.* Homewood, IL: Dow Jones-Irwin.

Public Health England (PHE) (2016) Making Every Contact Count (MECC): Consensus statement. Available at: https://assets.publishing.service.gov.uk/government/uploads/system/uploads/attachment_data/file/769486/Making_Every_Contact_Count_Consensus_Statement.pdf (accessed 28 January 2023).

Royal Society of Public Health (RSPH) (2015) Rethinking the public health workforce. Available at: https://www.rsph.org.uk/our-work/policy/wider-public-health-workforce/rethinking-the-public-health-workforce.html (accessed 28 January 2023).

Wakefield, A. (1999) MMR vaccination and autism. *Lancet* 354(9182): 949–950.

Welsh Government (2022) A healthier Wales: Our plan for health and social care. Available at: https://gov.wales/healthier-wales-long-term-plan-health-and-social-care (accessed 28 January 2023).

World Health Organization (WHO) (1986) The 1st International Conference on Health Promotion. Available at: https://www.who.int/teams/health-promotion/enhanced-wellbeing/first-global-conference (accessed 28 January 2023).

Index

NOTE: Page numbers followed by *f*, *b* and *t* indicate material in figures, boxes and tables respectively.

A

Abbey Pain Scale, 450
'ABC of doctors' core needs', 15
Abdominal pain, during pregnancy, 343–345, 344*f*
Abducens cranial nerve, 97*t*
Acalculous cholecystitis, 263
ACEIs. *see* Angiotensin-converting enzyme inhibitors
Acne vulgaris, 392–394, 393*t*
ACP. *see* Advance care plan
ACR. *see* Albumin creatinine ratio
Acral lentiginous melanoma, 410
ACS. *see* Acute coronary syndrome
ACTH. *see* Adrenocorticotrophic hormone
Actinic keratosis, 407
Active listening techniques, 31, 33*t*
Acute anxiety, 126–127
Acute coronary syndrome (ACS), 212, 213, 218, 219
Acute cough/bronchitis, 183–185
Acute kidney injury, 74
Acute limb ischaemia, 236
Acute skin conditions
    contact dermatitis, 386–387
    intertrigo, 387
    pityriasis rosea, 387–388
    urticaria, 388
Addison's disease, 78, 422, 423
Additional Roles Reimbursement Scheme (ARRS), 1, 9
Adenoma, 429

ADH. *see* Anti-diuretic hormone
Adjuvant analgesics, 469–470
Adrenal gland
    Addison's disease, 423
    aetiology, 422
    Cushing's syndrome, 424
Adrenocorticotrophic hormone (ACTH), 422, 423
Adults with Incapacity (Scotland) Act (2000), 61
Advance care plan (ACP), 441–443, 442*t*
Advanced Clinical Practitioners in Emergency Medicine, 7
Advice and Guidance (A&G) services, 224
AECAs. *see* Anti-endothelial-cell antibodies
Affect heuristic, and decision making, 57
Agitation, 445–446, 455–456
Alanine transaminase (ALT), 87, 88, 248*t*, 265
Albumin, 249*t*
Albumin creatinine ratio (ACR), 233, 234
Alcohol dependency syndrome, 261–262
Alcohol, Smoking and Substance Involvement Screening Tool - Lite (ASSIST-Lite), 134
Alcohol use disorder, 261–262
Alkaline phosphatase (ALP), 87–88, 249*t*, 265, 269, 270
Allergic conjunctivitis, 149*t*, 150
Allergic shiners, 162
Allergies, 185–187, 186*t*
ALP. *see* Alkaline phosphatase
Alpha-1 antitrypsin deficiency (A1AD), 262
ALT. *see* Alanine transaminase
Altered neurology, 99–100
Amitriptyline, 470

Index

Amoxicillin, 202, 347, 354
ANAs. *see* Anti-nuclear antibodies
Angina, 211–214
Angiotensin-converting enzyme inhibitors (ACEIs), 229, 235
Angiotensin receptor blocker (ARB), 229, 235
Angular cheilitis, 402
Ankle-brachial pressure index, 236
Antenatal care, for uncomplicated pregnancies, 340, 341f
Antepartum haemorrhage, 357
Anticholinergic medication, 111
Anticoagulation, atrial fibrillation, 215–217, 216t
Anti-cyclic citrullinated peptide (anti-CCP), 375
Anti-diabetic drugs, 428, 428t
Anti-diuretic hormone (ADH), 78, 424
Anti-endothelial-cell antibodies (AECAs), 270
Anti-nuclear antibodies (ANAs), 269
Antiretroviral (ARV) therapy, 329
Apixaban, 215
Aspartate aminotransferase (AST), 87, 88, 248t, 265
Aspirational pneumonia, 199
AST. *see* Aspartate aminotransferase
Asthma
    aetiology, 187
    history and examination, 188
    investigations, 188
    management, 188
    non-pharmacological treatment, 190
    pharmacological treatment
        in adults, 189, 189f
        in children, 189, 190f
    reviews, 191
Atrial fibrillation (AF), 214–217
Atypical pneumonia, 199
Autoimmune hepatitis, 267
Autonomic nervous system (ANS), 133

B

Bacterial conjunctivitis, 149t
Bacterial skin conditions
    cellulitis, 388–389
    erysipelas, 388–389
    folliculitis, 389–390
    hidradenitis suppurativa, 390
    impetigo, 391
    Lyme disease, 391–392
Bacterial vaginosis (BV), 295, 296
Balanoposthitis, 283, 284t–285t
Balint Groups, 43
BARD model, 40–41
Basal cell carcinoma, 408–409
Basophils, 71
Benign paroxysmal positional vertigo (BPPV), 159
Bereavement, 127–128
Beta blockers, 229
Better Births. *see* National Maternity Review
Bilirubin (Br), 88, 249t
Bio-psycho-social model, 33–34
Black and minority ethnic (BME) groups, 302
Blast cells, 71
Bleeding, in pregnancy
    after 24 weeks, 357
    early pregnancy, 355–356, 355b
Blepharitis, 148
Blood in stools, 250–251
Blood tests, 65
    case study, 92
    C-reactive protein, 256
    electrolytes, 76
        calcium levels, 83–85
        magnesium levels, 86
        potassium levels, 80–83
        sodium levels, 76–80
    erythrocyte sedimentation rate, 256
    full blood count, 68–69
        bone marrow, 68
        haemoglobin, 69
        mean cell volume, 69–70
        platelets, 68, 70–71
        red blood cells, 68
        white blood cells/WCC, 68, 71
    for hepatitis B, 266t
    inflammatory markers, 72–73
    liver function tests, 86–87
        alanine transaminase, 87
        albumen, 87
        alkaline phosphatase, 87–88
        aspartate aminotransferase, 87

Index

bilirubin, 88
gamma GT, 88
results to certain diagnoses, 88t, 89t
ordering and interpretation, principles of, 65–66
learning skills, 67
patient factors, 67
reference range, 66–67
renal function test, 73
thyroid function tests, 89
hyperthyroidism, 91
hypothalamic-pituitary-thyroid axis, 89, 90f
hypothyroidism, 90–91
TRH, 89
TSH, 89
urea
acute kidney injury, 74
chronic kidney injury, 75, 75t
renal function test, 73
BNF. see British National Formulary
Body fluids, 18
Bolam v Friern Hospital Management Committee (1957), 61
Bone marrow, 68
Bone marrow oedema, 376t, 377
Bornholm disease, 219
Borrelia burgdorferi, 391
Bowel habit, change in, 250–251
Bowel obstruction, 252
Brain naturetic peptide (BNP), 227
Braxton Hicks contractions, 344
Breaking bad news, 43–45, 44t
Breastfeeding, 314, 321
Breast pain
aetiology, 285–286
cyclical, 286
mastitis, 286–287
British National Formulary (BNF), 231, 354
Bronchiectasis, 191–192
Bronchiolitis, in children, 192–193
Bronchodilator reversibility (BDR), 188
Bulk-forming laxatives, 253
Burnout, occupational stress, 14
managing stress and, 15–17
recognition, 14–15
symptoms of, 14b

Bursitis, 376t, 377
BV. see Bacterial vaginosis

C

Calcium levels, in blood, 83
hypercalcaemia, 83–84
hypocalcaemia, 84–85
negative feedback loop, 83, 84f
Calgary-Cambridge consultation model, 39, 39f
Candida intertrigo, 387
Candidiasis, 181, 402–403
CAP. see Community-acquired pneumonia
Capillary blood glucose monitoring (CBGM), 426
Carbimazole, 430
Cardiovascular presentations
assessment, 210
auscultation, 210, 211f
case studies, 239–242
description of, 209
palpation, 210
in primary care
angina, 211–214
atrial fibrillation, 214–217
chest pain, 218–220
deep vein thrombosis, 220–222
fits, faints and funny turns, 222–225
heart failure, 226–229
hyperlipidaemia, 229–231
hypertension, 231–235, 232t
peripheral vascular disease, 235–236
pulmonary embolism, 237–239, 238t
Care Act (2014), 485
Career progression, for paramedics, 9
Care Inspectorate in Scotland, 12
Care Quality Commission, 10, 12
Catastrophic cardiac arrythmias, 81
Cefalexin, 354
Cellulitis, 388–389
Central cyanosis, 181
CHA_2DS_2-VASc score, 50, 215, 216t
Chest, auscultation of, 182, 182f, 183
Chest infection, during pregnancy, 345–347
Chest pain, 218–220
Chickenpox, 399t–401t
Childbirth, contraception after, 314

503

Index

Child in Need (CIN), 487–488
Child protection, 488
Child Protection-Information Sharing (CP-IS), 487
Child Protection Plan (CPP), 487, 488
Chlamydia, 323–324
Cholecystitis, 263
Cholestasis, 265–266
Cholesteatoma, 155
Chronic bronchitis, 193
Chronic fatigue syndrome (CFS). see Myalgic encephalomyelitis
Chronic hypertension, 348, 349
Chronic kidney injury, 75, 75*t*
Chronic obstructive pulmonary disease (COPD), 193–197, 195*f*, 196*f*, 262
Chronic pain
    consultation template, 463–465
    description of, 462
    epidemiology, 461–462
    medications, 467–468
        adjuvant analgesics, 469–470
        non-opioid analgesics, 468–469
        opioids, 471–472
    self-management of, 465–467, 466*f*
    treating in primary care, 461
Chronic skin conditions
    acne vulgaris, 392–394, 393*t*
    eczema, 394–395
    psoriasis, 396, 397*t*–398*t*
    rosacea, 398
    stasis/varicose eczema, 395
CIN. *see* Child in Need
Clinical commissioning group (CCG), 95
Clinically isolated syndrome (CIS), 113
Cluster headaches, 105–106
Cockcroft-Gault formula, 217
COCP. *see* Combined contraceptive pill
Coeliac disease, 251–252
Cognitive behaviour therapy (CBT) intervention, 133
Cognitive biases, in clinical practice, 57
Cognitive testing, 110
College of Paramedics, 6, 9
    career framework, 7–8, 8*f*
'Collusion of anonymity', 43

Combined contraceptive pill (COCP), 304, 308–311
COM-B model, 496
Community-acquired pneumonia (CAP), 200
Compression hosiery, 395
Computerised tomography pulmonary angiogram (CTPA), 238
Condoms, 313
Confusion, 100, 101*t*
Conjunctivitis, 181
    clinical features of, 148, 149*t*, 150
Constipation, 252–253
    for palliative and end-of-life care patient, 446–447, 447*t*
Consultation models
    BARD model, 40–41
    bio-psycho-social model, 33–34
    breaking bad news, 43–45, 44*t*
    Calgary-Cambridge model, 39, 39*f*
    easily missed diagnoses, 47, 47*t*
    FRAYED model, 41
    management plan formulation, 49–51, 50*t*
    Medical Model, 31–33, 32*f*
    most likely diagnosis, 45–46, 46*f*
    Murtagh's diagnostic model, 45
    Murtagh's Masquerades, 48, 48*t*
    narrative medicine, 40
    Neighbour's model, 36–39, 36*f*
    Pendleton's model, 35–36, 35*f*
    in practice, 43
    psychology of, 42–43
    red flags, 47–48
    safety netting, 51, 51*t*–52*t*
    serious pathology, 47
    telephone and video consultations, 41–42, 42*b*
    yellow flags, 49, 49*b*
Contact dermatitis, 386–387
Contact lens associated conjunctivitis, 149*t*
Continuous positive airway pressure (CPAP) therapy, 199
Contraception, 302–303
    after childbirth, 314
    breastfeeding, 314
    case study, 332–333

Index

combined contraceptive pill, 309–311
combined transdermal patch, 311–312
combined vaginal ring, 312–313
condoms, 313
contraceptive implant, 308
contraceptive injection, 306–307
emergency contraception (see Emergency contraception (EC))
examination, 305–306
female sterilisation, 314
FSRH UK Medical Eligibility Criteria, 303–304, 303t
health promotion, opportunities for, 314
history taking, 304–305
intrauterine contraceptive devices, 307
LARC, 306
legal and ethical requirements for, 315
ongoing, 321
in patients under 18 years, 315
progesterone-only pill, 308
sexually transmitted infections, 322
vasectomy, 313
Contraceptive implant, 308
Contraceptive injection, 306–307
Contraceptive transdermal patch, 311–312
Contraceptive vaginal ring, 312–313
COPD. see Chronic obstructive pulmonary disease
Copper intrauterine devices (Cu-IUDs), 307, 318–320
Corneal arcus, 210
Coronavirus disease (COVID-19), 200
symptoms, in pregnancy, 346b
thromboembolism, increases risk of, 237
unvalidated Roth Score during, 41
vaccination, 498
Costochondritis, 219
COXII inhibitors, 468
Cranial nerves, neurological examination of, 96, 96t–97t
C-reactive protein (CRP), 72, 73f, 164, 256, 375
Critical limb ischaemia, 236
Crohn's disease, 255–256
CRP. see C-reactive protein
Cu-IUDs. see Copper intrauterine devices

Cushing's syndrome, 422, 424
Cyclical breast pain, 286

D

Dacryocystitis, 148
D-dimer, 73
Decision-making theory
cycle of, 55, 55f
data-collection stage, 56
informed consent, 60–61
person-centred care, 60–61
risk and, 58
complexity and uncertainty, 59
perceived risk, 58–59
shared decision making, 60
stages, 55–56
theoretical approaches to, 56–57
Decontamination, of equipment, 20
Deep vein thrombosis (DVT), 220–222, 237
Dehydration, stages of, 253, 254t
Dehydroepiandrosterone, 423
Delayed onset muscle soreness (DOMS), 374, 375
Dental abscess, 170
Department of Health and Social Care, 17
Department of Health Northern Ireland (2020), 12
Depo-provera and Sayana Press, 306–307
Depression, 128–129
Dermatological presentations. see Skin conditions
Diabetes insipidus (DI), 424–425
Diabetes mellitus, 425–428, 428t
Diabetic ketoacidosis (DKA), 82, 426
Diagnostic momentum, 57
Diagnostic testing, for confusion, 101t
Diagnostic Triads, 46
Diarrhoea, 253–255, 254t, 255t
Direct oral anti-coagulants (DOACs), 215, 217, 222
Diuretic therapy, 235
Divergence of Care theory, 44, 44f
Dizziness, 158–159
DOACs. see Direct oral anti-coagulants
'Doctor as drug', 42–43
Domestic Abuse Act (2021), 481
DOMS. see Delayed onset muscle soreness

505

Index

Driver and Vehicle Licensing Agency (DVLA), 199
DR SAMOSA model, 41, 42b
Drug therapy, 235
Dry mucous membranes, 181
Dual process theory, 56
Duloxetine, 470
Duodenal ulcer, 257
Duty of candour, 11–12
    ethical duty, 13
    in primary care, in England, 12–13
    principles, 12
DVT. see Deep vein thrombosis
DVT Wells score, 221, 222t
Dying phase
    anticipatory medications, 456
    breaking bad news, 456–457
    defined, 454
    non-essential observations, 455
    signs and symptoms of, 454, 455t
    terminal restlessness/agitation, 455–456
Dysmenorrhea, 291–292
Dyspnoea, for palliative and end-of-life care patient, 447–448

E

Earache, 152–153
    otitis externa, 153–154, 154t
    otitis media, 155
Early pregnancy
    abdominal pain, 343–345, 344f
    bleeding, 288–289, 355–357, 355b
    chest infection, 345–347
    confirmation of, 287
    headaches, 347–349
    loss, 288–289
    miscarriage, 288–289
    nausea and vomiting, 349–351
    pruritis, 351–353
    termination of pregnancy, 287
    urinary tract infection, 353–354
Ear pain. see Earache
Ear presentations, 144
    case study, 174–175
    neurological examination, 145
    in primary care
        cholesteatoma, 155
        dizziness, 158–159
        earache, 152–155
        hearing loss, 156–157, 156t–157t
    Rinne test, 144
    Weber test, 144
EC. see Emergency contraception
Ectopic pregnancy, 288–289, 343
Ectroprion, 148
Eczema, 394–395
    stasis/varicose, 395
Edinburgh Claudication Questionnaire (ECQ), 235
eGFR. see Estimated glomerular filtration rate
Egophony, 182
Electrolytes, 76
Emergency contraception (EC), 315–316
    and breastfeeding, 321
    comparisons of, 319, 319t–320t
    consultation flow chart, 316f
    examination, 318
    history of, 316–317
    indications for, 316
    methods of, 318
    ongoing contraception, 321
    pregnancy test, 321
    regular use of, 321
    safeguarding, 317–318
    selection, 319, 321
    STIs, 321
Emphysema, 193
Employer responsibilities, for supervision, 10
Endocarditis, 219–220
Endocrine system
    case studies, 434–436
    description of, 421–422
    hypothalamus, 421
    pituitary gland, hormonal love letters from, 421, 422b
    in primary care
        adrenal disease, 422–424
        diabetes insipidus, 424–425

diabetes mellitus, 425–428, 428t
overactive thyroid disease, 429–431
parathyroid disease, 431–432
underactive thyroid disease, 432–434
Entropion, 148
Eosinophils, 71
Epilepsy, 111–112
Epistaxis, 160, 160b
Epworth Sleepiness Scale, 198
Erysipelas, 388–389
Erythrocytes, 68
Erythrocyte sedimentation rate (ESR), 72, 164, 256, 269, 375
Erythroderma, 411–412
ESR. see Erythrocyte sedimentation rate
Estimated glomerular filtration rate (eGFR), 75, 217
Exanthems, of childhood, 398, 399t–401t
Expected death, verification of, 457
Eye discharge, 148–150, 149t
Eye, ear, nose and throat (EENT) examination, 143
Eyelids, disorders of, 148
Eye movement desensitisation and reprocessing (EMDR) therapy, 133
Eye presentations, 144
  case study, 173–174
  in primary care
    eye discharge, 148–150, 149t
    eyelids, disorders of, 148
    loss of vision, 146–147, 146t, 147f
    red eye, 150, 151t, 152

F

Facial cranial nerve, 97t
Facial palsy, 101–102
Faculty of Sexual and Reproductive Healthcare (FSRH), 305, 310, 319, 321
Faecal specimen, 254, 255t
FBC. see Full blood count
Female genitalia, 279
Female genital mutilation (FGM), 295
Female sterilisation, 314
Fermentable oligosaccharides, disaccharides, monosaccharides and polyols (FODMAP) diet, 257

Fibroids, 289–290
Fibrous liver changes, 261
FICA Spiritual History Tool, 444, 444t
Fingertip unit (FTU), 395
Fits, faints and funny turns, 222–225
Flexural psoriasis, 397t
Focal seizures, 111
Folliculitis, 389–390
Fractional exhaled nitric oxide (FeNO) testing, 188
Frank's sign, 210
Fraser guidelines, for contraception, 315
FRAYED model, 41
Frenulum tears, 283
FSRH. see Faculty of Sexual and Reproductive Healthcare
FSRH UK Medical Eligibility Criteria (UKMEC), 303–304, 303t, 308
Full blood count (FBC), 68–69, 350, 375
  bone marrow, 68
  haemoglobin, 69
  mean cell volume, 69–70
  platelets, 68, 70–71
  red blood cells, 68
  white blood cells/WCC, 68, 71
Functional constipation, 252
Fungal skin infections
  angular cheilitis, 402
  candidiasis, 402–403
  oral candidiasis, 403
  pityriasis versicolor, 403–404
  tinea infection, 404–405, 405t

G

Gabapentin, 470
Gabapentinoids, 470
GAD score. see Generalised anxiety disorder score
Gamma GT(GGT), 88
Gastric ulcer, 257
Gastrointestinal (GI) presentations, 247
  case studies, 271–273
  in primary care
    bowel habit, change in, 250–251
    coeliac disease, 251–252

Index

Gastrointestinal (GI) presentations (*Continued*)
    constipation, 252–253
    diarrhoea, 253–255, 254*t*, 255*t*
    inflammatory bowel disease, 255–256
    irritable bowel syndrome, 256–257
    peptic ulcers, 257–258
    poor appetite, 258–259
    rectal bleeding, 259–260
    stoma issues, 260
Generalised anxiety disorder (GAD) score, 124, 128
Generalised seizures, 111
General Medical Council (GMC), 11, 15
General Practice Forward View (NHS England, 2016), 1
General practitioners (GPs), 1, 8
    indemnity schemes, 9
    national shortage of, 122
    training, 11
Genital herpes, 324–325
Genital warts, 325–326
Genitourinary and gynaecological presentations
    assessment
        abdominal, 278
        female genitalia, 279
        male genitalia, 279
        urinalysis, 279–280
    case studies, 296–298
    history of, 277–278
    in primary care
        breast pain, 285–287
        early pregnancy, 287–289
        pelvic pain/masses, 289–291
        penile pain and discharge, 283, 284*t*–285*t*
        testicle pain and swelling, 285
        urinary retention, 282–283
        urinary symptoms, 281
        urinary tract infection, 281–282
        vaginal bleeding (*see* Vaginal bleeding)
Genito-urinary medicine (GUM), 291
Gestational hypertension, 348, 349
Giant cell arteritis, 106–107
Gillick competence, 315
Glossopharyngeal cranial nerve, 97*t*
Glyceryl trinitrate (GTN), 212, 213
Gonorrhoea, 326–327, 326*t*
Gout, 376*t*, 377
Grave's disease, 429
GTN. *see* Glyceryl trinitrate
GUM. *see* Genito-urinary medicine
Guttate psoriasis, 398*t*
Gynaecological presentations. *see* Genitourinary and gynaecological presentations

H

Haematinics, 70
Haemochromatosis, 263–264
Haemoglobin (Hb), 69
Hallucinations, visual/auditory, 136–137
Hand, foot and mouth viral exanthems, 399*t*–401*t*
Hand hygiene, 18–20
Handwashing technique, 18, 19*f*
HAP. *see* Hospital-acquired pneumonia
HAS-BLED tool, 50
HbA1c blood test, 426–427
HCPC. *see* Health and Care Professions Council
Headaches, 102
    cluster, 105–106
    during pregnancy, 347–349
    giant cell arteritis, 106–107
    medication-overuse, 104–105
    migraines, 107–109, 107*t*
    primary, 102
    secondary, 102–103
    tension-type, 103–104
Head impulse, nystagmus and test of skew (HINTS) examination, 145, 159
Health and Care Professions Council (HCPC), 1, 2, 5, 61
    scope of practice, 6, 7
    Standards (2018c), 13
Health and Social Care Act 17, 60
Healthcare Inspectorate in Wales, 12
Health Education England (HEE), 2
    capabilities, 6–7
    frameworks and roadmaps, 9
Health Needs Assessment (HNA) questionnaire, 463, 464*b*, 465
Health promotion
    description of, 493–494
    immunisation programmes, 498–499

Index

MECC, 496–498
   opportunities for, 314
   in primary care, 495–496
   theories and models, 494
   UK policy, 494–495
Health protection unit (HPU), 327
Hearing loss, 156–157, 156t–157t
Heart failure, 226–229
Heavy menstrual bleeding (HMB), 292–293
Helicobacter pylori (HP/H. pylori), 258
HELLP syndrome, 343–344, 352, 353
Helman's Folk Model, 34, 40
Hepatic presentations, 247
   case studies, 271–273
   in primary care
     alcohol use disorder, 261–262
     alpha 1 antitrypsin deficiency, 262
     cholecystitis, 263
     haemochromatosis, 263–264
     hepatitis, 264–267
     NAFLD, 267–268
     pancreatitis, 268–269, 269t
     primary biliary cirrhosis, 269–270
     primary sclerosing cholangitis, 270
     Wilson's disease, 270–271
Hepatitis, 264–267
Hepatitis A virus, 265–266
Hepatitis B virus (HBV), 266, 266t, 327
Hepatitis C virus (HCV), 267
Hepatomegaly, 266
Hernias, examination of, 278
Herpes simplex virus, 325, 413–414
Herpes virus conjunctivitis, 149t
Herpes zoster opthalmicus, 415
Herpes zoster virus, 414–415
HG. see Hyperemesis gravidarum
HHS. see Hyperosmolar hyperglycaemic state
Hidradenitis suppurativa, 390
HMB. see Heavy menstrual bleeding
HNA questionnaire. see Health Needs Assessment questionnaire
Hoarse voice, 181
Hospital-acquired pneumonia (HAP), 200–201
Hospital Clerking Model, 31–33, 32f

Human immunodeficiency virus (HIV), 328–330
Human papilloma virus (HPV), 325
Hypercalcaemia, 83–84, 432, 452–453, 453f
Hyperemesis gravidarum (HG), 349, 350
Hyperkalaemia, 81–82, 423
Hyperlipidaemia, 229–231
Hypermagnesaemia, 86
Hypernatraemia, 79–80
Hyperosmolar hyperglycaemic state (HHS), 426, 428
Hyperparathyroidism, 431
Hypertension, 231–235, 232t
   in pregnancy, 347, 348
Hyperthyroidism, 91, 429
Hypocalcaemia, 84–85
Hypoglossal cranial nerve, 97t
Hypokalaemia, 80–81, 228
Hypomagnesaemia, 86
Hyponatraemia, 76–79, 228, 423
Hypothalamic-pituitary-thyroid (HPT) axis, 89, 90f
Hypothyroidism, 90–91
   sub-clinical, 434

I

IBD. see Inflammatory bowel disease
IBS. see Irritable bowel syndrome
ICP. see Intrahepatic cholestasis of pregnancy
IDDM. see Insulin-dependent diabetes mellitus
Ideas, Concerns and Expectations (ICE), 34, 34t, 49
Immunisation programmes, 498–499
Impetigo, 391
IMSAFE mnemonic, 37, 37t
Indemnity insurance, 9–10
Independent Domestic Violence Advisor (IDVA) form, 483–484
Independent Sexual Violence Advisor (ISVA), 317–318
Infection control
   blood and body fluids, 18
   hand hygiene, 18–20
Inflammatory bowel disease (IBD), 255–256
Inflammatory markers, blood tests, 72–73
Informed consent, in decision making, 60–61
Insulin-dependent diabetes mellitus (IDDM), 425, 428

Index

Intermittent claudication, 236
International normalised ratio (INR), 215, 217
Intertrigo, 387
Intrahepatic cholestasis of pregnancy (ICP), 351
Intranasal corticosteroids, 165
Intrauterine contraceptive devices (IUCDs), 307
Intrauterine system (IUS), 307
Intravenous drug users (IVDUs), 266
Invasive devices, 20–21
Iritis, 181
Iron deficiency anaemia, 257
Irritable bowel syndrome (IBS), 250, 256–257

J

Janeway lesions, 210
Joint Committee on Vaccination and Immunisation (JCVI), 346b
Joint stiffness, 374
Jugular venous pressure (JVP), 181

K

Korsakoff syndrome, 262

L

Laboratory tests. see Blood tests
Labour pain, 344
Labyrinthitis, 158, 159
LARC. see Long-acting reversible contraception
Last menstrual period (LMP), 317
Lentigo maligna melanoma, 410
Leucocytes, 71
Levonorgestrel, 318
Levonorgestrel intrauterine systems (LNG-IUS), 307
LFTs. see Liver function tests
Lhermitte's sign, 113
Liver function tests (LFTs), 86–87, 265, 267, 269, 270, 350
  alanine transaminase, 87
  albumen, 87
  alkaline phosphatase, 87–88
  aspartate aminotransferase, 87
  bilirubin, 88
  defined, 248
  gamma GT, 88
  primary care investigations, 248, 248t–249t
  results to certain diagnoses, 88t, 89t
  second-line tests for, 248, 250t
LNG-IUS. see Levonorgestrel intrauterine systems
Long-acting reversible contraception (LARC), 303, 304, 306
Loss of vision, 146–147, 146t, 147f
Low molecular weight heparin (LMWH), 222
Lung cancer, 197–198
Lyme disease, 391–392
Lymph nodes
  Inspect and palpate, 181
  neck examination for, 146
Lymphoma, 252

M

Magnesium levels, in blood, 86
Magnetic resonance cholangiopancreatography (MRCP), 270
Making every contact count (MECC), 342, 496–498
Malassezia fungus, 403
Male genitalia, 279
Malignant spinal cord compression (MSCC), 452
MASH. see Multi-agency Safeguarding Hub
Mastitis, 286–287
Mean cell volume (MCV), 69–70
Measles, 399t–401t
MECC. see Making every contact count
Medical Certificate of Cause of Death (MCCD), 457
Medical Model, 31–33, 32f
Medical Research Council dyspnoea scale, 180, 180t
Medication Authorisation and Administration Record (MAAR), 456
Medication-induced orthostatic hypotension, 225
Medication-overuse headaches, 104–105
Medicines and Healthcare products Regulatory Agency (MHRA), 112
Megaloblastic red blood cell, 69
Membership of the Royal College of General Practitioners (MRCGP), 11, 39

Index

Memory loss, 109–110
Menorrhagia, 292–293
Mental Capacity Act, 61
Mental capacity testing, in primary care, 122–123
Mental health presentations
   assessment
      clinical assessment tools, 124–126
      mental capacity testing, in primary care, 122–123
      Mental State Examination, 123
      principles of, 122
   case study, 138–140
   description of, 121–122
   in primary care
      acute anxiety, 126–127
      bereavement, 127–128
      depression, 128–129
      panic disorder, 129–130
      paranoid personality disorder, 130–131
      post-natal mental health issues, 131–132
      stress, 132–133
      substance misuse, 134
      suicidal ideation, 135–136
      visual/auditory hallucinations, 136–137
   social prescribing, importance of, 137
Mental State Examination (MSE), 123
Mental status, neurological assessment, 96
Men who have sex with men (MSM), 302
Migraines, 107–109, 107t
Mineralocorticoid receptor antagonists, 229
Minor injury presentations, 368–371
Miscarriage, 343, 355, 356
   early pregnancy, 288–289
Miscarriage Association, 356
Molar pregnancy, 343
Molluscum contagiousum, 399t–401t
Monocytes, 71
Monophonic airway, 182
Montgomery v Lanarkshire Health Board (2015), 61
Mouth
   dental abscess, 170
   oral cancer, 171–172, 172t
   pain, 171

MSK presentations. *see* Musculoskeletal presentations
Mucus in stools, 250–251
Multi-agency review, 491
Multi-agency Risk Assessment Conference (MARAC), 484
Multi-agency Safeguarding Hub (MASH), 483, 485f
Multiple sclerosis (MS), 112–114
Mumps, 166–167
Murtagh's diagnostic model, 45
Murtagh's Masquerades, 48, 48t
Muscle stiffness, 374
Musculoskeletal chest pain, 220
Musculoskeletal (MSK) presentations, 365
   assessment, 365
      history, 365–366
      inspection, 366
      movement, 367–368
      palpation, 366–367
   case studies, 378–380
   in primary care
      minor injury, 368–371
      pain, 371–372
      redness, 372–373
      spasticity, 373–374
      stiffness, 374–375
      swelling, 375–378, 376t
Myalgic encephalomyelitis (ME), 114–115
Myocarditis, 220

N

NAATs. *see* Nucleic acid amplification tests
NAFLD. *see* Non-alcoholic fatty liver disease
Nail psoriasis, 397t
Narrative medicine, consultation model, 40
Nasal flaring, 181
Nasal obstruction, 161
National Early Warning Score (NEWS), 338
National Health Service (NHS), 5, 16, 338, 342, 494
National Institute for Health and Care Excellence (NICE), 16, 114, 183, 214, 224, 227, 233, 250, 319, 347, 469

511

Index

National Institute for Health and Care Excellence (NICE) (*Continued*)
   identifies change in bowel habit, 250
   inpatient management, 351
   d-dimer, 238
   guidelines, 126, 256
   risk of stroke, 215
   stepped-care model, for depression, 129
   typicality, in angina, 212
National Maternity Review, 338
Naturalistic decision making (NDM), 56, 57
Nausea and vomiting (N&V), 349–351
   for palliative and end-of-life care patient, 448–449, 449*t*
NDM. *see* Naturalistic decision making
Neck swelling, 165, 166t
   mumps, 166–167
   sore throat, 167–168, 168*t*
Necrotising fascitis, 412
Nefopam hydrochloride, 468–469
Neighbour's consultation model, 36–39, 36*f*
Neisseria gonorrhoeae (N. gonococcus), 326
Neurological presentations
   assessment, 96
      coordination, 98
      cranial nerve examination, 96, 96*t*–97*t*
      gait, 98
      mental status, 96
      power, 98
      reflexes, 98
      sensory assessment, 98
      tone, 98
   case study, 116–118
   description of, 95–96
   long-term conditions
      epilepsy, 111–112
      multidisciplinary team and local services, 111
      multiple sclerosis, 112–114
      myalgic encephalomyelitis, 114–115
   in primary care
      altered neurology, 99–100
      confusion, 100, 101*t*
      facial palsy, 101–102
      headaches (*see* Headaches)

      memory problems, 109–110
Neuropathic pain, 469
Neutropenic sepsis, 451–452
Neutrophils, 71
NHS. *see* National Health Service
NHS England (2016), 122
NHS Long Term Plan, 1
NHS People Plan, 1
NICE. *see* National Institute of Health and Care Excellence
Nitrofurantoin, 354
Nodular melanoma, 410
Non-alcoholic fatty liver disease (NAFLD), 267–268
Non-alcoholic steatohepatitis (NASH), 267
Non-megaloblastic red blood cells, 70
Non-opioid analgesics, 468–469
Nonoxinol-9 chemical, 313
Non-steroidal anti-inflammatory drugs (NSAIDs), 220, 292, 468
Non-tuberculous mycobacteria (NTM), 191
Nose presentations, 145
   case study, 175
   in primary care
      epistaxis, 160, 160*b*
      nasal obstruction, 161
      rhinitis, 162
      sinusitis, 162–165, 163*t*
Novel oral anti-coagulants (NOACs), 215
NTM. *see* Non-tuberculous mycobacteria
Nucleic acid amplification tests (NAATs), 324, 326, 331

O

Obstetric cholestasis (OC), 351, 352
Obstetric presentations
   abortions, 342
   assessment, 338–339
   case studies, 358–360
   description of, 337–338
   early pregnancy issues
      abdominal pain, 343–345, 344*f*
      bleeding, 355–357, 355*b*
      chest infection, 345–347
      headaches, 347–349
      nausea and vomiting, 349–351

pruritis, 351–353
    urinary tract infection, 353–354
    pregnancy diagnosis, 339–342, 341f
    pregnancy loss, types of, 343
Obstructive sleep apnoea, 198–199
OC. see Obstetric cholestasis
Occupational stress, in primary care, 13
    burnout, 14
        managing stress and, 15–17
        recognition, 14–15
        symptoms of, 14
Oculomotor cranial nerve, 97t
Oesophageal varices, 261–262
Olfactory cranial nerve, 96t
OM. see Otitis media
Ophthalmia neonatorum, 149t
Opioids, 471–472
    therapeutic trial, 472
Optic cranial nerve, 96t
Oral cancer, 171–172, 172t
Oral candidiasis, 403
ORBIT score, 215–216, 216t
Orthostatic hypotension, 225
Osler's nodes, 210
Osteoarthritis (OA), 376t, 377
Osteomyelitis, 376t, 377
Otalgia. see Earache
Otitis externa, 153–154, 154t
Otitis media (OM), 155
Overactive thyroid disease, 429–431

P

Paediatric Assessment Triangle (PAT), 181
Pain
    cycle, of chronic pain, 465, 466f
    in musculoskeletal presentations, 371–372
    for palliative and end-of-life care patient, 449–451
Palliative and end-of-life care presentations
    assessment, 441
        advance care plan, 441–443, 442t
        history taking, 441–443
        psychosocial, 443
        religion and spirituality, 443–444, 444t
    care after death, 457
    case study, 458–459
    description of, 439–440
    dying phase, recognition and management of, 454–457, 455t
    oncological management
        hypercalcaemia, 452–453, 453f
        malignant spinal cord compression, 452
        neutropenic sepsis, 451–452
        superior vena cava obstruction, 454
    symptoms
        agitation, 445–446
        constipation, 446–447, 447t
        dyspnoea, 447–448
        nausea and vomiting, 448–449, 449t
        pain, 449–451
        total pain, 440, 440f
pANCAs. see Perinuclear antineutrophil cytoplasmic antibodies
Pancreatitis, 268–269, 269t
Panic disorder, 129–130
Paracetamol, 468
Paramedic responsibilities, for supervision, 11
Paranoid personality disorder (PPD), 130–131
Paraphimosis, 283
Parathyroid disease, 431–432
Parathyroid hormone (PTH), 83, 431, 432
Parathyroid hormone-related protein (PHTrp) secretion, 452
Parkinson's disease, 225
PBC. see Primary biliary cirrhosis
PE. see Pulmonary embolism
Peak expiratory flow rate (PEFR) readings, 188
Pelvic inflammatory disease (PID), 290–291
Pelvic pain/masses, 289, 295
    fibroids, 289–290
    pelvic inflammatory disease, 290–291
Pendleton's consultation model, 35–36, 35f
Penile pain and discharge, 283, 284t–285t
People living with HIV (PLWHIV), 329
PEP. see Post-exposure prophylaxis
Peptic ulcers, 257–258
Perceived risk, in decision making, 58–59
Pericarditis, 220
Perinuclear antineutrophil cytoplasmic antibodies (pANCAs), 270

513

Index

Peripheral nervous system (PNS), 133
Peripheral vascular disease (PVD), 235–236
Peritonitis, 258
Personal protective equipment (PPE), 21
    applying, 23–24, 23f
    aprons, 21
    eye protection, 21
    face masks, 22, 22t
    gloves, 22
    removing, 24f
Person-centred care, in decision making, 60–61
PE rule-out criteria (PERC) score, 237–238
Per vaginum (PV) bleeding, 295, 297–298
PE Wells score, two-level, 238, 238t
Phaeochromocytoma, 233
PHQ-9 tool, 124–125, 128
PID. see Pelvic inflammatory disease
Pityriasis rosea, 387–388
Pityriasis versicolor, 403–404
Placental abruption, 344
Plantar fasciitis, 369
Plaque psoriasis, 397t
Plasma viscosity (PV), 72, 73f
Platelets (Plt), 68, 70–71
Pneumonia
    aspirational, 199
    atypical, 199
    CAP, 200
    COVID-19, 200
    description of, 199
    HAP, 200–201
    history and examination, 201–202
    investigations, 202
    management of, 202–203
    viral, 201
PNS. see Peripheral nervous system
Point-of-care d-dimer tests, 237
Polyphonic airway, 182
Poor appetite, 258–259
POP. see Progesterone-only pill
Post-coital bleeding, 293, 295
Posterior vitreous detachment (PVD), 147
Post-exposure prophylaxis (PEP), 318, 328, 329
Postmenopausal bleeding, 293–294, 294t

Post-natal mental health issues, 131–132
Postpartum thyroiditis, 433
Post-traumatic stress disorder (PTSD), 133
Potassium levels, in blood, 80
    hyperkalaemia, 81–82
    hypokalaemia, 80–81
    pseudohyperkalaemia, 82
PPD. see Paranoid personality disorder
PPE. see Personal protective equipment
Pre-eclampsia, 343–344, 348, 352, 353
Pre-exposure prophylaxis (PrEP), 329–330
pregabalin, 470
Pregnancy loss, types of, 343
Pregnancy of unknown location (PUL), 343
Pregnancy-related presentations. see Obstetric presentations
PrEP. see Pre-exposure prophylaxis
Primary biliary cirrhosis (PBC), 269–270
Primary dysmenorrhoea, 291, 292
Primary headache, 102
Primary progressive MS (PPMS), 113
Primary sclerosing cholangitis (PSC), 255, 270
Prinzmetal's angina, 213
Professionalism, in paramedics, 5
    duty of candour, 11–12
        ethical duty, 13
        in primary care, in England, 12–13
        principles, 12
    infection prevention and control
        blood and body fluids, 18
        decontamination of equipment, 20
        hand hygiene, 18–20, 19f
        invasive devices, 20–21
        personal protective equipment, 21–24
        sharps management, 25
        SICPs, 17–18
        splash/inoculation injuries, 25
    occupational stress, in primary care, 13
        burnout, 14–15, 14b
        managing stress and burnout, 15–17
    scope of practice, 6
        career progression, 9
        core capabilities framework, 6–7
        indemnity insurance, 9–10
        titles, 7–8

Index

supervision, 10
    employer responsibilities, 10
    paramedic responsibilities, 11
    supervisor responsibilities, 11
Progesterone-only pill (POP), 304, 308
Prostatitis, 282
Protection, rest, ice, compression, elevation (PRICE), 370
Proton pump inhibitors (PPIs), 257
Pruritis, 269, 351–353
PSC. see Primary sclerosing cholangitis
Pseudohyperkalaemia, 82
Psoriasis, 396, 397t–398t
Psoriasis Area and Severity Index (PASI), 396
PTH. see Parathyroid hormone
PTSD. see Post-traumatic stress disorder
Pulmonary embolism (PE), 237–239, 238t
PV. see Plasma viscosity
PVD. see Peripheral vascular disease; Posterior vitreous detachment
Pyelonephritis, 343

Q
QRISK2 scoring tool, 230, 231

R
RA. see Rheumatoid arthritis
Ramsay Hunt syndrome, 415
RAPRIOP mnemonic, for formulating management plan, 50, 50t
Rashes, description of, 385
Rate control, in atrial fibrillation, 215
RCN. see Royal College of Nursing
Rebound headaches, 104–105
Recognition-primed decision theory, 57
Rectal bleeding, 259–260
Red eye, 150, 151t, 152
Red flags, 47–48
    for hypertensive emergency, 232
Redness, with musculoskeletal presentations, 372–373
Reflective listening cycle/techniques, 31, 33f, 33t, 40
Relapsing-remitting MS (RRMS), 113
Relative afferent pupillary defect (RAPD), 144

Relative rest, stiffness, 375
Remote Consultations Handbook (Abbs), 42
Renal function test, 73
Resilience, development of, 16, 16b–17b
Respiratory presentations
    assessment, 180–183
    case studies, 203–205
    patients management with, 179
    in primary care
        acute cough/bronchitis, 183–185
        allergies, 185–187, 186t
        asthma, 187–191, 189f, 190f
        bronchiectasis, 191–192
        bronchiolitis, in children, 192–193
        COPD, 193–197, 195f, 196f
        lung cancer, 197–198
        obstructive sleep apnoea, 198–199
        pneumonia, 199–203
Rheumatoid arthritis (RA), 376t, 377
Rheumatoid factor, swelling, 375
Rhinitis, 162
Rhythm control, in atrial fibrillation, 217
Rifabutin, 310
Rifampicin, 310
Ringworm. see Tinea infection
Rinne test, 144
Rosacea, 398
Roseola, 399t–401t
Royal College of General Practitioners (RCGP), 6, 11, 33–34, 41, 42
Royal College of Midwives (RCM), 346b
Royal College of Nursing (RCN), 477, 484
Royal College of Obstetricians and Gynaecologists (RCOG), 131, 346b
Rubella, 399t–401t

S
SAD PERSONS scale, 125, 135
Safeguarding
    adults
        concerns, 477, 478t–480t, 481
        MASH process, 485f
        name of, 488b
        principles, 477
        referral for, 475, 476f

515

Index

Safeguarding (*Continued*)
    reporting, 482–484, 483*f*
    system-based issues, 482
    training requirements, for healthcare professionals, 476, 476*f*
  children
    concerns identification, 484–487
    referral for, 475, 475*f*
    reporting, 487–490, 488*b*–490*b*
  documentation, 491
  emergency contraception, 317–318
  multi-agency review, 491
  serious case review, 491
Safety netting
  defined, 51
  types of, 51*t*–52*t*
Sarcomas, 376*t*, 378
Scabies, 386–406
Scalp psoriasis, 397*t*
Scarlet fever, 399*t*–401*t*
Scope of practice, 6
  career progression, 9
  core capabilities framework, 6–7
  indemnity insurance, 9–10
  titles, 7–8
Scottish Intercollegiate Guidelines Network (SIGN), 189
Sebaceous keratosis, 407
Secondary dysmenorrhoea, 291, 292
Secondary headache, 102–103
Secondary progressive MS (SPMS), 113
Section 17 (Child in Need), 487–488
Section 47 (Child Protection), 488
Section 17 of the Children Act (1989), 487–488
Selective serotonin reuptake inhibitor (SSRI), 133, 253
Self-care cycle, 466, 466*f*
Self-management, of chronic pain, 465–467, 466*f*
Septic arthritis, 376*t*, 377
Serious case review, 491
Severe acute respiratory syndrome coronavirus 2 (SARS-CoV-2), 200
Sexual assault, vaginal bleeding, 294

Sexually transmitted infections (STIs), 149*t*, 295, 302, 321, 322
  case study, 333–334
  in primary care
    chlamydia, 323–324
    genital herpes, 324–325
    genital warts, 325–326
    gonorrhoea, 326–327, 326*t*
    hepatitis B virus, 327
    human immunodeficiency virus, 328–330
    syphilis, 330
    trichomoniasis, 331, 331*t*
Shared decision making, 60
Sharps management, 25
Shingles, 38, 38*f*, 414–415
SIADH. *see* Syndrome of inappropriate anti-diuretic hormone
Sick-day rules, 423
SICPs. *see* Standard infection control precautions
Sidaway v Board of Governors of the Bethlem Royal Hospital (1985), 61
Sinusitis, 162–165, 163*t*
Skin cancer, 408
  malignant melanoma, 409–411
  non-melanoma
    basal cell carcinoma, 408–409
    squamous cell carcinoma, 409
Skin conditions
  acute
    contact dermatitis, 386–387
    intertrigo, 387
    pityriasis rosea, 387–388
    urticaria, 388
  bacterial
    cellulitis, 388–389
    erysipelas, 388–389
    folliculitis, 389–390
    hidradenitis suppurativa, 390
    impetigo, 391
    Lyme disease, 391–392
  case studies, 416–417
  chronic
    acne vulgaris, 392–394, 393*t*
    eczema, 394–395
    psoriasis, 396, 397*t*–398*t*

Index

rosacea, 398
    stasis/varicose eczema, 395
  description of, 384
  fungal
    angular cheilitis, 402
    candidiasis, 402–403
    oral candidiasis, 403
    pityriasis versicolor, 403–404
    tinea infection, 404–405, 405t
  history related to, 384–385
  lesions
    actinic keratosis, 407
    sebaceous keratosis, 407
  rash, description of, 385
  scabies, 386–406
  skin cancer (see Skin cancer)
  skin emergencies
    erythroderma, 411–412
    necrotising fasciitis, 412
    Stevens-Johnson syndrome, 412–413
    vasculitis, 413
  terminology, 385, 386t
  viral
    herpes simplex, 413–414
    shingles (herpes zoster), 414–415
  viral exanthems, with childhood, 398, 399t–401t
Skin emergencies
  erythroderma, 411–412
  necrotising fasciitis, 412
  Stevens-Johnson syndrome, 412–413
  vasculitis, 413
Slapped cheeked syndrome, 399t–401t
Snoring, 169
Social determinants of health, 231
Social prescribing services, 137
Sodium levels, in blood, 76
  hypernatraemia, 79–80
  hyponatraemia, 76–79
Sore throat, 167–168, 168t
Spasticity, in musculoskeletal presentations, 373–374
Speech and Language Therapy (SALT), 111
SPIKES protocol, for breaking bad news, 43, 44t
Spinal (accessory) cranial nerve, 97t

Spirometry, 188
Splash/inoculation injuries management, 25
Splinter haemorrhage, 210
Squamous cell carcinoma, 409
SSRI. see Selective serotonin reuptake inhibitor
Standard infection control precautions (SICPs), 17–18
The Standards of Conduct, Performance and Ethics, 13
Standards of Proficiency - Paramedics, 10, 11
Staphylococcus aureus, 388, 389, 391
Stasis eczema, 395
Steatorrhoea, 269
Stevens-Johnson syndrome, 412–413
Stiffness, in musculoskeletal presentations, 374–375
STIs. see Sexually transmitted infections
Stoma, 260
Streptococcus pyogenes, 388
Stress, 132–133
Stroke, in pregnancy, 349
Sub-clinical hypothyroidism, 434
Substance misuse, 134
Sudden-onset dyspnoea, 237
Suicidal ideation, 135–136
Superficial spreading melanoma, 410
Superior vena cava obstruction (SVCO), 454
Supervision, 10
  employer responsibilities, 10
  paramedic responsibilities, 11
  supervisor responsibilities, 11
Supervisor responsibilities, 11
Swelling, in musculoskeletal presentations, 375–378, 376t
Symphysio-fundal height measurement, 344, 344f
SynACTHen test, 423
Syndrome of inappropriate anti-diuretic hormone (SIADH), 78
Syphilis, 330
Systemic vasculitis, 413

T

Tachycardia, 237
T1DM. see Type I early onset diabetes mellitus

Index

T2DM. *see* Type II (2) diabetes mellitus
Telephone consultations, 41–42, 42b
Temporal arteritis, 106–107
Ten footsteps, chronic pain self-management, 467
Tension-type headache, 103–104
Termination of pregnancy (TOP), 287
Testicle pain and swelling, 285
Thiamine, 262
Thinking, Fast and Slow (Kahneman), 56
Throat presentations, 145
    case study, 175–176
    in primary care
        neck swelling, 165–168, 166t, 168t
        snoring, 169
        voice changes, 169–170
Thrombocytes, 70–71
Thyroid function tests (TFTs), 89, 350
    hyperthyroidism, 91
    hypothalamic-pituitary-thyroid axis, 89, 90f
    hypothyroidism, 90–91
    TRH, 89
    TSH, 89
Thyroiditis, 429
Thyroid peroxidase (TPO), 430, 433
Thyroid-stimulating hormone (TSH), 89, 422, 430, 433, 434
Thyroid storm, 429
Thyrotoxicosis, 429
Thyrotrophin releasing hormone (TRH), 89
Thyroxine, 422
Tietze's Syndrome, 219
Tinea capitis, 405t
Tinea corporis, 405t
Tinea cruris, 405t
Tinea Incognito, 405
Tinea infection, 404–405, 405t
Tinea pedis, 405t
TLOC. *see* Transient loss of consciousness
TPO. *see* Thyroid peroxidase
Transactional analysis, 43
Transference and counter-transference theory, 43
Transient ischaemic attack (TIA), 212
Transient loss of consciousness (TLOC), 224, 225
Treponema pallidum, 330
TRH. *see* Thyrotrophin releasing hormone

Trichiasis, 148
Trichomonas vaginalis, 331
Trichomoniasis, 331, 331t
Tricyclic antidepressants (TCAs), 470
Trigeminal cranial nerve, 97t
Trimethoprim, 354
Triple-diagnosis/triaxial model. *see* Bio-psycho-social model
Trochlear cranial nerve, 97t
TSH. *see* Thyroid-stimulating hormone
Two-week wait (2WW) rule, 407, 409, 411, 431, 432
Type I early onset diabetes mellitus (T1DM), 425–427
Type II (2) diabetes mellitus (T2DM), 425–428

U

UC. *see* Ulcerative colitis
UKMEC. *see* FSRH UK Medical Eligibility Criteria
UK policy, 494–495
Ulcerative colitis (UC), 255, 256, 270
Ulipristal acetate, 318
Underactive thyroid disease, 432–434
Unprotected sexual intercourse (UPSI), 266, 316, 321, 322
Urate, 375
Urea and electrolytes (U&Es), 229, 350
Urinalysis, 279–280
Urinary retention, 282–283
Urinary symptoms, 281
Urinary tract infection (UTI), 281–282
    during pregnancy, 353–354
Urine pregnancy test strips, 339
Ursodeoxycholic acid (UDCA), 270
Urticaria, 388
Uterine rupture, 344
UTI. *see* Urinary tract infection

V

Vaginal bleeding
    dysmenorrhea, 291–292
    female genital mutilation, 295
    heavy menstrual bleeding, 292–293
    post-coital bleeding, 293
    postmenopausal bleeding, 293–294, 294t

sexual assault, 294
   vaginal discharge, 295–297, 296t
Vaginal discharge, 295–297, 296t
Vaginal ring, 312–313
Vagus cranial nerve, 97t
Varicose eczema, 395
Vascular, Infection, Cancer, Endocrine (VICE), 47
Vasculitis, 413
Vasectomy, 313
Venlafaxine, 133
Vertigo, 158–159
Vestibular neuronitis, 158, 159
Vestibulocochlear cranial nerve, 97t
Video consultations, 41–42
Viral conjunctivitis, 149t, 150
Viral exanthems, with childhood, 398, 399t–401t
Viral pneumonia, 201
Viral skin infections
   herpes simplex, 413–414
   shingles (herpes zoster), 414–415
Visual/auditory hallucinations, 136–137

W
Weber test, 144
Wernicke-Korsakoff syndrome, 262
White blood cells, 68, 71
White cell count (WCC), 68, 71
WHO analgesic ladder, 450, 450f
Wilson's disease, 270–271
Workload, 13. *see also* Occupational stress, in primary care
World Health Organization (WHO), 102, 121, 128, 327

X
Xanthelasma, 210
Xanthomas, 210

Y
Yellow flags, 49, 49b